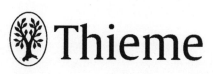

Atlas of Facial Nerve Surgeries and Reanimation Procedures

Madhuri Mehta, MS (ENT)
Director,
Department of ENT and Head and Neck Surgery,
N. C. Jindal Institute of Medical Sciences and Research,
Hisar, Haryana, India

Thieme
Delhi • Stuttgart • New York • Rio de Janeiro

Publishing Director: Ritu Sharma
Senior Development Editor: Dr Gurvinder Kaur
Director-Editorial Services: Rachna Sinha
Project Manager: Nidhi Chopra
Managing Director & CEO: Ajit Kohli

Thieme Medical and Scientific Publishers Private Limited.
A - 12, Second Floor, Sector - 2, Noida - 201 301,
Uttar Pradesh, India, +911204556600
Email: customerservice@thieme.in
www.thieme.in

Cover design: Thieme Publishing Group
Page make-up by RECTO Graphics, India

Printed in India by Nutech Print Services - India

5 4 3 2 1

ISBN: 978-93-92819-13-1
Also available as an e-book:
eISBN (PDF): 978-93-95390-15-6
eISBN (ePub): 978-93-95390-16-3

Dedicated to my teachers and mentors.

*Dedicated to my family members, who have always been there with me,
all though the journey of making this atlas and...*

...My son, Navroz.

A mediocre teacher tells, a good teacher explains, a superior teacher demonstrates, but a great teacher inspires...

Teachers, with their wisdom and experience, can shape us in the most exquisite way, and change us way beyond our own expectations. All my finest work has been inspired by such great teachers I worked with.

There is a famous saying, "When the pupil is ready, the master appears." And they truly appeared in my case, in the form of Prof. K.P. Morwani, Prof. Mario Sanna, Prof. M.V. Kirtane, and Dr. Satish Jain to name a few.

The first teacher in my life has been my father who taught me the basic values of honesty, hard work (relentless work), and commitment toward the profession. "Work is worship" is the motto I learnt from him.

My deep respect and reverence for my guru, teacher, and guide, Prof. K.P. Morwani, who taught me not only otology but the ideology of life as well. The transformation under his guidance was unimaginable. He was always supportive and encouraging and had all the patience while teaching new skills and techniques of surgeries. He has been there at every step of my learning. He awakened in me a special love for the facial nerve, which has been the main motivation for writing this book.

I had the good fortune of meeting Prof. Mario Sanna in one of the conferences in India. I had just been exposed to the vast field of lateral skull base surgery in those days. Prof. Sanna's mastery over the subject and his ultimate surgical skills motivated me. Then I had the great opportunity to visit his center "Gruppo Otologico" in Piacenza, Italy, and the 5 days' course changed my life and brought me where I am today. Dr. M.V. Kirtane has been another great teacher and master, who with his great skills and knowledge could guide me further in my journey of self improvisation. Actually he has been the one to encourage me in writing books and publications.

And finally my acknowledgment to the youngest teacher in my life, my son Dr. Navroz Mehta, who is pursuing postgraduation in otorhinolaryngology and is already in love with his subject. He has always been my best friend and the best critique as well. We have been together in every activity, be it painting, music, reading, and now the latest being "otorhinolaryngology." He taught me honesty, simplicity, and "walk the talk" philosophy. Thank you, son, for being there at every step and showing me the purpose of my life.

Madhuri Mehta

Contents

Foreword

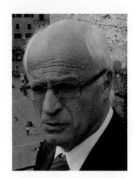

The facial nerve is a noble element that we must respect. Its disorder presenting as facial paralysis is always experienced as a tragedy by the patients and their family. Management of the facial nerve disorders is a challenge and is aimed to either prevent, as far as possible, or treat this debilitating pathology. This challenge is brilliantly taken up by Dr. Madhuri Mehta, demonstrating the extent of her medical art and her surgical skills in *Atlas of Facial Nerve Surgeries and Reanimation Procedures*.

After an update on fundamental knowledge in embryology, anatomy, physiopathology, etc., the different pathological situations are listed. Each of them has a clear and comprehensive description, followed by several perfectly illustrated cases placing the reader in the reality of the surgical act and its result. Such a collection of documents represents an enormous work and an immense experience that Dr. Madhuri Mehta makes available to us. The questions regarding how to preserve and how to repair the facial nerve receive both elaborative answers as well as an exhaustive description of the different surgical techniques involved.

This atlas is not only a book for the library of an otologist and head and neck surgeon, but above all a book to leave on your desk to be consulted at any time.

Professor Emeritus Jacques Magnan
University of Aix-Marseille
Marseille, France

Preface

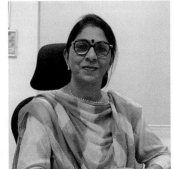

The path to perfection is endless and we may never be able to achieve it throughout our lives. But in the process, we will definitely attain excellence. And for a surgeon, precision or excellence is not a dispensable luxury, but a prerequisite, especially when the surgery involves facial nerve, the most important and the most vulnerable structure in the whole otology and lateral skull base.

For me, the facial nerve has always been a golden majestic lady with an air of supremacy around it. The enthusiasm to handle it during surgery is coupled with the intention to protect it in every situation. The fascination and fear go hand in hand. Many a times, the facial nerve has been sacrificed by surgeons on the altar of false presumption, limited experience, or overconfidence on their part.

In the pursuit to become a good otologist, my love, fascination, and strive for perfect facial nerve handling kept growing. The passion to learn and know everything about facial nerve grew so much, that I would gather knowledge from every authentic source describing the intricacies of the facial nerve. I wanted to know the minutest details about the nerve and its every fiber.

Of course, it has been a difficult task and a great challenge to understand and master its anatomy and placement in the temporal bone. For me, surgery on or around the facial nerve is the ultimate test of our surgical skills as an otologic surgeon.

I could understand that the management of the facial nerve does not mean just a good surgical hand, but it includes learning, observing, evaluating, treating, and last but not the least, keeping post-treatment records in a case of facial palsy. This learning about the anatomy of the facial nerve, its location, and surrounding important structures and landmarks can only be achieved through regular training in temporal bone dissection courses. In cadaver temporal bone dissection, we can expose and see the complete course of facial nerve as it takes different turns and curves, changes its orientation from the base of skull till its terminal branches, reaching up to the facial mimic muscles. It is better to damage the facial nerve in a cadaver than to give permanent, life-long deformity to the patient's face. Other than the surgical anatomy of facial nerve, one must understand the pathology leading to facial palsy or paresis.

The evaluation of a case of facial palsy needs to be learnt well, as it includes extensive systematic analysis for evaluating the cause, extent, and duration of facial palsy. The detailed evaluation forms an important aspect to be learnt as it helps us in deciding the corrective measures which includes medical as well as surgical management, assessing chances of post-treatment recovery of the facial nerve, and finally counseling the patient regarding the extent and duration of recovery after treatment. Then comes the surgical skills and experience of the surgeon. The interesting fact I came across in the process of all my learning was that, many times a well-performed surgery does not give the desired results, and at times, when we are not expecting good recovery, the patient may show so and surprise us. So, important lesson learnt here was to not get demotivated by results not being up to the mark; the important thing is to perform the surgery/procedure to your best ability and according to the protocols and record your work so that the pursuit for perfection continues. My philosophy is that with our sincere efforts, the patients can be served well.

The question may arise, "When so much literature about facial nerve is already available, where is the need for another book?" The answer is that, though there are multiple books on facial nerve, but in this ever-changing and progressing science, the principles and ideas which seemed right might have become obsolete. Many new improvisations and techniques keep evolving over time. Also, there is no single right way of performing facial nerve surgery as many surgeons have added variations in surgical techniques producing great results. This atlas has been written to provide a newer and comprehensive insight into the facial nerve and its management. This is the journey of an otologist, who wants to share the acquired knowledge with the rest of the world. The aim of writing this atlas is to add my perception and improvisations to the already available literature on the facial nerve. I have learned that techniques could be different, but the only thing consistent is the result on the face of the patient.

Another thing that prompted me to develop this atlas is my creative and artist instinct. Had I not been a surgeon, I would definitely have been a painter or a musician. The artistic instinct made me draw different aspects of the facial nerve as I see it and click detailed photography of the facial nerve in different situations. Pictures of preoperative facial deformity and postoperative recovery on the face which are often found missing in other monograms, make the most highlighting point of this atlas. It was a herculean task though, to collect the immense data, put it together along with the hand drawn diagrams, and produce it in the present form. My sincere efforts have been to truly present the outcomes of the extensive management procedures, be it medical or surgical, in a simplified yet detailed manner. It has taken me around 3 years to collect data and all the preoperative, operative and postoperative pictures, draw all the diagrams to make the understanding of steps easy, and finally weave them together meticulously and put in this atlas. The aim has been to share all the knowledge and techniques with my otologist colleagues and friends.

Madhuri Mehta, MS (ENT)

Acknowledgments

To my mother who left for heavenly abode very early, but whose love has always surrounded me and has been my motivating force.

To my father who always motivated me to learn something new every day, and perform each day better than the previous one. He taught me to challenge my own boundaries and limitations and keep progressing towards newer horizons.

My deepest gratitude and thanks to my team in ENT department at N.C. JIMS, without whom I could not have dreamt of writing this book. The team includes Mr. Krishan Kumar, Mrs. Neeru, Mrs. Sushila, Ms. Poonam, Mr. Deepak, Mr. Tejveer, Mr. Rakesh, Mr. Devender, Mrs Pinki, Mrs Suman, Mr. Suresh, Mr. Sunil, Mr. Sanjay, and the rest. I got their support in every sense and at every stage, which helped me to sail through the difficult and impossible times while writing this book. There were times when it seemed almost impossible to finish the mammoth task of completing the atlas. Those were the times when they were there, rock solid, besides me and chipped in all their presence and support, and finally this atlas could see the light of day.

And finally, my deepest love, reverence, and gratitude to my dear son Navroz, whose presence is divine in my life, who is the reason for all my happiness and success.

Madhuri Mehta, MS (ENT)

Note from the Author

I would like to thank our contributors, listed below, for offering valuable content to the book:

For devising and contributing the technique "Transzygomatic Anterior Attic Technique for Decompressing Facial Nerve"
K.P. Morwani, MS (ENT)
Head
Department of ENT and Skull Base Surgery
Nanavati Super Speciality Hospital
S. L. Raheja Hospital, Mumbai;
Senior ENT Consultant
Hinduja Healthcare
Mumbai, Maharashtra, India

For contributing the chapter "Management of Facial Nerve in Lateral Skull Base Surgery"
Narayan Jayashankar, DORL, DNB (ENT), MNAMS
Consultant Otorhinolaryngologist and Skull Base Surgeon
Nanavati Super Speciality Hospital
Mumbai, Maharashtra, India

For contributing the chapter "Facial Nerve in Cochlear Implantation"
Milind V. Kirtane, MS, DORL, FNAMS, DSc (Hon)
Professor Emeritus
Seth GS Medical College & KEM Hospital;
ENT Consultant
P. D. Hinduja Hospital
Saifee Hospital
Breach Candy Hospital
SRCC Hospital
Mumbai, Maharashtra, India

For contributing cadaveric images of facial nerve
Rahul Agrawal, DLO, DNB
ENT Surgeon & Cochlear Implant Surgeon
Agrawal Hospital & Research Institute
Gwalior, Madhya Pradesh, India

1 Embryology and Development of Facial Nerve

Introduction

The facial nerve is developmentally derived from the second pharyngeal, or branchial arch. The second pharyngeal arch is also called the hyoid arch because it contributes to the formation of the lesser horn and upper body of the hyoid bone (the rest of the hyoid is formed by the third arch). The facial nerve supplies motor and sensory innervation to the muscles which are also derived by the second pharyngeal arch, including the muscles of facial expression, the posterior belly of the digastric, stylohyoid, and stapedius. The motor division of the facial nerve is derived from the basal plate of the *embryonic pons*, while the sensory division originates from the cranial neural crest.

The anterior two-thirds of the tongue is derived from the first pharyngeal arch, which gives rise to fifth cranial nerve (CN). So the lingual branch of the mandibular division (V3) of CN V carries nontaste sensation (pressure, heat, texture) from the anterior part of the tongue via general visceral afferent fibers, whereas the taste sensation from the anterior two-thirds is carried by the chorda tympani branch of CN VII via special visceral afferent fibers.

The facial nerve with its complex course, branches, and its relationship with the surrounding structures develop during the first 3 months of prenatal life, although the nerve is not fully developed before 4 years of life. So, to clearly understand the embryological developmental pattern of facial nerve along with its surrounding structures, it can be divided into categories based on gestational weeks of the embryo.

0 to 4 Weeks of Gestation

The facial nerve development starts as a "facioacoustic primordium or crest" attached to the metencephalon, just rostral to the otic vesicle after the third week of gestation. It is a collection of neural crest cells which finally becomes facial nerve (CN VII). At this stage it is just a collection of neural tissue without any branches or ganglia.

In the 4th week (**embryo size 4.8 mm**), the facial nerve divides into two branches. The main branch becomes the main trunk of facial nerve and it terminates into mesenchyme. The smaller branch becomes the chorda tympani nerve. It travels anteriorly to the first pharyngeal pouch and enters the mandibular arch.

At size 6 mm, the nerve approaches the epibranchial placode, and appearance of the large, dark nuclei of neuroblasts mark the development of the geniculate ganglion (**Fig. 1.1**).

Weeks 5 to 6 of Gestation: 8 to 18 mm

At **7 mm of embryo length**, the branches in the form of greater superficial petrosal nerve and the ganglion in the form of geniculate ganglion start to appear. The chorda tympani enters the mandibular arch and terminates near a branch of the mandibular nerve, which finally becomes the lingual nerve.

At **8-mm size stage**, facial nerve motor nucleus is developed.

In the **5th week** (**10-mm length**) itself, the facial nerve gives off another branch in the form of postauricular branch, very close to chorda tympani, which travels to the posterior digastric premuscle mass. At this stage, the facial nerve completely separates from acoustic nerves along with appearance of small nervus intermedius, which becomes a separate entity approximately in the **7th week**.

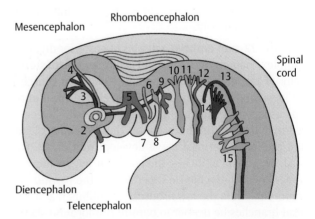

Fig. 1.1 Illustration shows the development of brain, spinal cord, and cranial nerves in a 5-week-old embryo. The cranial nerves are depicted as: 1. Olfactory; 2. optic; 3. oculomotor; 4. trochlear; 5. trigeminal sensory; 6. trigeminal motor; 7. abducens; 8. facial; 9. vestibulocochlear; 10. glossopharyngeal; 11. vagus; 12. cranial accessory; 13. spinal accessory; 14. hypoglossal; 15. cervical I, II, III, and IV.

At **14-mm** size embryo, the greater superficial petrosal nerve and the geniculate ganglion are fully developed. The greater superficial petrosal nerve while developing courses anteriorly lies on the lateral aspect of the developing internal carotid artery where it is joined by the deep petrosal nerve and both continue as a single nerve called "the nerve of the pterygoid canal." It terminates in the tissue that will become the future pterygopalatine ganglion.

In the middle of the 6th week (16- to 17-mm length), a branch arises from the anterior aspect of the geniculate ganglion and courses posteroinferiorly to the superior ganglion of glossopharyngeal nerve. The chorda tympani and lingual nerves finally reach the developing submandibular ganglion.

As far as the development of facial muscles is concerned, it goes along with the development of facial nerve. When the embryo is between **10 to 18 mm** in length, the mesenchymal tissue starts differentiating into the posterior digastric complex (the stapedius muscle, the stylohyoid muscle, and the posterior belly of the digastric muscle).

Weeks 7 to 9 of Gestation: 18 to 58 mm

At **18-mm length**, the nervus intermedius enters into the brainstem between the facial nerve motor root and vestibulocochlear nerve. The chorda tympani and lingual nerves unite to become one nerve to enter the submandibular gland.

By the time the embryo is **19-mm long**, all of the peripheral branches of developing facial nerve lie close to the deep surfaces of the myoblastic laminae that will form the facial muscles. At the end of the 7th week, all peripheral branches have got segregated and can be identified separately.

In the **22-mm embryo**, muscles of posterior digastric complex, namely, the stapedius muscle, the posterior belly of the digastric muscle, and stylohyoid muscles, are developing. A branch which developed from anterior aspect of geniculate ganglion in the 6th week is reduced to a communication as the tympanic plexus and the lesser petrosal nerve develop from CN IX. Out of all peripheral branches, the temporal, zygomatic, and upper buccal branches lie superficial to the parotid primordium, while the lower buccal, mandibular, and cervical branches lie deeper to parotid primordium, as the parotid gland itself is in the stage of development. Many of the facial muscles have developed at this time as well, including frontalis, zygomaticus major and minor, buccinators, and depressor anguli oris.

At the same time (**around 18-mm embryo length**), the parotid gland has begun to develop from the parotid bud, appearing as an evagination from the lateral oral cavity area. At this stage, it is called parotid primordium.

In the 8th week (32- to 49-mm length), the fallopian canal (FC) starts developing around the facial nerve in the form of a sulcus. The facial muscles, namely, the orbicularis oculi, the levator anguli oris, and the orbicularis oris muscles, develop by week 8 as well.

In the 9th week (50- to 60-mm length), rest of the facial muscles, namely, auricularis anterior, corrugator supercilii, platysma, and levator labii superioris alaeque nasi muscles, appear.

Weeks 10 to 15 of Gestation: 58- to 80-mm Length

Most of the peripheral branches of the facial nerve are developed at this stage. Extensive communications form between developing facial nerve and branches of the trigeminal nerve and also between the nervus intermedius, the VIII nerve and the motor root of the VII nerve. The vertical course of facial nerve starts developing at this stage and its location at this stage is far anterior to the external and middle ear structures than it is seen in the adult.

Weeks 11 to 15 of Gestation: 80- to 146-mm Length

The third branch from geniculate ganglion, namely, external petrosal nerve, arises from distal to the geniculate ganglion and courses with a branch of the middle meningeal artery. Branches also arise from the facial nerve between the stapedius and the chorda tympani nerves. All these branches along with those of CNs IX and X provide sensory innervation to the external auditory canal. These branches also develop communication with the zygomaticotemporal nerve. Communications develop with the lesser occipital and transverse cervical nerves, which are the branches of cervical nerves. The horizontal portion of the facial nerve at this stage lies close to the developing otic capsule.

At 14 or 15 weeks of gestation, the geniculate ganglion is fully developed, and relationship of facial nerve to middle ear structures is fully developed.

Week 16 of Gestation Till Birth

As the enlargement and development of middle ear is in progress, the facial nerve remains more superficial and anterior in relation to the auricle than it is in the adult. All important communicating branches of facial nerve are developed at this stage.

By 26 weeks, with the ossification and growth of the outer layer of periosteal bone of FC, the closure of the sulcus starts at this stage.

By 35 weeks, the geniculate ganglion separates from the epitympanic rim.

At birth, the facial nerve has completely developed into a consistent structure. Its anatomy and location approximate with that of the adult; however, at its exit through the stylomastoid foramen (SMF) it is still superficially located. The deeper location of exit of facial nerve at SMF occurs along with the parallel development of mastoid tip which goes on till about 4 years of age.

Development of the Fallopian Canal

The FC enclosing the intratemporal part of facial nerve courses from the internal acoustic meatus (IAM) to the SMF. The intratemporal part of facial nerve includes the labyrinthine (LS), tympanic (TS), mastoid segments (MS), and two genus of the facial nerve. The development of the FC can be divided into three stages: before 16 weeks of gestation, from 16 to 21 weeks of gestation, and from 22 to 25 weeks of gestation.

Before 16 weeks of gestation, when the otic capsule is still in cartilaginous form, its perichondrium divides to enclose the facial nerve. So, at this stage, FC is cartilaginous on its medial wall and condensed mesenchymal on its lateral aspect. The FC along with the facial nerve passes posteriorly from the geniculate ganglion, runs horizontally, lying superior to the stapes, and then takes a turn inferiorly around the developing round window toward the SMF. At this stage, the FC is dehiscent from labyrinthine to tympanic segment. The final position and complete covering of FC is decided by the normal development of otic capsule (stapes and labyrinth).

At the early stage of development, the labyrinthine portion lies in a sulcus on the superior aspect of the otic capsule between the developing cochlea and superior semicircular canal. As this position of FC is always constant, so there are least chances of developing dehiscence in labyrinthine segment.

The development of the tympanic portion of the FC depends on a direct apposition between the developing facial nerve and the otic capsule, so bony dehiscence in tympanic portion is a possibility if there is any abnormal development of otic capsule.

The development of otic capsule starts from the otic placode, which invaginates to form the otic pit and, subsequently, the otic vesicle during the **4th week of gestation**. This period of development coincides with the development of FC which runs as a sulcus along the lateral aspect of the otic capsule. The common origin of the stapes and facial nerve from the hyoid arch explains the association between malformed stapes and facial nerve aberrations. The stapes bone has dual origin in a way that, the head and crura of stapes are of neural crest origin, along with the central part of footplate, whereas the outer ring of the footplate is mesoderm in origin. This part of stapes connects to the surrounding mesodermal annular ligament, which makes the movement of stapes possible. This part of the stapes is, therefore, derived and intricately linked with otic capsule. The direct contact of facial nerve with the otic capsule during development may explain why the tympanic segment is most prone to dehiscence and anomalous positioning.

The mastoid segment of the FC along with the mastoid process begin to develop from the surrounding mesenchyme from around **15 weeks of gestation.**

At **16 to 21 weeks of gestation**, ossification of the otic capsule occurs along with the development of facial sulcus. A superior and inferior rim develop from the facial sulcus and start growing toward each other to form the future FC.

At **22 to 25 weeks of gestation**, complete ossification of the superior and inferior rims takes place leading to formation of complete bony FC. The superior rim contributes to most of the circumference of the canal and the inferior rim contributes to the rest. Incomplete fusion can lead to dehiscence of the canal, the commonest being the posterior aspect of the tympanic segment of the FC, superior to the stapes and oval window (OW). Other segments of the FC where dehiscence can be seen are processus cochleariformis, vertical segment, and lateral to the genu of the facial nerve. In case there is bony dehiscence in the vertical part of the mastoid segment, there can be associated lateral displacement of the facial nerve as it descends toward the SMF. It is commonly seen in case of aural atresia where the second genu and mastoid segment may get displaced anteriorly and laterally making the facial nerve more susceptible to iatrogenic trauma.

Facial Nerve Aberrations and Anomalies

Aberration or anomalies of the facial nerve can be associated with either normal facial nerve functioning or facial palsy. It can occur with or without malformations of the ear, or in conjunction with various syndromes which include abnormalities involving other organs in the body.

Associated anomalies of the ear include anomalous pinna, external auditory canal, and/or middle ear (including ossicles) and internal ear. Ossicular deformity can be in the form of abnormal long process of incus (rudimentary and medially rotated), stapes suprastructure malformation, fixed or absent footplate, atresia or stenosis of the OW, or absence of both stapes and OW. The common aberrations of facial nerve observed are classified into the following:

Facial Nerve Dehiscence:

1. Nerve at normal anatomic location

This is the commonest aberration or anomaly involving the FC. The dehiscence is found in 25 to 55% of all temporal bones. The commonest site is the tympanic portion and more so in its posterior part just superior to stapes.

Case 1

Case of congenital cholesteatoma with intact tympanic membrane (**Fig. 1.2**). The cholesteatoma found to be involving middle ear, attic, antrum, and mastoid (**Fig. 1.3**). After complete clearance of cholesteatoma from mastoid and middle ear (**Fig. 1.4**), the tympanic segment of facial nerve was found dehiscent in its posterior part, just superior to stapes (**Fig. 1.5**).

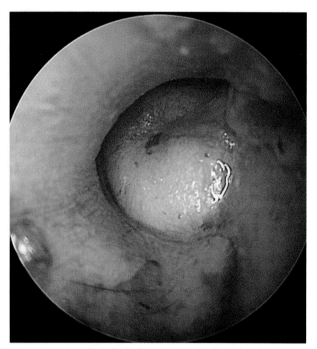

Fig. 1.2 Congenital cholesteatoma with intact tympanic membrane in left ear.

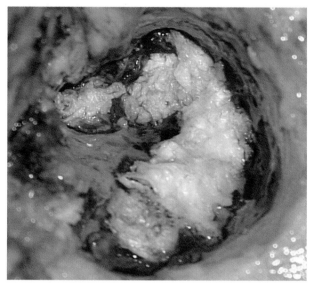

Fig. 1.3 Tympanomeatal flap lifted, cholesteatoma found extending beyond middle ear into attic, antrum and up to mastoid tip with necrosis of ossicles. Inside out canal wall down mastoidectomy already performed and whole cholesteatoma sac has been exposed in all dimensions without disturbing its continuity.

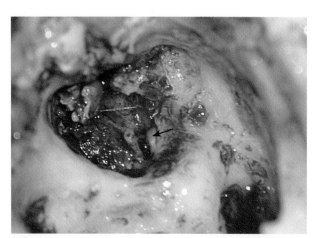

Fig. 1.4 The cholesteatoma sac has been removed in toto from mastoid cavity till middle ear. The Facial nerve horizontal segment seems dehiscent (*black arrow*).

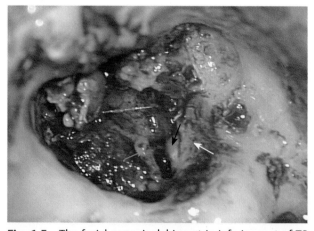

Fig. 1.5 The facial nerve is dehiscent in inferior part of TS (*black arrow*), and has intact fallopian canal in rest of the segments (*white arrow*), with the stapes (*blue arrow*).

2. With anteroinferior displacement of facial nerve

Following the dehiscence of facial nerve, the second most common aberration of facial nerve is displacement, including hanging over the OW partially or completely obliterating it, bifurcation and crossing over up to the promontory. In case the facial nerve anomaly is a part of a syndrome involving development of ear and other organ systems, the time of growth arrest is to be predicted, as the arrested development of both facial nerve and the organ must have happened at the same time during development (like in middle ear malformations). That way the surgeon can predict location of anomalous facial nerve, which helps in right treatment and avoidance of iatrogenic trauma to the facial nerve.

There are two theories explaining the coexistence of facial nerve displacement with middle ear deformities. According to the theory given by Gerhardt and Otto, the anterior displacement of the facial nerve happens due to underdevelopment and shortening of the first branchial arch, which in turn becomes the cause of the second branchial arch to over-shift in a rostral direction. The facial nerve, being the nerve of the second branchial arch, follows this shift. *According to this theory, facial nerve displacement is secondary to underdevelopment of first branchial arch.*

According to Jahrsdoerfer, the stapes develops later than the facial nerve. The extrinsic forces (e.g., hyoid arch shifting) displace the nerve anteroinferiorly before the stapes has fully developed. So migration of the facial nerve in an anterior direction is already in progress while the stapes is still forming and may prevent the development of the footplate and OW, causing either absence of one or both stapes crura, or the crura may be small and the rudimentary stapes may be free-hanging. *So according to Jahrsdoerfer's theory, the abnormal development of the facial nerve is the cause of malformation in stapes or OW, rather than the reverse* (Gerhardt and Otto, 1981; Jahrsdoerfer, 1988).

- **Covering the oval window partially or completely**

Congenital anomaly includes low lying (anteroinferior) facial nerve in its tympanic segment, with/without dehiscence, with abnormal stapes supra structure and footplate, and footplate is incompletely or completely obscured by low lying facial nerve.

Case 2

Case of a 15-year-old girl with right-sided hearing loss, pure tone audiometry (PTA) showing moderate conductive hearing loss with Carhart notch, and impedance showing As type tympanogram on right side. Facial nerve was found to be functioning normally. Intraoperative findings are short, medially rotated long process of incus with rudimentary suprastructure of stapes (only posterior crus and head formed) (**Figs. 1.6** and **1.7**). Tympanic segment of facial nerve found low lying, completely obscuring OW area with complete absence of OW and footplate (**Fig. 1.8**).

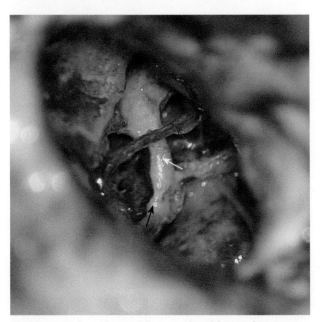

Fig. 1.6 Right side: Middle ear after lifting of tympanomeatal flap. Incus has rudimentary long process (*white arrow*) and incompletely developed stapes suprastructure (only posterior crus and head present) (*black arrow*); chorda tympani visible (*red arrow*).

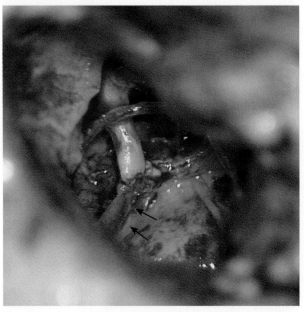

Fig. 1.7 Congenital anomaly of the ossicular chain short and medially rotated long process of incus with rudimentary stapes suprastructure) with doubtful anteroinferior displacement of TS of facial nerve (*black arrows*).

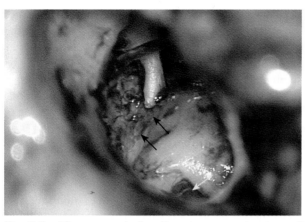

Fig. 1.8 After removal of rudimentary suprastructure of stapes, low-lying facial nerve in its tympanic segment is seen covering the footplate completely (*black arrows*). Round window is depicted by *yellow arrow*.

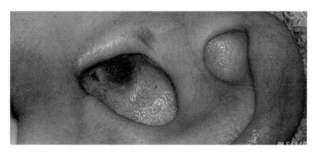

Fig. 1.9 Congenital deformity of pinna on right side.

- **Crossing over the promontory**

When facial nerve is located even further inferiorly, it can be found crossing the promontory. This usually happens in situations where there is associated anomaly involving pinna, external auditory canal, and/or middle ear (including ossicles).

Case 3

Case of congenital deformity of pinna on right side (**Fig. 1.9**), with atresia of external auditory canal. Patient presented with cholesteatoma involving middle ear and mastoid but with normal facial nerve functioning Intraoperative finding showed inferiorly placed facial nerve reaching up to middle of promontory (**Fig. 1.10**). Stapes suprastructure and footplate were nonexistent (**Figs. 1.11** and **1.12**). Such cases are the most difficult to manage. As facial nerve is so much low lying, there is considerable risk of causing iatrogenic injury to facial nerve and hearing cannot be improved through traditional ossiculoplasty. Modified radical mastoidectomy (canal wall down mastoidectomy) with prosthesis like BAHA or bone bridge implant is the technique of choice.

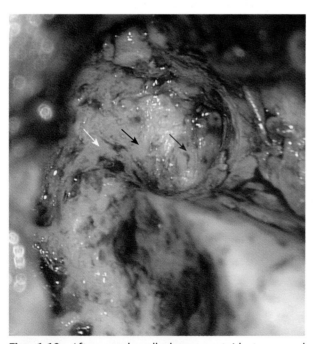

Fig. 1.10 After canal wall down mastoidectomy and complete removal of cholesteatoma. On examination, no oval window could be visualized. Location of normal oval window is shown by *black arrow*. Ampula of lateral semicircular canal location shown by *white arrow*. Low-lying facial nerve could be visualized in middle of promontory (*red arrow*).

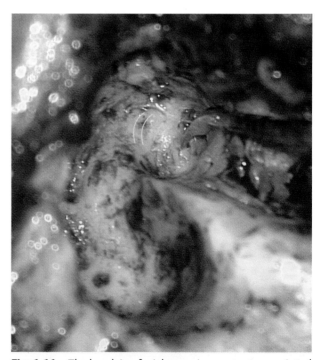

Fig. 1.11 The low-lying facial nerve in promontory pointed out with sickle knife. The normal location of TS and second genu facial nerve marked with *yellow lines*.

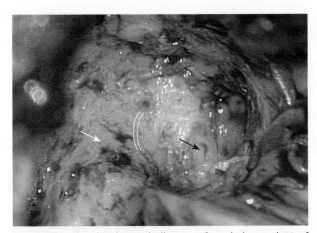

Fig. 1.12 The thin bony shell over inferiorly located TS of facial nerve is removed to confirm its presence (*red arrow*). *White arrow* depicts the location of ampulla of lateral semicircular canal, *yellow lines* show the actual location of normally present TS.

3. Bifurcation at different segments

The bifurcation of facial nerve can involve any of the segments. If the nerve is bifid in its horizontal segment, it may lie encircling the OW. The OW may be obliterative with or without the abnormality in suprastructure of stapes.

Case 4

Case of post head injury facial nerve palsy on left side. Computed tomography (CT) scan was performed to visualize the fracture line. High-resolution computed tomography (HRCT) scan of temporal bone shows facial nerve becoming bifid in its mastoid segment, second genu up to tympanic segment (**Fig. 1.13**). The radiological images corelated with the surgical findings (**Figs. 1.14** and **1.15**).

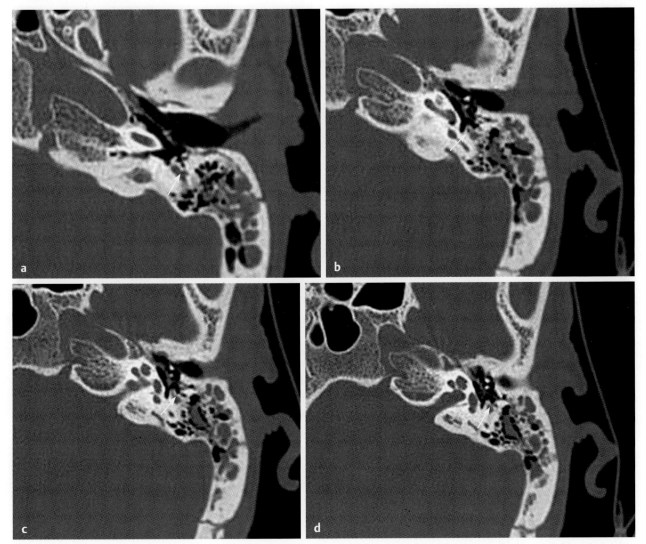

Fig. 1.13 High-resolution computed tomography (HRCT) scan of temporal bone **(a, b)** Axial cut showing bifid facial nerve in its mastoid segment (*white arrow*). **(c, d)** Axial cut showing bifid facial nerve (*white arrow*) till second genu.

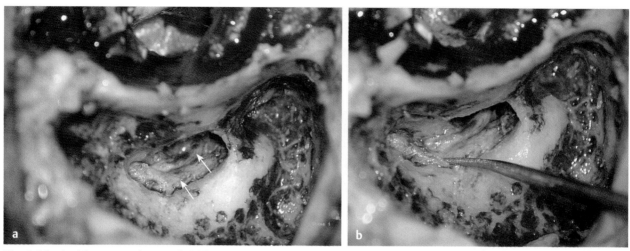

Fig. 1.14 **(a, b)** Pictures showing bifid facial nerve in its vertical part reaching up to the second genu (*white arrows*).

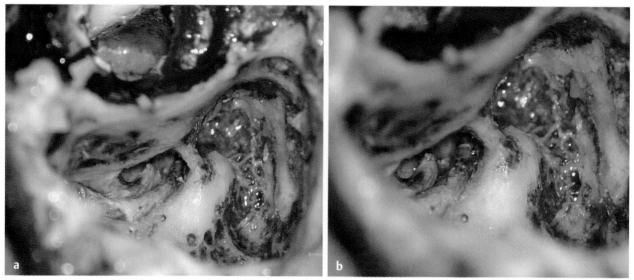

Fig. 1.15 **(a, b)** Pictures showing duplication of vertical part of facial nerve and continuity of one segment as the tympanic segment and the second segment ending at stapes.

Case 5

A case of facial nerve neuroma involving facial nerve in its LS, TS and MS up to the SMF. Along with radiological finding of neuroma the axial cuts of HRCT of temporal bone show bifid facial nerve in its MS in the inferior part (**Fig. 1.16**). operative findings showed bifid facial nerve in lower part of its mastoid segment, anterior segment was involved by tumor whereas the posterior segment was free of tumor (**Figs. 1.17** and **1.18**).

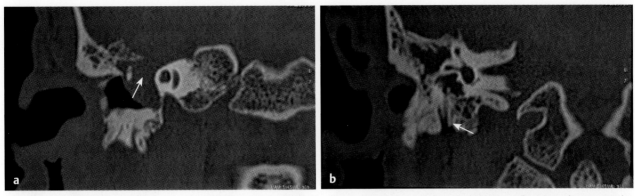

Fig. 1.16 **(a)** High-resolution computed tomography (HRCT) of temporal bone axial cuts showing soft tissue density in the first genu area and labyrinthine segment eroding through tegmen tympani (*white arrow*). **(b)** HRCT showing bifid facial nerve in its mastoid segment close to stylomastoid foramen (SMF) (*white arrow*).

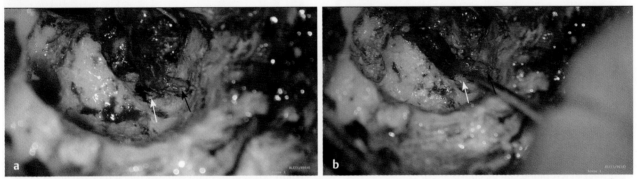

Fig. 1.17 **(a, b)** Pictures depicting bifid facial nerve in lower part of mastoid segment close to stylomastoid foramen (SMF). Anterior segment seems involved by facial nerve neuroma (*black arrows*). The posterior segment seems healthy and free of disease (*white arrows*).

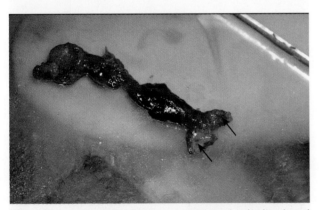

Fig. 1.18 Excised facial nerve specimen (with distal end bifid) (*black arrows*) for histopathology.

4. Concomitant malformation of stapes

Congenital deformity of middle ear, mastoid, and external auditory canal (EAC) is a common finding associated with facial nerve aberrations. Concomitant malformations of stapes and OW with aberrant facial nerve placement are also a common finding. Commonest malformation is that of stapes, followed by atresia/stenosis of OW. Very few cases can have absence of both stapes and OW.

Among malformations of stapes, isolated fixation of footplate is the least severe.

Case 6

A patient presented with hearing loss in left ear since many years. On examination, congenital deformity of pinna was noted on left side (**Fig. 1.19**). PTA showed moderate conductive hearing loss on left ear Impedance showed As type of tympanogram Intra-operative findings were bifid facial nerve in its tympanic segment with rudimentary stapes with obliterative and fixed footplate, surrounded both superiorly and inferiorly by the two segments of bifid facial nerve (**Fig. 1.20**).

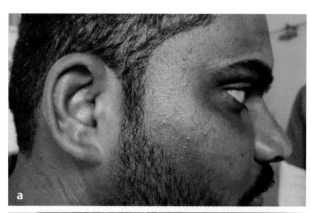

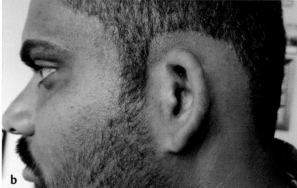

Fig. 1.19 **(a)** Right ear showing normal pinna. **(b)** Slight deformity in left pinna can be appreciated.

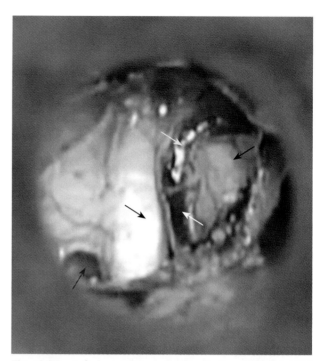

Fig. 1.20 Left ear. Intra-operative finding showed bifid facial nerve in its TS, one part inferior to footplate and other superior to footplate (*black arrows*). Rudimentary stapes (only head and posterior crus present) depicted by *white arrow*. Medially rotated long process of incus marked by *yellow arrow* and round window marked by *red arrow*.

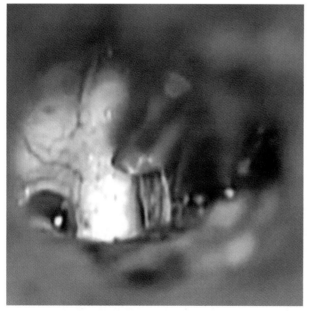

Fig. 1.21 Rudimentary suprastructure of stapes being removed.

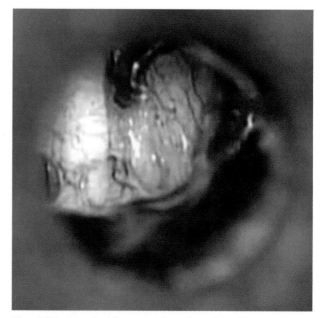

Fig. 1.22 Fixed obliterative footplate found between two segments of bifid facial nerve.

■ Congenital Facial Paralysis

Facial nerve paresis or palsy at the time of birth can either be congenital or acquired and must be evaluated before we plan the management.

Acquired

One in 2,000 live births suffer from unilateral facial palsy out of which almost 90% recover spontaneously. Approximately 75 to 80% of palsies in newborns are related to birth trauma.

Most of the cases of unilateral facial paresis or palsy are due to trauma at birth in the form of either forceps delivery, prolonged labor, pressure over mastoid and ear leading to ecchymosis over mastoid, or hemotympanum causing temporary facial nerve injury in any of its segment, most commonly in its tympanic, mastoid, or extratemporal segment. Early diagnosis is important to define etiological factor, which if traumatic must be addressed at the earliest. Although most cases of posttraumatic facial weakness improve on their own, in very rare situations, surgery and facial nerve repair may be required.

Investigations required are CT scan, electromyography (EMG), and evoked electromyography (EEMG).

If the cause is traumatic, treatment is taken up as early as possible, whereas if it is not traumatic, treatment is generally delayed.

Congenital

The presence of bilateral facial paralysis, other cranial nerve deficits, or other anomalies suggests a developmental etiology and facial palsy in such cases is part of different syndromes involving other parts of the body.

Most of the syndromes involving facial nerve are manifested at the time of birth only. Very few may present later in life.

Many hereditary and congenital malformations may be associated with abnormal facial nerve anatomy in the presence of normal nerve function. The otolaryngologist must be familiar with that abnormal anatomical location so as to avoid any iatrogenic injury to facial nerve.

■ Clinical Application

The knowledge about development of facial nerve, FC, and the surrounding structures is very important for the treating surgeon as while planning for management, it allows the surgeon to predict the anatomy of the deformed ear and location of facial nerve on the basis of its usual embryologic development at the time when the arrest occurred. Presence of anomalies in other organ systems also point toward the fetal age at which developmental arrest happened. A systematic correlation of all anomalies should be done clinically and radiologically, so that when opting for surgery, the location of facial nerve is well demarcated.

There are two situations to be managed in cases of facial nerve aberrations with ear malformations. First is surgery for the purpose of hearing improvement with management of congenital deformity of ear and congenital cholesteatoma if required and the second is rehabilitation for facial nerve palsy.

- **Surgery for Hearing Improvement**

Elective surgeries include stapedotomy with piston implantation, labyrinthectomy, labyrinthotomy + total ossicular replacement prosthesis (TORP) implantation, bone anchored hearing aid and Vibrant Soundbridge (VSB) implantation, and cochlear implantation.

The anatomical relationship between the aberrant facial nerve and the stapes/OW plays a key role in hearing restoration. If the stapes/FP is not or only partially blocked by the facial nerve, adjustable and nonadjustable prostheses with variable heights and designs, including partial ossicular replacement prosthesis (PORP), total ossicular replacement prosthesis (TORP), and piston, may be implanted based on the integrity and mobility of the stapes. In such cases we may need to displace the low-lying segment slightly upwards (the nerve is almost always dehiscent in its inferior quadrant in such cases) to expose the FP for fixation of hearing prosthesis. In case of bifurcation of the facial nerve, piston can be easily implanted through the fixed footplate of stapes because it is not blocked by the divergent branches of facial nerve. Both Teflon and titanium implant provide good biological compatibility and hearing improvement. Counseling of the patient is very important in such cases as there are chances of temporary facial nerve palsy/paresis post surgery, which the patient may not perceive well if not explained before surgery.

When the aberrant facial nerve blocks the stapes/OW completely, or the OW is absent, classic ossicular chain restoration is not possible. Unless until we make our diagnosis before surgery, we may need to abort it due to severe malformation. We must counsel our patient regarding the choice of treatment in such cases. Fenestration with prosthesis is one choice for hearing improvement. The right location for fenestra is a topic of debate. Some advocate fenestra in the vestibule above the facial nerve. Ugo Fisch advocated fenestration of the scala vestibule below the facial nerve. The optimal location of fenestration is controversial. Recently, Yang and his colleagues reported three cases with OW atresia and malformed facial nerve that were treated with the scala tympani drill-out technique combined with TORP implantation. They regarded the initial part of scala tympani as the optimal location of fenestration, corresponding to the promontory wall anteroinferior to the RW membrane (not the niche). At this location, vibration through the fenestration can be best conducted to the perilymph in the scala tympani. Anterosuperior to the RW membrane should be avoided (Yang et al, 2016).

Regardless of the location, fenestration increases the risk of labyrinthitis.

The second choice can be hearing aids and implants which is a good choice as it avoids opening the inner ear and/or provide better audiological benefits. There are three main types: active middle ear implants, active bone conduction implants, and passive bone conduction implants. All three types of implants improve speech perception, speech recognition, signal-to-noise ratio, and directional hearing. Decision to choose the right implant depends on the extent of malformation, so it becomes important to make our diagnosis clear before any final decision. For that imaging in the form of HRCT of temporal bone is mandatory. Imaging assessment of middle ear structures includes the relationship between facial nerve and stapes/OW. It helps in selecting the optimal treatment strategy of hearing improvement along with the right choice of prosthesis (**Fig. 1.4**).

- **Management of Facial Nerve Palsy**

In syndromic ear, usually the treatment is delayed by the surgeon or the patient presents late. The atrophy or non-development of facial muscles has already set in, so the usual repair or reconstruction of facial nerve is never the treatment of choice. Also, it is very difficult to surgically treat the facial nerve aberration, as the nerve development is arrested. So the best management in such cases has to be facial nerve reanimation in the form of static or dynamic reconstruction of facial function which will be discussed in subsequent chapters along with specific situations.

Bibliography

1. Baxter A. Dehiscence of the fallopian canal. An anatomical study. J Laryngol Otol 1971;85(6):587–594
2. Dickinson JT, Srisomboon P, Kamerer DB. Congenital anomaly of the facial nerve. Arch Otolaryngol 1968;88(4):357–359
3. Durcan DJ, Shea JJ, Sleeckx JP. Bifurcation of the facial nerve. Arch Otolaryngol 1967;86(6):619–631
4. Frenzel H. Hearing rehabilitation in congenital middle ear malformation. In: Lloyd SKW, Donnelly NP, eds. Advances in Hearing Rehabilitation. Karger Publishers; 2018. Vol. 81. pp. 32–42
5. Fowler EP Jr. Variations in the temporal bone course of the facial nerve. Laryngoscope 1961;71:937–946
6. Gerhardt HJ, Otto HD. The intratemporal course of the facial nerve and its influence on the development of the ossicular chain. Acta Otolaryngol 1981;91(5–6):567–573
7. Glastonbury CM, Fischbein NJ, Harnsberger HR, Dillon WP, Kertesz TR. Congenital bifurcation of the intratemporal facial nerve. AJNR Am J Neuroradiol 2003;24(7):1334–1337
8. Gupta S, Mends F, Hagiwara M, Fatterpekar G, Roehm PC. Imaging the facial nerve: a contemporary review. Radiol Res Pract 2013;2013:248039
9. Hasegawa J, Kawase T, Hidaka H, Oshima T, Kobayashi T. Surgical treatment for congenital absence of the oval window with facial nerve anomalies. Auris Nasus Larynx 2012;39(2):249–255
10. Inagaki T, Kawano A, Ogawa Y, et al. Stapes fixation accompanied with abnormal facial nerve pathway. Auris Nasus Larynx 2014;41(3):313–316
11. Jahrsdoerfer RA. The facial nerve in congenital middle ear malformations. Laryngoscope 1981;91(8):1217–1225
12. Jahrsdoerfer RA. Embryology of the facial nerve. Am J Otol 1988;9(5):423–426
13. Kieff DA, Curtin HD, Healy GB, Poe DS. A duplicated tympanic facial nerve and congenital stapes fixation: an intraoperative and radiographic correlation. Am J Otolaryngol 1998;19(4):283–286
14. Liu J, Chuah JH, Murugasu E. Facial nerve bifurcation in congenital oval window atresia. Otol Neurotol 2017;38(4):e13–e14
15. Liu Y, Yang F. Scala tympani drill-out technique for oval window atresia with malformed facial nerve: A report of three cases. J Otol 2015;10(4):154–158
16. McRackan TR, Carlson ML, Reda FA, Noble JH, Rivas A. Bifid facial nerve in congenital stapes footplate fixation. Otol Neurotol 2014;35(5):e199–e201
17. Murai A, Kariya S, Tamura K, et al. The facial nerve canal in patients with Bell's palsy: an investigation by high-resolution computed tomography with multiplanar reconstruction. Eur Arch Otorhinolaryngol 2013;270(7):2035–2038
18. Sando I, English GM, Hemenway WG. Congenital anomalies of the facial nerve and stapes: a human temporal bone report. Laryngoscope 1968;78(3):316–323
19. Som PM, Curtin HD, Liu K, Mafee MF. Current embryology of the temporal bone, Part II: the middle and external ears, the statoacoustic and facial nerves, and when things go developmentally wrong. Neurographics 2016;6(5):332–349
20. Sprinzl GM, Wolf-Magele A. The bonebridge bone conduction hearing implant: indication criteria, surgery and a systematic review of the literature. Clin Otolaryngol 2016;41(2):131–143
21. Yang F, Liu Y, Sun J, Li J, Song R. Congenital malformation of the oval window: experience of radiologic diagnosis and surgical technique. Eur Arch Otorhinolaryngol 2016;273(3):593–600
22. Hao J, Xu L, Li S, Fu X, Zhao S. Classification of facial nerve aberration in congenital malformation of middle ear: Implications for surgery of hearing restoration. J Otol 2018;13(4):122–127

23. Nager GT. Pathology of the ear and temporal Bone. Philadelphia: Lippincott Williams & Wilkins; 1993: 147–164

24. Marquet J. Congenital malformations and middle ear surgery. J R Soc Med 1981;74(2):119–128

25. Basek M. Anomalies of the facial nerve in normal temporal bones. Ann Otol Rhinol Laryngol 1962; 71:382–390

26. Nager GT, Proctor B. The facial canal: normal anatomy, variations and anomalies. II. Anatomical variations and anomalies involving the facial canal. Ann Otol Rhinol Laryngol Suppl 1982;97:45–61

27. Romo LV, Curtin HD. Anomalous facial nerve canal with cochlear malformations. AJNR Am J Neuroradiol 2001;22(5):838–844

28. Remley KB, Swartz JD, Harnsberger HR. The external auditory canal. In: Swartz JD, Harnsberger HR, eds. Imaging of the Temporal Bone. 3rd ed. New York: Thieme; 1997:16–46

29. Zeifer B, Sabini P, Sonne J. Congenital absence of the oval window: radiologic diagnosis and associated anomalies. AJNR Am J Neuroradiol 2000;21(2):322–327

30. Booth TN, Vezina LG, Karcher G, Dubovsky EC. Imaging and clinical evaluation of isolated atresia of the oval window. AJNR Am J Neuroradiol 2000;21(1):171–174

31. Celin SE, Wilberger JE, Chen DA. Facial nerve bifurcation within the internal auditory canal. Otolaryngol Head Neck Surg 1991;104(3):389–393

32. Curtin H, May M. Double internal auditory canal associated with progressive facial weakness. Am J Otol 1986;7(4):275–281

33. Raine CH, Hussain SS, Khan S, Setia RN. Anomaly of the facial nerve and cochlear implantation. Ann Otol Rhinol Laryngol Suppl 1995;166:430–431

34. Sperber GH. Craniofacial embryology. 4th ed. Oxford: Wright; 1989:49, 62–64

35. Sataloff RT. Embryology of the facial nerve and its clinical applications. Laryngoscope 1990;100(9):969–984

2 Anatomy of the Facial Nerve

Introduction

Facial nerve (CN VII) is one of the longest cranial nerves with the most intricate and tortuous route throughout its course. It carries approximately 10,000 fibers out of which 7,000 fibers are motor fibers innervating the facial muscles with each fiber carrying impulse to around 25 muscle fibers. The rest 3,000 fibers are parasympathetic and sensory in nature.

The nerve provides innervation to the muscles of facial expression, middle ear, tongue, and salivary and lacrimal glands, and the facial nerve functions like eye closure, smiling, swallowing, and taste form an important part of human expression and communication.

Suffering from facial paralysis can be emotionally as well as functionally devastating to the patient. The psychological trauma caused by functional compromise and aesthetic facial deformity can lead to social alienation of the patient. To manage such situations, a detailed knowledge about the facial nerve anatomy, its right location, course, and function is mandatory. The extra-axial anatomy of facial nerve from cerebellopontine angle (CPA) till its termination in facial muscles and glands will be discussed and explained in detail in this chapter, but pathway from the cortex to the brainstem, being very complex, will be just briefly mentioned, only to make an understanding about the rest of the pathway of facial nerve till its peripheral course.

Anatomy of Facial Nerve

Facial nerve, the seventh cranial nerve, embryologically develops from the second branchial arch. It is a mixed nerve containing four different types of fibers, namely, general somatic afferent (GSA) fibers, special visceral afferent (SVA) fibers, general somatic efferent (GSE) fibers, and general visceral efferent (parasympathetic secretomotor) (GVE) fibers.

The whole set of nerve fibers is organized into two roots. One is the motor root which is known as "the facial nerve" and the other root is named as "the nervous intermedius."

There are four major functions of facial nerve. The GSAs (general sensory fibers) carry cutaneous sensation from the skin over the mastoid and lateral surface of pinna, the external auditory meatus, and the tympanic membrane. The SVA fibers (special sensory fibers) carry taste information from the anterior two-thirds of the tongue. The GSE fibers (motor fibers) which constitute the main facial nerve innervate the muscles of facial expression and muscles in the *scalp* (which are derived from the *second pharyngeal arch*), the *stapedius muscle*, the posterior belly of the *digastric muscle*, and the stylo-hyoid muscle. The GVE fibers (parasympathetic secreto-motor fibers) innervate and supply the *lacrimal gland*, the salivary glands, and the mucous membranes of the *nasal cavity*, and both *hard* and *soft palates*. The facial nerve carries GSE fibers (motor fibers) only whereas the nervus intermedius carries descending parasympathetic GVE fibers from the superior salivatory nucleus and ascending GSA, and SVA fibers from the geniculate ganglion (GG).

The complete course of facial nerve can be divided into three segments, namely, intracranial, intratemporal, and extratemporal segments (**Figs. 2.1** and **2.2**).

Intracranial Segment

It is further divided into three parts, namely, supranuclear, nuclear, and infranuclear segments.

Supranuclear Segment

This includes both voluntary and involuntary motor pathways. The voluntary pathway (which includes voluntary responses like smiling on command) starts from motor cortex, travels through internal capsule, extrapyramidal system, midbrain, and reaches up to brainstem (pons) (**Fig. 2.1**). The upper motor neuron (UMN) of the facial nerve is located in the primary motor cortex of the frontal lobe (anterior to the central fissure in the precentral gyrus). The axons from the UMN are then carried through the fascicles of corticobulbar tract to the posterior part of the internal capsule from where they continue further into the brainstem (midbrain, pons, and medulla oblongata) where after passing through the midbrain, they synapse in the facial nerve nucleus

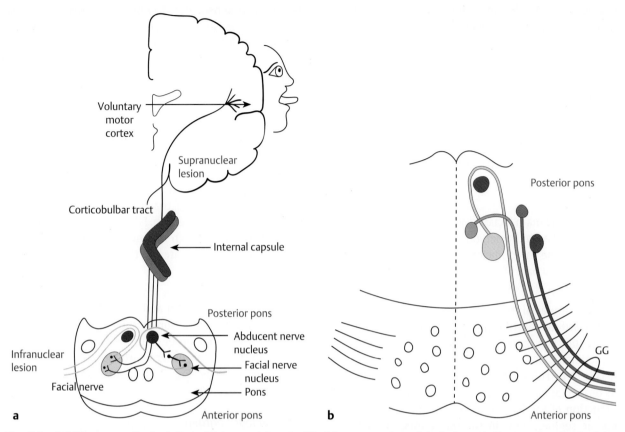

Fig. 2.1 **(a)** Diagrammatic depiction of intracranial part of facial nerve nucleus: it includes voluntary motor cortex, internal capsule, pons, and origin of facial nerve in facial nerve nucleus. Cut section of pons shows: *yellow nucleus* as facial nerve nucleus and *red nucleus* as abducent nerve nucleus.It also shows location of supra nuclear and infranuclear lesions. **(b)** The level of pontomedullary junction of midbrain where the facial nerve (*yellow colored*) loops around the abducent nucleus (*red colored*). The superior salivatory nucleus (SSN) and lacrimatory nucleus (LN) are *green colored*. Nucleus of tractus solitarius (NTS) is *blue colored* and sensory nucleus is *purple colored*. Nerve tracts are: *purple* (general somatic afferent fibers, GSAs), *blue* (special visceral afferent fibers, SVA), *yellow* (general somatic efferent fibers, GSEs), and *green* (general visceral efferent fibers GVE). GG is geniculate ganglion.

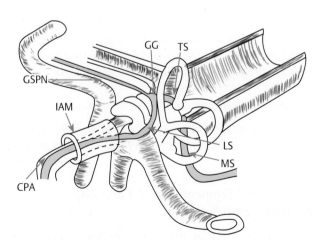

Fig. 2.2 Showing diagrammatic depiction of facial nerve from CPA till SMF. CPA, cerebellopontine angle; GG, geniculate ganglion; GSPN, greater superficial petrosal nerve; IAM, internal auditory meatus; LS, labyrinthine segment; MS, mastoid segment; TS, tympanic segment.

situated in the pons (**Fig. 2.1**). The facial nucleus contains the cell bodies of the facial nerve lower motor neurons (LMNs). It is divided into dorsal and ventral parts. The neurons in the dorsal part innervates the muscles of the upper face, whereas neurons in the ventral part innervate muscles of the lower face. The dorsal part receives input from both the left and right cerebral hemispheres. So muscles of the upper part of the face is supplied by both sides of the cerebral hemispheres. The ventral part of the facial nucleus receives input from contralateral side only, leading to the lower part of the face receiving input from contralateral cerebral hemisphere only (**Fig. 2.1**). Thus, the upper part of the face has both crossed and uncrossed fibers and the lower part of the face has crossed fibers only. This explains why an ipsilateral supranuclear lesion (UMN lesion) to the facial nerve results in contralateral facial paralysis but with bilateral sparing of the muscles of the upper part of the face, whereas a LMN lesion to the facial nerve results in ipsilateral facial palsy (entire face on the same side).

The involuntary motor pathways are not as well understood as the voluntary pathways, as they appear complicated due to the multisynaptic pathways involved in it connecting to various parts of the brain. These pathways use extrapyramidal system for producing involuntary, spontaneous, emotion-induced facial movements and the additional synaptic junctions for this lie in the hypothalamus, basal ganglia, and midbrain.

Nuclear Segment

It consists of the main facial nerve motor nucleus within the pons along with the nervous intermedius connected to the rest of the three nuclei. The main motor nucleus lies in the caudal part of pons, anterolateral to abducent nerve nucleus (CN VI nucleus) (**Fig. 2.1**).

Axons from facial motor nucleus run dorsally/posteriorly toward the fourth ventricle, loop around the CN VI nucleus, and then travel anterolaterally to emerge from the junction of pons and medulla (pontomedullary junction) (**Fig. 2.1**). This loop around the abducens nerve (CN VI) is termed as "internal genu." The first genu formed at the junction of the labyrinthine segment (LS) with the tympanic segment (TS) in the intratemporal part has been named the "external genu."

The facial motor nucleus is responsible for the voluntary movements of the facial muscles, the auricular muscles, the posterior belly of the digastric muscle, the stapedius muscle, and the stylohyoid muscle. The emotional facial expressions are under the control of involuntary motor pathway already described above.

The motor fibers from facial nucleus are joined by those of nervus intermedius, which contains sensory, special sensory, and parasympathetic fibers connected to rest of the three nuclei. These three nuclei are the nucleus of tractus solitarius (NTS), superior salivatory nucleus (SSN), and lacrimatory nucleus (LN) (**Fig. 2.1**).

The parasympathetic pathway: The SSN and LN are the two parasympathetic nuclei of the facial nerve and are located in lower pons. The efferent input to SSN is from hypothalamus. The input is also from the NTS which carries and delivers information regarding taste to the SSN. The SSN finally supplies the minor salivary glands of the nose, paranasal sinuses, and palate, and the sublingual and submandibular salivary glands. The efferent input to LN is from two sources. One is from hypothalamus (emotional response), and the other is from sensory trigeminal nerve (reflex lacrimation secondary to eye irritation) and it supplies the lacrimal glands.

The special sensory and general sensory pathways: The special sensory and general sensory pathways are through the NTS and sensory nucleus, respectively. The NTS, located posterolateral to the motor nucleus and parasympathetic nuclei in the pons, receives taste information mainly from anterior two-thirds of the tongue through the SVA. These taste fibers are carried first in the chorda tympani nerve. From the chorda tympani, the fibers reach the GG where they synapse with the first-order neurons. From here the taste fibers travel and synapse in NTS (second-order neuron) in the pons. Axons of the second-order neurons cross to the contralateral side and ascend to the thalamus, where they synapse with the third-order neuron. Fibers from the third-order neurons ascend through the internal capsule and reach the center for taste located in the sensory cortex in the postcentral gyrus.

General sensory fibers from the skin over mastoid bone and pinna, external auditory canal, and tympanic membrane carry sensation to the GG where they synapse with the first-order neurons which further synapse with the second-order neuron located in the spinal trigeminal nucleus (**Fig. 2.1**), located posterolateral to facial motor nucleus.

Infranuclear Segment

It lies in the CPA (**Figs. 2.2** and **2.3**) It is also known as CPA or cisternal segment. The segment starts from its point of exit at pontomedullary junction to its entrance at the porus of internal auditory meatus (IAM) and its total length is around 15 to 17 mm. This segment is devoid of epineurium, covered by pia mater and cerebrospinal fluid (CSF) only. At the exit from brainstem, the nerve lies lateral and rostral to the abducens nerve (CN VI) and medial and caudal to vestibulocochlear nerve (CN VIII). It is joined by nervus intermedius, which lies lateral to it. The facial nerve with nervus intermedius and vestibulocochlear nerve (CN VIII) travels laterally through the CPA to reach the porus of IAM. This segment has no branches.

Intratemporal Segment

It is further divided into four segments, namely, meatal segment, labyrinthine segment, tympanic segment, and mastoid segment.

Meatal (IAM) Segment (Figs. 2.3 and 2.4): 8–10 mm, Zero Branch

The passage of facial nerve with nervus intermedius through the IAM is accompanied by CN VIII. From porus (medial end) to the fundus (lateral end) of IAM, the length of the segment is around 8 to 10 mm and it does not

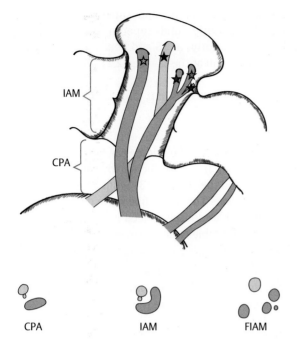

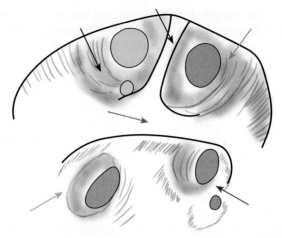

Fig. 2.3 Diagrammatic depiction of CPA and meatal segment of cranial nerve (CN) VII. The facial (CN VII) (*yellow color*) and vestibulocochlear (CN VIII) (*orange color*) nerves exit the brainstem at the CPA and enter the IAM together. In the CPA, the CN VII lies anteroinferior to CN VIII whereas in IAM, CN VII lies anterosuperior to CN VIII. The relationship of the facial nerve (*black star*) with respect to the superior vestibular nerve (SVN) (*green star*), inferior vestibular nerve (IVN) (*red star*), cochlear nerve (CN) (*blue star*), and the singular nerve (SN) (*purple star*) is depicted. CPA, cerebellopontine angle; FIAM, fundus of IAM; IAM, internal auditory meatus.

Fig. 2.4 At the fundus of internal auditory meatus (FIAM), the internal auditory meatus (IAM) is divided into superior and inferior compartments by a horizontal transverse bony crest called "crista falciformis" (*orange arrow*). The superior compartment of the FIAM is divided by a vertical bony prominence termed as "Bill's bar" (*purple arrow*) into anterior and posterior parts. The anterior part (*black arrow*) contains facial nerve and nervous intermedius and posterior part (*green arrow*) contains superior vestibular nerve. The inferior compartment contains: cochlear area anteriorly (*blue arrow*) which contains the cochlear nerve, inferior vestibular area posteriorly (*red arrow*) which contains the saccular nerve, and singular nerve in singular foramen posteroinferiorly.

have any branch here. From the exit at fundus the nerve continues as the LS. The relationship between the three nerves, namely, the facial nerve, nervus intermedius, and vestibulocochlear nerve (CN VIII), changes in IAM; near the brainstem, the facial nerve lies anteroinferior to the vestibulocochlear nerve. As they move through the CPA, and IAM, the facial nerve becomes anterosuperior to the CN VIII with the sensory root (nervus intermedius) between them (**Figs. 2.3** and **2.4**). The vestibulocochlear nerve divides into vestibular and cochlear nerves in the IAM.

The vestibular nerve further divides into superior and inferior vestibular nerves. The positioning of the nerves after division of vestibulocochlear nerve in the IAM becomes as follows:

The facial nerve lies in the anterosuperior quadrant and the cochlear nerve occupies the anteroinferior quadrant. The superior vestibular nerve occupies the posterosuperior quadrant whereas the inferior vestibular nerve lies in posteroinferior quadrant (**Figs. 2.3** and **2.4**).

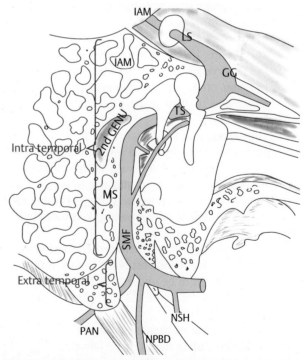

Fig. 2.5 Illustration depicting the course of the facial nerve in the fallopian canal (from internal auditory meatus [IAM], till stylomastoid foramen [SMF]) with branches in the neck. GG, geniculate ganglion; LS, labyrinthine segment; PAN, posterior auricular nerve; TS, tympanic segment.

At the fundus, the IAM is divided into superior and inferior compartments by a horizontal transverse bony crest called "crista falciformis." The superior compartment of the FIAM is divided by a vertical bony prominence termed as "Bill's bar" into anterior and posterior parts. The anterior part contains facial nerve and nervus intermedius and posterior part contains superior vestibular nerve which is formed by the confluence of utriculoampullary nerve (confluence of utricular, superior, and lateral ampullary nerve).

The inferior compartment contains cochlear area anteriorly which contains the cochlear nerve, inferior vestibular area posteriorly which contains the saccular nerve, and singular foramen posteroinferiorly which transmits the posterior ampullary nerve (**Fig. 2.3**). The meninges including pia, arachnoid, and dural layers covering the facial nerve reach up to the fundus of IAM from where the facial nerve pierces the dura and merges with nervus intermedius to form a single nerve named as "the facial nerve." In few cases, the meninges covering the facial nerve may extend along with the nerve till the GG.

Surgical Relevance

- Knowledge of the anatomy of the facial nerve and its orientation and relationship with surrounding structures in the CPA area and IAM is mandatory to avoid causing iatrogenic trauma to the facial nerve while performing surgeries for resection of tumors in lateral skull base area.
- The lesions involving structures other than the facial nerve in the CPA and IAM can cause compression, stretching, or involvement of the facial nerve due to their anatomical closeness to the facial nerve.
- The segment of the facial nerve from the brainstem to the fundus of the IAC is covered only by a thin layer of glia. With such a thin covering, the nerve is vulnerable to trauma due to surgical procedures but resistant to stretching or compression during growth of slow growing skull base tumors like acoustic neuroma.
- The changing relation between the facial nerve and the cochlear and vestibular nerves in the CPA and IAM need to be understood to avoid traumatizing the facial nerve during tumor removal in lateral skull base.
- The extension of meningeal layers covering the facial nerve up to the GG in certain cases can help viral inflammatory process to spread from one segment to another segment of the facial nerve.

After its exit from the fundus of IAM, the course of the facial nerve is through the fallopian canal. It passes anterolaterally between and superior to the cochlea (located anteriorly) and superior semicircular canal (located posteriorly) as LS and bends posteriorly creating the first genu at the GG (**Fig. 2.2**).

The Labyrinthine Segment (Fig. 2.2):3–4 mm, Two Branches from GG

The LS starts from the fundus of IAM and ends in the GG in the medial wall of the middle ear. It is covered by bony fallopian canal. It is both the narrowest (0.5–0.7 mm in diameter) and the shortest (3–5 mm length) segment of the facial nerve. The nerve fibers are devoid of epineurial layer and are loosely placed in this segment, which makes it vulnerable to any form of trauma or pressure.

The LS is bounded anteriorly by basal turn of cochlea, posteriorly by superior semicircular canal (**Fig. 2.2**), inferiorly by the vestibule, and superiorly by tegmen tympani separating it from the middle cranial fossa. The LS ends in the GG.

Clinical Relevance

- The part of the LS just after its exit from the fundus of IAM is the narrowest (the cross-sectional area is around 0.68 mm[2)]) due to the presence of an arachnoid band around it along with a sudden bent (around 132 degrees angle) and sudden reduction in diameter of bony canal from the IAM to the labyrinthine canal.
- This creates a bottleneck here, making it more vulnerable to compression.
- Due to the narrow diameter of the labyrinthine canal, the ratio of thickness of the facial nerve to the inner diameter of labyrinthine canal becomes different from the rest of the segments. The facial nerve occupies up to 83% of the labyrinthine canal's cross-sectional area compared to 73% occupancy in the tympanic portion and around 64% occupancy in the mastoid segment (MS).
- Arterial supply to the LS is single (without the anastomosing arterial arcades) unlike the rest of the segments which have double blood supply.
- The internal diameter of the main artery supplying this segment is quite less than in other segments, making the ratio of spatial occupancy of the vessels to the canal and to the nerve itself very small compared with that of the rest of the segments in the fallopian canal. Due to the reduced space for the nerve as well the artery supplying it, in the labyrinthine canal, any inflammation leading to edema of the nerve in this segment can easily lead to ischemia of the nerve making it more vulnerable for facial palsy than the other segments.

- Due to these anatomical compromises, the LS is considered to be the most vulnerable segment for getting strangulated post Bell's palsy or trauma.
- The angle at the junction of the labyrinthine and tympanic segments (first genu) is very acute (90–110 degrees), leading to nerve getting injured due to shearing forces or transection post trauma, in transverse fractures of temporal bone.

The Geniculate Ganglion (Two Branches)

The GG is located at the anterior third part of the first genu and is related to the point from where the greater superficial petrosal nerve (GSPN) arises. It is situated between the cochlea medially and the tympanic cavity laterally, just inferior to the middle cranial fossa dural plate. Further, it lies posterolateral to internal carotid artery and anteromedial to lateral semicircular canal. Although it is a sensory ganglion, it contains sensory, special sensory, motor, and parasympathetic nerve fibers out of which, sensory nerve cell bodies (first-order neuron) are located in GG only. It carries special sensory nerve fibers for taste from the anterior two-thirds of the tongue through chorda tympani and from the roof of the palate through the GSPN. The sensory nerve fibers carry external ear sensation through the posterior auricular branch. Motor and parasympathetic fibers of CN VII pass through the GG without synapsing (**Figs. 2.2** and **2.5**).

Sensory and parasympathetic inputs are carried into the GG via the nervus intermedius. Motor fibers are carried via the facial nerve proper. The greater superficial petrosal nerve (GSPN), which carries sensory fibers as well as preganglionic parasympathetic fibers, emerges from the anterior aspect of the ganglion. It starts from the anterior aspect of the GG. It contains the GVE (parasympathetic secretomotor) fibers meant for the mucous glands of oral cavity, nose, pharynx, and lacrimal gland. It moves in anteromedial direction to exit the temporal bone and enters into the middle cranial fossa. From here, the GSPN (carrying the preganglionic fibers) travels through the foramen lacerum, combines with the deep petrosal nerve (carrying sympathetic postganglionic fibers from the superior cervical ganglion) to form the nerve of the pterygoid canal (Vidian nerve), which then passes through the pterygoid canal (Vidian canal) to enter the pterygopalatine fossa. Here the parasympathetic fibers synapse with postganglionic neurons in pterygopalatine ganglion. Branches from this ganglion then go on to provide parasympathetic innervation to the mucous glands of the oral cavity, nose and pharynx, and the lacrimal gland.

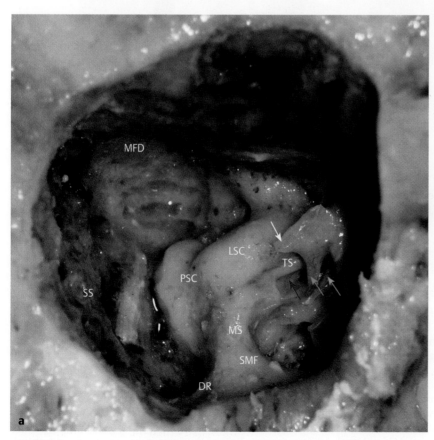

Fig. 2.6 **(a)** The course of the facial nerve in the fallopian canal in natural position. The figure shows the tympanic segment (TS) and mastoid segment (MS) of the facial nerve and the relationship of the facial nerve with the incudostapedial joint (*green arrow*) and short process of incus (*white arrow*), oval window (*red arrow*), lateral semicircular canal (LSC) and posterior semicircular canal (PSC), and the digastric ridge (DR). GG, geniculate ganglion; LS, labyrinthine segment; MS, mastoid segment; NPBD, nerve to posterior belly of digastric muscle; NSH, nerve to stylohyoid muscle; PAN, post auricular nerve; SMF, stylomastoid segment; TS, tympanic segment. (*Continued*)

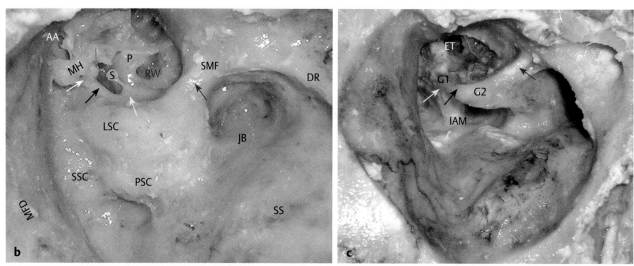

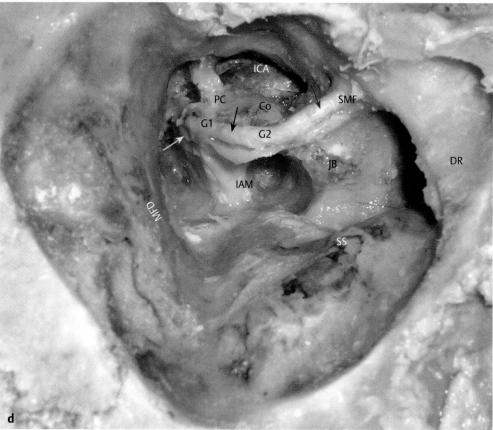

Fig. 2.6 (*Continued*) **(b)** Picture showing the surgical position of temporal bone. Canal wall down mastoidectomy performed; all mastoid air cells cleared. Semicircular canals exposed and course of the facial nerve in the fallopian canal defined. MS is shown with *red arrow*; TS is shown with *black arrow*; the second genu is shown with *yellow arrow*; the first genu is shown with *white arrow*. In the middle ear, the incus has been removed to expose the TS and the first genu. The different structures in the vicinity of facial nerve are: stylomastoid foramen (SMF), digastric ridge (DR), jugular bulb (JB), sigmoid sinus (SS), middle fossa dura (MFD), lateral semicircular canal (LSC), posterior semicircular canal (PSC), superior semicircular canal (SSC), anterior attic (AA), malleus head (MH), stapes (S), promontory (P), round window (RW), and processus cochleariformis (*green arrow*). **(c)** Skeletonization of the facial nerve from the SMF till porus of IAM after drilling away the semicircular canals and vestibule (labyrinthectomy). MS is shown with *red arrow*; TS is shown with *black arrow*; LS is shown with *yellow arrow*. G1, first genu; G2, second genu; ET, Eustachian tube opening; IAM, internal auditory meatus. **(d)** Picture showing skeletonization of complete course of intratemporal facial nerve, right side. MS is shown with *red arrow*; TS is shown with *black arrow*; LS is shown with *yellow arrow*. G1, first genu; G2, second genu; IAM, internal auditory meatus. Rest of the surrounding important structures: stylomastoid foramen (SMF), digastric ridge (DR), jugular bulb (JB), sigmoid sinus (SS), middle fossa dura (MFD), cochlea (Co), internal carotid artery (ICA), and processus cochleariformis (PC), (*Continued*)

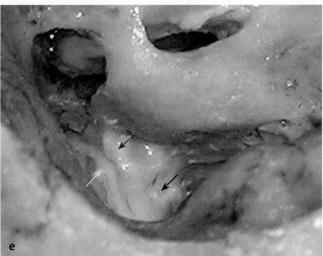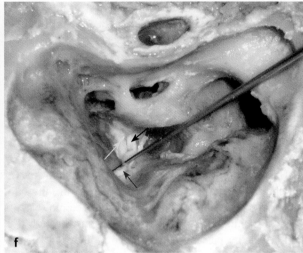

Fig. 2.6 (*Continued*) **(e)** Picture showing close-up view of the IAM after removing the covering bone, but still covered with dural layer. The different nerves visible in IAM after separating the covering dura are: superior vestibular nerve occupying posterosuperior quadrant (*red arrow*), inferior vestibular nerve occupying the posteroinferior quadrant of IAM (*black arrow*), and facial nerve occupying anterosuperior quadrant of IAM (*yellow arrow*). The cochlear nerve is not visible as it is hidden beneath the inferior vestibular nerve. **(f)** Picture showing the anterior compartment of IAM after detaching the superior and inferior vestibular nerves. The contents in the anterior compartment are facial nerve in anterosuperior quadrant (*yellow arrow*) and cochlear nerve in anteroinferior quadrant (*black arrow*). Detached superior and inferior vestibular nerves (*red arrow*).

The external petrosal nerve is the second branch which may be absent at times. It provides sympathetic innervation to the middle meningeal artery.

The lesser petrosal nerve is the third branch from the GG. This branch carries parasympathetic fibers associated with the glossopharyngeal nerve (CN IX) to the parotid gland.

The GG lies covered in fallopian canal, but in around 15% of cases it may only be covered with thin sheath making it vulnerable to injury.

Tympanic Segment (Fig. 2.6): 8–11 mm, Zero Branches

At the first genu the facial nerve takes a sharp turn posteriorly to become the TS. The angle the TS makes with the first genu is around 90 degrees. From here it courses in posterolateral direction along the medial wall of the middle ear, passing above the tensor tympani tendon and processus cochleariformis. The landmark for identifying the TS are "Cog" superiorly and processus cochleariformis inferiorly. The TS ends at the second genu just beneath the short process of incus, making an angle of 95 to 125 degrees with the second genu and here it is situated anteromedial to the ampulla of the lateral semicircular canal and superior to the oval window. The whole length of the TS is around 8 to 11 mm. The posterior end of the TS lies just above the pyramidal eminence which lodges the stapedial muscle.

Surgical Relevance

- As dehiscence of the bony facial canal is found most commonly in the TS, there is a risk of causing trauma to the nerve in this segment while performing middle ear surgery leading to immediate or delayed facial paralysis.
- The relationship of the facial nerve to the oval window, semicircular canals, and annulus puts the nerve at risk while performing steps for canal wall up or canal wall down mastoidectomy, ossiculoplasty, or posterior tympanotomy.

Mastoid Segment (Fig. 2.6) 8–15 mm, Two Branches

From the second genu the nerve turns inferiorly as the MS. The MS extends from the second genu to the stylomastoid foramen (SMF), running in the bony fallopian canal. An important landmark for tracing the second genu is the pyramid in which the stapedial muscle is located. The second genu lies just a few millimeters posterior to the posterior edge of the pyramid. The facial nerve while descending first lies anteromedial to the lateral semicircular canal and further inferiorly lies anterolateral to posterior semicircular canal and lateral to the annulus. The lower part of the MS lies on the lateral surface of the jugular bulb bisecting it, just anterior to the digastric ridge which is again an important landmark for tracing the facial nerve at the level of the SMF. The nerve exits at the SMF to become extratemporal segment.

The MS gives two branches. The first branch is the nerve to stapedius which is also the most proximal motor branch of facial nerve. It arises from the nerve at the level of the pyramid process and supplies the stapedius muscle which originates and fills the hollow of the pyramid. The insertion of the muscle is either on the capitulum or the neck of the stapes on its posterior side. The function of stapedius muscle is to protect the hearing apparatus and prevent excessive movement of stapes when it is exposed to loud sounds.

The second branch is the chorda tympani nerve which arises from the distal part of the MS, usually 4 to 8 mm above the SMF (though the distance may vary). After branching off the facial nerve it runs through the middle ear by passing between the malleus and incus (lateral to the long process of incus and medial to the neck of malleus) and re-emerges anterior to the middle ear cavity by passing through the petrotympanic fissure (canal of Hugier) to reach the infratemporal fossa. Here it joins the lingual nerve (a branch of trigeminal nerve).

It carries the GVE fibers (parasympathetic fibers) to the sublingual and submandibular gland and the SVA fibers (taste fibers) from the anterior two-thirds of the tongue. The GVE fibers (preganglionic fibers) of the chorda tympani join with the lingual nerve in the infratemporal fossa, and form submandibular ganglion. In the ganglion, the parasympathetic fibers synapse with the postganglionic cells which further innervate the submandibular and sublingual salivary glands. The SVA fibers (taste fibers) pass through the chorda tympani to innervate the tongue and relay taste information from the anterior two-thirds of the tongue.

Surgical Relevance

As the MS descends inferiorly from the second genu, it takes a sudden posterolateral turn toward the lateral semicircular canal putting the nerve at risk of injury during mastoid and middle ear surgery.

Important Measurements

The anterior part of the TS of the facial nerve lies above and medial to the cochleariform process at a distance of around 2 mm. The mean distance between the posterior border of the oval window and the MS of the facial nerve is around 4 mm. This is an important distance to keep in mind while performing canaloplasty or exposing the sinus tympani for clearance of disease medial to fallopian canal in retrotympanum area. This is also important to be considered while performing posterior tympanotomy for cochlear implantation. As already mentioned earlier, the chorda tympani nerve arises from the facial nerve at around 4 to 8 mm proximal to the SMF. The mean distance of the facial nerve at the second genu to the outer

cortex of mastoid is around 21.6 mm, whereas the mean distance of the facial nerve at the SMF to the outer cortex is 12.8 mm. The distance between the ampullary end of the horizontal semicircular canal and the second genu of the facial nerve is 2 mm. The second genu may have a normal course, or rarely may present as a lateral hump or posterolateral bulge below the horizontal semicircular canal.

The Extracranial Segment: 15–20 mm, Eight Branches, Three in the Neck and Five on the Face

At the Stylomastoid Foramen (SMF)

The facial nerve exits the temporal bone at the SMF which is located at the anterior border of the digastric ridge. In newborn babies and children up to 4 years of age, the facial nerve at the exit lies very superficial, just deep to the subcutaneous tissue underlying the skin. After 4 years of age, as the mastoid tip develops and tympanic bone thickens, the facial nerve takes a deeper position. In the adults, at the SMF, the facial nerve lies protected by the mastoid tip, tympanic plate, ascending ramus of mandible, and fascia between the cartilaginous external auditory canal and parotid. As the nerve exits at the SMF, it runs parallel and slightly superior to the superior margin of posterior belly of digastric, and gives two or three branches (**Fig. 2.6a**) in the neck before it bifurcates into terminal branches on the face. These are:

- The first branch is the posterior auricular nerve (PAN) which supplies the intrinsic muscles of ear and occipital belly of occipitofrontalis muscle.
- The second branch (motor branch) is the nerve to the stylohyoid (NSH) muscle and the posterior belly of digastric (NPBD). In place of single branch, it can present as two separate branches to supply the two muscles separately. The action of the stylohyoid muscle is to initiate swallowing action by drawing the hyoid bone in a posterior and superior direction and elevating the tongue. The digastric muscle including both anterior and posterior bellies is involved in any complex jaw action such as speaking, swallowing, chewing, and breathing.

Localization of the facial nerve trunk (FNT) (i.e., the portion of the facial nerve between the SMF and pes anserinus) may be required during various surgical interventions such as parotid surgery and repair for facial trauma or facio-masseteric and facio-hypoglossal anastomosis. For that, certain landmarks are used which should have consistent location and be easy to palpate. The most important landmarks used in practice are:

- Tragal pointer: The anterior part of tragus points anteroinferiorly and deep to superficial surface of the preauricular area. It takes a bluntly pointed shape on its medial aspect and is thus called "pointer." The facial nerve at its exit at the SMF lies approximately 1 to 1.5 cm inferior and deeper to tragal pointer.

- Tympanomastoid suture line: It is palpable as a hard ridge deep to the cartilaginous part of the EAC. The facial nerve emerges around 3.5 mm deeper to its outer edge.
- Posterior belly of digastric muscle: It is the most easily identifiable and very consistent landmark for identification of facial nerve at the SMF. After lateral retraction of sternocleidomastoid muscle, the posterior belly of digastric muscle can be identified as it inserts on digastric ridge on the mastoid bone. The FNT lies approximately 8 mm above and parallel to the upper border of the digastric muscle near its insertion.

Surgical Relevance

- In children younger than 4 years the facial nerve lies relatively superficial at its exit from the SMF as explained earlier. Postauricular incisions in pediatric patient must be carefully planned and modified in a way that it runs till upper half of post aural groove and does not reach lower down.
- The nerve must be identified by its anatomical location and surrounding landmarks.
- Just distal to the SMF the nerve is crossed by occipital artery and venus plexus, which may bleed briskly. Meticulous hemostasis is achieved by using bipolar cautery.
- While performing facio-masseteric or facio-hypoglossal anastomosis or anterior transposition of facial nerve extra length or maximum extent of facial nerve can be released by cutting off the branches it gives in the neck to avoid stretch on the facial nerve.

At Pes Anserinus and Face

After giving off branches in the neck, the facial nerve turns anterolaterally in the retromandibular fossa and crosses the lateral surface of styloid process to enter the parotid gland. The parotid gland is not supplied by the facial nerve (innervated by glossopharyngeal nerve). In the substance of parotid gland, the nerve crosses the external carotid artery and posterior facial vein (retromandibular vein) and divides at the posterior border of ramus of mandible into two primary branches, **temporofacial** and **cervicofacial** trunks (**Fig. 2.9**). The length of facial nerve from the SMF to its bifurcation is around 2 cm. Both branches run through the substance of parotid gland usually passing lateral to the retromandibular vein (which is formed by the confluence with the posterior branch of posterior facial vein just below the apex of the parotid gland) and further divide into the temporal, zygomatic, buccal, marginal mandibular, and cervical branches. The facial nerve branches like a tree into its five terminal branches which finally innervate the muscles of facial expression (mimetic muscles). As the terminal branches emerge from the outer margins of parotid, they become very superficial. They run just deep to the skin, subcutaneous tissue, and superficial musculoaponeurotic system (SMAS). On their way to the facial muscles, the terminal branches intermingle with each other through network of very fine nerve filaments. It may seem that the axons are mixing with each other, but finally all axons reach their appropriate specific facial muscle groups. These rich interconnections between all the branches are the reason for the continuity and specificity in facial expressions. The branches innervate the specific muscles from their deeper side other than three muscles which are buccinator, levator angularis oris, and mentalis, where the nerve enters from the lateral or superficial surface.

■ Mimetic Muscles

All mimetic muscles are paired muscles other than orbicularis oris which is a single muscle. These facial muscles develop from the second *pharyngeal arch* and all are supplied by the facial nerve. They are also called "the muscles of facial expressions." Contrary to the other skeletal muscles which due to their origin and insertion on bone serve to move bones, the mimetic muscles, due to their insertion directly into the overlying skin of face (though they originate from the bones or fibrous structures of skull), serve to manipulate the skin and soft tissues of the face. The specific location and attachments of the facial muscles directly to the skin enable them to produce expressions of emotions and movements on the face, like smiling, laughing, grinning, frowning etc., through their contraction.

*There are five groups of mimetic muscles (**Fig. 2.7**):*

1. Scalp group: Occipitofrontalis and epicranial aponeurosis: This muscle has two parts, frontalis and occipital belly. Both are joined by epicranial aponeurosis. The frontalis part is supplied by the temporal branch of the facial nerve, whereas the occipital part is supplied by post auricular branch of facial nerve. In frontalis part, when its forehead attachment is fixed, the contraction of the frontalis muscle pulls the scalp forwards and wrinkles the forehead creating an expression of frown. If its aponeurotic attachment is fixed, the frontal belly elevates the eyebrows and skin of the forehead, creating an expression of surprise. In occipital part, when the nuchal attachment of the muscle is fixed, the occipital

part retracts the scalp. When the aponeurotic attachment is fixed, the muscle moves the scalp anteriorly.

2. Periorbital group:

- Orbicularis oculi (orbital, palpebral, and lacrimal parts): Contraction of the orbital part pulls the skin of the forehead and cheek toward the nose and causes tight closure of the eyes with contraction of skin around the eyes. This movement is for protecting the eye. The action of the palpebral part causes gentle closing of eyelids specifically for blinking or sleeping. The action of lacrimal part facilitates the flow of tears through the *lacrimal apparatus.*
- Corrugator supercilli: Its contraction pulls the eyebrows medially and downwards and creates vertical wrinkles over the glabella, leading to expression of frowning.

3. Nasal muscle group:

- Procerus: The contraction of procerus depresses the medial ends of the eyebrows and wrinkles the skin over the glabella creating expression of frowning in reaction to exposure to bright light.
- Nasalis (lateral and alar parts): The contraction of lateral part compresses the nasal aperture, and contraction of its alar part dilates the AICA (anterior cerebellar artery) nostrils. These actions are either part of normal or deep breathing or for expressing anger.
- Depressor septi nasi: It depresses the nose.

4. Buccolabial or oral muscle group:

- Orbicularis oris (labial and marginal parts): This is the only nonpaired single mimetic muscle that surrounds the mouth and forms most of the lips. Both parts originate from modiolus, a fibromuscular structure on both the lateral sides of the mouth. Modiolus is important because many facial muscles converge to attach to it and it is also used for attaching the facial slings used as static procedure for facial reanimation. A bilateral contraction of the complete orbicularis oris muscle brings the lips together and seals the mouth. If only certain parts of the muscle contract, it produces different movements like pout, puckering, twisting etc. All these movements help in expressing certain human emotions and help in creating speech.
- Levator labii superioris alequae nasi: Its contraction elevates and everts the upper lip, as well as deepens and increases the depth of the nasolabial furrow.
- Levator labii superioris: In coordination with other buccolabial muscles its contraction helps to elevate and evert the upper lip, deepening the nasolabial

furrow and thus helps in achieving certain facial expressions, such as smiling, grinning, and anger.

- Levator anguli oris: Contracting together with the risorius and zygomaticus major and minor, it elevates the angles of the lips for producing a smile.
- Zygomaticus major: The coordinated movement or contraction of zygomaticus major with other muscles mentioned above produces smile by elevating and everting the angle of the mouth.
- Zygomaticus minor: In a synergistic action with other muscles its contraction leads to elevation and eversion of the upper lip to produce a variety of facial expressions such as smiling, frowning, or grimacing.
- Depressor labii inferioris: As the name suggests, its contraction helps in pulling the lower lip inferomedially along with the fibers of platysma.
- Depressor anguli oris: Its action depresses the angle of the mouth for expressing feelings of sadness or anger. It also helps in opening the mouth during speaking or eating.
- Risorius: Due to its action of pulling the angles of the mouth superolaterally to produce a smile, this muscle is also known as "smiling muscle."
- Mentalis: Its contraction depresses and everts the lower lip, creating wrinkles on the skin of the chin. Its action contributes in activities like drinking, or creating facial expressions of sorrow, anger, and doubt.
- Buccinator: Its contraction pulls back the angle of the mouth and flattens the cheek area against the teeth, which aids the teeth during chewing. By keeping the food in the correct position when chewing, the buccinator assists the muscles of mastication. It also helps in actions like smiling and whistling. The suckling reflex of neonates is aided by the action of this muscle.
- Platysma: Although it is a big muscle, contraction of its different parts produces different actions. The contraction of the lateral fibers attaching to the modiolus lowers the corners of the mouth and lower lip, while contraction of its medial attachment on the mandible depresses the mandible which helps in opening the mouth.

5. Auricular muscle group:

- Anterior auricular muscles: It pulls ear forwards or anteriorly.
- Posterior auricular muscles: It pulls ear backwards or posteriorly.
- Superior auricular muscles: It raises the ear upwards.

The movements of the ear produced by these muscles are not very significant and just form a part of other actions like smiling and yawning.

The facial muscles not only regulate the movements of face, but also makes it more expressive. Because of these muscles the face is able to convey emotions and psychological state of mind and develop a nonverbal communication between two persons.

The names of different facial muscles are: (1) Frontalis medial and lateral; (2) depressor supracilii; (3) corrugator supercili; (4) orbicularis oculi: pretarsal portion; (5) orbicularis oculi: preseptal portion; (6) orbicularis oculi: orbital portion; (7) procerus; (8) levator labii superioris alaeque nasi; (9) compressor nasi; (10) dilator nasi; (11) depressor septi; (12) levator labii superioris; (13) zygomaticus minor; (14) zygomatic major; (15) risorius; (16) orbicularis oris; (17) depressor anguli oris; (18) depressor labii; (19) mentalis; and (20) platysma (**Fig. 2.7**).

Branches and Their Supply to Different Facial Muscles

- Temporal branch (frontal branch) is the first terminal branch which leaves the parotid gland at its upper pole, just anterior to superficial temporal

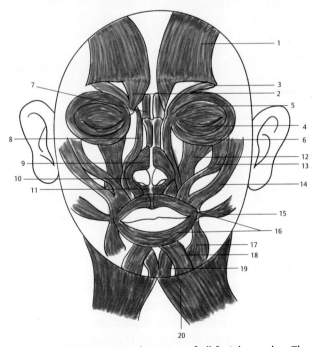

Fig. 2.7 Diagrammatic depiction of all facial muscles. The orange lines are the imaginary lines for dividing the face into three parts, upper, mid, and lower face. The names of different facial muscles are: (1) Frontalis medial and lateral; (2) depressor supracilii; (3) corrugator supercili; (4) orbicularis oculi: pretarsal portion; (5) orbicularis oculi: preseptal portion; (6) orbicularis oculi: orbital portion; (7) procerus; (8) levator labii superioris alaeque nasi; (9) compressor nasi; (10) dilator nasi; (11) depressor septi; (12) levator labii superioris; (13) zygomaticus minor; (14) zygomatic major; (15) risorius; (16) orbicularis oris; (17) depressor anguli oris; (18) depressor labii; (19) mentalis; and (20) platysma.

artery. It crosses lateral to the periosteum of zygomatic process, runs directly upwards, traverses the temporal region lying underneath the temporoparietal fascia, and divides into anterior temporal branch which innervates the frontalis, superior part of orbicularis oculi, corrugator supercilii, and procerus, and posterior temporal branch innervates anterior and superior auricular muscle.

- Zygomatic branch emerges from the parotid at its anterosuperior border and after crossing zygomatic arch innervates the inferior part of orbicularis oculi.
- Buccal branches are more than one in number, and may arise from both temporofacial and cervicofacial branches of facial nerve and innervate the muscles, namely, the nasalis, procerus, depressor septi, risorius, zygomaticus major and minor, levator labi superioris, levator labii superioris alaque nasi, levator anguli oris, orbicularis oris, and buccinator muscles.
- Marginal mandibular branch emerges from the parotid gland at its lower pole, runs below the angle of the mandible under the platysma, but superficial to the deep cervical fascia, passes through the upper part of digastric triangle, turns up and forward across the body of the mandible to reach and supply muscles of the lower lip, namely, the depressor anguli oris, depressor labii inferioris, and mentalis muscles.

Surgical relevance: As the marginal mandibular nerve travels along the inferior border of the mandible just beneath the platysma muscle fibers, it may get traumatized during an open approach to submandibular region. The surgeon has to take utmost care to avoid injuring this branch while making incision in this area. The incision is made in single go, up to the platysma, approximately 1.5 cm below the inferior border of the body of the mandible. Injury to the marginal mandibular nerve leads to paralysis of muscles of the lower lip of that side. The correction of resultant deformity may require complex surgical procedures like transfer of anterior belly of digastric muscle.

- Cervical branch emerges from the posterioinferior surface of the gland and innervates the platysma.

There are two categories of branches of facial nerve: The first category consists of branches of distribution which have already been explained above. Along with that, there are branches of communication with the surrounding nerves in the vicinity.

- Branches of distribution includes:
  - ➤ Branches within the temporal bone:
    1. Nerve to stapedius.
    2. Chorda tympani.

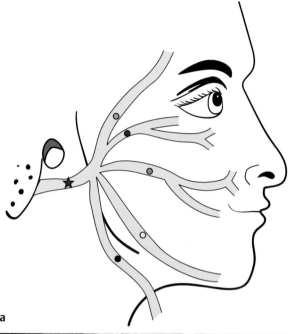

Fig. 2.8 **(a)** Diagrammatic depiction of terminal branches of facial nerve: *blue star* shows the main trunk; *blue dot* shows the temporal branch; *red dot* shows the zygomatic arch; *green dot* shows the buccal branch; *yellow dot* shows the marginal mandibular branch; *black dot* shows the cervical branch. **(b)** Exposure of the main facial nerve trunk after its exit from the stylomastoid foramen (SMF) and its temporofacial and cervicofacial divisions; main focus on cervicofacial trunk and its terminal branches. **(c)** Temporofacial division and its further branches. PD, parotid duct; RMV, retromandibular vein.

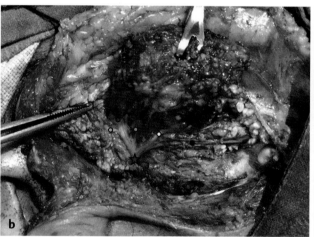

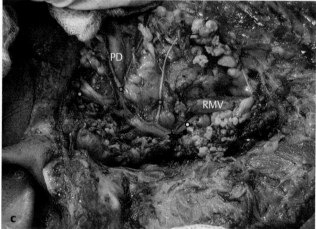

> Branches in the neck:
>   1. Posterior auricular.
>   2. Nerve to stylohyoid.
>   3. Nerve to digastric.
> Branches on the face:
>   1. Temporal.
>   2. Zygomatic.
>   3. Buccal.
>   4. Marginal mandibular.
>   5. Cervical.
- Branches of communication with adjacent cranial and spinal nerves include:
>   In IAM: CN VII connects with CN VIII.
>   At GG: It is connected with sphenopalatine ganglion via GSPN, with the otic ganglion by a branch which joins the lesser superficial petrosal nerve and with the sympathetic on middle meningeal artery.

> In fallopian canal: With auricular branch of vagus nerve (CN X).
> At its exit at SMF: With glossopharyngeal nerve (CN IX), vagus nerve (CN X), great auricular nerve, and auriculotemporal nerve.
> Behind the pinna: With lesser occipital nerve.
> On the face with the trigeminal nerve.
> In the neck: With the cutaneous cervical branch.

Surgical Relevance

- As the facial nerve has multiple branches of communications with other cranial nerves (CNs V, X, XI, and XII) and parasympathetic and sympathetic nerves along its course, it can cause referred pain syndromes in head and neck pathologies.
- Persisting function of mimetic muscles even after complete denervation of facial nerve have been a

cause of debate for many years. These intercommunicating branches are found to be the reason for the residual function of mimetic muscles of face following an apparently complete denervation of facial nerve post injury or even after nonfunctioning of facial nerve in long-term facial nerve palsy (>2 years).

- A sound knowledge of the anatomy of the extratemporal facial nerve is important so as to enable safe dissection through the planes of the face during surgical procedures on face and neck.

■ Blood Supply of Facial Nerve

The blood supply to the facial nerve in its different segments is through multiple sources (**Fig. 2.9**). It begins with the Rolandic branch of middle cerebral artery, which is a paired artery and branches from internal carotid artery, supplying the motor cortex area for facial nerve functioning.

The facial nucleus in the pons receives blood supply from a combination of the anterior inferior cerebellar artery (AICA), which is a branch of basilar artery, and the short and long circumferential arteries.

The facial nerve in the IAM is supplied by labyrinthine artery (internal auditory artery) which is a branch of the AICA. It enters in the IAM, in close association with the facial and vestibulocochlear nerves.

The blood supply to the labyrinthine part is from the superficial petrosal artery, a branch of middle meningeal artery which arises from mandibular branch of maxillary artery which is one of the terminal branches of external carotid artery. The petrosal artery runs laterally with the GSPN to enter the middle ear (**Fig. 2.2**). At the GG level, the artery divides into an ascending branch which supplies the region proximal to the GG (labyrinthine part) and a descending branch which continues along the facial canal below the horizontal part of the facial nerve to anastomose with the stylomastoid artery. So, the nerve in the fallopian canal including the GG, horizontal part, and second genu area is supplied by the superficial petrosal artery.

The MS is supplied by stylomastoid artery, a branch of posterior auricular artery which again is a branch of external carotid artery. It enters the facial canal through the SMF, and lies on the anteromedial aspect of the nerve. The artery loops around the nerve and divides into several branches. From the convexity of the loop, two branches arise, one accompanies the facial nerve and ascends in superior direction and the other divides into branches which pierce the posterior meatal wall and accompanies the auricular branch of the vagus

nerve. The main ascending branch first lies on the medial aspect of the facial nerve as far as the second genu and then loops around the inferior aspect of the bend to reach the inferomedial surface of the horizontal part of the nerve. It anastomoses directly with the superficial petrosal artery to form a complete arterial arcade in the facial canal. From the arcade, branches are given to the nerve close to the origin of the chorda tympani and the second genu. A few branches run along the posterior canal wall to supply mastoid air cells.

So, the blood supply to the intratemporal part of the facial nerve is through three arteries with overlapping territories, which makes each segment of the facial nerve to have dual blood supply, except the LS which has single blood supply. There are no anastomoses between the arterial systems immediately proximal to the GG which is the LS.

Venous drainage, in similar pattern as arterial supply, is into the venae comitantes of the superficial petrosal and stylomastoid veins.

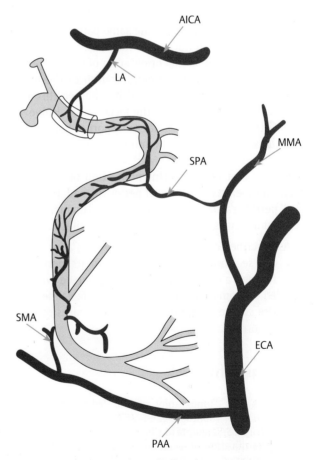

Fig. 2.9 Vascular supply to the facial nerve. Abbreviations: AICA, anterior inferior cerebellar artery; LA, labyrinthine artery; SPA, superficial petrosal artery; MMA, middle meningeal artery; SMA, stylomastoid artery; ECA, external carotid artery; PAA, posterior auricular artery.

These finer branches of arteries and tributaries of veins lie within the loose connective tissue of the epineurium, which covers the facial nerve between the periosteum of facial canal wall and the nerve sheath.

The extratemporal portion of the facial nerve receives its blood supply from the branches of the stylomastoid, posterior auricular, superficial temporal, and transverse facial arteries.

Surgical Relevance

The overlapping of arteries in all parts other than labyrinthine part, which has a single blood supply, makes the labyrinthine portion more susceptible to vascular compromise secondary to any inflammatory change as compared to other areas.

■ Spatial Orientation of Facial Nerve

Lots of studies and researches have been conducted to demonstrate the spatial orientation of the facial nerve in its extra-axial course from the brainstem to its terminal branches persisting in the same pattern as it is in the cortex and facial nucleus in the pons. Some studies favor the theory of spatial orientation of the nerve and suggest a discrete compartmentalization of the axons existing in the motor cortex and maintained throughout the peripheral course of the facial nerve. However, recent studies using retrograde transport of horseradish peroxidase (HRP) within the motor axons[12] and axonal degeneration studies using Marchi and Osmium stain[13] suggested that no compartmentalization of the motor axon group exists in the facial nerve. Instead, the fibers to all peripheral branches are lying mixed up in the facial nerve at all levels before peripheral branching occurs.

As described earlier, the facial nerve has a very complex course from the motor cortex to its peripheral branches and a clinician has to be well versed with the detailed anatomy and orientation of the facial nerve in its entire course before dealing with the cases of facial nerve disorders.

Bibliography

1. Harris WD. Topography of the facial nerve. Arch Otolaryngol 1968;88(3):264–267
2. Saha S, Pal S, Sengupta M, Chowdhury K, Saha VP, Mondal L. Identification of facial nerve during parotidectomy: a combined anatomical & surgical study. Indian J Otolaryngol Head Neck Surg 2014;66(1):63–68
3. Kukwa A, Czarnecka E, Oudghiri J. Topography of the facial nerve in the stylomastoid fossa. Folia Morphol (Warsz) 1984;43(4):311–314
4. Sunderland S, Cossar DF. The structure of the facial nerve. Anat Rec 1953;116(2):147–165
5. Fisch U, Esslen E. Total intratemporal exposure of the facial nerve. Pathologic findings in Bell's palsy. Arch Otolaryngol 1972;95(4):335–341
6. Nakashima S, Sando I, Takahashi H, Fujita S. Computer-aided 3-D reconstruction and measurement of the facial canal and facial nerve. I. Cross-sectional area and diameter: preliminary report. Laryngoscope 1993;103(10):1150–1156
7 Hunt JR. On herpetic inflammation of the geniculate ganglion. A new syndrome and its complications. J Nerv Ment Dis 1907;34:73–96
8. Rouviere H, Delmas A. Nerfs de la tet et du cou. In: Anatomie Humaine: Descriptive Topographique et Functionnelle. Paris: Masson; 1985:276
9. Hitselberger WE, House WF. Acoustic neuroma diagnosis. External auditory canal hypesthesia as an early sign. Arch Otolaryngol 1966;83(3):218–221
10. Wilhelmi BJ, Mowlavi A, Neumeister MW. The safe face lift with bony anatomic landmarks to elevate the SMAS. Plast Reconstr Surg 2003;111(5):1723–1726
11. Davis RA, Anson BJ, Budinger JM, Kurth LR. Surgical anatomy of the facial nerve and parotid gland based upon a study of 350 cervicofacial halves. Surg Gynecol Obstet 1956;102(4):385–412
12. Baker DC, Conley J. Avoiding facial nerve injuries in rhytidectomy. Anatomical variations and pitfalls. Plast Reconstr Surg 1979;64(6):781–795
13. Pitanguy I, Ramos AS. The frontal branch of the facial nerve: the importance of its variations in face lifting. Plast Reconstr Surg 1966;38(4):352–356
14. Stuzin JM, Wagstrom L, Kawamoto HK, Wolfe SA. Anatomy of the frontal branch of the facial nerve: the significance of the temporal fat pad. Plast Reconstr Surg 1989;83(2):265–271
15. Gosain AK, Sewall SR, Yousif NJ. The temporal branch of the facial nerve: how reliably can we predict its path? Plast Reconstr Surg 1997;99(5):1224–1233, discussion 1234–1236
16. Bell C. On the nerves, giving an account of some experiments on their structure and functions, which leads to a new arrangement of the system. Trans R Soc Lond 1821;3:398–424
17. Bell C. The nervous system of the human body. 2nd ed. London: Longman; 1830
18. Crosby EC, Dejonge BR. Experimental and clinical studies of the central connections and central relations of the facial nerve. Ann Otol Rhinol Laryngol 1963;72:735–755
19. Lang J. Anatomy of the brainstem and the lower cranial nerves, vessels, and surrounding structures. Am J Otol 1985;(Suppl):1–19
20. Anson BJ, Harper DG, Warpeha RL. Surgical anatomy of the facial canal and facial nerve. Ann Otol Rhinol Laryngol 1963;72:713–734
21. Basek M. Anomalies of the facial nerve in normal temporal bones. Ann Otol Rhinol Laryngol 1962;71: 382–390
22. Kudo H, Nori S. Topography of the facial nerve in the human temporal bone. Acta Anat (Basel) 1974;90(3): 467–480

23. Yadav SP, Ranga A, Sirohiwal BL, Chanda R. Surgical anatomy of tympano-mastoid segment of facial nerve. Indian J Otolaryngol Head Neck Surg 2006;58(1):27–30

24. Anson BJ, Donaldson JA, Warpeha RL, Rensink MJ, Shilling BB. Surgical anatomy of the facial nerve. Arch Otolaryngol 1973;97(2):201–213

25. Adkins WY, Osguthorpe JD. Management of trauma of the facial nerve. Otolaryngol Clin North Am 1991;24(3):587–611

26. Rulon JT, Hallberg OE. Operative injury to the facial nerve. Explanations for its occurrence during operations on the temporal bone and suggestions for its prevention. Arch Otolaryngol 1962;76:131–139

27. Sullivan JA, Smith JB. The otological concept of Bell's palsy and its treatment. Ann Otol Rhinol Laryngol 1950;59(4):1148–1170

28. Haynes DR. The relations of the facial nerve in the temporal bone. Ann R Coll Surg Engl 1955;16(3):175–185

29. Proctor B, Nager GT. The facial canal: normal anatomy, variations and anomalies. I. Normal anatomy of the facial canal. Ann Otol Rhinol Laryngol Suppl 1982;97:33–44

30. Proctor B. The anatomy of the facial nerve. Otolaryngol Clin North Am 1991;24(3):479–504

31. Botman JW, Jongkees LB. Endotemporal branching of the facial nerve. Acta Otolaryngol 1955;45(2):111–114

32. Guild SR. Natural absence of part of the bone wall of the facial canal. Laryngoscope 1949;59(6):668–673

33. Hough JV. Malformations and anatomical variations seen in the middle ear during the operation for mobilization of the stapes. Laryngoscope 1958;68(8):1337–1379

34. Beddard D, Saunders WH. Congenital defects in the fallopian canal. Laryngoscope 1962;72:112–115

35. Fowler EP Jr. Variations in the temporal bone course of the facial nerve. Laryngoscope 1961;71:937–946

36. Kettel K. Surgery of the facial nerve. Arch Otolaryngol 1966;84(1):99–109

37. Green JD Jr, Shelton C, Brackmann DE. Iatrogenic facial nerve injury during otologic surgery. Laryngoscope 1994;104(8 Pt 1):922–926

38. Nager GT, Proctor B. Anatomic variations and anomalies involving the facial nerve. Otolaryngol Clin North Am 1928;24:531

39. Kullman GL, Dyck PJ, Cody DT. Anatomy of the mastoid portion of the facial nerve. Arch Otolaryngol 1971;93(1):29–33

40. May M. Anatomy of the facial nerve (spatial orientation of fibers in the temporal bone). Laryngoscope 1973;83(8):1311–1329

41. May M. Anatomy for the clinician. In: May M, Schaitkin BM, eds. The Facial Nerve. 2nd ed. New York: Thieme; 2000:19–56

42. Podvinec M, Pfaltz CR. Studies on the anatomy of the facial nerve. Acta Otolaryngol 1976;81(3–4):173–177

43. Sabini P, Wayne I, Quatela VC. Anatomical guides to precisely localize the frontal branch of the facial nerve. Arch Facial Plast Surg 2003;5(2):150–152

44. Dingman RO, Grabb WC. Surgical anatomy of the mandibular ramus of the facial nerve based on the dissection of 100 facial halves. Plast Reconstr Surg Transplant Bull 1962;29:266–272

45. Seckel BR. Facial Danger Zones: Avoiding Nerve Injury in Facial Plastic Surgery. Saint Louis: Quality Medical Publishers; 1993

46. Freilinger G, Gruber H, Happak W, Pechmann U. Surgical anatomy of the mimic muscle system and the facial nerve: importance for reconstructive and aesthetic surgery. Plast Reconstr Surg 1987;80(5):686–690

47. Happak W, Burggasser G, Liu J, Gruber H, Freilinger G. Anatomy and histology of the mimic muscles and the supplying facial nerve. Eur Arch Otorhinolaryngol 1994:S85–S86

48. Freilinger G, Happak W, Burggasser G, Gruber H. Histochemical mapping and fiber size analysis of mimic muscles. Plast Reconstr Surg 1990;86(3):422–428

49. Happak W, Liu J, Burggasser G, Flowers A, Gruber H, Freilinger G. Human facial muscles: dimensions, motor endplate distribution, and presence of muscle fibers with multiple motor endplates. Anat Rec 1997;249(2):276–284

50. Conley JJ. Symposium: Facial nerve rehabilitation. Accessory neuromuscular pathways to the face. Trans Am Acad Ophthalmol Otolaryngol 1964;68:1064–1067

51. Banfai P. [Applied anatomy of the facial nerve. I. Nuclei, supranuclear connections and peripheral nerve (author's transl)] [in German]. HNO 1976;24(8):253–264

52. Graeber MB, Bise K, Mehraein P. Synaptic stripping in the human facial nucleus. Acta Neuropathol 1993;86(2):179–181

53. Bischoff EPE. Microscopic Analysis of the Anastomosis between the Cranial Nerves [Sacks EJ, Valtin EW, eds]. Hanover, NH: University Press of New England; 1977:181

54. Norris CW, Proud GO. Spontaneous return of facial motion following seventh cranial nerve resection. Laryngoscope 1981;91(2):211–215

55. Graeber MB, López-Redondo F, Ikoma E, et al. The microglia/macrophage response in the neonatal rat facial nucleus following axotomy. Brain Res 1998;813(2):241–253

56. Saha S, Pal S, Sengupta M, Chowdhury K, Saha VP, Mondal L. Identification of facial nerve during parotidectomy: a combined anatomical & surgical study. Indian J Otolaryngol Head Neck Surg 2014;66(1):63–68

57. Gupta S, Mends F, Hagiwara M, Fatterpekar G, Roehm PC. Imaging the facial nerve: a contemporary review. Indian J Otolaryngol Head Neck Surg 2014;66(1):63–68

58. May M. Anatomy of the facial nerve (spatial orientation of fibers in the temporal bone). Laryngoscope 1973;83(8):1311–1329

59. Myckatyn TM, Mackinnon SE. A review of facial nerve anatomy. Semin Plast Surg 2004;18(1):5–12

60. Hellekant G. Vasodilator fibres to the tongue in the chorda tympani proper nerve. Acta Physiol Scand 1977;99(3):292–299

61. Rao A, Tadi P. Anatomy, head and neck, chorda tympani. 8.StatPearls [Internet]. Treasure Island, FL: StatPearls Publishing; 2021

3 Facial Nerve Unit: Structure, Lesions, and Repair

Introduction

Facial nerve is a bundle of axons arranged in the form of a "cable." Through these axons, the electrochemical impulses are transmitted to target tissue which can be either muscle or secretory glands. The structure of facial nerve consists of:

- Cellular part:
  - ➤ Neuron with its cell body, dendrites, and myelinated axons
  - ➤ Myelin sheath with Schwann cells encasing the axons
- Connective tissue:
  - ➤ Epineurium (outermost layer)
  - ➤ Perineurium (middle layer)
  - ➤ Endoneurium (inner layer)
  - ➤ Blood vessels

Anatomy of a Neuron

Neurons, like other cells, have a cell body (soma) with a nucleus located in it. Multiple short branches (protrusions) extend from the soma. These are called dendrites. The dendrites and cell body are involved in neuronal functions like receiving and processing incoming neural information.

A separate single long process called axon extends from the other side of the stoma. The center of each axon is composed of axoplasm, which is the cytoplasmic extension of the nerve cell body. It comprises several physiologically distinct zones that aid in transport of nutrients and essential biochemical components from the nerve cell body to the terminal axon and neuromuscular terminals. There is a cell membrane called axolemma that surrounds the axoplasm. The axon is surrounded by myelin sheath and Schwann cells. The myelin sheath is a double spiral of lipoprotein that is adjoining to the plasma membrane of the body of Schwann cells. The myelin sheath develops from Schwann cell itself. Each Schwann cell and its associated myelin encase a histologically distinct zone of axon (internode zone) (**Fig. 3.1**). Gaps appear between two internodes and are referred to as nodes of Ranvier (**Fig. 3.1**). Enveloping the Schwann cell–axon unit is the basement membrane. This structure serves as a histologic demarcation between the neural and connective tissue elements of the facial nerve. Immediately adjacent to the basement membrane is the endoneurium.

The distal end of the axon splits up into multiple terminals. Each terminal synapses with a dendrite or cell body of another neuron. The cell in which the axon terminal is sending information is called the presynaptic cell (sending cell), while the cell in which the dendrites are receiving information are called the postsynaptic cell (receiving cell). An action potential arriving at the axon terminal triggers the release of neurotransmitter from the presynaptic cell which diffuses through the synapse to the other side and binds to receptors on the membrane of the dendrites of postsynaptic cell (**Fig. 3.2**).

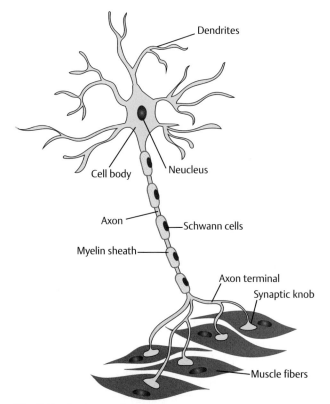

Fig. 3.1 Anatomy of neuron.

The synaptic connections between neurons and skeletal muscle cells are called neuromuscular junctions, through which the action potential is transmitted to the muscle. This action potential can carry an excitatory or inhibitory signal.

A single postsynaptic cell can receive inputs from many presynaptic neurons through dendrites and in the same manner it can make synaptic connections on numerous postsynaptic neurons via different axon terminals.

■ Facial Nerve Structure

Within a nerve, each axon is surrounded by a layer of connective tissue called endoneurium. The axons are

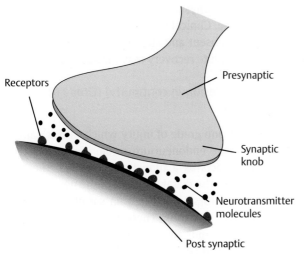

Fig. 3.2 Synaptic connection.

bundled together to form groups called fascicles. Each fascicle is packed in a layer of connective tissue called perineurium and finally all fascicles are wrapped in a connective tissue layer called epineurium (**Fig. 3.3**).

Endoneurium, which surrounds each nerve fiber, provides protection and tubular structure for regeneration. Perineurium has fibrils (characteristic of collagen type III) which provide tensile strength to the nerve and protect it from infection. The perineurium along with the endoneurium forms the blood–nerve barrier as it encircles the fascicles. Epineurium, which surrounds the entire nerve, has two layers, outer and inner layers. The outer layer has connective tissue with tightly packed fibrils (characteristic of collagen type I). The inner epineurium contains small amount of adipose tissue and the vessels supplying and coursing through the nerve. The extraordinary property of facial nerve to undergo elastic deformation without rupture is due to the tensile strength and elastic properties of the epineurium only.

Fascicles in the facial nerve are not arranged in single uninterrupted strands. They undergo multiple divisions and fusion with other fascicles leading to multiple plexuses along the course of the nerve trunk. Two types of fascicles are found in the facial nerve. Simple fascicles are those that are composed of fibers that supply purely to a particular set of muscle or cutaneous area. Compound fascicles are those which are composed of axons from several different fascicles in varying combinations and proportions. This property allows for the integration of various funicular components that distribute to innervate specific anatomical regions. It proves that unless complete transection of a nerve trunk takes place, after any trauma, partial function of the nerve may sustain.

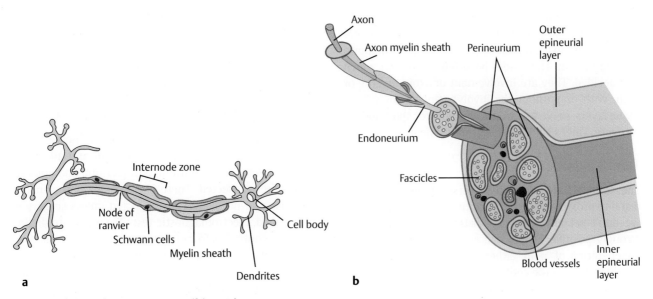

a   b

Fig. 3.3   (a) Single axon anatomy. (b) Facial nerve structure.

The vascular supply courses through all these layers to reach the facial nerve fibers. The vascular supply is by small arterioles arranged into an extensive capillary network. These nutrient arterioles while coursing toward the facial nerve are enclosed first in mesoneurium which is the connective tissue sheath around the nerve trunk and is continuous with the underlying epineurium. The epineurial sheath contains the extrinsic blood vessels, whereas internal plexuses lie in the epineurium, perineurium, and endoneurium. Multiple anastomoses between branches of perineurial and axon vessels ensure adequate collateral vascular supply in instances of segmental interruption.

Mechanism of Injury to Facial Nerve

Facial nerve could be injured due to any of the following insults:

- Stretch/traction
- Laceration/transection
- Crush/compression
- Ischemia
- Radiation
- Electrical injury
- Thermal injury

Facial Nerve Reaction to Trauma/ Neuropathy

Trauma to facial nerve causes inflammation and degeneration of the nerve fibers resulting in impairment of the conductivity of impulses through it.

The nerve injury can be either due to systemic conditions or local pathologies. The pathophysiology of nerve injury related to local pathology has been classified into grading system. The grades have few factors on which it is decided. They are involvement of axon, myelin, or both, with or without the involvement of connective tissue layers, nerve functionality, ability for spontaneous recovery, Tinel's sign, and electrophysiological studies.

Tinel's Sign

The surgeon taps along the course of the nerve in a distal to proximal direction. Positive Tinel's sign is when we don't get any sensation distal to site of injury. A strongly positive Tinel's sign signifies injury of axons. Regeneration of axon, either spontaneous or repair, is confirmed when the centrifugally moving Tinel's sign is persistently stronger than that at the suture line. In an unsuccessful repair, Tinel's sign is stronger at the suture line than at the growing point.

Grading of Nerve Injury

There are various classification systems defining the grades of nerve injury. The most important ones are discussed below.

Seddon's Classification

In 1943, Sir Herbert Seddon classified the injuries into three grades:

Neuropraxia (transient block) (Fig. 3.4)

Here the injury is in the form of contusions or compression after a blunt trauma. There is temporary conduction block with demyelination at the site of injury. All layers including the axon and endoneurium are intact.

There is only physiological interruption of transmission of impulse. Clinically, there is sensory dysfunction. Tinel's sign is absent and electrophysiologic studies are negative. Complete recovery may take up to 3 weeks.

Axonotmesis (lesion in continuity) (Grade II) (Fig. 3.4)

This is the second grade of injury which causes damage to axon but the endoneurium remains intact. So, the endoneurium acts as a tube through which the axon can regenerate. The distal segment of the nerve releases chemotactic factors, which help in sprouting from the proximal parts of axons. These factors released from distal ends also guide the sprouting axons to the appropriate direction and destination. Clinically, motor and/or sensory dysfunction is present and Tinel's sign is positive at the site of injury. Electrophysiologic study reveals decreased nerve conduction velocity and denervation changes with fibrillation of target muscles. These denervation changes are temporary and reinnervation takes place slowly with appearance of muscle unit potential on electrodiagnostic testing.

Neurotmesis (complete division of nerve) (Fig. 3.4)

It is the third and the most severe form of nerve injury where the nerve is completely divided and all layers (axon, myelin, endoneurium, perineurium, and epineurium) are transected. There is no conduction of nerve impulse and no recovery is expected unless surgery is performed. Electrodiagnostic tests are unable to distinguish axonotmesis from neurotmesis. This classification is quite simple but distinction of different categories is not that clear. Further distinction of injury involving different layers (which helps in deciding for surgical technique and has prognostic value) has been described by Sir Sydney Sunderland classification.

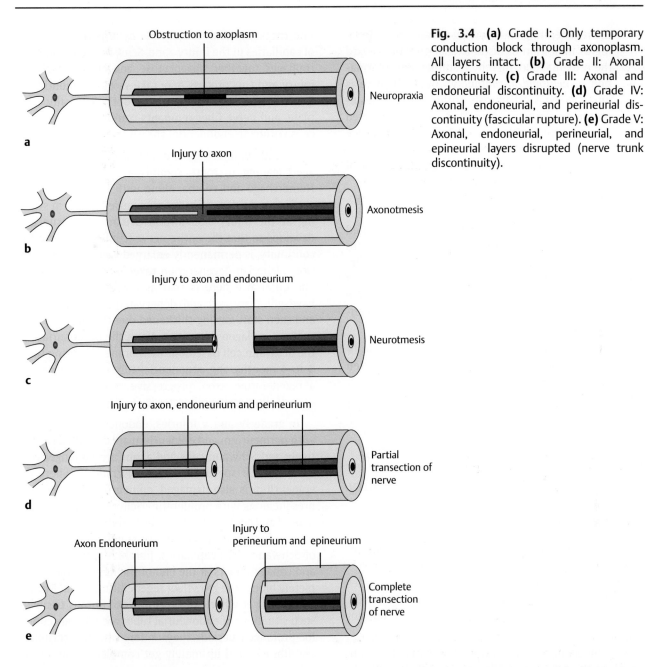

Obstruction to axoplasm

Neuropraxia

a

Injury to axon

Axonotmesis

b

Injury to axon and endoneurium

Neurotmesis

c

Injury to axon, endoneurium and perineurium

Partial transection of nerve

d

Axon Endoneurium

Injury to perineurium and epineurium

Complete transection of nerve

e

Fig. 3.4 (a) Grade I: Only temporary conduction block through axonoplasm. All layers intact. **(b)** Grade II: Axonal discontinuity. **(c)** Grade III: Axonal and endoneurial discontinuity. **(d)** Grade IV: Axonal, endoneurial, and perineurial discontinuity (fascicular rupture). **(e)** Grade V: Axonal, endoneurial, perineurial, and epineurial layers disrupted (nerve trunk discontinuity).

Sir Sydney Sunderland Classification (Fig. 3.4)

This classification is based on the injury to various structures of facial nerve:

- Grade I: It is same as neurapraxia.
- Grades II and III correspond to axonotmesis as described above. Grade III injury is more severe as compared to grade II injury, because in grade II injury, although the axon and myelin sheath are damaged, the endoneurium tube is still intact, whereas in grade III, the endoneurium is also damaged. But in both grades, fascicular continuity is maintained. While recovery in grade II is fast due to conduit support of endoneurium, it takes long time (over many months) for complete recovery in grade III with conservative treatment, so surgical intervention is at times required to release the entrapped nerve.
- Grade IV: This also comes under category of axonotmesis. Along with damage to axon, myelin sheath, and endoneurium, there is damage to perineurium as well, and as their connective tissue sheaths are disrupted, the regenerating axons get misdirected and are unable to reach the destination and innervate the required nerve endings or set of muscle fibers. So, the recovery of nerve functioning is quite erratic and, often, incomplete. Also, hemorrhage at the time of injury and fibrous tissue which develops at the site of injury entraps

the regenerating and growing nerve ending, leading to inhibition of distal axonal growth, toward the proximal end, thereby resulting in the formation of *neuroma-in-continuity*. Although there is interspersed focal fibrosis within *a neuroma-in-continuity*, the action potentials may be conducted through preserved axons which may produce minimal muscular contractions upon stimulation (if more fibers are involved) or almost normal functioning (if the neuroma involves few fibers).

- Grade V: This corresponds to stage of neurotmesis. Here all layers including axon, myelin, endoneurium, perineurium, and epineurium are disrupted leading to complete nerve discontinuity. Due to complete transection of the nerve, the regenerating axon fails to find a connection, and it forms end on neuroma. In grade V, Tinel's sign is negative beyond the level of injury and muscle unit potentials are completely absent.

Electrodiagnostic testing cannot differentiate grade IV and V injuries and functional recovery is not expected without surgery.

- Grade VI includes variable combination of any of the above five categories.

Degenerative and Regenerative Processes in Response to Nerve Injury

Degeneration

Neural response starts at the injury site with degenerative changes followed by regeneration of nerve fibers.

The changes are mild or absent in grade I injuries as there is no true injury but a conduction block only. So, degeneration or regeneration processes do not take place.

In grade II injuries (axonotmesis) proximal to the site of injury, the cell body swells up and nucleus moves to periphery of stoma due to increased metabolic activity. Distal to the injury site, calcium-mediated process known as *Wallerian degeneration* takes place (**Fig. 3.5**). In this, the primary histological change involves damage to both axons and myelin sheath, which begins within hours of injury. By 48 to 96 hours post injury, axonal continuity is lost and conduction of impulses stops. Schwann cells play an important role in Wallerian degeneration. They initially become active within 24 hours of injury by multiplying in number and exhibiting nuclear and cytoplasmic enlargement to assist first in the degeneration and later in regeneration of axon. It helps in degeneration by removing the degenerated axonal and myelin debris and then pass it on to macrophages which have migrated into the injury site through the hyperpermeable walls of capillaries in the injury zone. Schwann cells and macrophages together phagocytose and clear the site of injury and this process may take weeks to months. By 5 to 8 weeks, the degenerative process is usually complete, and nerve fiber remnants composed of Schwann cells within an endoneurial sheath are all that remain.

In grade III injuries, the endoneurium also gets damaged leading to more significant reaction to injury. Hemorrhage and edema, along with fibroblasts proliferation, and a dense fibrous scar cause a fusiform swelling at the injury site. Interfascicular scar tissue also develops so that the entire nerve trunk, which is left in continuity, is permanently enlarged. Distal to the injury site, Wallerian degeneration takes place as in grade II. The difference here is that as the endoneurial tubes have got disrupted and denervated, they first shrink and then start getting thickened due to collagenization process (collagen deposition along the outer surface of the Schwann cell basement membrane). If during these 3 to 4 months, the endoneurial tube does not receive a regenerating axon, progressive collagenization and fibrosis ultimately obliterates it.

In grade IV and V injuries, endoneurial tubes along with perineurium and epineurium are disrupted respectively and Schwann cells and axons are no longer confined in their specific fascicles. In grade V, where the epineurium is also damaged, epineurial fibroblasts are present along with proliferating Schwann cells and perineurial and endoneurial fibroblasts at the injury site. This cellular proliferation leads to a swollen mass consisting of Schwann cells, capillaries, fibroblasts, macrophages, and collagen fibers at the end of the nerve, which completely blocks the growth of regenerating axons. Most of the axons get whorled in this mass of fibrous tissue. In such situations, if endoneurial tubes are left unoccupied for prolonged periods they undergo further shrinkage and fibrosis, and ultimately get completely blocked by collagen fibers.

Nerve Regeneration

Regeneration usually starts after the degenerative changes have taken place or slight overlapping may be there. In grade I and II injuries, restoration of function happens early via reversal of conduction block or late via axonal regeneration. Functional recovery is complete. Both morphological and physiological changes are fully reversible.

In higher grades of injuries in which endoneurial tubes are disrupted, regenerating axons do not have a sheath to keep them confined. They may disperse into surrounding tissue or different endoneurial tubes,

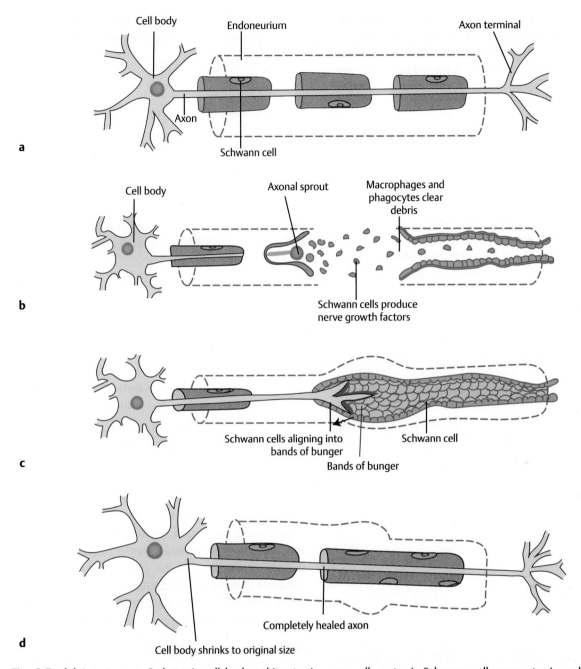

Fig. 3.5 **(a)** Intact axon. *Red star* is cell body, *white star* is axon, *yellow star* is Schwann cell, *green star* is endoneurium, and terminal is axon. **(b)** Postinjury changes: Cell body swelling due to increased metabolic activity; changes at injury site: macrophages and phagocytes clear debris, axonal sprout, and Schwann cells produce nerve growth factors. **(c)** Schwann cells align into bands of bunger to guide the growing axonal sprout. **(d)** Completely healed axon. Cell body shrinks to original size.

thus failing to reinnervate the right set of muscles. Neurological recovery is compromised, generally to a degree proportional to the severity of the injury.

The regeneration takes months to get completed and takes place at different levels which includes the cell body, the proximal axonal segment between the cell body and the injury site, the injury site, the distal segment between the injury site and the end organ itself.

Fibrosis at any of these levels can cause delay in regeneration. The steps are:

Cell body retains its normal size with return of the nucleus to the cell center.

Axoplasm of proximal axonal segment starts regenerating at the axon tip as growth cones. It starts as early as 24 hours post trauma in mild injury and may take weeks after severe injuries. The growth cone encounters the debris of Wallerian degeneration in the distal segment. This debris does not appear to impede regeneration due to the secretion of protease that can help dissolve material blocking its path. Stacks of Schwann cell processes representing collapsed endoneurial tubes start piling up and forming columns known as "bands of Büngner," which guide the sprouting axons from proximal part during reinnervation.

The regenerative process may persist for at least 12 months after injury. The distal regeneration rate is slower if the endoneurial tubes have been disrupted because axon sprouts must first find their way into the tubes before advancing. Regenerating axonal sprouts follow the original Schwann cells to the denervated motor end plates to re-form neuromuscular junctions (**Fig. 3.5**). The multiplied stacks of Schwann cell processes representing collapsed endoneurial tubes start piling up and forming columns known as "bands of Büngner" which guide the sprouting axons from proximal part during reinnervation. Remyelination develops and it involves alignment of Schwann cells and encircling of the axon to form a multi-lamellated sheath. This process begins within 2 weeks of the onset of axonal regeneration and results in myelinated axons quite as the originals except with shortened internodes which over time increases progressively to normal dimensions.

The rate of axonal regeneration is generally estimated to be 1 mm per day and can be either measured by an advancing Tinel's sign or functional recovery. Axonal regeneration is not synonymous with return of function which is quite slower than the regeneration of axons and takes as long as 1 year.

▣ Traumatic Neuromas

Traumatic neuromas occur in response to injury (laceration/penetration) to the nerve and indicate axonotmesis or neurotmesis (grades II to V). They are benign nonneoplastic overgrowth of nerve fibers along with myelin sheath and Schwann cells.

Histopathology

Post injury, after clearance of debris by macrophages, there occurs shrinkage of neural sheaths, and overproliferation of endoneurium and Schwann cells from proximal end to neural reinnervation. If regenerating and proliferating end meets scar tissue, continuous proliferation leads to the formation of neuroma. This traumatic neuroma consists of haphazard arrangement of small nerve fascicles containing axons, Schwann cells, and perineurial cells with surrounding fibrosis. There is no distinctive myelin sheath. There are reactive changes,

such as capillary and myofibroblastic proliferation. The different varieties of traumatic neuroma are:

- Neuroma-in-continuity
- End on neuroma

Neuroma-in-Continuity (Figs 3.6–3.11): Neuroma along the Nerve Line

On gross inspection, it appears as a bulge of thickened tissue on an intact nerve. The surrounding tissue and the layers of the nerve may be intact; however, some of the fascicles do get disrupted and undergo Wallerian degeneration. The regenerating axons grow out of their endoneurial sheath but are still covered with the epineurial layer.

Neuroma-in-continuity is classified into different categories: (1) fusiform, (2) bulbous, (3) lateral, (4) dumbbell, and (5) neuroma after nerve repair.

Fusiform Neuroma (Fig. 3.6)

A fusiform neuroma is located on one side of nerve and indicates very minimal tissue damage, and integrity of fascicles is mostly maintained in the area of injury.

It usually forms after blunt trauma (compression or traction) and is characterized by an intact perineurial sheath (endoneurial sheath is usually disrupted) with increased fibrous tissue deposition and collagen formation at injury site from chronic irritation of the intact nerve. This finally leads to neuroma formation. In such cases, careful dissection, separation of fibrotic tissue, and releasing the entrapped nerve fibers can enhance the nerve regeneration. But the recovery may not be complete if neuroma-in-continuity is involving more fibers. And at times the surgical procedure may itself lead to further scarring.

Bulbous Neuroma (Fig. 3.7)

It has more severe nerve damage than fusiform, although the nerve continuity may be maintained. The procedure performed is decompression of nerve by drilling away the bony fallopian canal followed by removal of fibrous tissue around the neuroma and opening up the sheath of facial nerve on both sides of neuroma. Usually, neuroma resection is not needed.

Lateral Exophytic Neuroma (Fig. 3.8)

It forms if the axon, the perineurium, and the fascicles are partially disrupted and a neuroma forms on the surface of the nerve (**Fig. 3.9**). Lateral neuromas also indicate minimal damage with near-normal functioning of nerve.

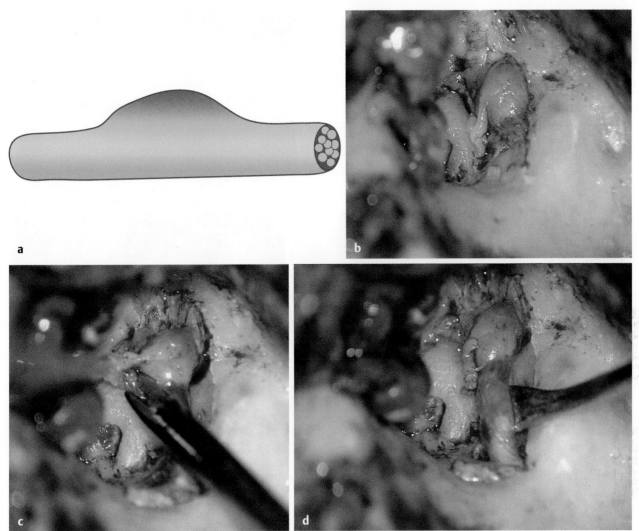

Fig. 3.6 **(a)** Fusiform neuroma, diagrammatic depiction. **(b)** Fusiform neuroma involving lateral half of horizontal segment of facial nerve. Fibrous layer can be seen surrounding neuroma. **(c)** After decompressing the nerve on both sides of neuroma, fibrous layer is being gently separated from around neuroma and in the vicinity of nerve. **(d)** After the epineurial layer covering the neuroma and few millimeters of nerve on each side of neuroma are incised, fusiform neuroma with healthy functional facial nerve on either side is visualized.

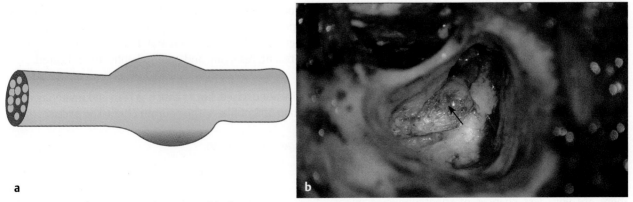

Fig. 3.7 **(a)** Diagrammatic depiction of bulbus neuroma-in-continuity. **(b)** Left ear, revision mastoidectomy showing post iatrogenic trauma, bulbous neuroma formation, in mastoid segment formation of bulbus neuroma-in-continuity (*black arrow*).

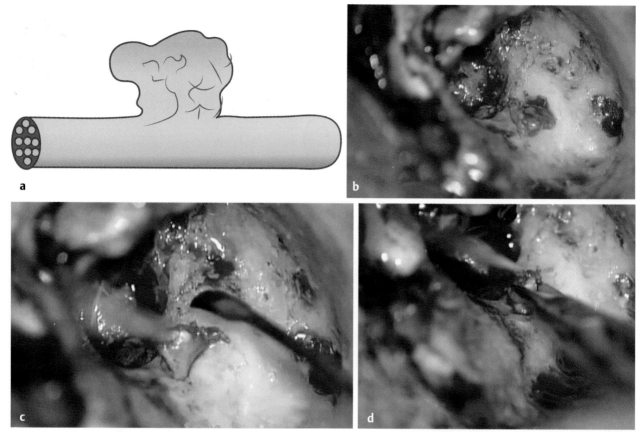

Fig. 3.8 **(a)** Diagrammatic depiction of exophytic neuroma. **(b)** Left ear, Revision mastoidectomy, showing exophytic neuroma-in-continuity in the mastoid segment of facial nerve. **(c)** Intact fallopian canal around exophytic neuroma. **(d)** Slight trimming is needed without disturbing the intact nerve fibers as the patient has normal facial nerve functioning in such cases.

Dumbbell-Shaped Neuromas (Figs. 3.9–3.12)

These suggest widespread damage with very less chances for spontaneous recovery. Excision of the neuroma and neurorrhaphy is indicated in these cases. In dumb bell shaped neuroma, there is a reactive neuroma formation in the proximal part followed by collegenized fibrotic segment distal to it. Further distal to fibrotic segment there is a small neuroma formation along the length of facial nerve giving the whole neuroma a dumb bell shaped neuroma.

Neuroma after Nerve Repair

These are commonly seen in nerve repairs where the cut ends of two nerves with mismatched fascicular patterns are reapproximated.

Consistency of neuroma is equally important. If consistency of neuroma is soft, there is a greater chance for spontaneous healing. But if the neuroma is firm, and lots of fibrosis has occurred at the point of injury, then there are very less chances of spontaneous recovery, as regenerating axons cannot grow through fibrosed neurotubules.

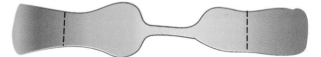

Fig. 3.9 Diagrammatic depiction of dumbbell-shaped neuroma.

Extent of injury plays an important role. If the injury does not exceed 50% of the width of the nerve trunk, spontaneous recovery may occur without surgical intervention. However, if greater than 50% involvement is present, resection and neurorrhaphy are indicated.

So, the principle is that neuroma-in-continuity is usually not excised, but in case it is firm and involving more than 50% of fibers, the neuroma has to be excised.

End on Neuroma

> ➤ It forms in grade V nerve injury (neurotmesis) where the nerve is completely transected. In such a case, complete resection of neuroma is performed along with a cuff of nerve tissue beyond the neuroma. This is followed

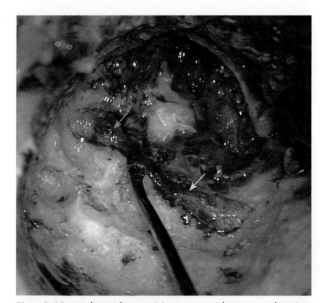

Fig. 3.10 right side, revision mastoidectomy showing dumb bell shaped neuroma formation post iatrogenic trauma to nerve which is extending from 1st genu up to MS Beyond reactive neuroma in the proximal part (*blue arrow*), the collegenized fibrotic segment (*black arrow*) followed by a small neuroma formation (*yellow arrow*) distal to it can be visualized. The normal facial nerve beyond the dumb bell neuroma (*red arrows*) can be visualized on both sides of neuroma. The whole neuroma with the fibrosed nerve that is collapsed and collagenized at the distal end, leading to complete blockage of nerve impulse along with distal small neuroma needs to be excised before any repair work.

by grafting across the nerve defect. Maximum recovery expected after grafting is up to grade III (House-Brakmann's Scale) and takes almost 1.5 to 2 years or even up to 5 years in few cases for optimal recovery (**Fig. 3.13**).

Important definitions relevant to facial nerve paresis or palsy:

1. Facial palsy: it includes facial paresis, complete flaccid (grade VI) facial paralysis and post paralytic facial palsy
2. Flaccid Facial palsy: Complete absence of facial movement and tone both during rest and volitional activity and involuntary emotional expressions(grade VI facial palsy)
3. Facial synkinesis: The facial synkinesis can be defined as the abnormal involuntary facial movement which takes place along with voluntary reflex activity of a different set of facial muscles, which do not normally act together, on the same or the contralateral side of the face.
4. Post paralytic facial nerve syndrome: this syndrome comprises facial synkinesis, facial muscles rigidity, spasm, pain and contractures.
5. Post paralytic facial palsy: it comprises varying degree of post paralytic syndrome disorders which include zonal synkinesis, hypoactivity and hyperactivity.

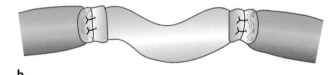

a

b

Fig. 3.11   The illustrations showing **(a)** The unhealthy and fibrotic part of nerve along with neuroma excised. **(b)** The big defect is repaired with interposition graft.

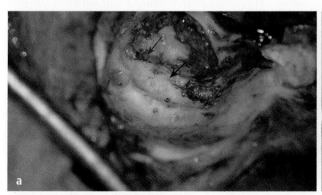
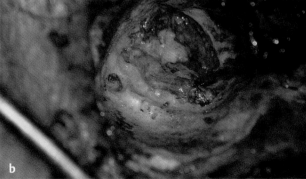

a
b

Fig. 3.12   The actual surgical pictures showing **(a)** The defect after removal of affected part of nerve (*black arrow*) with two cut ends (*red arrows*). **(b)** Interposition graft sutured between two cut ends.

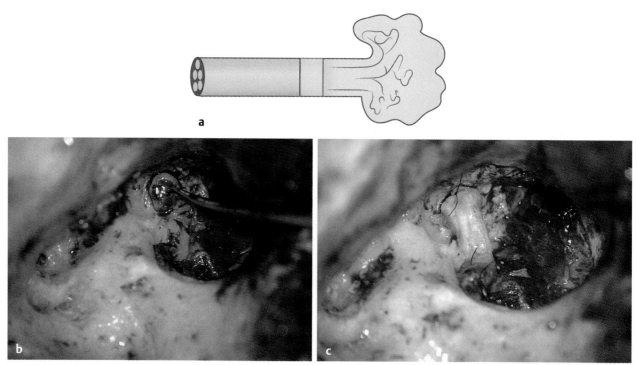

Fig. 3.13 **(a)** Diagrammatic depiction of End on neuroma. The *blue line* shows where the first cut is to be made. The *orange line* shows the second cut to remove cuff of nerve beyond the neuroma. Both specimens are to be sent for histopathology. **(b)** Right ear, canal wall down mastoidectomy showing end on neuroma involving the first genu. **(c)** Interposition graft between two cut ends of facial nerve (after excision of neuroma).

Recovery of Different Grades

The fundamental of nerve injury is that if the cell body is damaged, cell cannot regenerate but if the axon is damaged, the cell can regenerate.

- Grade I: Full spontaneous recovery; time of recovery is from one to three weeks.
- Grade II: Full spontaneous recovery; time of recovery is up to 6 months approximately.
- Grade III: Spontaneous recovery is partial. Although surgery is not required, but at times surgical procedure (neurolysis) to release the regenerating fibers from the fibrosis is required.
- Grades IV and V: Spontaneous recovery is not possible. Surgery in the form of nerve repair, graft, or nerve transfer is performed. Recovery takes few months to up to 2 to 5 years.
- Garde VI: Recovery and type of surgery performed depend on the combination of set of injuries.

Basic Techniques of Nerve Surgery

Decompression/Neurolysis

Decompression is drilling the fallopian canal and exposing the site of injury along with healthy nerve for a few millimeters beyond the site of injury, on both sides, opening the nerve sheath and releasing nerve fibers from intraneural and extraneural scar tissue, so as to improve the functional recovery closest to normal. Neurolysis involves meticulously releasing any scar or constricting tissue around or within a nerve (**Fig. 3.14**).

Nerve Repair

It involves reapproximating the healthy fibers of the cut ends of nerve with end-to-end repair (**Figs. 3.15–3.17**). At times, after trimming the lacerated ends of transected facial nerve there may develop a gap between the two ends. If the gap is up to 8 mm, end-to-end repair can still be achieved after rerouting of facial nerve in its proximal or distal end depending upon the site of injury. Rerouting may lead to some loss of blood supply to the rerouted segment but it saves two anastomotic sites (neurorrhaphies). The advantage of single neurorrhaphy is better coaptation and vascularity and no conduit or tube to support the regeneration is required. Optimal regeneration is expected as there is least chance of mismatch of regenerating fibers or collateral microsprouting outside the epineurium. It can be primary (within 1 week) or secondary (>1 week) repair depending on the condition of trauma site and time of presentation of the patient to the surgeon. The repair should be free of tension. In case there is fallopian canal to support the anastomotic

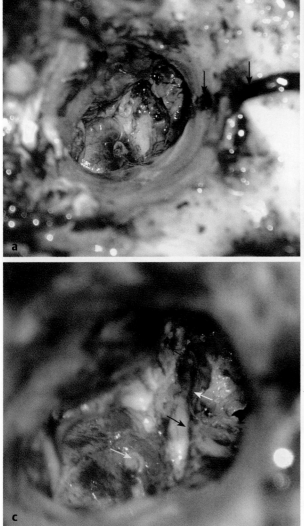

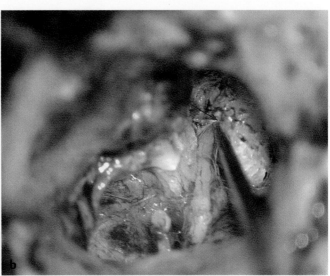

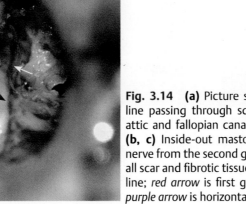

Fig. 3.14 **(a)** Picture showing left ear, post-traumatic fracture line passing through squamous temporal bone reaching up to attic and fallopian canal in the first genu and labyrinthine area. **(b, c)** Inside-out mastoidectomy with decompression of facial nerve from the second genu to labyrinthine portion and removing all scar and fibrotic tissue around the nerve. *Black arrow* is fracture line; *red arrow* is first genu; *white arrow* is labyrinthine portion; *purple arrow* is horizontal segment; *yellow arrow* is stapes.

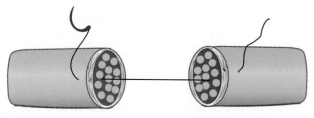

Fig. 3.15 Diagrammatic representation of suturing from epineurium to epineurium (*black arrow*).

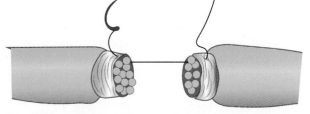

Fig. 3.16 Diagrammatic representation perineurium-to-perineurium suturing after stripping away the epineurium for few millimeters on both sides.

site, no soft tissue bed is required. Otherwise a pedicled muscle flap is placed to support and provide vascularity to the anastomotic site (**Fig. 3.17**).

The suturing can be:

- Epineurium to epineurium: Performed in cases of fresh trauma. The cut ends of the nerve should be sharp, without lacerated ends. Minimal two

epineurial sutures to maintain the alignment of two ends are placed with 8-0 or 9-0 monofilament ethilon (**Fig. 3.15**).

- Perineurium to perineurium: It involves stripping away the epineurium at the cut ends of nerve. It is performed in old injuries where the epineurium is stripped along with any fibrotic scar tissue at the injury site. After exposing perineurium on both

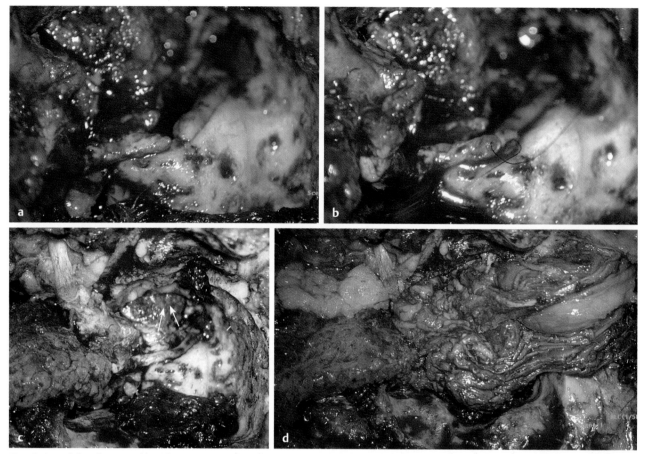

Fig. 3.17 **(a)** Left ear, subtotal petrosectomy with iatrogenic trauma to facial nerve in vertical part. Fresh cut ends of facial nerve are reapproximated. As no gap is present between two cut ends, nerve repair (end to end) is performed. **(b)** Suturing with 8-0 monofilament ethilon, epineurium to epineurium. **(c)** Healthy bed for the anastomosed nerve is created with pedicled postaural and sternocleidomastoid muscle to support and provide vascularity to the nerve and prevent the displacement of facial nerve stumps (*white arrows*). **(d)** Adequate soft tissue coverage with pedicled split temporalis muscle flap to provide vascularity to the healing nerve.

sides, the suturing is performed from perineurium to perineurium. Minimum two sutures are placed. Maximum 4-5 sutures can be placed in an end to end approximated nerve endings. Care is to be taken to avoid trauma to nerve fibers. Presence of neuroma is to be checked on both sides (**Fig. 3.16**).

- Fascicular: Only performed in big nerves and not performed for facial nerve repair (**Fig. 3.17**).

Suturing versus Fibrin Glue

The suture used is 8-0 or 9-0 monofilament ethilon. At least two sutures are to be applied between two cut ends. Fibrin glue is a nontoxic alloplastic material used to keep the cut ends of nerve approximated and glued to each other, without blocking axon regeneration. The common components of glue are fibrinogen, thrombin, and calcium chloride. It has low tensile strength. The coaptation of nerve tissue achieved by applying glue eliminates tissue trauma, eliminates tension on suture, and improves alignment of fascicles. It can be used alone or in combination with sutures. Outcome is equivalent.

Nerve Grafting

In extensive injury, loss of nerve tissue may result in a nerve gap making approximation of cut ends impossible. In case the gap is >5 mm even after rerouting or the rerouting is not possible, the next procedure of choice is interposition nerve grafting for optimal return of function. A sensory nerve (great auricular or sural nerve) is used to bridge this segmental gap between the two cut ends of facial nerve, although the limitation in such procedure is that there are two neurorrhaphies (anastomosis), which make the recovery time longer (up to 2–5 years) and maximum recovery of up to grade III or II only. The proximal and distal nerve stumps are realigned to both ends of cable graft using epineurial or perineurial sutures, with or without fibrin glue reinforcement. The different variations in nerve grafting can be full-thickness interposition grafting, partial-thickness interposition grafting, and double grafting.

Greater Auricular Nerve

Greater auricular nerve (GAN) is a sensory nerve that remains the first choice as grafting material due to its comparable diameter to facial nerve (axonal density per square millimeter is comparable with facial nerve) due to its proximity to facial nerve, being in the same surgical field, and due to the fact that the functional deficit is minimal (sensory loss of inferior two-thirds of the auricle and over the angle of the mandible).

GAN Harvest

GAN is a sensory branch of superficial cervical plexus, arises from C2 and C3 spinal roots, to fuse into the main trunk before emerging onto the mid-body of the sternocleidomastoid (SCM) muscle, lying just deep to platysma, before dividing into anterior and posterior branches. The anterior branch supplies to the skin of parotid gland and anteroinferior aspect of the pinna. The posterior branch reaches the postaural area to supply posteroinferior aspect of pinna.

The most important landmarks to locate GAN:

- The line drawn between angle of mandible (gonion) and mastoid tip (**Fig. 3.18**) is bisected by GAN at right angle.
- Erb's point (one-third of the distance either from the mastoid process or the external auditory canal to the clavicular origin of the sternomastoid muscle): From this point, GAN runs over the sternocleidomastoid muscle in posteroinferior to anterosuperior direction.
- The nerve runs parallel and 1 to 2 cm posterior to the external jugular vein.

In an adult almost 8 to 9 cm of nerve can be harvested. Extra length can be harvested by dissecting the nerve behind the posterior end of SCM muscle. As the nerve is superficially placed, just deep to the investing layer of deep fascia covering the SCM muscle, so the elevation of skin flap should be within the subcutaneous layer. After exposing the whole length of the great auricular nerve, harvesting is performed with watchmaker's forceps, without undue traction and pressure over nerve. All the loose areolar tissue around nerve is dissected sharply. Reversing the polarity of the nerve before grafting is optional; this is facilitated by placing the suture at one end. Edges of harvested nerve are cut bevel-shaped (**Fig. 3.18**).

Sural Nerve

Sural nerve, which is also a sensory nerve, can be used if GAN is not available (revision or long-standing facial nerve palsy or injury to facial nerve in its extratemporal segment, after its bifurcation). It is also used where a longer graft is required (intracranial-to-extracranial grafting or cross-face nerve grafting). It is far away from the operative field so a two-team approach is needed.

Its advantage over the GAN is that it is longer than the GAN and has a number of branches, which makes it better suited for larger defects and for grafting more than one peripheral branch. Another favorable point is its thickness which matches well with the facial nerve diameter. The donor site morbidity (sensory loss on the lateral border of the foot) is also minimal.

Sural Nerve Harvest

The sural nerve (S1, S2) is a sensory nerve of the lower limb and arises in the posterior compartment of the leg (calf region). it is formed by the union of two smaller sensory nerves: the medial cutaneous nerve (branch of tibial nerve) and lateral sural cutaneous nerve (branch of common fibular nerve), that supply the lower posterolateral part of the leg, lateral part of ankle, and lateral part of the dorsum of the foot. The sural nerve leaves the tibial nerve in the popliteal fossa and descends between the two heads of gastrocnemius and pierces the fascia in the middle of the back of leg. Here, it is joined by the sural communicating branch of the common peroneal nerve. In the lower leg, the sural nerve can be located between lateral malleolus and Achilles tendon just posterior to small saphenous vein. It passes down to the posterolateral side of leg and onto dorsal aspect of lateral side of foot.

Steps for sural nerve harvesting are (**Fig. 3.19**):

- A curvilinear incision is made behind the lateral malleolus.
- Identify the nerve approximately 2 cm behind the lateral malleolus, and lying immediately posterior to the small saphenous vein. Place vessel loop around nerve, spread up and down the nerve to create more length.
- Multiple small incisions can be made along the course of sural nerve for harvesting a longer graft. By gently pulling the nerve at the distal incision, the locations of proximal incisions can be determined.
- After the necessary exposure, dissect the medial sural cutaneous nerve proximally to just below the popliteal fossa and harvest around 30 to 35 cm of

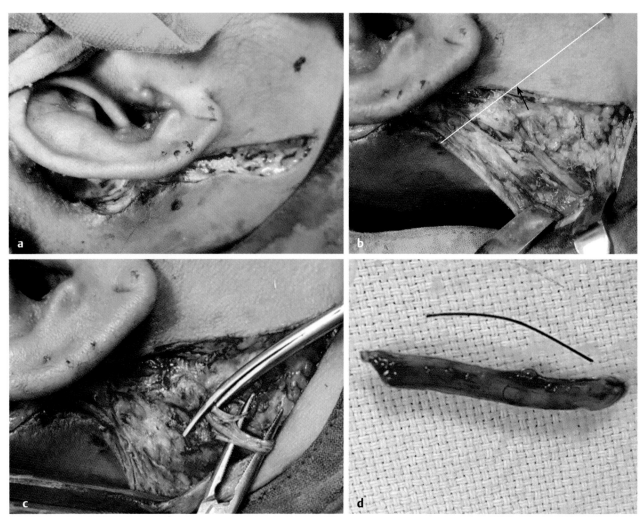

Fig. 3.18 **(a)** Postaural incision extended anteroinferiorly up to hyoid bone. The points on angle of jaw (gonion) and mastoid tip are marked with blue dots. **(b)** Greater auricular nerve (GAN) bisects (*black arrow*) line joining the mastoid tip and angle of jaw (*white line*). **(c)** GAN graft is being harvested. **(d)** The size of graft is longer than the actual gap between the two cut ends as measured with a piece of ethilon suture. Both the edges are cut sharply in beveled shape to have maximum surface area for the axons to grow.

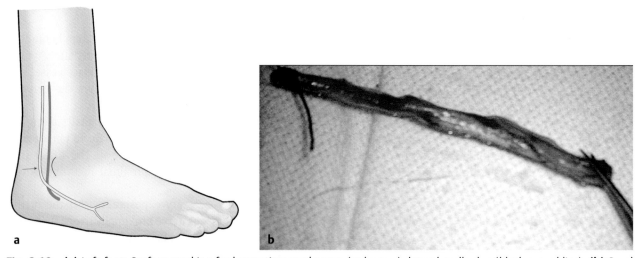

Fig. 3.19 **(a)** Left foot: Surface marking for harvesting sural nerve (*red arrow*), lateral malleolus (*black curved line*). **(b)** Sural nerve harvested. The edge being cut sharp and bevel-shaped.

the nerve for grafting by transecting at the proximal end. The donor site is closed with subcutaneous sutures of 4-0 vicryl, and the skin is closed with 3-0 nylon or staples.

The other technique is through a single incision with an instrument named stripper to go around nerve to harvest the complete graft through single stab incision.

The different types of nerve repair are:

1. Full-thickness interposition graft

The key points are:

- The edges of the facial nerve stumps and the cable graft are cut sharp and in a beveled manner to have maximum surface area and indirectly maximum fibers to approximate with each other.
- The cut ends of healthy facial nerve stumps (after trimming of the unhealthy margins) as well as that of cable graft are to be reapproximated in a way that maximum fibers grow through the cable graft conduit to reach and innervate the appropriate muscle group.
- Trimming of the nonessential branches of facial nerve as well as the cable graft so as to avoid the growth of nerve fibers through them.
- Reverse the ends of cable graft (rotating the donor nerve graft so that its distal end is sutured to the proximal end of facial nerve). This is to maximize the number of useful tubules through which the new nerve will grow and minimize the possibility of new nerve fibers growing out ineffectively through small branches that have been cut. This theory though has been challenged lately. The genetic theory says that at the time of embryogenesis, the growing or regenerating facial nerve fibers are genetically programmed to reach their appropriate set of muscle group. So, while performing repair, the fibers are going to finally more or less reach the appropriate muscle territory regardless of the orientation of nerve fibers.

- The cable graft should be at least 10 to 15% more than the length required (lying in "S" or "C" shape after final suturing), so as to allow shrinkage and avoid tension on suture line.
- The diameter of nerve graft should be equivalent or slightly bigger than the diameter of the nerve stump to maximize the potential for successful grafting procedures. Inadequate graft diameter may predispose to incomplete axonal regrowth owing to an insufficient number of Schwann tubes provided by the graft.
- The two ends of facial nerve should be freed up for few millimeters on both sides. Then either epineurium-to-epineurium or perineurium-to-perineurium suturing is performed. For suturing from perineurium to perineurium, the epineurium at the cut end is stripped back (on both facial nerve stump and cable graft ends) for a few millimeters and perineurium and endoneurium are exposed. The two anastomotic sites are then approximated and matched without tension in a bony or soft tissue bed and suture applied entering through perineurium and out of endoneurium of facial nerve stump to get through endoneurium and out of perineurium on the cable graft side. The same is repeated on the second anastomotic site. This helps in well-matched approximation of ends which allows maximum number of axons to pass through the nerve graft.
- Minimum 2 to upto 5 sutures are to be placed between the two approximated ends (**Fig. 3.20**).

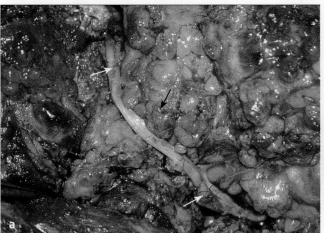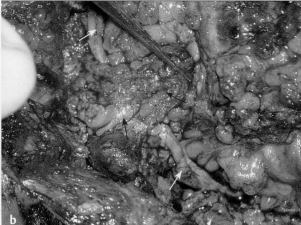

Fig. 3.20 (a, b) Right side face: Facio-masseteric anastomosis with cable graft sutured in between. Parotid gland tissue is providing support from beneath the anastomotic sites (*black arrow*) and superficial lobe of parotid provides soft tissue coverage on lateral side (*red arrows*). *White arrows* are neurorrhaphies.

As already explained, there are two anastomotic sites (two neurorrhaphies) when we perform interposition nerve grafting, so the recovery takes a very long time (up to 2 years approximately) and not better than grade III or II (HBS). The presence of neuroma should always be checked and if present should be excised along with an extra cuff of facial nerve beyond it. The nerve graft does not become a part of regenerating nerve, but acts as a distal nerve stump which goes through Wallerian degeneration to provide conduit for axonal regeneration.

For a seamless regeneration, few important prerequisites are:

- Healthy tissue bed as revascularization initially happens through this tissue bed around the anastomotic sites, in the first 4 to 5 days
- Healthy nerve ends
- No undue tension
- Adequate soft tissue coverage

- Graft length should be optimal, as a short graft will cause tension at suture line and if too long, may cause delay in regeneration

2. Partial-thickness interposition grafting

In case there is partial transection of facial nerve, which usually happens in iatrogenic trauma, a partial-thickness graft is used, maintaining the continuity of intact fibers. The only prerequisite is that the intact fibers should be healthy and functional. Before going ahead with grafting, all unhealthy fibers with necrotic and fibrotic tissue should be cleared and removed (**Fig. 3.21**).

3. Double grafting

In case the thickness of cable graft is less than the nerve trunk, it will create mismatch between the two, leading to regeneration of lesser fibers (**Fig. 3.22a**). So in place of single graft, two cable grafts are sutured to the wide endoneurial surface of the proximal and distal recipient facial nerve to make maximum nerve fibers to grow

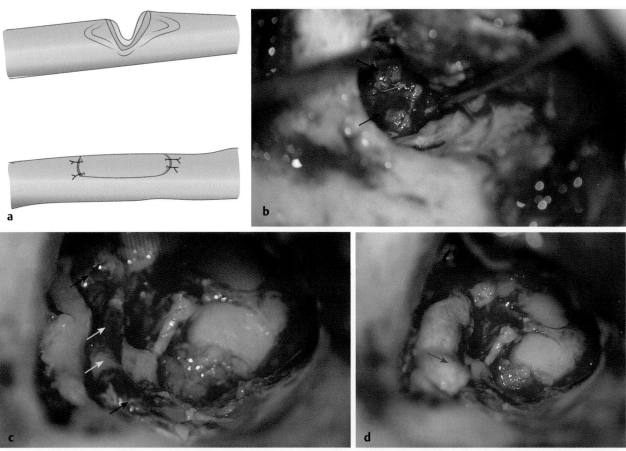

Fig. 3.21 **(a)** Diagrammatic depiction of iatrogenic trauma to partial thickness of facial nerve along with partial-thickness nerve grafting. **(b)** Right ear, revision inside-out atticotomy. Iatrogenic injury in previous surgery caused partial-thickness damage to horizontal segment. Cut ends of damaged facial nerve (*black arrow*) visualized. *Green arrow* is stapes. **(c)** After trimming of lacerated margins, a gap is there between the two cut ends with almost 50%-thickness in nerve continuity visible (*yellow arrow*). **(d)** Partial-thickness cable grafting (*red arrow*) between the two cut ends is performed.

through them (more axon surface match to the proximal stump) (**Fig. 3.22b**). In case the proximal end is wide but the distal end is smaller in diameter, the cable graft can be doubled up and the bend is cut partially in a horizontal manner so that it approximates with the distal end properly (**Fig. 3.22c**). The stump of the facial nerve is cut sharp in bevel shape to have maximum number of axons available for growth.

Double grafting is also performed in cases of trauma or a lesion affecting the nerve at the stylomastoid foramen (SMF) after its bifurcation into its terminal branches. The two divisions of cable graft can be sutured to upper and lower branches of facial nerve (**Fig. 3.23**). For double grafting, as more length of graft is required, sural nerve is the nerve of choice for grafting.

Nerve Transfer

Nerve transfer with a cranial nerve is performed in cases where the proximal stump is not available.

The motor nerves used for coaptation with distal facial nerve stump are:

- Hypoglossal nerve
- Nerve to masseter

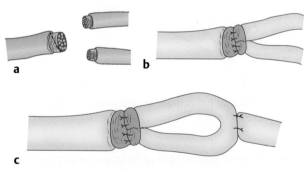

Fig. 3.22 **(a)** Illustration showing double grafts and facial nerve stump. The cut end of facial nerve stump is bevel-shaped so as to have wider surface area and more axons to grow through the cable graft. **(b)** double graft anastomosis performed on proximal side. **(c)** On distal side, the bent surface of cable graft is cut partially on outer surface to approximate with the distal stump of facial nerve.

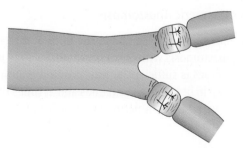

Fig. 3.23 Double grafting for lesions causing disruption of facial nerve after its bifurcation into two terminal branches on face.

Hypoglossal nerve has been the nerve of choice since long but in last few years, the masseter nerve is becoming a better choice for the neural input for the reasons discussed below.

Facio-hypoglossal Anastomosis

Classical End-to-End Facio-hypoglossal Anastomosis

Transection of the entire thickness of hypoglossal nerve distal to ansa cervicalis and transection of facial nerve at its exit from SMF are performed. Coaptation of full-thickness stump of hypoglossal nerve to the main trunk of the facial nerve is performed (**Fig. 3.24**).

Advantage
The full-thickness coaptation and single neurorrhaphy make the regeneration closest to normal.

Disadvantage
Paralysis and atrophy of the ipsilateral tongue due to its denervation lead to speech and swallowing impairment.

Hemi End-to-End Facio-hypoglossal–Jump Nerve Anastomosis

This technique is an improvisation on the classical technique designed to preserve the functioning of hypoglossal nerve. It involves partial sectioning of hypoglossal nerve rather than complete transection, thus avoiding tongue atrophy. An end-to-side anastomosis is performed between the partially sectioned surface of hypoglossal nerve and cable graft which acts as a jump graft, which is sutured on the other side with distal stump of facial nerve in an end-to-end manner. The hypoglossal nerve is sectioned partially in its 30% thickness. The nerve opens up in a wedge-shaped manner making it possible to house the graft on the proximal surface of the wedge for the end-to-side nerve suture (**Fig. 3.25**).

The advantage over end-to-end anastomosis is that the functioning of ipsilateral hypoglossal nerve can be preserved.

Disadvantage
As it is not possible to bring together hypoglossal and facial nerve without using interposition graft, the nerve has to grow through two neurorrhaphies, making recovery time longer. So a further modification to this technique is hemi end-to-end facio-hypoglossal anastomosis.

Hemi End-to-End Facio-hypoglossal Anastomosis
To avoid the use of cable graft, extra length of facial nerve is attained by mobilizing the mastoid segment of the facial nerve as far as the second genu, and transecting it there rather than at its exit at stylomastoid foramen (SMF). In such situation, the distal longer stump of the facial nerve can now be directly sutured to partial-thickness cut fibers of the hypoglossal nerve

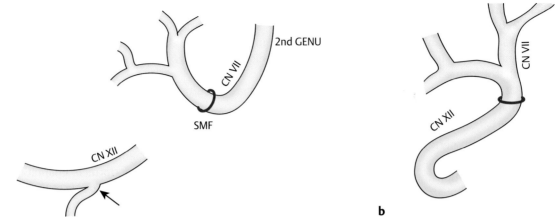

Fig. 3.24 **(a, b)** Diagrammatic depiction of facio-hypoglossal anastomosis. Facial nerve CN (VII) is transected at its exit from stylomastoid foramen (SMF) and hypoglossal nerve is transected distal to ansa cervicalis (*black arrow*). Both facial and hypoglossal nerves are coapted in full thickness.

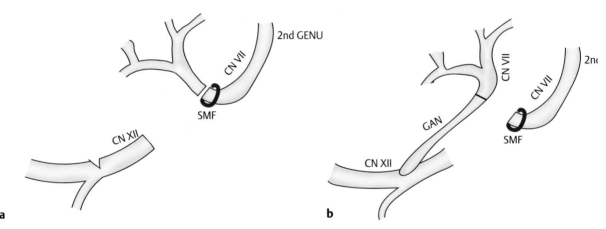

Fig. 3.25 **(a, b)** Illustration showing steps of hemi end-to-end facio-hypoglossal jump graft anastomosis technique. GAN, greater auricular nerve; SMF, stylomastoid foramen.

in an end-to-side anastomosis, without using any cable graft in between. The length of the mastoid part of facial nerve is approximately 15 to 18 mm and from its exit at SMF to its bifurcation is around 16 to 20 mm, so total length attained becomes around 35 mm. The length of hypoglossal nerve from close to internal jugular vein to its turn toward the tongue is around 31.6 mm, which is attained by transecting the facial nerve at the second genu. The use of interposition graft is thus avoided, and nerve fibers regenerate through one neurorrhaphy only, making it easy for nerve to regenerate faster.

Procedure

- Additional cortical mastoidectomy is performed.
- Facial nerve followed back from SMF and traced up to the second genu.

- Complete transection of facial nerve at the second genu and distal stump released till its bifurcation in parotid gland (**Fig. 3.26**).
- An end-to-side anastomosis is performed between the partially sectioned surface of hypoglossal nerve and distal stump of facial nerve over single neurorrhaphy.

Facio-masseteric Anastomosis

Use of masseter nerve can be in the form of direct end-to-end anastomosis with facial nerve stump if the length of both nerves is sufficient or interposition graft in case there is gap in between the cut ends and at times the gap can be covered by transacting facial nerve at 2nd genu and utilising the whole length of mastoid segment for

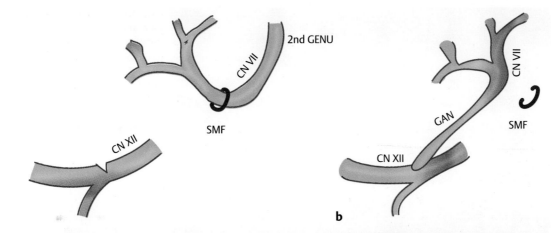

Fig. 3.26 (a, b) Illustration showing steps of hemi end-to-end facio-hypoglossal anastomosis. GAN, greater auricular nerve; SMF, stylomastoid foramen.

end to end anastomosis, if its available. Use of interposition graft can delay the recovery by few months and improvement in grade of functioning can never be up to grade I.

Advantages Over Facio-hypoglossal Anastomosis

- As it is anatomically located in the same surgical field, dissection is relatively easy due to proximity.
- Unlike facio-hypoglossal anastomosis, where the patient has difficulty in the first stage of deglutition and articulation for a long time, this anastomosis does not cause any restriction of function. The donor deficit is very minimal and not clinically relevant as there are other muscles for mastication available.
- Better nerve for producing spontaneous effortless smile as it is the natural function of masseter muscle supplied by masseter nerve.
- There is early reinnervation and improved symmetry.
- Its use is not contraindicated in patients with lower cranial nerve deficits or palsies or in patients susceptible to develop multiple cranial nerve deficits (neurofibromatosis type II).

Disadvantages

- It is quite close to temporal and zygomatic branches of the facial nerve, which can get injured while locating the masseter nerve.
- Unless the surgeon is well versed with the surgical anatomy of masseter nerve, it may take a long time and at times difficult to locate the nerve.

Anatomy of Masseter Nerve

It originates as a branch from the anterior division of mandibular branch of trigeminal nerve (CN V). It leaves the mandibular nerve shortly after its entrance into the infratemporal fossa. The nerve passes over the lateral pterygoid muscle and leaves the infratemporal fossa through the sigmoid notch, accompanied by the masseteric artery. Distance from the notch to its entry into the masseter muscle is an average of 32 mm, so almost 3.2 cm of the nerve can be released as stump for motor transfer. The nerve is located in the plane between the middle and deep lobes of masseter muscle and enters from medial surface of masseter.

Surface Marking of Masseter Nerve

- Approximately 3.06 cm anterior to tragus
- Approximately 1.6 cm inferior to zygomatic arch inferior margin
- Around 1.5 cm deep to superficial muscular aponeurotic system (SMAS)
- The nerve bisects the subzygomatic triangle
- It is in close proximity to zygomatic branch of facial nerve, forming an angle of 50 degrees with zygomatic nerve while descending (**Fig. 3.27**)

Subzygomatic triangle is an important landmark to locate masseter nerve. Its three sides (limbs) are (**Fig. 3.28**):

- Superior limb: Zygomatic arch inferior margin
- Posterior limb: Vertical line through temporomandibular (TM) joint anterior margin
- Inferoanterior limb: Frontal branch of facial nerve

The masseter nerve bisects this triangle.

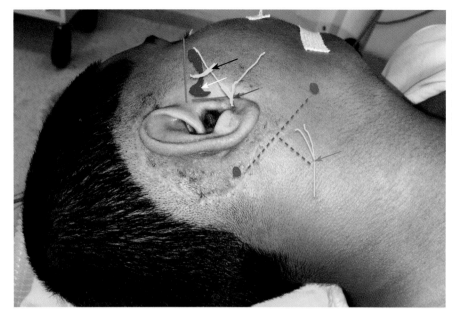

Fig. 3.27 Picture showing the surface marking for locating masseter nerve. Greater auricular nerve (GAN) (*blue arrow*), facial nerve (*red arrow*), masseter nerve (*black arrow*), sigmoid notch (*white arrow*), and *green* outlines are for lower border of zygomatic arch and line along the anterior margin of temporomandibular joint.

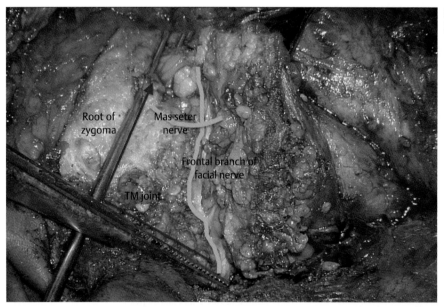

Fig. 3.28 Picture demonstrating the boundaries of subzygomatic triangle.

Procedure

An end-to-end anastomosis is performed between the full-thickness stump of masseter nerve and full-thickness distal stump of facial nerve transected at SMF, over single neurorrhaphy. In case the length of facial nerve is not sufficient to fill the gap, the extra length can be achieved by performing cortical mastoidectomy and transecting the facial nerve at the second genu rather than at SMF. The details of the procedure with images and the cases have been taken up in details in chapter number 8 titled 'Short duration flaccid facial palsy with proximal stump unavailable'.

Pearls

- The most important factor which matters for nerve repair is timing. Excellent results are obtained if repair is performed within 30 days. Window period is 30 days to 6 months.
- In case of end to end grafting, the proximal and distal irregular or fibrotic ends to be cut sharply till the healthy ends are reached, even if it means increasing the gap between the ends.
- The excision of neuroma, fibrotic, or unhealthy ends is more important than the size of the gap.

- In case there is neuroma formation, the % involvement of nerve fibres is important. If the neuroma is involving full thickness of the nerve, it should be excised, but if it involves less than 50% of fibers, decompression on both sides of the neuroma with clearing of the fibrotic tissue and incising the nerve sheath on both sides of the neuroma suffice.
- In case of dumb bell neuroma, reactive neuroma at the proximal end and the collagenized fibrotic segment on the other side is to be addressed.
- Endoneurium on both cut ends should be well approximated. For that the epineurial layer on both ends are to be stripped back to expose perineurium and endoneurium. For clean cutting of irregular ends, the epineurium must be stripped back.
- Endoneurium match on the cross-sectional surface area of both ends to be achieved.
- In case of cable grafting, Cable graft should be slightly longer than the actual gap for suturing without tension.
- Endoneurial surface of cable graft should match with the cut ends of facial nerve on both sides. If cable graft surface area is smaller, then use double cable graft on that side.
- The suturing between cut ends of nerve is epineurium to epineurium in fresh trauma and perineurium to perineurium in old injury.

■ Facial Nerve in Tumors

Facial nerve involvement can be different in different tumors. The nerve may show evidence of neural invasion even when the clinical presentation is not there as in cases of adenocystic carcinoma of the parotid. In the same way, in cases of facial nerve neuroma, the tumor involves the Schwann cells only but the compression by neuroma may cause compression and necrosis of facial nerve fibers though the patient may not clinically show it. In such cases the patient is to be counseled and educated about the chances of postsurgery facial nerve palsy that happens in such cases. The facial nerve repair, in such situations should be performed in the same stage whenever possible with technique customized accordingly. A delay of 3 months or more can lead to formation of fibrosis and scar at the cut ends which can lead to nonviability of stumps of facial nerve. Then it becomes difficult to give optimal results to the patient.

Whereas in tumors like pleomorphic adenoma or other benign tumors of parotid gland, the patient may show signs of facial paresis even when the microscopic picture is showing just compression of few fibers.

Such cases are going to improve remarkably after removing the tumor and sparing the nerve.

Factors Affecting the Outcome of Nerve Repair

Intrinsic factors (beyond the control of surgeon):

- Health and age of the patient
- State of tissue nutrition
- Time since injury
- Injury factor:
  - ➢ Type of injury
  - ➢ Level of injury
  - ➢ Condition of nerve ends
  - ➢ Length of gap
- Time of surgery
- Delay in repairing

This information can be gathered from history and physical examination and may aid in prognostic evaluation.

Extrinsic factors (depend on clinical management):

- Understanding of anatomy and physiology of facial nerve and temporal bone
- Surgical factors:
  - ➢ Technique
  - ➢ Selection of right procedure
  - ➢ Proficiency of the surgeon
  - ➢ Selection of instruments and suture material

Before undertaking cases of facial nerve injury or neuropathy, a surgeon must spend a long time in temporal bone lab to acquire sufficient knowledge about the anatomy of facial nerve and the temporal bone, the surgical techniques and their right application, and proficiency to perform the right surgical procedures to treat and not cause further irreparable damage to facial nerve. Regarding special instruments to handle and repair the facial nerve, mostly these are ophthalmic instruments which usually suffice. The special instruments are ophthalmic needle holder, two pair of jeweler's forceps, 4" strabismus scissors, 4" iris scissors, a mouse-tooth Adson forceps, and a razor blade holder, double-edge razor blades or scalpel blade, and suture material (8-0 or 9-0 monofilament ethilon suture).

Tissue dissection should be clean and along the anatomical planes of separation. If exposure requires separation of muscle tissue, the muscle should be split in the direction of its fibers and if this is not possible, then at its ligamentous attachment. Suturing is to be performed at the end of surgical procedure. All through the surgery, hemostasis is to be maintained with minimal tissue damage, since bleeding and tissue debris can lead to excessive scarring, leading to less optimal results. Hemostasis around facial nerve is achieved by using bipolar cautery on soft tissue and dry diamond burr on bleeding from bone. For bleeding from the facial nerve sheath use gelfoam soaked in adrenaline and for bleeding from thinned fallopian canal bony shell over facial nerve, gentle pressure of a diamond burr in static position at the bleeding point will suffice.. Constant lavage of the surgical site with saline is mandatory for avoiding thermal damage caused by moving burr, for clearing tissue debris, and to have better visibility of microscopic structures.

After the nerve is exposed, it is to be mobilized from the surrounding tissues for reapproximating the ends and applying sutures or glue for repair. Each nerve is surrounded by an adventitious tissue (mesoneurium) that contains collateral vessels. To avoid compromising on the blood supply of facial nerve, separate only few millimeters of nerve from surrounding tissue. If there is bony fallopian canal beneath the nerve, the bony bed gives support to the repaired nerve and anastomotic site. In case there is no bony bed supporting the anastomotic site or sites, pedicled muscle flap is used as a healthy vascular bed to provide support and vascularity to the anastomotic site (revascularization initially happens through tissue bed around the anastomotic sites) and as soft tissue coverage of the anastomotic site from outside.

All these steps put together in the right way can result in maximum potential for successful return of clinical function.

Postsurgery Care

On postsurgery day 1, the dressing is removed in most of the cases, except in cases where lateral skull base surgery has been performed, where the dressing is kept for 5 days. Supervised physiotherapy is started after 3 to 4 weeks of surgery. Once the facial muscles start regenerating, muscle strengthening exercises are started.

Nerve Regeneration Evaluation

As the nerve begins to grow, the nerve recovery is monitored using Tinel's sign. When the nerve is lightly tapped, the patient feels an electric tingling sensation in the region where nerve is regenerating.

Conclusion

The facial nerve is a bundle of nerve fibers surrounded by connective tissue component. As the axon of nerve fiber does not have the capacity to synthesize macromolecules, it depends on perikarya (cell body with stoma) to supply these substances. Any interruption in the continuity of axon due to any of the reasons such as injury, inflammation, edema, or compression leads to certain specific changes in different parts of nerve fibers. These degenerative changes are followed by regenerative changes. The ability of an injured nerve to regenerate is dependent upon the degree of continuity remaining in the nerve trunk following injury. In general, neuropraxic lesions have a greater probability of regeneration than axonotmesic or neurotmesic lesions. The supporting structures and Schwann cells remain intact in milder injury; thus a "lesion in continuity" is present. The prognosis is more favorable for injury of milder degree.

In facial nerve repair, the motor function of facial mimic muscles is the only end point to be considered, so the prerequisites for successful intervention are anatomical reconstitution of neuronal pathway and sufficient retention of viable facial muscle fibers to allow reinnervation.

Time of intervention and technique of facial nerve surgery are two important factors that influence the functional outcome.

Keeping the principles of nerve regeneration in view, the best results can be obtained from facial reanimation techniques by performing the nerve repair at the earliest with minimal time gap between time of injury and intervention.

The basic techniques of nerve reconstruction include primary repair, interposition grafting, motor nerve transfers from the neighboring cranial nerves, and cross-facial nerve grafting. Decompression or direct repair between two cut ends of facial nerve carried out in tension-free manner can optimize recovery of nerve up to grade I, whereas, when the gap between the two ends is >5 mm, interposition grafting, even after rerouting or II, can achieve recovery of facial nerve up to grade III at the maximum. Motor nerve transfer performed in end-to-end manner between the cranial nerve and facial nerve results in recovery of up to grade I, whereas any interposition graft used between cut ends of the cranial nerve and facial nerve can not improve facial nerve functioning upto grade I.

With time, new and novel techniques for suturing, grafting, crossing, and implanting nerves along with transferring regional muscles and grafting free muscle grafts are evolving (to be discussed in the successive chapters).

Above all, right instruments and skillful hands behind them can make all the difference for optimal results.

Bibliography

1. Jowett N. A General Approach to Facial Palsy. Otolaryngol Clin North Am 2018;51(6):1019–1031
2. May M, Schaitkin BM, eds. Microanatomy and pathophysiology of facial nerve. In: Facial Paralysis. Thieme; 2002
3. May M, Schaitkin BM, eds. Nerve repair. .In: Facial Paralysis. Thieme; 2002
4. Mannarelli G, Griffin GR, Kileny P, Edwards B. Electrophysiological measures in facial paresis and paralysis. Oper Tech Otolaryngol-Head Neck Surg 2012; 23(4):236–247
5. The American Laryngological, Rhinological and Otological Society, Inc. The Laryngoscope. Lippincott Williams & Wilkins; 2008
6. Principles of Peripheral Nerve Repair
7. Chapter 65 Marc R. Raffe
8. Biology of Nerve Repair and Regeneration
9. Miloro M, Larsen P, Ghali GE, Waite P. Peterson's Principles of Oral & Maxillofacial Surgery. 2nd ed. BC Decker; 2004
10. Kruger G. Textbook of Oral and Maxillofacial Surgery. 6th ed. St. Louis: Mosby; 1984
11. Mackinnon SE. Nerve Injury and Repair. Washington University School of Medicine
12. Osbourn A. Peripheral nerve injuries and repair. Review of surgeries
13. Yavuzer R, Ayhan S, Latifoğlu O, Atabay K. Turnover epineural sheath tube in primary repair of peripheral nerves. Ann Plast Surg 2002;48(4):392–400
14. Payne SH. Nerve repair and grafting in the upper extremity. J South Orthop Assoc 2001;10(3):173–189
15. White H, Rosenthal E. Static and dynamic repairs of fascial nerve injuries. Oral Maxillof Surg Clin North Am 2013;25(2):303–312
16. Miloro M, Ruckman P 3rd, Kolokythas A. Lingual nerve repair: to graft or not to graft? J Oral Maxillofac Surg 2015;73(9):1844–1850

4 Facial Palsy: Evaluation and Diagnosis

Introduction

Facial palsy is a debilitating condition and can cause severe functional and cosmetic sequel leading to extreme mental trauma to the patient. In many cases recovery is spontaneous and complete, whereas others may need medical and/or surgical intervention to improve the outcome. Objective measurements are valuable tools that can help identify candidates for intervention which can be either medical or surgical. They also help in deciding when to perform surgery, which surgical technique to choose for optimal results, and how to rightly counsel and prepare the patient for the outcome. A detailed assessment with objective measurement along with management strategy has to be developed for every case of facial palsy. The assessment can be divided into three headings:

- Evaluation (described in this chapter).
- Management strategy. Surgical rehabilitation techniques.
- Outcome tracking.

Management strategy and outcome tracking are described in Chapter 5.

Evaluation

Step-by-step preoperative evaluation is very important to decide the right management. In patients with palsy, a detailed history, standardized clinical examination including analysis of face at rest and during voluntary movements of face (frowning, wrinkling forehead by lifting eyebrows, eye closure, nose wrinkling, showing the teeth, dropping of angle of the mouth, pursing the lips) along with topographic, radiological, audiological, and electrodiagnostic tests are performed for right evaluation.

History

A detailed history of facial palsy includes:

- Onset, degree, and duration: Accurate information about the time of onset and degree of palsy is mandatory as a sudden-onset, immediate, complete palsy has different etiologies (trauma, viral infections), whereas a slowly progressing, delayed palsy points toward a chronic disease or situation. Delayed, incomplete palsy will mainly require conservative treatment, whereas immediate, complete palsy will definitely require surgical intervention. Duration of facial nerve palsy is equally important as long-term palsy can lead to facial musculature atrophy, and the surgical technique and choice of graft become totally different than what we use for short duration palsy.

- The time period between facial palsy and patient's first visit to otologist is very important because, if a few months have already passed before the patient's first visit to the clinician, the period of wait and watch with conservative management is already over, and a surgical repair or reconstruction may be the first line of treatment. But if the patient has reached the surgeon within hours or days of palsy, there may be a role for conservative treatment.

- Unilateral or bilateral palsy will point toward the etiology.

- Alteration in taste or lacrimation: This guides the treating physician in making clinical judgment about the level of injury or lesion in facial nerve.

- Symptoms of underlying or associated diseases.

- **Past history:** In case of suspected Bell's palsy, if there is a history of recurrent episodes of facial palsy in the past, the patient is investigated to rule out some other pathology like facial nerve tumor.

- A surgery in the past may be the cause for iatrogenic facial nerve palsy.

Physical Examination

Step-by-step clinical examination for further classification of etiology, location of disease, severity of lesion, and functional deficits is required:

- Complete ear, nose, and throat (ENT) examination.
- Neurological examination.
- Clinical analysis of face at rest and during voluntary movements (**Fig. 4.1**): Photography and videography to document appearance of face at rest and during seven volitional facial movements (wrinkling forehead by lifting eyebrows, eye closure on

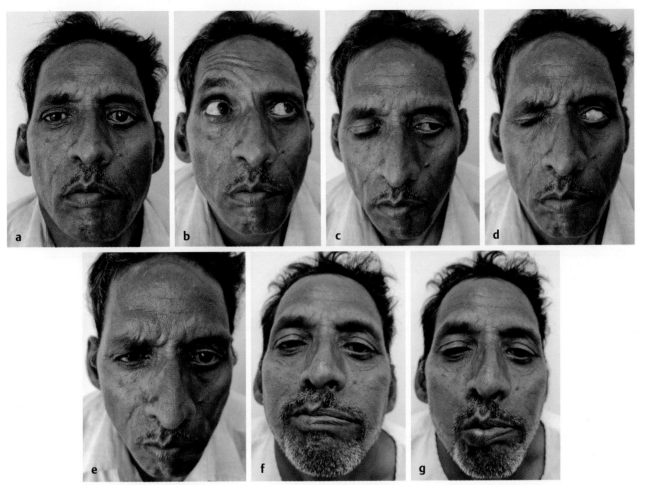

Fig. 4.1 Clinical analysis of face **(a)** at rest, **(b)** wrinkling forehead by lifting eyebrow, **(c)** eye closure on light effort, **(d)** eye closure on full effort, **(e)** smile, **(f)** lower lip depression, and **(g)** puckering of lips.

light and full effort, nose wrinkling, smile, lower lip depression, and puckering of lips).

- Grading of facial palsy depending on House-Brackmann's/Sunny Brook's grading system.
- Central or peripheral facial paralysis.
- Complete head and neck examination.
- Evaluation of lower cranial nerves functioning.

Ideal Characteristics of Grading System for Facial Palsy

- There should be accurate regional scoring of facial function on the face.
- Facial nerve functions, both in static and dynamic state, are to be taken into consideration.
- Secondary sequelae of facial paralysis also need to be assessed.
- The grading system should have low inter- and intraobserver variability.
- It should be sensitive to prognostic changes progressing over time.

- It should be easy and convenient for the clinician to conduct it in routine.

Since 1955, many grading systems have been proposed to assess facial nerve function, but the most universally accepted classification till date is House-Brackmann's grading system.

House-Brackmann's Grading System (1985)

House-Brackmann's grading system (HBGS) was originally described in 1985. Till date, it is the most convenient and user-friendly classification which provides clinicians with a standardized method of assessing patients with facial paralysis and monitoring their clinical course. The grades are from I to VI. It measures the function of the five terminal branches of the facial nerve, namely, temporal, zygomatic, buccal, marginal mandibular, and cervical branches. The grading system proposed includes a six-point scale, with Grade I representing normal and Grade VI representing total, flaccid paralysis (**Table 4.1**). Although they initially suggested

Table 4.1   House-Brackmann's facial grading system

Grade	Description	Characteristics	
I	Normal	Normal facial function in all areas	
II	Mild dysfunction	Gross:	Slight weakness noticeable on close inspection; may have very slight synkinesis
		At rest:	Normal symmetry and tone
		Motion:	Forehead: moderate to good function
		Eye:	Complete closure with minimal effort Mouth: slight asymmetry
III	Moderate dysfunction	Gross:	Obvious but not disfiguring difference between two sides; noticeable but not severe synkinesis, contracture, and/or hemifacial spasm
		At rest:	Normal symmetry and tone
		Motion:	Forehead: slight to moderate movement
			Eye: complete closure with effort
			Mouth: slightly weak with maximum effort
IV	Moderately severe dysfunction	Gross:	Obvious weakness and/or disfiguring asymmetry
		At rest:	Normal symmetry and tone
		Motion:	Forehead: none
			Eye: incomplete closure
			Mouth: asymmetric with maximum effort
V	Severe dysfunction	Gross:	Only brely perceptible motion
		At rest:	Asymmetry
		Motion:	Forehead: none
			Eye: incomplete closure
			Mouth: slight movement
VI	Total paralysis	No movement	

that a grading score can be correlated with an eight-point scale from direct measurements of the movement of the eyebrow and corner of the mouth and comparing the results with those on the unaffected side, but finally they devised a much simpler method of assigning grades based on the six-point scale from simple clinical observation. In this system, three situations are compared and divided into six grades. These are: gross observation, observation of the face at rest, and observation of voluntary facial movements. Although the classification is very simple and comfortable for clinical use, it has few limitations also. When the three components of the grade do not fall into the same grade level, they are assigned the more severe grade. That way the accuracy of the classification becomes doubtful. The different grades are:

- Grade I: Normal facial movement in all parts of the face with no weakness or synkinesis.
- Grade II: Normal symmetry at rest, mild dysfunction, slight weakness on close inspection with possible slight synkinesis, complete closure of eye.
- Grade III: Moderate dysfunction, obvious but not disfiguring difference between the sides; there can

be noticeable but not severe synkinesis, contracture, and/or hemifacial spasm; eye can be completely closed with effort.
- Grade IV: Normal tone at rest, moderately severe dysfunction, obvious weakness or asymmetry with movement, incomplete closure of eye.
- Grade V: Asymmetry at rest, severe dysfunction, only barely perceptible motion; the forehead has no motion, the eyelids cannot close completely, and the mouth can move only slightly with maximum effort.
- Grade VI: Complete paralysis with no movement.

Facial Nerve Grading System 2.0 (2009)

To overcome the limitations of original (House-Brackmann) (HB) scale, 15 years later, a revised version named Facial Nerve Grading System 2.0 was introduced with few improvements. Face is divided into four separate regions and are scored from 1 to 6 based on degree of movement. The additional feature is measuring synkinesis which is scored on a scale of 0 to 3. In addition, the total summed score of 4 to 24 is converted to a HB scale grade. Interobserver reliability is quite high in this system (**Table 4.2**). Four facial zones (eyebrow, eye, nasolabial folds, and oral) are graded according to the variation in movement and the level of synkinesis and given marks. The sum total of all the marks is then categorized into grades and converted into HB scale.

Sunny Brook's Facial Grading System (SFGS)

It was introduced in 1996 by Ross and colleagues and is another reliable scale for grading facial palsy (**Table 4.3**). The system is divided into three sections—resting symmetry, symmetry of voluntary movements, and

Table 4.2 Modified House-Brackmann's grading system

Facial zone	Movement (%)	Movement score	Synkinesis (quantity)	Synkinesis score	Total score	Grade
Eyebrow	100	1	None	0	4	I
Eye	>75	2	Slight	1	5–9	II
Nasolabial fold	>50	3	Obvious	2	10–14	III
Oral	<50	4	Disfiguring	3	15–19	IV
	Poor	5			20–23	V
Whole face	None	6			24	VI

Table 4.3 Sunny Brook's Facial Grading System (SFGS)

Resting symmetry score (RSS)	Voluntary movement score (VMS)	Synkinesis score (SS)
In comparison to contralateral side: **Eye opening** 1. Normal = 0 2. Narrow = 1 3. Wide = 2 4. Eyelid surgery = 3 **Nasolabial fold prominence** 1. Normal = 0 2. Less prominent = 1 3. Absent = 2 4. More prominent = 1 **Angles of mouth** 1. Normal = 0 2. Drooping = 1 3. Pulled up = 2 **RSS = Total × 5**	Degree of facial muscle activity in comparison to contralateral side: **Forehead wrinkling by raising eyebrows** 1. No movement (gross asymmetry) = 1 2. Slight movement (severe asymmetry) = 2 3. Initiated movement with mild excursion (moderate asymmetry) = 3 4. Movement almost complete (mild asymmetry) = 4 5. Movement complete (normal symmetry) = 5 **Gentle eye closure** Same grades from 1 to 5 **Smile** Same grades from 1 to 5 **Snarl/lifting of nose** Same grades from 1 to 5 **Puckering of lips** Same grades from 1 to 5 **VMS = Total × 4**	Involuntary muscle contractions associated with each expression: 1. None (no synkinesis) = 0 2. Mild (slight synkinesis) = 1 3. Moderate (obvious synkinesis) = 2 4. Severe (disfiguring synkinesis/mass movement of a group of muscles) = 3 **SS = Total**
Composite Score = VMS − RSS − SS		

synkinesis. The benefits of this scale are summed up in the following points:

- The scale is quite objective and reliable.
- It is quantitative; so it can measure the gradient of all movements.
- It is sensitive to clinical changes over time.
- It describes the patient's facial functions in detail.

The three factors taken into consideration for grading are:

- Resting symmetry score (RSS).
- Voluntary movements score (VMS).
- Synkinesis score (SS).

Resting Symmetry Score (RSS)

It evaluates the face at rest compared to the normal side. Evaluation is graded with the use of point scales.

- Eye: Normal (0), Narrow (1), Wide (1), Eyelid surgery (1).
- Cheek: Normal (0), Absent (2), Less pronounced (1), More pronounced (1).
- Mouth: Normal (0), Corner dropped (1), Corner pulled up/out (1).

Score: Total sum is multiplied by 5.

Voluntary Movement Score (VMS)

The five standard expressions on the face are measured and they reflect the motor function of the five peripheral branches of the facial nerve. By measuring the expressions, it evaluates the degree of maximal excursion of facial muscles compared to the normal side. The responses are graded with the use of point scales:

- Unable to initiate movement (1).
- Initiates slight movement (2).
- Initiates movement with mild excursion (3).
- Movement almost complete (4).
- Movement complete (5).

Score: Total sum × 4.

Synkinesis Score (SS)

It evaluates the degree of synkinesis associated with each voluntary movement, and the degree is converted into scores depending upon point scale.

- None: No synkinesis (0).
- Mild: Slight synkinesis (1).
- Moderate: Obvious but not disfiguring synkinesis (2).
- Severe: Disfiguring synkinesis/gross mass movement of several muscles (3).

Sunny Brook's facial grading system (SFGS) total score is calculated by the following formula:

- RSS is multiplied by 5.
- VMS is multiplied by 4.
- SS is taken as it is.
- The total score is derived by subtracting the RSS and SS from VMS:
- VMS – RSS – SS = Composite score.
- Composite score: 0 (complete facial palsy) to 100 (normal).

Advantages of SFGS

- It is very simple and easy to use.
- It quantifies the recovery in different parts of the face.
- It does not require special equipment.
- As its sensitivity to clinical changes is very accurate, so it can be used as prognostic tool.

Disadvantages of SFGS

- It is less prevalent than House-Brackmann's classification.
- Symmetry at rest is not scored.

Topographic Evaluation

It is the evaluation through certain tests to determine the anatomical level of a peripheral lesion.

Inclusion criteria: Patients with head injury with proven intratemporal lesion with immediate complete facial paralysis or delayed-onset paralysis not responding to conservative management with Glasgow coma scale (GCS) of more than 3.

Exclusion criteria: Patients with head injury due to gunshot or missile injuries with GCS of more than 4 at the time of presentation but who loses consciousness or subsequently do not regain consciousness; patients whose investigations could not be performed; patients suffering from any concomitant major illness like diabetes, hypertension etc.; patients suffering from any ear disorder prior to injury; and patients associated with cerebrovascular accidents.

Following tests are done for topographical evaluation of facial nerve palsy:

- Schirmer's test: It is a test for lesion at or proximal to the geniculate ganglion.
  It tests the function of greater superficial petrosal nerve (GSPN), which is responsible for lacrimation. In this test, 5-mm strips of filter paper are placed in inferior fornix for 5 minutes and the length of paper moistened is compared between the two eyes.
  Assessment is done as follows: In case of >75% unilateral decrease in lacrimation or bilateral decrease in lacrimation (<10 mm for both sides

in 5 minutes), the test is considered positive for lesion proximal to GSPN.

- Stapedius reflex test: It is a test for lesion proximal to stapedial muscle.

    It tests the nerve to stapedius muscle through impedance audiometry. Nonfunctioning of nerve to stapedius can cause ipsilateral hyperacusis (hypersensitive to sound). Impedance audiometry can record the presence or absence of stapedius muscle contraction to sound stimuli of 70 to 100 dB above hearing threshold. An absent reflex or a reflex less than half the amplitude is due to a lesion proximal to stapedius nerve.

- Salivation test: It tests for lesion proximal to chorda tympani which leads to reduced salivation and loss of taste on the ipsilateral two-thirds of the tongue.

    For salivation testing, either physical taste examination is performed with solution of salt, sugar, citrate, or quinine, or electrical stimulation or electrogustometry test is performed where electric stimulation compares amount of current required for a response on each side of the tongue.

    It is considered normal when the difference <20 µA between the two sides. Threshold difference of more than 25% is considered positive for lesion proximal to chorda tympani nerve.

    These tests have lost significance over time because of their false positive and negative results.

Tuning Fork Test and Pure Tone Audiometry Test

These tests are performed to evaluate the level and type of hearing loss associated with facial palsy.

Radiological Investigations

Imaging plays a very important role in evaluation of the anatomical course of the facial nerve and its various anomalies and lesions. The two most important modalities are computed tomography (CT) scan and magnetic resonance imaging (MRI). CT and MRI have complementary roles for evaluating facial nerve palsy. CT scan evaluates the bony details including fractures, dehiscence, anomalous location of fallopian canal, bony destruction due to disease, and periosteal reaction to disease. MRI, on the other hand, evaluates the soft tissue abnormalities around the facial nerve, as seen in inflammatory diseases, tumors or malignancy, and anomalous course of the nerve. For evaluation of tumor of facial nerve, both MRI and high-resolution CT (HRCT) are performed.

Keeping this in mind, imaging should be customized according to the suspected pathology and clinical localization of the lesion involving or compressing the nerve.

Supranuclear lesions require standard brain MRI and nuclear lesions in brainstem require high-resolution, T2-weighted MRI sequences. Lesions in cisternal part, internal auditory meatus (IAM), and labyrinthine portion require both high-resolution, T2-weighted and contrast-enhanced, T1-weighted MRI images through the IAM. For assessing geniculate ganglion, tympanic segment, mastoid segment, and its exit at stylomastoid foramen, both high-resolution CT of temporal bone and skull base and MRI are required. Soft tissue CT with contrast or MRI can be used to evaluate areas of the distal course of the facial nerve within the parotid and soft tissues of the face.

HRCT of Temporal Bone

HRCT of the temporal bone best visualizes the course of the nerve within the fallopian canal up to the stylomastoid foramen (**Fig. 4.2**). It is useful in evaluating the anatomical course, abnormal location, and caliber of nerve in different pathologies like congenital atresia of external auditory canal (EAC) or middle ear. It also evaluates any dehiscence, fracture, erosion, or destruction of fallopian canal. Also, it can demonstrate the relationship of facial nerve with surrounding structures like ossicles, cochlea, and vestibule which cannot be seen on MRI. This helps in planning for the surgery in that patient.

HRCT scan is performed in axial, coronal, and sagittal planes, but a special cut in Posh's or Stenver's reformat is added in specialized condition like semicircular canal (SCC) dehiscence. Contrast-enhanced CT is performed in case there is suspicion of neoplasm or vascular abnormalities.

Magnetic Resonance Imaging

MRI is performed to evaluate soft tissue facial nerve abnormalities, so it is not of much utility in evaluating the intratemporal segment covered by bony fallopian canal (**Fig. 4.3**). MRI is more useful for visualizing facial nerve from the brainstem to the fundus of the IAM and then on the face after its exit from stylomastoid (SM) foramen. In the neck and face, its utility is in evaluating the involvement of facial nerve in parotid tumors and malignancies. The sequences required are: T1-weighted sequence (3-mm axial cuts) of skull base and whole brain; noncontrast, T2-weighted sequence (5-mm axial cuts); an axial constructive interference in the steady state (CISS) sequence (heavily T2-weighted sequence, 0.6 mm) from the occipital bone to superior petrous ridge; axial, 5-mm, whole-brain, postcontrast fluid-attenuated inversion recovery (FLAIR) and T1-weighted sequences; a coronal, 4-mm, postcontrast, T1-weighted sequence of the IAM; and an axial, 3-mm, T1-weighted, fat-saturated sequence of the IAM.

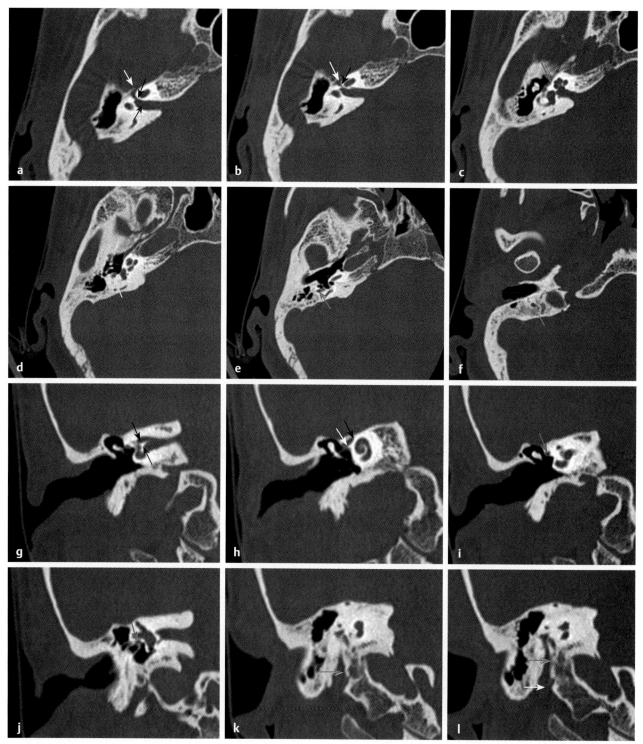

Fig. 4.2 **(a)** Computed tomography (CT) of temporal bone, axial image, showing facial nerve (FN) in internal auditory meatus (IAM) (*red arrow*), labyrinthine segment (*black arrow*), and geniculate ganglion (*white arrow*). **(b)** CT of temporal bone, axial image, showing FN in geniculate ganglion (*white arrow*). **(c)** CT of temporal bone, axial image, showing tympanic segment (*green arrow*) coursing back from geniculate ganglion toward the second genu. **(d)** CT of temporal bone, axial image, showing the second genu (*yellow arrow*). **(e)** CT of temporal bone, axial image, showing mastoid segment (*blue arrow*). **(f)** CT of temporal bone, axial image, showing mastoid segment (*blue arrow*). **(g)** CT of temporal bone, coronal image, showing labyrinthine segment (*black arrow*) with Bill's bar (*red arrow*). **(h)** The first genu (*white arrow*) and labyrinthine segment (*black arrow*) both in single cut. **(I, j)** CT of temporal bone, coronal image, showing tympanic segment (*green arrow*) in fallopian canal. **(k, l)** CT of temporal bone, coronal image, showing mastoid segment (*blue arrow*) in fallopian canal coursing vertically within temporal bone and exiting via stylomastoid foramen (*white arrow*).

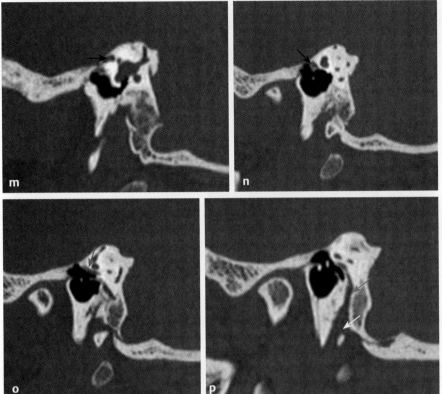

Fig. 4.2 (*Continued*). **(m, n)** CT of temporal bone, sagittal image, showing labyrinthine segment (*black arrow*). **(o, p)** CT of temporal bone, sagittal image, showing tympanic segment (*green arrow*) and the second genu (*yellow arrow*) continuing into mastoid segment (*blue arrow*) coursing vertically within temporal bone and exiting via stylomastoid foramen (*white arrow*).

In high-resolution, T2-weighted or CISS images, the normal facial nerve appears as a hypointense linear structure extending from the brainstem to the IAM, anterior to the vestibulocochlear nerve, surrounded by T2 hyperintense cerebrospinal fluid, whereas the proximal extracranial portion of the facial nerve after its exit from stylomastoid foramen in the parotid gland is best visualized with axial, high-resolution, T1-weighted image. MRI is not preferred for intratemporal part of facial nerve as the labyrinthine, tympanic, and mastoid segments of the facial nerve are not well visualized in noncontrast images. But once the gadolinium contrast is used, the normal facial nerve faintly enhances in the geniculate ganglion, tympanic, and mastoid segments.

Ultrasound

Ultrasound has been lately utilized to predict outcome of facial nerve in Bell's palsy.

It is performed between 2 and 7 days of onset of paralysis in patients with Bell's palsy. Facial nerve diameter is measured proximally at the stylomastoid foramen, distally just proximal to the pes anserinus, and midway between these two points. The average diameter of the facial nerve is calculated using these three measurements and then compared with blink reflex studies and nerve conduction studies. A normal ultrasound measurement on the affected side had a 100% positive predictive value for normal facial function recovery at 3 months, whereas an abnormal facial nerve ultrasound predicts incomplete or no recovery.

Diffusion Tensor Tractography

It is a new modality for three-dimensional visualization of facial nerve fibers, which can clearly show the demarcation plane between facial and vestibulocochlear nerve. It can evaluate and lower the risk of facial nerve injury during surgery for vestibular schwannomas, as it is difficult to distinguish between the facial nerve and the tumor on MRI. Both the facial nerve and the schwannoma have similar signal intensities, and larger tumors cause thinning of the facial nerve, making the nerve even more difficult to identify. Also, there is absence of intervening cerebrospinal fluid between the schwannoma and the facial nerve. In these cases, diffusion tensor (DT) tractography may be useful for assessing facial nerve course and displacement.

Electrodiagnostic Tests

These are mainly used to determine the severity and prognosis of a facial nerve lesion and are performed in:

- Idiopathic facial palsy (Bell's palsy).
- Post-traumatic facial nerve palsy.
- Hemifacial spasm.

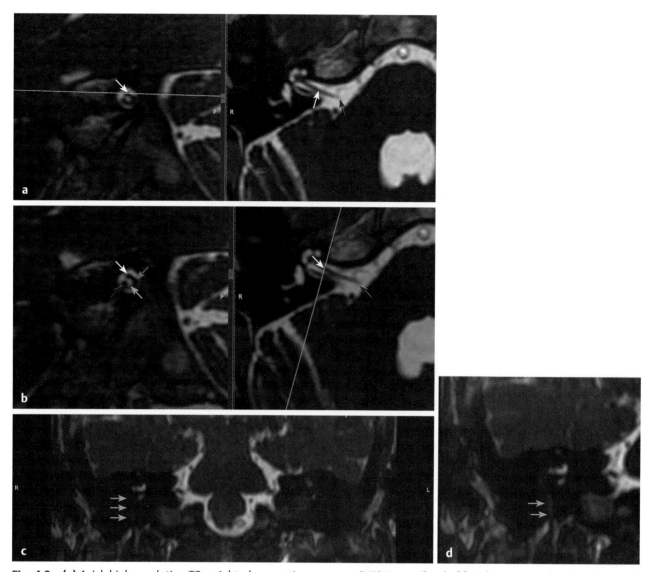

Fig. 4.3 **(a)** Axial, high-resolution T2-weighted magnetic resonance (MR) image (level of facial nerve correlated with sagittal oblique view of left side) shows cisternal segment (*red arrow*) emerging from root exit zone in cerebellopontine angle and entering internal auditory meatus (IAM) to become canalicular segment (*white arrows*). **(b)** High-resolution, T2-weighted MR image in sagittal oblique view in left-sided image (level of facial nerve correlated with axial view of right-sided image) shows canalicular segment of facial nerve (*white arrows*) along with cochlear (*purple arrow*), superior (*orange arrow*), and inferior vestibular nerve (*light blue arrow*). **(c, d)** High-resolution, T2-weighted MR image in coronal view showing mastoid segment (*blue arrows*).

- Neoplastic lesions of parotid where infiltration of facial nerve is suspected. In patients with malignant parotid tumor presenting with facial paresis, electrodiagnostic tests can show signs of nerve degeneration. This may be the first sign of a malignant lesion and may guide the surgeon in the preoperative period to do surgical planning and counseling of the patient about the facial palsy.
- These tests can also be helpful in clearly differentiating a central facial palsy from an incomplete peripheral facial palsy that spares the upper face.

The tests include nerve excitability test (NET), maximum stimulation test (MST), electroneurography (ENoG), electromyography (EMG), and intraoperative nerve monitoring.

- **Nerve excitability test:** It measures the minimal current required to stimulate muscle movement when applied to a branch of facial nerve. A difference of 3.5 mA or greater between two sides is thought to be significant.
- **Maximum stimulation test:** In this the strength and duration of stimulation is gradually increased

from 1 to 5 mA. In MST, facial movement of the paralyzed side is compared with the contralateral side at the stimulation level where the greatest amplitude of facial movement is seen on the normal side.

Both NET and MST are dependent upon the cooperation of the patient and on the examiner's subjective evaluation of the electrically elicited facial movement. So the reliability becomes less. These limitations are overcome by ENoG test popularized by Fisch and Esslen in 1972.

- **Electroneurography**

Electroneurography (ENoG) analyses the evoked compound muscle action potential (CMAP) of a specific facial muscle after transcutaneous stimulation of the main trunk of the facial nerve. This stimulation is performed with a bipolar stimulator placed at facial nerve's exit from the stylomastoid foramen. The response is recorded with the a pair of surface electrodes placed on the target muscle which is either nasolabial fold or nasalis muscle on both normal and affected sides. Stepwise increased levels of electrical current of up to 50 mA are given and response of muscle is noted (**Fig. 4.4**).

The test is performed on both sides of the face, first on the healthy side of the face and then on the affected side. In case of degeneration of nerve fibers, there is decrease or loss of the CMAP. The response of the CMAP on the affected side is compared to the CMAP of the healthy side and expressed as percentage (amplitude of the paralyzed side divided by the amplitude of the normal side).

A side difference of 30% or bigger is considered pathologic. For prognosis, a side difference of 70 to 95% is considered to be relevant. Surgical intervention is the treatment of choice in case of immediate paralysis with >90% degeneration. ENoG can also predict long-term

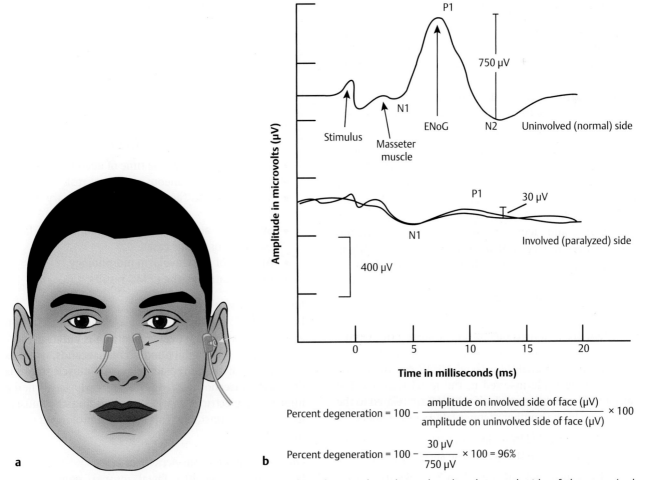

Electroneuronography (ENoG) Analysis

Analysis: "Significant degeneration in facial nerve response"

$$\text{Percent degeneration} = 100 - \frac{\text{amplitude on involved side of face (μV)}}{\text{amplitude on uninvolved side of face (μV)}} \times 100$$

$$\text{Percent degeneration} = 100 - \frac{30\ \mu V}{750\ \mu V} \times 100 = 96\%$$

Fig. 4.4 **(a)** Electroneurography (ENoG) procedure explained. Recording electrodes placed on each side of the nose (*red arrow*). Stimulator placed in front of the ear (*yellow arrow*). **(b)** Reporting of ENoG.

prognosis of facial function, but it is not a complete test in itself to differentiate between Grades II to V of nerve injury. It has to be performed and interpreted in combination with EMG.

Scheduling and interpreting ENoG depend on the site of lesion and the onset of an acute palsy. For example, if the injury site is away from stylomastoid foramen, located more proximally, it will take about 72 hours for Wallerian degeneration to reach the extratemporal nerve distal to the Stylomastoid Foramen (SMF) where the nerve is stimulated. As abnormal ENoG report relies on Wallerian degeneration, it should be always performed after 3 days. For the next 5 to 6 days, the response to ENoG starts building up and remains till 21 days as nerve degeneration is complete by then. The reading will show no change after 21 days. So ENoG is helpful for predicting recovery within the time window of 3 to 21 days. The first ENoG is performed at about 3 days after the onset of nerve injury and then monitored every 3 to 5 days. Early signs of denervation on ENoG are a poor prognostic sign because they predict a more severe nerve injury. Surgical intervention is needed when ENoG degenerates by 90% and no volitional EMG is recorded.

- **Electromyography (EMG)**

EMG is the recording of motor unit action potentials (MUAPs). MUAPs are the spikes in electrical activity generated when a motor unit (MU) gets activated. **Each MU consists of the neuron and its axon, which have multiple synaptic junctions that are affiliated with corresponding muscle fibers. These synaptic junctions are called neuromuscular junctions.**

Each neuromuscular junction and muscle fiber generates a small electrical potential when activated. The synchronized discharge arising from the neuromuscular junctions of all the axons combines to form the larger MUAP which is then detected by EMG testing which can detect and demonstrate quantitative or qualitative changes in electrical activity of the muscle MUs in the resting state, following direct or indirect electrical stimulation, or during voluntary or reflex MU activation. In this test, the signals are not compared with that of opposite side.

There are two methods for performing EMG, needle EMG (nEMG) and surface EMG (sEMG). nEMG is the method used to analyze a facial MUAP recorded from a needle electrode inserted in the facial muscles. The amplitude and duration of facial MUAP are related to the reduction in the number of innervated muscle fibers.

sEMG is recorded from the skin surface. sEMG records the sum of MUAP in the area of the surface electrode.

EMG is most helpful from 2 to 3 weeks to up to 3 months after the onset of the palsy. Scheduling and interpreting the responses are equally important as in ENoG. When the infratemporal facial nerve fibers are injured, it takes about 10 to 14 days before degeneration reaches the facial muscle, whereas if the nerve lesion is more distal, degeneration reaches the affected muscles earlier, so the right time for first EMG is 10 to 14 days after injury. Therefore, the time frame for conducting EMG is 2 to 3 weeks to 3 months after the onset of a facial nerve injury. EMG is also helpful in monitoring for regeneration if reinnervation occurs. EMG should be used and interpreted in combination with clinical examinations.

Needle EMG (nEMG)

Two or more needles are used for the synchronous analysis of several muscles. A reference surface electrode is placed at a myoelectric inactive location of the body such as the area of the bony manubrium sterni. Bipolar concentric needle electrodes are used to record muscle responses from the mimetic muscles innervated by the four motor branches of the facial nerve that contribute to facial expression. These four muscles are frontalis, orbicularis oculi, orbicularis oris, and mentalis. The concentric needle electrode is inserted into the frontalis muscle in the forehead, in the orbicularis oculi near the lateral canthus of the eye, in the perioral muscles for orbicularis oris, and finally into the mentalis muscle in the chin (**Fig. 4.5**).

If a patient is able to elicit volitional EMG, a complete nerve transection is effectively ruled out. Therefore, it is possible to use EMG to rule out a Grade VI injury immediately after the onset of injury.

The recording sequence are as follows:

- Insertion activity at the time of needle insertion.
- Pathologic spontaneous activity at rest.
- Volitional EMG (activity during voluntary muscle movement).
- Synkinetic activity in cases of long-term facial palsy or postrepair cases.
- Analysis of the waveform morphology.
- Interpretation of the nEMG results.

Insertion Activity

In a normal healthy facial muscle, normal insertion activity in response to needle insertion is bursts of electrical activity for several hundred milliseconds, whereas in case of scar tissue replacing normal muscle, there is decreased insertion activity. During early facial nerve injury, the electrical charges surrounding the muscle membrane are unstable. This leads to a prolonged insertion activity.

Pathologic Spontaneous Activity at Rest

In the normal healthy facial muscle, nonpathologic spontaneous electrical activity is present at rest.

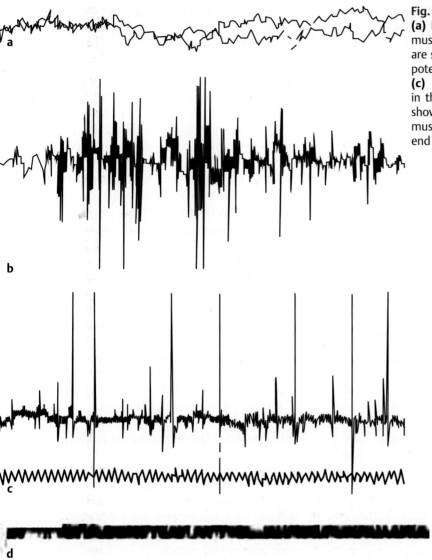

Fig. 4.5 Electromyography responses. **(a)** Normal response. In a normal resting muscle, biphasic or triphasic potentials are seen every 30 to 50 ms. **(b)** Fibrillation potential indicating denervated muscle. **(c)** Polyphasic pattern signifying muscle in the process of regeneration. **(d)** Graph showing electrical silence indicating severe muscle atrophy and degradation of motor end plate.

A denervated facial muscle will show pathologic spontaneous activity in the form of unstable electrical charges during the phase of ongoing nerve injury. This presents as fibrillation potentials (**Fig. 4.5b**), complex repetitive discharges, and sharp positive waves and is diagnostic of nerve injury.

Spontaneous activity, if present for a long time, indicates a poor prognosis for nerve recovery. If nerve starts regenerating, it sends new electrical impulses to the muscles and pathologic spontaneous activity decreases and disappears about 2 to 4 weeks after the nerve injury. Decreasing of fibrillation potential means recovery has started, whereas the persistence of fibrillation in a malignant tumor shows the infiltration of disease to the nerve and holds a bad prognosis for nerve recovery. Pathologic action potential persists until the nerve is completely destroyed.

Volitional EMG (Activity during Voluntary Muscle Movement)
In this, the patient is asked to perform the action of four mimic muscles where electrodes are placed like frowning for the frontalis muscle, closing the eye for the orbicularis oculi muscle, showing the teeth for the zygomatic muscle etc. The patient is asked to fully contract the muscle and the presence or absence of any voluntary MU potentials is recorded. The number of impaired facial nerve fibers is directly proportional to a decrease in the EMG pattern.

The electrophysiological configuration of MUs is normally not changed in patients with neurapraxia. The duration of MUs and the number of their potential phases are found to be increased in patients with axonotmesis or neurotmesis. If a patient is able to elicit a normal volitional EMG, a complete nerve transection is effectively ruled out. Hence, although it cannot differentiate between Grades II to V, it can rule out total transection if test is found normal. If the facial nerve regenerates, spontaneously or after nerve repair, facial axons reinnervate the target muscles. A typical sign of reinnervation is polyphasic regeneration potentials but with greater amplitudes than normal and a prolonged duration (**Fig. 4.5c**), whereas an electrical silence signifies severe muscle atrophy and degeneration of motor end plate.

Synkinetic Activity

The regenerating axons may not find the right fascicle and join another fascicle connecting to a separate set of mimetic muscles. This can finally result in synkinesis (involuntary movement of one facial muscle during voluntary movement of another facial muscle). Abnormal nerve regeneration can also lead to more nerve fibers than normal to get activated which can cause a strong resting tone and movements (hyperkinetic syndrome). During nEMG, the synkinetic activity can be shown by placing the needle electrode in one muscle and having the patient move another facial muscle.

Analysis of the Waveform Morphology

A normal facial MU is biphasic or triphasic, with a downward positive spike and an upward negative spike with an amplitude of 200 to 500 mV and duration of 5 to 7 ms. It can become polyphasic if the action potential is recorded very close to the motor end plate.

Interpretation of the nEMG Results

The electrophysiological findings should be categorized into neurapraxia, axonotmesis, and neurotmesis.

Neuropraxia: In a patient with acute facial palsy, if nEMG beyond 10 to 14 days shows normal insertion activity, no pathological spontaneous activity, and a single action potential during voluntary contraction, neurapraxia should be suspected.

Axonotmesis and neurotmesis: If pathological spontaneous activity occurs, either axonotmesis or neurotmesis should be suspected.

Only an nEMG reporting will not be sufficient to segregate the two situations.

In a normal resting muscle, biphasic/triphasic potentials are seen every 30 to 50 ms. Muscle that has been denervated displays fibrillation potentials, while muscle that is in the process of reinnervation demonstrates polyphasic potentials. Electrical silence in a patient with long-standing facial paralysis indicates severe muscle atrophy and degradation of motor end plate. In such cases, nerve repair or grafting does not work but muscle transfer procedure is required.

The utility of EMG is more in long-standing facial nerve palsy cases, where the surgical technique needs to be decided based on availability of viable facial muscles capable of useful function after reinnervation.

Reinnervation: If voluntary contraction produces polyphasic regeneration potentials, it indicates reinnervation. If the lesion site is located in the temporal bone or at the main trunk of the peripheral facial nerve, it can take 3 to 6 months to see the first regeneration potentials. That means that the EMG showing regeneration precedes the clinical signs of recovery. Actual muscular movement in these situations will not be seen until 5 to 9 months after injury.

So, through EMG, as reinnervation can be detected about 2 to 3 months before clinical presentation of recovery.

EMG can be used to determine:

- If a nerve in question is **in continuity** (volitional activity recorded).
- Evidence of **degeneration** (fibrillation after 10–14 days).
- Early signs of **reinnervation** (polyphasic innervation potentials after 4–6 weeks).
- Detection of the functioning of facial muscles in cases of long duration facial palsy.

Intraoperative Nerve Monitoring (IONM)

IONM is a relatively recent inclusion in the list of electrodiagnostic tests for facial nerve functioning in various procedures and its routine use has not yet been established as a standard procedure in otologic surgery. It is utilized more for tracing facial nerve in lateral skull base and parotid surgery. The different indications for IONM are:

- For tracing facial nerve when it is not clearly visible in the surgical field (otologic procedures like post-traumatic cases, cochlear implantation, congenital anomalies of ear, revision or extensive disease, acoustic neuroma surgeries, or parotid surgery).
- For early identification of facial nerve continuity.
- For tracing the anomalous course of facial nerve.
- For tracing the course and recording the viability of nerve.
- For evaluating facial nerve function at the end of operation.
- For prognosis of nerve recovery.

Procedure

The nerve monitoring system monitors EMG activity from multiple facial muscles depicting different zones of the face (**Fig. 4.6**).

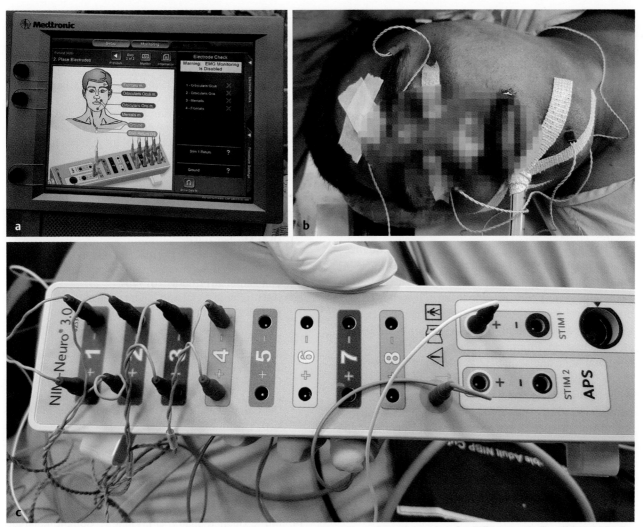

Fig. 4.6 **(a)** Nerve monitoring machine with color touch screen monitor with color coding for different muscles. **(b)** Application of electrodes in specific muscles according to color coding. **(c)** Electrodes connected to the Compound Muscle Action Potential (CMAP) recording system.

Electrode Placement

The electrodes are placed in the muscles supplied by facial nerve. Four electrodes are placed in frontalis, orbicularis oculi, orbicularis oris, and mentalis muscles (color-coded placement) which are then connected to the monitor. The ground electrodes are placed over the sternum. When the facial nerve is stimulated by the surgeon, all the electrodes get stimulated and a Compound Muscle Action Potential (CMAP) is recorded from the monitored facial muscles which is plotted on an oscilloscope with a loudspeaker which emits a sound and also produces an impulse on the monitor indicating that the main nerve and the branches are intact. The visual alerts on the color touch screen monitor and audio feedback help to minimize trauma to the nerve.

Gentle mechanical stimulation will create the sound called "bursts" on the machine. Mechanical stretching or thermal stimulation produces a trail of discharges called "trails." It gives instant feedback regarding the location of facial nerve and a warning when the surgeon is unknowingly close to the nerve. It can also confirm the continuity of facial nerve at the end of the procedure. Surgeons can use monopolar and bipolar stimulating probes and dissection instruments to assist in early nerve identification and confirmation. These tools may be used to locate, identify, and map the facial nerve and branches, as well as verify nerve function and integrity.

Conclusion

Each patient presenting with facial palsy must go through detailed evaluation for right diagnosis, treatment, and optimal recovery of facial nerve.

Based on the detailed history and physical examination which also includes facial nerve and lower cranial nerve examination, the treating surgeon must carefully assess the situation and lesion and choose appropriate tests for finalizing the diagnosis.

Topographical evaluation has lost its relevance over time due to high chances of false positive or negative results which are mostly due to extension of inflammation on both sides of site of injury. Radiological investigations, which include both CT scan and MRI, need to be customized according to the suspected pathology and clinical localization of the lesion involving or compressing the nerve. Supranuclear lesions require standard MRI of the brain, and nuclear lesions in brainstem require high-resolution, T2-weighted MRI sequences. Lesions in cisternal part, internal auditory meatus (IAM), and labyrinthine portion require both high-resolution, T2-weighted and contrast-enhanced, T1-weighted MRI images through the IAM. For assessing geniculate ganglion, tympanic segment, mastoid segment, and its exit at stylomastoid foramen, both high-resolution CT of temporal bone and skull base and MRI are required. Soft tissue CT with contrast or MRI can be used to evaluate areas of the distal course of the facial nerve within the parotid and soft tissues of the face. Modalities like ultrasound (for predicting outcome of facial nerve in Bell's palsy) and diffusion tensor tractography (for localization of facial nerve in tumors of IAM) are being utilized lately, adding to the armamentarium of battery of tests.

The electrodiagnostic tests which include ENoG and EMG are used to determine the severity and prognosis of a facial nerve lesion and are performed in lesions like idiopathic facial palsy (Bell's palsy), post-traumatic facial nerve palsy, hemifacial spasm, and neoplastic lesions of parotid where infiltration of facial nerve is suspected. These tests guide the surgeon in choosing the right surgical technique and counseling the patient regarding the outcome.

An important and valuable modality, intraoperative nerve monitoring, which is used in very few centers around the world, needs to be included in the armamentarium of management of facial palsy or involvement.

Bibliography

1. Lo YL, Fook-Chong S, Leoh TH, et al. High-resolution ultrasound in the evaluation and prognosis of Bell's palsy. Eur J Neurol 2010;17(6):885–889
2. Taoka T, Hirabayashi H, Nakagawa H, et al. Displacement of the facial nerve course by vestibular schwannoma: preoperative visualization using diffusion tensor tractography. J Magn Reson Imaging 2006;24(5):1005–1010
3. Raghavan P, Mukherjee S, Phillips CD. Imaging of the facial nerve. Neuroimaging Clin N Am 2009;19(3):407–425
4. Cisneros A, Orozco JRW, Nogues JAO, et al. Development of the stapedius muscle canal and its possible clinical consequences. Int J Pediatr Otorhinolaryngol 2011;75(2):277–281
5. Liu L, Arnold R, Robinson M. Dissection and exposure of the whole course of deep nerves in human head specimens after decalcification. Int J Otolaryngol 2012;2012:418650
6. May M, Schaitkin BM. The Facial Nerve. 2nd ed. New York, NY, USA: Thieme; 2000
7. Curtin HD, Sanelli PC, Som PM. Temporal bone: embryology and anatomy. In: Som PM, Curtin HD, eds. Head and Neck Imaging. Vol. 2. 4th ed. St. Louis, Mo, USA: Mosby; 2003
8. Al-Noury K, Lotfy A. Normal and pathological findings for the facial nerve on magnetic resonance imaging. Clin Radiol 2011;66(8):701–707
9. Jäger L, Reiser M. CT and MR imaging of the normal and pathologic conditions of the facial nerve. Eur J Radiol 2001;40(2):133–146
10. Veillona F, Ramos-Taboada L, Abu-Eid M, Charpiot A, Riehm S. Imaging of the facial nerve. Eur J Radiol 2010;74(2):341–348
11. Crawford SC, Harnsberger HR, Swartz JD. The facial nerve (cranial nerve VII). In: Swartz JD, Harnsberger HR, eds. Imaging of the Temporal Bone. New York, NY, USA: Thieme; 1998
12. Nager GT, Proctor B. Anatomic variations and anomalies involving the facial canal. Otolaryngol Clin North Am 1991;24(3):531–553
13. Yellon RF, Branstetter BF IV. Prospective blinded study of computed tomography in congenital aural atresia. Int J Pediatr Otorhinolaryngol 2010;74(11):1286–1291
14. Mu X, Quan Y, Shao J, Li J, Wang H, Gong R. Enlarged geniculate ganglion fossa: CT sign of facial nerve canal fracture. Acad Radiol 2012;19(8):971–976
15. Brodsky JR, Smith TW, Litofsky S, Lee DJ. Lipoma of the cerebellopontine angle. Am J Otolaryngol 2006;27(4):271–274
16. Isaacson B, Telian SA, McKeever PE, Arts HA. Hemangiomas of the geniculate ganglion. Otol Neurotol 2005;26(4):796–802
17. De Foer B, Vercruysse JP, Spaepen M, et al. Diffusion-weighted magnetic resonance imaging of the temporal bone. Neuroradiology 2010;52(9):785–807
18. Yorgancılar E, Yildirim M, Gun R, et al. Complications of chronic suppurative otitis media: a retrospective review. Eur Arch Otorhinolaryngol 2013;270(1):69–76
19. Chen DQ, Quan J, Guha A, Tymianski M, Mikulis D, Hodaie M. Three-dimensional in vivo modeling of vestibular schwannomas and surrounding cranial nerves with diffusion imaging tractography. Neurosurgery 2011;68(4):1077–1083
20. Kennedy PG. Herpes simplex virus type 1 and Bell's palsy—a current assessment of the controversy. J Neurovirol 2010;16(1):1–5
21. Lanser MJ, Jackler RK. Gadolinium magnetic resonance imaging in Bell's palsy. West J Med 1991;154(6):718–719

22. Pickuth D, Heywang-Köbrunner SH. Neurosarcoidosis: evaluation with MRI. J Neuroradiol 2000;27(3):185–188

23. Vanzieleghem B, Lemmerling M, Carton D, et al. Lyme disease in a child presenting with bilateral facial nerve palsy: MRI findings and review of the literature. Neuroradiology 1998;40(11):739–742

24. Salvinelli F, Casale M, Vitaliana L, Greco F, Dianzani C, D'Ascanio L. Delayed peripheral facial palsy in the stapes surgery: can it be prevented? Am J Otolaryngol 2004;25(2):105–108

25. Gianoli GJ. Viral titers and delayed facial palsy after acoustic neuroma surgery. Otolaryngol Head Neck Surg 2002;127(5):427–431

26. Brackmann DE, Fisher LM, Hansen M, Halim A, Slattery WH. The effect of famciclovir on delayed facial paralysis after acoustic tumor resection. Laryngoscope 2008;118(9):1617–1620

27. Verzijl HTFM, Valk J, de Vries R, Padberg GW. Radiologic evidence for absence of the facial nerve in Möbius syndrome. Neurology 2005;64(5):849–855

28. Silverman IE, Liu GT, Volpe NJ, Galetta SL. The crossed paralyses. The original brain-stem syndromes of Millard-Gubler, Foville, Weber, and Raymond-Cestan. Arch Neurol 1995;52(6):635–638

29. Eggenberger E. Eight-and-a-half syndrome: one-and-a-half syndrome plus cranial nerve VII palsy. J Neuroophthalmol 1998;18(2):114–116

30. Saia V, Pantoni L. Progressive stroke in pontine infarction. Acta Neurol Scand 2009;120(4):213–215

31. Bassetti C, Bogousslavsky J, Barth A, Regli F. Isolated infarcts of the pons. Neurology 1996;46(1):165–175

32. Cattaneo L, Saccani E, De Giampaulis P, Crisi G, Pavesi G. Central facial palsy revisited: a clinical-radiological study. Ann Neurol 2010;68(3):404–408

33. Kim JYS. Facial nerve paralysis. In: Narayan D, ed. Medscape Reference. 2012

34. Nentwich LM, Veloz W. Neuroimaging in acute stroke. Emerg Med Clin North Am 2012;30(3):659–680

35. Spencer BR Jr, Digre KB. Treatments for neuro-ophthalmologic conditions. Neurol Clin 2010;28(4):1005–1035

36. Boghen D, Tozlovanu V, Iancu A, Forget R. Botulinum toxin therapy for apraxia of lid opening. Ann N Y Acad Sci 2002;956:482–483

37. Ahmadi N, Newkirk K, Kim HJ. Facial nerve hemangioma: a rare case involving the vertical segment. Laryngoscope 2013;123(2):499–502

38. Friedman O, Neff BA, Willcox TO, Kenyon LC, Sataloff RT. Temporal bone hemangiomas involving the facial nerve. Otol Neurotol 2002;23(5):760–766

39. Künzel J, Zenk J, Koch M, Hornung J, Iro H. Paraganglioma of the facial nerve, a rare differential diagnosis for facial nerve paralysis: case report and review of the literature. Eur Arch Otorhinolaryngol 2012;269(2):693–698

40. Garden AS, Weber RS, Morrison WH, Ang KK, Peters LJ. The influence of positive margins and nerve invasion in adenoid cystic carcinoma of the head and neck treated with surgery and radiation. Int J Radiat Oncol Biol Phys 1995;32(3):619–626

41. Malata CM, Camilleri IG, McLean NR, et al. Malignant tumours of the parotid gland: a 12-year review. Br J Plast Surg 1997;50(8):600–608

42. Ross BG, Fradet G, Nedzelski JM. Development of a Sensitive Clinical Facial Grading System. Otolaryngology-Head and Neck Surgery. 1996;114(3):380–386

5 Facial Palsy: Management Strategy, Surgical Rehabilitation Techniques, and Outcome Tracking

Introduction

A standardized approach for management of facial nerve palsy needs to be developed, taking into consideration all factors like cause, site, extent, and duration of facial palsy. Once it is clear that surgical management is the treatment of choice, counseling of the patients is done and they should be educated about the possible outcomes of surgical management. A good managment strategy ensures achievement of maximum functioning of facial nerve post treatment.

The aim of surgical reconstruction is to restore the function of all mimic musculature to the optimum level, which means restoration of frontal frowning, wrinkling of forehead while lifting the eyebrow, closure of the eye with light and full effort, a symmetric nasolabial fold, and the ability to smile symmetrically.

Factors Affecting Management of Facial Nerve Palsy

Management of a case of facial nerve palsy depends upon few very important factors which are described below.

Etiology of Facial Nerve Palsy

There are different etiologies leading to facial nerve palsy. but the important thing is that, etiology may be different, but the cause for facial palsy remains disruption anywhere in the neural pathway from the facial motor cortex to the facial muscles. Knowing the etiology though helps us in determining whether the facial nerve function can recover spontaneously with conservative treatment, or any surgical intervention will be required. It also guides us in deciding the surgical approach and technique to be followed in a specific case. The fact remains that out of all cases of facial nerve palsy, only a minority of the patients actually require surgical management. In acute phase, it is mostly managed conservatively so as to give time to individual's chance of spontaneous functional recovery. Whereas in chronic cases, surgery is indicated in all patients who have not benefitted with medical line of management, as there can be incomplete recovery if waited too long on conservative management. The various etiologies for facial nerve palsy are:

- **In its intracranial route, the facial nerve can be affected by:**
  - Iatrogenic injury
  - Neoplastic lesions
  - Congenital anomalies like
    1. Moebius syndrome where the facial nerve is absent
    2. Absence of motor units
- **In its intratemporal part, the facial nerve (due to its long tortuous route) can be affected by:**
  - Trauma in the form of
    1. Fractures of temporal bone
    2. Penetrating injuries
  - Iatrogenic injuries
  - Cholesteatoma
  - Neoplastic
    1. Facial neuroma
    2. Acoustic neuroma
    3. Meningiomas
    4. Hemangiomas
  - Infections
    1. Herpes zoster oticus
    2. Acute otitis media
    3. Chronic otitis media
    4. Malignant otitis externa
    5. Tubercular mastoiditis
  - Idiopathic
    1. Bell's palsy
    2. Melkersson-Rosenthal syndrome
  - Congenital
- **The extratemporal segment gets affected by:**
  - Trauma, which can be
    1. Blunt injury
    2. Penetrating injury
    3. Lacerated wounds of face
  - Iatrogenic injuries

> Neoplasm
> 1. Parotid tumors
> 2. Tumors of the external and middle ear
> 3. Facial nerve neuroma
> 4. Metastatic lesions
> Congenital absence of facial musculature

For convenience, the whole list of etiologies can be divided into:

- Idiopathic
- Traumatic
- Neoplastic
- Inflammatory
- Congenital

Idiopathic facial paralysis (Bell's palsy) is one of the commonest causes for facial nerve palsy. It is a viral induced inflammation of the nerve that causes edema and vascular compromise leading to facial paralysis. Most of the patients regain function spontaneously, thus not requiring any surgical intervention. Very few select cases who have not improved over a long time (>4 months) may require decompression of facial nerve.

Traumatic facial paralysis (post-traumatic or iatrogenic injury) is the next most common etiology for sudden-onset facial palsy. The traumatic injury can involve any segment, so it is managed accordingly. Indication for surgery depends on the severity of the nerve lesion, i.e., blunt trauma leading to nondegenerative neuropraxia will not need surgical reconstruction, whereas disruption leading to degenerative neurotmesis will need surgery.

In iatrogenic injuries, the site and the grade of injury help the surgeon in deciding the approach to manage the palsy, which can range from simple decompression, nerve grafting, nerve transfer to dynamic or static procedures. Iatrogenic injury in skull base surgeries, like acoustic neuroma, may cause loss of proximal stump of facial nerve leading to its nonavailability for repair. In such cases, the primary nerve is replaced with another motor nerve like hypoglossal or masseter nerve (motor nerve transfer), whereas trauma involving segment distal to internal auditory meatus (IAM) can be repaired with a cable graft between proximal functional stump and the distal segment of facial nerve.

Neoplastic lesions in the intracranial or intratemporal part can lead to compression of facial nerve lying in the vicinity. In the intracranial part, they can be acoustic neuroma or certain brain tumors. In intratemporal part, it can be paragangliomas, meningiomas, or malignancies. Any tumor in the course of the facial nerve from the brainstem to the periphery can cause facial palsy or surgical treatment of the tumor itself can be the reason for facial palsy. In such circumstances, the surgery of the primary disease is combined with surgical reconstruction of the facial nerve in the same stage for maximum recovery of facial nerve function. Other tumors involving extratemporal part of facial nerve can be parotid tumors, mostly malignant. In such tumors, the facial nerve, if entrapped in primary disease, needs to be sacrificed. In that situation, sural nerve with branches can be used as cable graft which can be anastomosed between the proximal stump and peripheral disease-free branches of facial nerve intraoperatively only. In case the terminal branches are also involved in the malignancy, second-stage cross-face nerve grafting, free muscle with neurovascular transplant, or temporalis muscle transplant with upper eyelid implants are the procedures of choice.

Inflammatory and infectious causes of facial nerve palsy are usually postviral infections, e.g., herpes zoster (Ramsay Hunt syndrome), mumps, coxsackie virus, and mononucleosis, which are usually self-limiting. Bacterial infections include complicated otitis media, skull base osteomyelitis, Lyme disease, and sarcoidosis. In the infections which are self-limiting, the recovery of facial nerve function takes place over few months. However, few situations like complicated otitis media, tubercular mastoiditis, or skull base osteomyelitis can involve and cause irreversible loss of functioning of facial nerve. In such situations, the affected segment of facial nerve may need to be excised and grafted with cable graft. Grafting in such cases are performed in the second stage due to prevailing chronic resistant bacterial infection.

Congenital facial palsy is most uncommon, Moebius syndrome being the commonest of all. As there is nondevelopment of facial nerve, the facial rehabilitation in such cases can only be achieved by the procedure of free muscle (gracilis) grafting with neurovascular anastomosis followed by either cross-face nerve grafting in single or two stages or anastomosis with masseter nerve, a branch of mandibular division of trigeminal nerve.

Degree and Time of Onset of Paralysis

The degree of palsy along with the time of onset of palsy are two most important factors which help in deciding the right management. In cases of post-traumatic facial palsy, if it is immediate complete (Grade VI HB) palsy with computed tomography (CT) scan showing a transverse fracture line, involving the whole thickness of fallopian canal, surgical intervention is to be performed at the earliest. Whereas if the patient has incomplete facial palsy (less than Grade VI) with delayed onset and the CT scan shows longitudinal fracture line, reaching only up to the lateral wall of fallopian canal, conservative management will suffice in most of the cases.

Duration of Paralysis

The time period between the onset of paralysis and the first visit to the otologist is also to be taken into account when deciding for surgical management. No surgical procedure should be attempted when spontaneous recovery is possible.

The question arises regarding how long and till what time shall the surgeon wait for spontaneous recovery to happen without any residual nonreversible defects or faulty regeneration.

We categorize all situations of facial palsy according to onset and status of facial nerve and facial musculature into two categories:

Category 1: Includes situations where facial nerve is intact and there is only conduction block

Acute onset

In cases of acute-onset facial palsy due to iatrogenic injury, post trauma, or infections, if the patient has reached or is already with the clinician, the clinician assesses the patient for establishing the diagnosis in the time period between 1 and 14 days, along with starting the conservative treatment and scrutinizes for candidacy for early surgical intervention.

Patients with incomplete facial palsy or paresis, after idiopathic, iatrogenic, or post-traumatic injury, are candidates for conservative therapy for at least 3 to 4 months. The conservative management includes corticosteroids, antiviral, antibiotics, and specific treatment for any comorbidities. Most of the cases improve and reach complete recovery in 4-6 months. The first sign of recovery in such patients starts showing in 2 months. In case of complete grade VI palsy, if there is no change in grade of facial palsy or not the slightest improvement after 4 months, the case is assessed again and the patient is considered for surgical intervention. Its the author's surgical experience that even when, the nerve is intact, the hypertrophic mucosa around nerve at the injury site starts compressing the nerve, if its dehiscent or the bony shell around it has got breeched due to trauma, leading to ischemia and fibrosis which can cause irreversible changes in nerve if surgical intervention is delayed maximum by more than 6 months. Research says that there is an eightfold decrease in axon diameter over 3 months due to its shrinkage along with gradual thickening of the collagen in endoneural sheath surrounding the axon (collagenization). So, the earliest repair of nerve encourages axons to grow through the collapsing tubes, thus reinflating them and avoiding the blockage to growth through collagenization.

The acute-onset Grade VI facial palsy may follow resection of tumors like acoustic neuroma, paragangliomas, or parotid tumors due to compression or stretching of facial nerve, even when the facial nerve is viable and its continuity has been maintained during surgical procedure. In such situations, there are chances of spontaneous recovery, with return of full movements expected between 6 and 12 months. The wait and watch policy in such cases can be followed comfortably for up to 1 year, and with close watch even up to 2 years, if the surgeon is sure and the video recording of surgery shows that the nerve is intact. While waiting for nerve to recover, temporary static procedure like tarsorrhaphy for avoiding exposure keratitis or upper eyelid implant for normal eye closure can be added. A close follow-up is needed in such cases every 3 months to reassess the situation and go ahead with surgical intervention if needed.

Chronic cases

In a post-traumatic, iatrogenic facial paralysis, when it is uncertain whether nerve is intact or not, the waiting period is up to 3 to 4 months, after which, post hemorrhage and edema, fibrosis develops and thickens around the site of injury entrapping the facial nerve leading to ischemia and fibrosis of nerve itself. If the patient has reached the clinician after 3 to 4 months of onset of Grade VI facial palsy, further waiting can reduce chances of recovery of useful functioning of the facial nerve. Waiting for too long may lead to only partial recovery or faulty recovery in the form of synkinesis, hyperkinesis, etc.

In cases of idiopathic facial palsy (Bell's palsy), if the patient is not recovering in 3 months (grade VI facial palsy persisting), surgical intervention may be required. Also, in such cases, imaging is performed to rule out facial nerve tumor or any other tumor in the vicinity of facial nerve compressing it leading to its palsy.

In cases of tumor removal with sparing of facial nerve (nerve continuity is to be absolutely confirmed), if no recovery or progress is observed for up to 12 months, the case should surely be taken up for surgical exploration and intervention. 12 months is the waiting time. After which, the atrophy of facial muscles may start progressing. If there is any doubt, the waiting is reduced to up to 3 months and reassessment is considered. In case the patient is visiting the clinician after a period of 1 year or more after surgery, or the surgery has been conducted some where else, and the detailed surgery notes are not available, the clinician immediately should go ahead with the repair but associate it with static and dynamic procedures like upper eyelid implant, lower eyelid tightening, facial slings and muscle transfer etc .

Category 2: Includes situations where the facial nerve is not intact. It is subdivided into two groups.

Facial nerve not intact with viable facial musculature

Once there is surety that the nerve has got transacted as in cases of iatrogenic trauma or the CT scan is favoring transection of facial nerve along with electroneurography (ENoG) report of >90% in cases of post-traumatic immediate complete facial palsy, then no time should be wasted in observation as such cases require urgent surgical intervention.

Also, in a case where no recovery is seen during the waiting period of 3 to 4 months in post-traumatic or postiatrogenic injury to facial nerve, the case is assessed again for any trauma to facial nerve which could have been missed in previous assessment, and the case is taken up for exploration and surgical intervention.

In facial nerve tumor removal, once injury to facial nerve is confirmed, immediate intraoperative repair of facial nerve in the same stage is considered, which may be end-to-end repair, interposition nerve grafting, or nerve transfer. These are associated with static procedure like upper eyelid implant and fascia lata slings as it is going to take at least 1 year for recovery to start. No time should be wasted in observation.

The ideal time for nerve grafting is within 30 days to up to 3 months following injury, as beyond 6 months the results are not very encouraging. If the continuity of nerve is doubtful, the latest to wait is up to 4 months.

Facial nerve not intact with nonviable musculature

In cases where facial musculature has either atrophied due to long-term facial palsy or not viable due to congenital absence or is unlikely to get innervated as terminal peripheral branches of facial nerve is infiltrated with tumor or damaged due to injury, nerve repair or nerve transfer is not the procedure of choice. The only choice that remains is dynamic or static procedures in the form of upper eyelid implant, facial slings, free muscle (gracilis) transfer with neurovascular anastomosis, masseter muscle transfer, or temporalis muscle elongation.

The right cut off time for considering the nonviability of facial musculature is a point of discussion. In the author's experience, cases of iatrogenic injury with long-term facial palsy (>3 years) could be improved by performing primary procedures like decompression, nerve repair, interposition grafting, or nerve transfer, although the primary procedure was always accompanied with static or dynamic procedures. In situations other than iatrogenic trauma, the electromyography (EMG) test can guide the clinician regarding the viability of facial muscles in a long-term facial palsy.

Beyond 12 months, fibrosis of the nerve, the motor end plate, and atrophy of the muscle all ensue as the time passes. The treating surgeon is in a race against this inevitable process. Thus, a repair performed 18 months after the onset of paralysis is sure to have a poorer chance of success than a repair that has been performed earlier.

Patient's Age and General Condition

Age plays an important role in presentation or recovery from facial palsy. In young children even with transected facial nerve, the face may show a decent symmetry at rest with eye closure. It is usually because of excellent tissue elasticity and subcutaneous fat giving the face a normal look. But, due to the same factors, the nerve transfer or muscle transfer is difficult as the planes are not well demarcated. Whereas in elderly patients, the sagging of tissue has already taken place due to loss of elasticity of tissue and fat, making the defect look exaggerated. In such cases, muscle or nerve transfer and face lift procedures are easy to perform because of the clearer planes due to loss of fat.

In addition, the patient's age influences clinical decision-making and results of the surgical repairs. In an elderly patient, slower nerve regeneration is expected, and the result of repair is likely to be poorer than could be achieved in a younger patient. If the patient's life expectancy is short, one may elect to perform an adjunctive procedure that produces an immediate improvement (e.g., upper eyelid implant, a dynamic muscle transfer or elongation or Botulinum toxin injections) rather than a nerve repair that, even in the best of circumstances, takes long time to show results.

In elderly patients, waiting may be appropriate in specific situations, like ill health of the patient, immunocompromised situation, or oncologic issues.

General condition of the patient plays an important role in recovery of facial functioning. A chronically ill, immunocompromised patient or a patient with malignancy who already has received radiotherapy will have delayed and limited recovery, even if the surgeon has performed excellent surgery. Facial nerve repair may be contraindicated in situations where patient's general health status prevents elective surgery.

In malignancies, planned radiation therapy is not a contraindication to facial nerve repair. Regeneration of nerve function has been demonstrated despite subsequent ablative doses of radiation.

Management Strategy and Surgical Rehabilitation Techniques

Once it is clear that surgical management is the treatment of choice, counseling of the patients is done and they should be educated about the possible results after surgery. Both the patient and the surgeon should appreciate that once facial nerve is damaged, there is no chance to restore the normal facial nerve functioning completely because although the voluntary movement will improve dramatically, the involuntary movements may remain deficient.

The aim of surgical reconstruction is to restore the function of all mimic musculature to as optimal as possible, which means restoration of frontal frowning, wrinkling of forehead while lifting the eyebrow, closure of the eye with light and full effort, a symmetric nasolabial fold, and the ability to smile symmetrically.

The surgical repair of the nerve should be followed by training the patient in postoperative period for symmetrical facial movement with good tone of functioning muscles, and avoiding complications like synkinesis,

dyskinesis, hyperkinesis with hypoactivity or hyperactivity or mass moment syndrome.

For deciding the timing of the surgical intervention and technique in that specific situation, the two most important factors are duration of palsy and presence or absence of proximal stump of facial nerve as is shown in **Flowchart 5.1**. Using these parameters, all surgical rehabilitation techniques can be divided into different categories.

Selection of the Optimal Surgical Concept

The facial palsy can be graded in to acute facial palsy (<3 weeks duration), intermediate duration facial palsy (3 weeks to 2 yr) and chronic facial paralysis (>2 yr with EMG -ve) and the surgical techniques can be divided as follows:

- Facial palsy of short and intermediate duration (less than 2 years or 2–3 years with EMG positive) with proximal stump available:
  - ➢ Facial nerve decompression
  - ➢ Facial nerve end-to-end repair
  - ➢ Facial nerve repair with cable graft

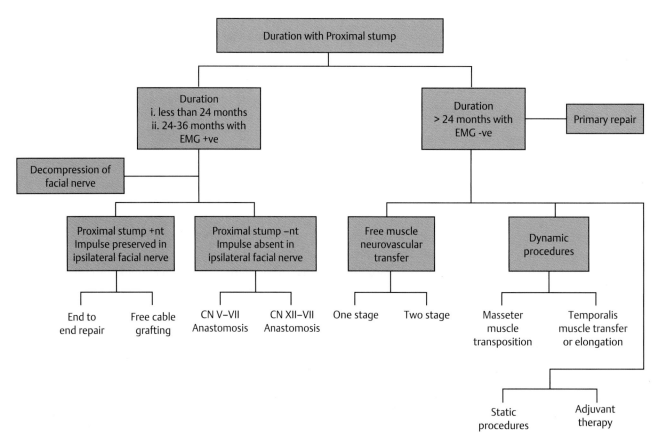

Flowchart 5.1 Algorithm showing the surgical management strategy and facial rehabilitation techniques for a case of facial palsy. EMG, electromyography. Note: +nt denotes "present" while -nt denotes "absent."

- Facial palsy of short and intermediate duration (less than 2 years or 2–3 years with EMG positive) with proximal stump unavailable:
  - ➢ Cranial nerve (CN) transfer (facio-masseteric or facio-hypoglossal anastomosis)
  - ➢ CN VII–VII cross-face graft
- Facial palsy of long duration (>2 years with EMG negative) with proximal and distal portion of facial nerve available:
  - ➢ Primary facial nerve repair with adjuvant static or dynamic procedures
- Facial palsy of long duration (>2 years with EMG negative) with proximal or distal portion of facial nerve unavailable, or the facial nerve is not developed (Moebius syndrome) or mimic muscles got atrophied due to long-term facial nerve palsy:
  - ➢ Free muscle neurovascular transfer witheither masseter nerve transfer in one stage or cross-face nerve graft, single- or two-stage surgery
  - ➢ Muscle transposition or dynamic transplant
    1. Temporalis muscle
    2. Masseter muscle
    3. Anterior digastric muscle transfer
  - ➢ Static procedures
  - ➢ Adjuvant procedures

All surgical and non surgical techniques can be summed up as follows:

- Decompression with or without incising the nerve sheath
- Direct end-to-end repair
- Interposition cable grafting
- Motor nerve transfer (facio-masseteric or facio-hypoglossal anastomosis)
- Cross-face nerve grafting
- Dynamic reanimation of face:
  - ➢ Masseter muscle transposition or temporalis muscle transfer or elongation
  - ➢ Free muscle (gracilis) with neurovascular bundle transfer
  - ➢ Anterior digastric muscle transfer
- Static reanimation of face:
  - ➢ Brow ptosis correction
  - ➢ Tarsorrhaphy
  - ➢ Upper eyelid implant
  - ➢ Static facial slings
  - ➢ Lower eyelid tightening—lateral tarsal strip procedure with or without medial tendon plication
  - ➢ Contralateral depressor labii inferioris (DLI) resection
  - ➢ Ipsilateral depressor anguli oris (DAO) resection
- Adjuvant therapy:
  - ➢ Botulinum toxin injections
- ➢ Physiotherapy
- ➢ Mirror biofeedback and neuromuscular retraining
- ➢ All techniques are described in detail in Chapters 6–9.

Outcome Analysis

Outcome measurement is the most relevant part in completing the whole schedule of management of facial nerve palsy, and unless until we do it accurately following certain protocols, the whole management strategy may become futile. The outcome analysis should include clinician's as well as patient's perspective regarding recovery of facial nerve functioning as well as the measurement of complications like synkinesis, hyperkinesis, or mass movement syndrome.

Outcome can be measured depending on various parameters:

- Patient's perspective
- Clinician's assessment through scale systems
- Third person's assessment/objective assessment tools
- Spontaneous smile assessment

Patient's Perspective

While treating for facial palsy, patients' specific aesthetic and functional concerns along with their expectations are to be taken into consideration and management should be decided accordingly. It is important to gauge the motivation of the individual patient before going ahead with the surgical management because this will influence the quality of the outcome.

During recovery phase also, the patient's perspective becomes important. As facial nerve palsy has a profoundly devastating effect on the psyche of the patient, once the patient is progressing toward regaining facial nerve function, the improvement has to be assessed from his or her point of view as well. While showing improvement on different scales and grading systems, it is equally important to see how the patient is perceiving it.

For that, we must educate our patients before surgery regarding the slow progress even after best management, and how their journey and progress are going to be throughout the treatment and recovery period. In the author's experience, unless the patient is educated about the chances of complete/incomplete recovery of facial palsy, percentage of improvement of different parts of face, the long period it takes for recovery, and last but not the least, the not-so-good recovery of the involuntary emotional expression before patient is taken up for surgery, patient usually feels less satisfied even with the best possible results for that given situation.

The various scales developed over the time are:

- Facial Disability Index
- Facial Clinimetric Evaluation Scale (FaCE)
- Synkinesis Assessment Questionnaire (SAQ)

Out of the three, FaCE is the best scale. It is composed of 15 questions with five-point scale responses ranging from 1 (worst) to 5 (best). The basis for calculation are: facial movement, facial comfort, oral function, eye comfort, lacrimal control, and social function. Total scoring is done from 0 (worst) to 100 (best). As it does not include parameters for calculating synkinesis, the SAQ has been developed separately, which is a nine-point questionnaire, with five-point Likert scale responses. The total score ranges from 20 (worst) to 100 (best). It relates to the patient's perception of facial synkinesis. When combined, both SAQ and FaCE give complete coverage of the patient's perception.

Clinician's Analysis and Grading

Usual clinical analysis by the surgeon includes grading of voluntary movements of the face (frowning, wrinkling forehead by lifting eyebrows, eye closure, nose wrinkling, showing the teeth, dropping of the angle of the mouth, pursing the lips) before and at different stages after management of facial palsy. These systems are based on clinical judgment based on various factors.

The effective grading system is based on measures that are objective, sensitive to changes happening over time, and easy to implement. Many staging systems failed as they were time consuming, required expensive equipment, and were very complex to perform and apply in clinical practice.

Ideal characteristics of a grading system for facial palsy include regional scoring of a facial function, static and dynamic measures, and secondary sequelae of facial paralysis, if any. Then there should be low interobserver and intraobserver variability, which makes it more reliable. It should be sensitive to track changes happening over time. And lastly, it should be convenient for clinical use. The most prevalent and widely followed grading systems have been described in details in Chapter 4.

Objective Assessment Tools

Other than clinician's and patients perspective there should ideally be some objective assessment tools in order to exactly measure the treatment outcomes and these standard objective tools can then guide us to evaluate the treatment options further. These objective tools have been described in details in literature, though in usual practice we don't use then so frequently. Simple photography of face at rest and during seven volitional movements is the most commonly used objective tool, though literature suggests at least 13 different photographic assessment methods. These are MEEI Facegram, Emotrics, Videography including 3D videography etc. Simple videography of face at rest, and during volitional facial movements at different stages before and after surgical intervention and associated development of synkinesis is another very informative tool which gives a very objective view of the treatment outcome. Restoring the basic functions, achieving more complex facial functions like emotional expression and attractiveness as defined by both the clinician and layperson should be the aim. The outcome measurement should not only be from clinicians' perspective but some objective assessment tools should be developed.

Clinical photography and videography are the simplest and most important tools which can measure and keep the record of the facial palsy grade in preoperative time and different stages of improvement in postsurgery or postconservative management. The face is pictured and videographed in different movements like face at rest, wrinkling forehead by lifting eyebrows, eye closure with light and full effort, nose wrinkling for nasolabial fold, smile, dropping of the angle of the mouth, puckering of the lips.

Preoperative Photography

Fig. 5.1 shows Grade VI facial palsy of the left side. The tarsorrhaphy was performed by an ophthalmologist before the first visit to otologist.

Surgery performed was decompression of facial nerve at geniculate ganglion and labyrinthine segment on left side.

Postoperative Photography

Fig. 5.2 shows 1 month postoperative results showing recovery to Grade V.

Fig. 5.3 shows 3 months postoperative pictures showing recovery to Grade IV.

Fig. 5.4 shows 6 months postoperative pictures showing recovery to Grade III.

Fig. 5.5 shows the postoperative pictures after 1 year. Recovery up to Grade II achieved.

Fig. 5.6 shows 2 years postoperative results. Recovery up to Grade I achieved.

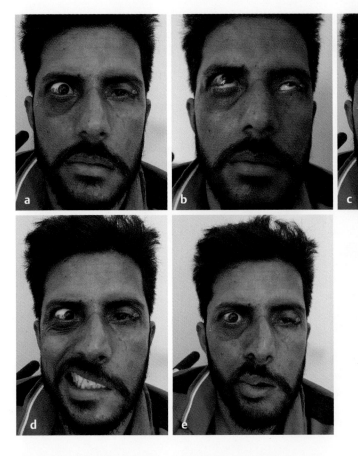

Fig. 5.1 Post injury, left-sided facial nerve palsy of Grade VI. **(a)** Face at rest. **(b)** Unable to wrinkle the forehead. **(c)** Inability to close the eye. **(d)** Inability to lift the angle of mouth. **(e)** Inability to purse the lips on left side. Tarsorrhaphy already performed on the left side.

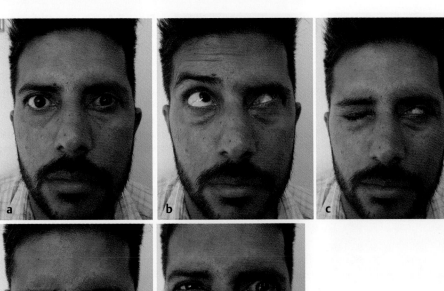

Fig. 5.2 One month postoperative pictures, left side: **(a)** perceptible facial asymmetry at rest, **(b)** inability to wrinkle the forehead, **(c)** inability to close the eye lightly, **(d)** inability to close eye on tight closure, **(e)** barely perceptible maintaining of the angle of mouth.

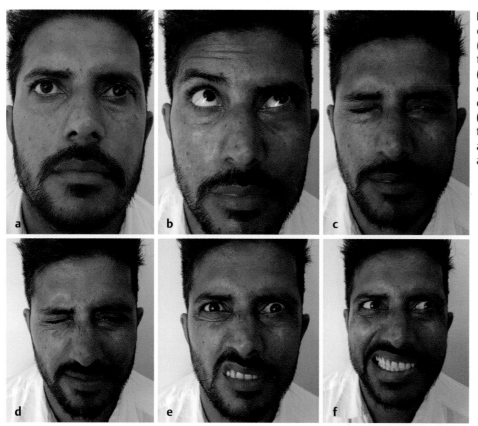

Fig. 5.3 Three months postoperative pictures, left side: **(a)** face at rest, **(b)** inability to wrinkle the forehead, **(c)** incomplete closing of eye on light closure, **(d)** incomplete closing of eye on tight closure, **(e)** incomplete wrinkling of the nose, nasolabial fold has appeared, **(f)** ability to hold angle of mouth.

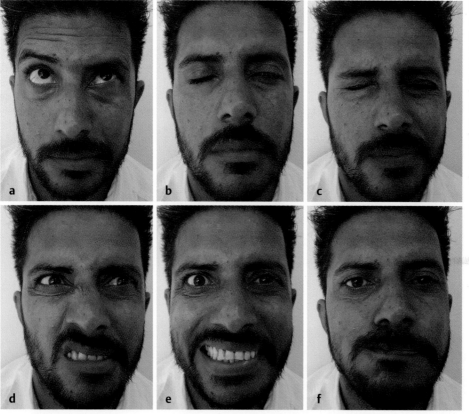

Fig. 5.4 Six months postoperative pictures, left side: **(a)** wrinkling of forehead appearing, **(b)** closure of eye on light closing, eyelid wrinkles still not appeared, **(c)** eye closing with tight closure along with synkinetic lifting of angle of mouth, **(d)** wrinkling of nose with nasolabial fold improved by 50%, **(e)** lifting of angle of mouth to almost 80%, **(f)** ability to fill air with lips pursed.

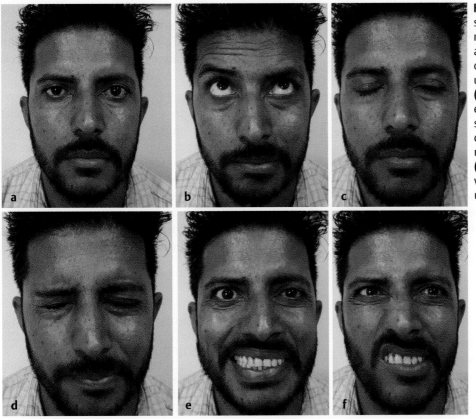

Fig. 5.5 18 months post surgery: **(a)** normal tone at rest, **(b)** wrinkles at forehead appearing, **(c)** closure of eye on light closing (wrinkling of upper eyelid skin appeared), **(d)** complete closure of eye on tight closure with synkinesis improved, **(e)** almost complete lifting of the angle of mouth improved up to 80%, **(f)** wrinkling of nose present with nasolabial fold recovering up to 75%.

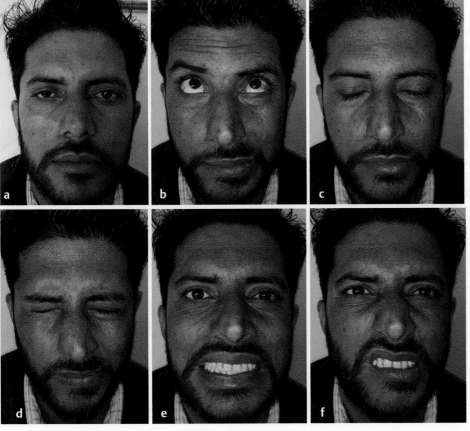

Fig. 5.6 Two years post surgery, left side: **(a)** normal tone at rest, **(b)** forehead wrinkles appeared, **(c)** complete closure of eye on light closure (wrinkling of upper eyelid skin present), **(d)** complete closure on tight closing with synkinesis improved, **(e)** angle of mouth lifting up to 100%, **(f)** nasolabial fold on wrinkling nose improved to 100%.

Spontaneous Smile Analysis

The voluntary smile can be easily executed and measured; the involuntary smile, which is also called true or emotional, is difficult to measure. It is considered the most desirable outcome of smile reanimation surgery by both the surgeon and the patient. Though there are ways to elicit a spontaneous smile, which are based on making the patient laugh or spontaneously smile, but to measure the spontaneous smile there is no tool. many a times the treating clinician can while conversing with patient determine the sponteneity on patient's face which help them in measuring the recovery of spontaneous expressions post surgical intervention. Tools and techniques like Spontaneous smile assay, Time stamping and synchronicity and Automated machine learning alalysis are the few mentioned in literature.

◼ Conclusion

Treating facial palsy is not a procedure, but a whole program, which includes participation of both the clinician and the patient along with detailed analysis of pretreatment situation and final outcome achieved. Not a single step out of this whole program should be missed as the outcome may not be up to clinician or the patient;s satisfaction.

Other than restoring the basic functions of facial nerve, achieving more complex facial functions like emotional expression and attractiveness as defined by both the clinician and layperson should be the aim. The surgical procedures which include primary repair, motor nerve transfer and multiple dynamic and static procedures are decided depending upon two important factors naming duration of palsy and availability of proximal and or distal stump. Once the right surgical technique or procedure has been performed, post management outcome tracking is to be measured with different tools, the most important ones being Patient's perspective, clinician's assessment through scaling systems, third person's assessment and spontaneous smile assessment. The literature says that cases with long duration facial palsy (>2 years) do not improve by performing primary surgeries on facial nerve like nerve decompression, grafting, or nerve transfer because of the long-term denervation of the facial muscles leading to atrophy of muscle fibers and motor end plates. It is a very interesting observation in author's cases though, that, revision surgery for long-standing facial nerve palsy could produce rewarding results even after a gap of >3 years. So the author's philosophy is that in all primary or revision cases of iatrogenic or post-traumatic facial palsy or revision middle ear surgery, with facial palsy of long-term duration, re-exploration and primary repair in the form of decompression, end-to-end repair, or cable grafting should always be performed along with static procedures like upper eyelid implant and fascia lata slings.

The recovery has been observed even up to 3 years as the facial muscles have been found viable up to that duration. The facial muscle fibers remain receptive to reinnervation for a period of up to 2 years, and during that period the facial musculature develops innervation from nerve fibers in the vicinity (i.e., trigeminal nerve fibers). So many a times, the facial muscles remain innervated through branches of other nerves in viscinity and primary repair procedures may give good results even after 3 years in such cases.

Bibliography

1. Dusseldorp JR, van Veen MM, Mohan S, Hadlock TA. Outcome tracking in facial palsy. Otolaryngol Clin North Am 2018;51(6):1033–1050
2. Lo YL, Fook-Chong S, Leoh TH, et al. High-resolution ultrasound in the evaluation and prognosis of Bell's palsy. Eur J Neurol 2010;17(6):885–889
3. Taoka T, Hirabayashi H, Nakagawa H, et al. Displacement of the facial nerve course by vestibular schwannoma: preoperative visualization using diffusion tensor tractography. J Magn Reson Imaging 2006;24(5):1005–1010
4. Raghavan P, Mukherjee S, Phillips CD. Imaging of the facial nerve. Neuroimaging Clin N Am 2009;19(3):407–425
5. Cisneros A, Orozco JRW, Nogues JAO, et al. Development of the stapedius muscle canal and its possible clinical consequences. Int J Pediatr Otorhinolaryngol 2011;75(2):277–281
6. Liu L, Arnold R, Robinson M. Dissection and exposure of the whole course of deep nerves in human head specimens after decalcification. Int J Otolaryngol 2012;2012:418650
7. May M, Schaitkin BM. The Facial Nerve. 2nd ed. New York, NY; Thieme; 2000
8. Curtin HD, Sanelli PC, Som PM. Temporal bone: embryology and anatomy. In: Som PM, Curtin HD, eds. Head and Neck Imaging. Vol. 2. 4th ed. St. Louis, MO: Mosby; 2003
9. Al-Noury K, Lotfy A. Normal and pathological findings for the facial nerve on magnetic resonance imaging. Clin Radiol 2011;66(8):701–707
10. Jäger L, Reiser M. CT and MR imaging of the normal and pathologic conditions of the facial nerve. Eur J Radiol 2001;40(2):133–146
11. Veillona F, Ramos-Taboada L, Abu-Eid M, Charpiot A, Riehm S. Imaging of the facial nerve. Eur J Radiol 2010;74(2):341–348
12. Crawford SC, Harnsberger HR, Swartz JD. The facial nerve (cranial nerve VII). In: Swartz JD, Harnsberger HR,

eds. Imaging of the Temporal Bone. New York, NY: Thieme; 1998

13. Nager GT, Proctor B. Anatomic variations and anomalies involving the facial canal. Otolaryngol Clin North Am 1991;24(3):531–553

14. Yellon RF, Branstetter BF IV. Prospective blinded study of computed tomography in congenital aural atresia. Int J Pediatr Otorhinolaryngol 2010;74(11): 1286–1291

15. Mu X, Quan Y, Shao J, Li J, Wang H, Gong R. Enlarged geniculate ganglion fossa: CT sign of facial nerve canal fracture. Acad Radiol 2012;19(8):971–976

16. Brodsky JR, Smith TW, Litofsky S, Lee DJ. Lipoma of the cerebellopontine angle. Am J Otolaryngol 2006;27(4): 271–274

17. Isaacson B, Telian SA, McKeever PE, Arts HA. Hemangiomas of the geniculate ganglion. Otol Neurotol 2005;26(4):796–802

18. De Foer B, Vercruysse JP, Spaepen M, et al. Diffusion-weighted magnetic resonance imaging of the temporal bone. Neuroradiology 2010;52(9):785–807

19. Yorgancılar E, Yildirim M, Gun R, et al. Complications of chronic suppurative otitis media: a retrospective review. Eur Arch Otorhinolaryngol 2013;270(1):69–76

20. Chen DQ, Quan J, Guha A, Tymianski M, Mikulis D, Hodaie M. Three-dimensional in vivo modeling of vestibular schwannomas and surrounding cranial nerves with diffusion imaging tractography. Neurosurgery 2011;68(4):1077–1083

21. Kennedy PG. Herpes simplex virus type 1 and Bell's palsy—a current assessment of the controversy. J Neurovirol 2010;16(1):1–5

22. Lanser MJ, Jackler RK. Gadolinium magnetic resonance imaging in Bell's palsy. West J Med 1991;154(6): 718–719

23. Pickuth D, Heywang-Köbrunner SH. Neurosarcoidosis: evaluation with MRI. J Neuroradiol 2000;27(3): 185–188

24. Vanzieleghem B, Lemmerling M, Carton D, et al. Lyme disease in a child presenting with bilateral facial nerve palsy: MRI findings and review of the literature. Neuroradiology 1998;40(11):739–742

25. Salvinelli F, Casale M, Vitaliana L, Greco F, Dianzani C, D'Ascanio L. Delayed peripheral facial palsy in the stapes surgery: can it be prevented? Am J Otolaryngol 2004;25(2):105–108

26. Gianoli GJ. Viral titers and delayed facial palsy after acoustic neuroma surgery. Otolaryngol Head Neck Surg 2002;127(5):427–431

27. Brackmann DE, Fisher LM, Hansen M, Halim A, Slattery WH. The effect of famciclovir on delayed facial paralysis after acoustic tumor resection. Laryngoscope 2008;118(9):1617–1620

28. Verzijl HTFM, Valk J, de Vries R, Padberg GW. Radiologic evidence for absence of the facial nerve in Möbius syndrome. Neurology 2005;64(5):849–855

29. Silverman IE, Liu GT, Volpe NJ, Galetta SL. The crossed paralyses. The original brain-stem syndromes of Millard-Gubler, Foville, Weber, and Raymond-Cestan. Arch Neurol 1995;52(6):635–638

30. Eggenberger E. Eight-and-a-half syndrome: one-and-a-half syndrome plus cranial nerve VII palsy. J Neuroophthalmol 1998;18(2):114–116

31. Saia V, Pantoni L. Progressive stroke in pontine infarction. Acta Neurol Scand 2009;120(4):213–215

32. Bassetti C, Bogousslavsky J, Barth A, Regli F. Isolated infarcts of the pons. Neurology 1996;46(1):165–175

33. Cattaneo L, Saccani E, De Giampaulis P, Crisi G, Pavesi G. Central facial palsy revisited: a clinical-radiological study. Ann Neurol 2010;68(3):404–408

34. Kim JYS. Facial nerve paralysis. In: Narayan D, ed. Medscape Reference. 2012

35. Nentwich LM, Veloz W. Neuroimaging in acute stroke. Emerg Med Clin North Am 2012;30(3):659–680

36. Spencer BR Jr, Digre KB. Treatments for neuro-ophthalmologic conditions. Neurol Clin 2010;28(4): 1005–1035

37. Boghen D, Tozlovanu V, Iancu A, Forget R. Botulinum toxin therapy for apraxia of lid opening. Ann N Y Acad Sci 2002;956:482–483

38. Ahmadi N, Newkirk K, Kim HJ. Facial nerve hemangioma: a rare case involving the vertical segment. Laryngoscope 2013;123(2):499–502

39. Friedman O, Neff BA, Willcox TO, Kenyon LC, Sataloff RT. Temporal bone hemangiomas involving the facial nerve. Otol Neurotol 2002;23(5):760–766

40. Künzel J, Zenk J, Koch M, Hornung J, Iro H. Paraganglioma of the facial nerve, a rare differential diagnosis for facial nerve paralysis: case report and review of the literature. Eur Arch Otorhinolaryngol 2012;269(2):693–698

41. Garden AS, Weber RS, Morrison WH, Ang KK, Peters LJ. The influence of positive margins and nerve invasion in adenoid cystic carcinoma of the head and neck treated with surgery and radiation. Int J Radiat Oncol Biol Phys 1995;32(3):619–626

42. Malata CM, Camilleri IG, McLean NR, et al. Malignant tumours of the parotid gland: a 12-year review. Br J Plast Surg 1997;50(8):600–608

43. Jowett N. A general approach to facial palsy. Otolaryngol Clin North Am 2018;51(6):1019–1031

44. Dusseldorp JR, van Veen MM, Mohan S, Hadlock TA. Outcome tracking in facial palsy. Otolaryngol Clin North Am 2018;51(6):1033–1050   45.   Ishi L. Dey J, boahene KDO, et al. The social distraction of facial paralysis objective measurment of social attention using eye tracking. Laryngoscope 2016; 126(2): 334-9

46. Guarin D, Dusseldrop JR, Hadlock TA, et al. Automated facial measurements in facial palsy: a machine learning approach. JAMA Facial plast surg2018; 20(4): 335-7

47. Hadlock T, Urban LS. Towards a universal automated facial measurment tool in facial reanimation. Arch Facial Plast Surg 2012; 14(4): 277-82

6 Evaluation and Management of Acute Facial Palsy

Introduction

Acute facial palsy (AFP) is a grave situation and may be associated with severe morbidity if not treated in time. It can have different etiologies. The commonest ones are idiopathic (Bell's palsy [BP]), herpes zoster oticus, acute otitis media (pediatric group), post-traumatic, iatrogenic, and granulomatous disease of middle ear and mastoid. Some rare viral infections such as dengue, COVID-19, mumps, Epstein–Barr virus, cytomegalovirus, HIV, polio, tetanus, and diphtheria and very rarely Lyme's disease may present with AFP. Initial evaluation should be as early as possible and it is good for patients if they visit the clinician at the earliest, so that no important sign is missed on examination. The different situations are described further in this chapter.

Idiopathic

Pathophysiology

Idiopathic or BP, suspected to be caused by herpes simplex virus (HSV), is an acute paralysis of one side of the face, although in rare situations, it can involve both sides of the face (Chapter 14 titled "Bilateral Facial Palsy"). It accounts for almost 75% cases of AFP.

HSV reactivation in the geniculate ganglion is thought to be the cause of BP. After primary infection which takes place through saliva, the virus lies latent in the geniculate ganglion. Later in life, reactivation of the virus causes inflammation of nerve which is found mostly in labyrinthine portion (various theories endorsing this fact) causing perineural edema from retention of fluid which makes the nerve swell up and lead to its mechanical compression within the bony fallopian canal covering the facial nerve. The different factors making labyrinthine portion most vulnerable are:

- The medial part of the labyrinthine segment (LS), where the nerve exits from the internal auditory meatus (IAM) and enters the fallopian canal, is called "meatal foramen," and it is the narrowest (minimum cross-sectional area is around 0.68 mm^2) part of the fallopian canal.
- The LS is surrounded by dense arachnoid band at meatal foramen. This arachnoid band along with a sudden bent (around 132 degrees angle) decreases the diameter of bony canal from the IAM to labyrinthine canal and creates a bottle neck here, making medial end of the LS more vulnerable to compression (**Fig. 6.1**).
- The subarachnoid space which surrounds the facial nerve in IAM (**Fig. 6.1**) extends along the LS up to the geniculate ganglion. There is no epineurial layer surrounding the LS. The epineurium (**Fig. 6.1**) starts at the geniculate crest (spine of bone separating the LS from tympanic segment [TS] of the facial nerve). Absence of epineurial layer further makes the LS more vulnerable to inflammatory changes during a viral infection.
- The LS ends at the first genu (geniculate ganglion) at the level of geniculate crest (GC). Geniculate ganglion may be dehiscent and attached to the dura of the middle cranial fossa. The dehiscence makes the facial nerve vulnerable to any postinflammatory edema of the nerve at and beyond the geniculate ganglion in both directions.
- The narrow dimensions of the whole labyrinthine canal make the facial nerve to occupy up to 83% of the labyrinthine canal cross-sectional area compared with around 64% of the more distal segments.

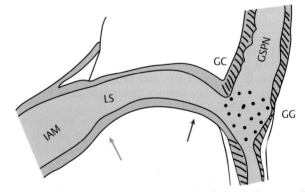

Fig. 6.1 Illustration showing IAM with a bent at the meatal foramen and the narrow canal surrounding the LS (*green arrow*). The next bent of fallopian canal at the junction of the LS and first genu is also visible (*red arrow*). Subarachnoid layer is continuing around the LS (*grey thick layer*) and epineurium starting at the first genu (*striped layer*). GC, geniculate crest; GG, geniculate ganglion; GSPN, greater superficial petrosal nerve; IAM, internal auditory meatus; LS, labyrinthine segment.

- Arterial supply to the LS is single (without anastomosing arterial arcades) unlike the rest of the segments which have dual blood supply.
- In the LS, the internal diameter of the main artery is found to be less than four-tenths of the diameters in the other segments of the facial canal. That makes the ratio of spatial occupancy of the vessels to the canal and to the nerve itself extremely small. The facial nerve itself gets very little space. In any inflammatory situation, edema of the nerve in this segment can make it more vulnerable than the other segments. Further ischemia after inflammatory edema in this segment may result in nerve palsy.
- At the first genu there is an acute angle (90–110 degrees) formed with the LS, which again makes inflammation getting trapped in this area.

Due to all these reasons, labyrinthine portion of the facial canal is considered to be the site of pathogenesis of BP. This inflammation can traverse in both directions leading to ischemia of nerve in other segments later on in untreated cases or disease not improving even after medical management.

Clinical Presentation

BP usually presents with sudden acute onset of unilateral or rarely bilateral facial weakness, which can culminate into complete facial palsy (FP). It often happens within a period of few hours. There can be preceding viral illness in certain cases. The motor deficit involves both the upper and lower parts of the affected side of the face. It is usually a mononeuropathy and if there is association with other cranial nerve palsies, one should suspect some other etiology and workup the case accordingly. Along with FP, the patient may complain of ipsilateral earache, numbness of the face, tongue, and ear, hyperacusis, tinnitus, loss of taste or dystaste, and decreased lacrimation.

Bell's phenomenon or the visible upward movement of the eye on attempted closure of the eyelid due to palsy of the orbicularis oculi is usually present. The phenomenon is named after the Scottish anatomist, surgeon, and physiologist Charles Bell.

Maximal weakness reaches within 2 days and starts resolving on its own or after a course of steroids and antiviral drugs in 3 to 4 weeks.

■ Infection

Ramsay Hunt Syndrome

AFP can be associated with varicella zoster virus (VZV) infection in the body. This condition is also known as Ramsay Hunt syndrome (RHS). RHS is caused by VZV reactivation in the geniculate ganglion and is the most common confirmed infective cause for facial nerve palsy (FNP). The classic triad consists of ipsilateral FNP, vesicles in the auditory canal, and otalgia. There can be associated acute sensorineural hearing loss also.

Clinical Presentation

The patient usually presents with unilateral facial weakness associated with vesicular lesions in the ipsilateral ear, hard palate, or anterior two-thirds of the tongue. It is usually associated with otalgia or vertigo or both. These patients have more painful lesions and palsy than that with BP.

FNP can be the first sign of AIDS, or may occur with late phase of HIV infection.

Acute Otitis Media

Acute otitis media leading to AFP is mostly seen in pediatric age group. There usually is dehiscent facial nerve in these cases and any inflammation of exposed facial nerve can lead to its strangulation, ischemia, and palsy. It can be easily localized on high-resolution computed tomography (HRCT) of temporal bone.

Skull Base Osteomyelitis

The infection begins as otitis externa of the external auditory canal (EAC), spreading further to the temporal bone and skull base. Facial nerve is the most common neural structure getting involved in skull base osteomyelitis. Its presentation is usually acute and an indicator of extensive spread of disease. This topic has been explained in details in Chapter 11 titled "Facial Nerve in Infections."

Post COVID-19 AFP

Lately, post–COVID-19 AFP has been diagnosed as an entity. The patient can present with acute-onset complete facial nerve palsy along with acute sensorineural hearing loss. These patients have immunocompromised state, leading to reactivation of virus in the body. This topic has been explained in details in Chapter 11 titled "Facial Nerve in Infections."

Lyme's Disease

Neuropathy associated with Lyme's disease is caused by *Borrelia burgdorferi*. It is a known cause of FNP in endemic regions. It is more common in children younger than 10 years of age. Presumptive diagnosis should be made in patients presenting with AFP associated with induration and erythema of the face, particularly in the summer.

Post-traumatic/Iatrogenic

Facial nerve injury can happen with both blunt and penetrating craniofacial trauma. Road traffic accidents are the commonest cause of temporal bone fractures. This topic has been explained separately in Chapter 12 titled "Management of Post-traumatic Facial Nerve Palsy."

Iatrogenic facial nerve injury may be caused accidentally during middle ear and mastoid surgery, or lateral skull base surgery. Mobilization, manipulation, deliberately sacrificing, or unknowingly injuring the nerve are few of the causes for the iatrogenic FP. This topic has been explained separately in Chapter 13 titled "Management of Iatrogenic Facial Nerve Palsy."

Neoplastic

Facial nerve palsy may be due to tumor of the facial nerve itself (though it presents rarely as AFP) or through direct compression, stretching, or infiltration of the nerve by a tumor in the vicinity. The topic has been taken up separately in Chapter 15 titled "Management of Facial Nerve Schwanomma".

Autoimmune or Systemic Causes

Disease like Guillain-Barre syndrome (GBS), multiple sclerosis, amyloidosis, granulomatosis with polyangiitis (GPA), and Wegener's granulomatosis have presentation of AFP as recurrent or bilateral AFP.

Granulomatous Diseases

FNP is the most frequent neurological presentation of sarcoidosis. There is usually a bilateral, asymmetric involvement of the parotid gland in these cases. Tuberculosis in temporal bone can also be a cause for AFP.

History, duration, and pattern of presentation of AFP can guide us toward management policy. **Fig. 6.2** depicts percentage and time taken for recovery of facial nerve in different situations. **Fig. 6.2a** shows recovery from BP.

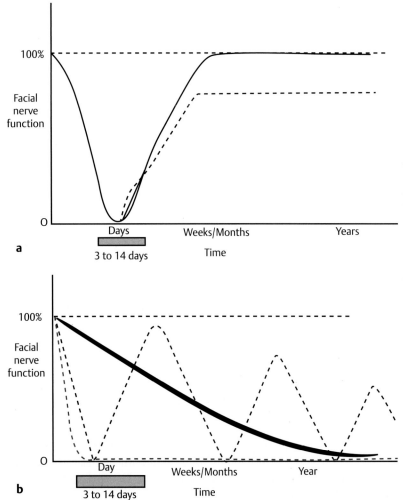

Fig. 6.2 (a) The graph shows percentage and time taken for recovery of acute facial palsy (AFP) in Bell's palsy (BP). *Continuous black line* shows complete recovery of facial nerve function in most of the patient's postviral or idiopathic AFP. The *dotted black line* shows minority of postviral or idiopathic AFP with incomplete recovery (not recovering up to grade I House Brackmann's scale). The time of recovery starts after almost 14 days. **(b)** *Thin red line* showing post-traumatic AFP leading to total loss of facial nerve function immediately or within days after trauma and may stay like this for days, months, or years, if not treated. The *dotted wavy pattern* depicts intermittent AFP in cases of vascular malformations, Melkersson–Rosenthal syndrome (MRS) or granulation disease or facial nerve tumor. The *thick black line* depicts AFP related to tumor in vicinity. The slow progression from weakness to complete facial palsy may take a long time unlike post injury where there is sudden complete loss of facial function.

Fig. 6.2b shows presentation and recovery from other different situations.

Evaluation

Accurate clinical history, comprehensive examination of ear, nose, throat, and facial nerve, head and neck including parotid area, and ophthalmological and neurological examination (multidisciplinary approach) will guide in establishing the cause for AFP which can be due to any of the above explained etiologies. Whether the palsy is unilateral or bilateral (this topic discussed in detail in Chapter 14 titled "Bilateral Facial Palsy"), or there is some secondary cause and whether it is upper or lower motor neuron lesion is also to be ruled out.

History

It includes history of any exposure to viral infection, outdoor activity with rash over body, vesicles over pinna and EAC, trauma, surgery in recent past, tumor of head and neck and parotid, diabetes, tuberculosis or sarcoidosis, and any autoimmune disease like Wegener's granulomatosis.

Physical Examination

Thorough physical examination is important for proper evaluation and it includes the following:

- Ear, nose, and throat examination.
- Ophthalmological examination.
- Head and neck examination.
- Neurological examination.
- Examination of facial nerve function according to House-Brackmann's or Sunnybrook's scale on the affected side and compared with the normal side.
- Examination of parotid area.

Ophthalmologic Examination

Ophthalmologists play an important role in the multidisciplinary team involved in the evaluation and rehabilitation of these patients. Baseline visual acuity, pupillary reactions, sensitivity of the cornea, Schirmer's test (though over time it has lost its relevance), and optic disc evaluation are performed. Bell's phenomenon is another important finding in cases of complete grade VI facial palsy.

Otological Examination

Vesicles around the ear suggest RHS. Inflammation or pus from the ear may indicate skull base osteomyelitis.

Tenderness of the mastoid may suggest infection spreading from the middle ear.

Oral Examination

The sensation of taste of the anterior two-thirds of the tongue and the function of salivary glands are not frequently tested as there can be false positive or negative reports due to inflammation of nerve in both directions, beyond the actual site of injury or lesion. Simply ask the patient about it or place small amounts of sugar, salt, vinegar, and quinine for evaluation.

Associated Diseases

Parotid swelling may suggest a malignant or inflammatory mass.

Neurologic Examination

Assessment of all cranial nerves is important.

Ocular Movements

Associated ipsilateral VI nerve palsy may suggest a pontine or petrous apex lesion.

Evaluation of Facial Nerve

Examination of the face at rest, during speech, and voluntary, emotional, and involuntary movements is conducted, and extent of the facial weakness noted. The detailed examination of the face has been explained in Chapter 4 titled "Preoperative Evaluation and Diagnosis."

Documentation

Photography and videography on day 1 when the patient visits the clinician for the first time and on all the follow-up visits are mandatory.

Outcome Documentation

Photography, videography, audiometry, and subjective and objective assessments of the recovery are to be documented at different intervals of recovery phase.

Routine Laboratory Investigation and Diagnostic Imaging

This is not indicated in patients with new-onset AFP, but should be performed in patients with risk factors, atypical cases, cases associated with certain other features suggesting a systemic disease, recurrent AFP, or in case of grade VI FP persisting beyond 3 months.

Laboratory Investigations

These include specific tests for the disease the patient is suffering from like complete blood count (CBC),

C-reactive protein (CRP), blood sugar and HBA1C, antinuclear antibodies (ANA), tests for vasculitis like antineutrophil cytoplasmic antibody (ANCA), PR3, and tests to rule out tuberculosis, sarcoidosis, and amyloidosis in case the clinical features direct toward that.

Radiological Imaging

Computed tomography (CT) and/or magnetic resonance imaging (MRI) with contrast is performed only in case where complete FP does not improve within 3 months, in case of recurrent episodes of AFP, or in case of confirmed disease like tumor, trauma, skull base osteomyelitis, tuberculosis, malignancy, etc.

Electrodiagnostic Testing

It is considered only in cases of acute complete (grade VI) FP of idiopathic origin, in confirmed cases of BP, or in non-displaced temporal bone fractures. Electroneuronography (ENoG) and electromyography (EMG) are the two tests performed. Acute, immediate surgical decompression is indicated in patients with ENoG showing >90% degeneration in comparison with normal side and EMG showing absent voluntary motor unit action potential within 4 to 14 days of onset of FP (not to be performed before 4 days of acute onset of FP because it takes 3 days for Wallerian degeneration to occur).

■ Management

Many factors are involved in determining the appropriate treatment for the patient with AFP, for example, age of the patient, the underlying cause, estimated period of nerve palsy, anatomical manifestations, severity of symptoms, and objective clinical examination.

Once the complete evaluation is done and correct diagnosis is made, general and specific management is started.

There is a specific treatment for facial nerve rehabilitation and multidisciplinary treatment for depending upon the etiology.

The treatment discussed below is specific for facial nerve rehabilitation.

Medical Therapy

- Corticosteroids are the mainstay of medical treatment. It is given in every patient unless contraindicated in some associated systemic disease. High dose steroids can reduce the neural inflammation and secondary ischemia leading to early recovery of facial nerve function with less chances of postpalsy synkinesis. Prednisolone is given in the dose of 1 to 1.5 mg/kg/day for 10 days, preferably in injectable form, followed by tapering dose till few weeks depending on recovery of facial nerve functioning.
- Antiviral medication in the form of either acyclovir in the dose of 400 mg five times a day or valacyclovir 1 g twice daily for 7 days. Contraindications to antiviral medications include any immunocompromised state, liver or kidney disease, or pregnancy.
- Eye care: The earliest treatment is to protect the exposed cornea. The exposure and damage to the cornea depend on the degree of nerve lesion, on the extent of lagophthalmos (inability to close upper eyelid), lower eyelid ectropion, and the quality of Bell's phenomenon (it is the movement of the eyeballs in an upward direction when the eyelids are forcibly closed). It is a normal reflex that protects the eyeball against sudden potential trauma. In BP, as the eyelids fail to close, this movement is clearly visible, along with the presence or absence of corneal sensitivity. The earliest therapy includes protective glasses, intensive lubrication with natural tears (preservative-free) along with eye drops in daytime and ointment along with taping of the eyelids at night.

  In case of suspected delayed recovery, tarsorrhaphy, scleral contact lenses, and upper eyelid implants are different procedures used to protect the cornea till self-recovery or surgical correction is achieved. Once the cornea is protected, longer term planning for eyelid and facial rehabilitation is considered. Spontaneous complete recovery of postinfective or idiopathic FP occurs in up to 70% of cases. Long-term complications if not treated at the right time can be in the form of nonrecovery or minimal recovery of facial functions and aberrant regeneration in different forms like synkinesis, abnormal lacrimation while eating (known as crocodile tears), corneal ulceration, and permanent visual impairment.
- Physiotherapy: Physiotherapy treatment includes exercises to improve and maintain the function of the facial muscles till the actual recovery takes place. It also prevents the contractures leading to tightening and rigidity of the facial muscles. Facial neuromuscular retraining and mime therapy (mirror stimulation of the facial expression) form an important part of physiotherapy. Electrical neural muscular stimulation is only performed in very early stage and should be avoided in later stage as it can lead to motor synkinesis.

For physiotherapy exercises, the patient must sit in front of the mirror. Each exercise is to be repeated 5 to 10 times. The following are different exercises for idiopathic and postviral infection AFP.

Exercises Involving Movements of Eyebrow

- Raise the eyebrows and wrinkle the forehead and hold them in the raised state directly or with the help of finger for 10 to 15 seconds.
- Rub the affected side forehead and eyebrow with the fingertips in an upward direction.
- Make a frowning expression and try to draw both eyebrows close.

Exercises Involving Eye Movements

- Keep both eyes open without raising the eyebrows.
- Perform light and forceful closure of eyelids.
- Keeping neck straight, look downwards with the eyes.
- Closing the upper eyelid with finger, lift the affected side eyebrow with another finger. This helps in relaxing the affected eyelid muscles.
- Alternatively close and open one eye at a time.

Exercises Involving Lip and Oral Cavity

- Curl both upper and lower lips like a pout/puckering movement.
- Squeeze and release alternatively.
- Smile lightly without showing teeth.
- Smile by showing the teeth by stretching both the lips to the maximum on both sides.
- Move both lips in downwards direction.
- Practice speaking certain vowels like AA, OO, EE, and UU.
- Blow out the cheeks by filling air in them and hold like this for 10 seconds.
- Try chewing your food by involving both the sides of your mouth.

Exercises Involving Nose

- Wrinkle up the nose.
- Perform forceful exhalation through one nostril by closing the other after deep inhalation.

Exercises Involving Neck and Chin for Stretching of Platysma

- Make tilting movements with head first on sideways and then backwards and forwards.
- Do forwards and backwards movement with chin.

Surgical Management

Indications for surgical management are:

- In post-traumatic cases, if the patient has consulted the clinician within 72 hours of onset of AFP, and the ENoG is showing >90% nerve degeneration as compared to normal side (not to be performed before 4 days of acute onset of FP because it takes 3 days for Wallerian degeneration to occur) along with EMG showing absent voluntary motor unit action potential within 4 to 14 days of onset of FP is a case for surgical decompression of facial nerve on the affected side.
- Cases of post-traumatic, postviral, or idiopathic AFP not recovering till 3 months (4 months is the uppermost limit) with or without medical treatment are the candidates for surgical management. Almost all cases of incomplete AFP (postviral or idiopathic) show complete recovery whereas almost 60% of cases with complete AFP show complete recovery without the need of surgical decompression, rest 40% may not improve up to grade I (HBs). That is why a safe time limit of up to 3 months is decided, after which irreversible changes in the form of collagenization (in cases of post-traumatic AFP) and ischemia and fibrosis (in case of BP or postviral AFP) take place. Maximum wait should be up to 4 months after which radiological imaging is to be carried out to confirm the diagnosis and decide for the surgical management, according to the cause. If the patients present late to the clinician (after 4 months of onset of FP), they should be explained about chances of less than complete recovery even after surgery.
- In the rest of the cases where the AFP is associated with some systemic disease as well, the surgical treatment is decided accordingly.

Counseling of the patient becomes very important in such cases. The patient and the attendants are educated in detail about the risk and benefits of surgery. They are made aware about the long recovery time taken even after surgery, the chances of suffering from surgical and postsurgery complications like hearing loss, iatrogenic trauma to facial nerve, injury to inner ear, synkinesis, etc.

Surgical Management for Bell's Palsy

As explained above, the meatal foramen and the labyrinthine portion of the facial canal are the site of pathogenesis of BP. So, the surgical procedure is to be designed in a way that it must be directed toward the LS without causing any trauma to surrounding structures. In case the patient has come very late to the surgeon (more than 6 months), the inflammation might have spread beyond the labyrinthine segment on both sides so decompression must include every segment which seems inflammed or affected. The illustration in **Fig. 6.10** explains how decompressing the facial nerve, by drilling away the bony fallopian canal in the first genu, LS, and meatal foramen area, relieves the compression of the facial nerve leading to normal neuronal flow.

The techniques performed by the author, to address the LS and first genu area directly and if needed extended up to stylomastoid foramen, are:

- Post aural, inside-out technique.
- Post aural/end aural, transzygomatic anterior attic technique.

Case 1

A 36-years-old patient presented with sudden-onset complete facial palsy (grade VI House-Brackmann's scale (HBS)] on the left side of face (both upper and lower compartments) since 10 days (**Fig. 6.3**). There were associated vesicles in left pinna (**Fig. 6.3f**), which were painful. On examination, bilaterally tympanic membrane were found intact. HRCT of temporal bone shows normal facial nerve dimensions and location from the IAM till stylomastoid foramen (**Fig. 6.4**).

The patient was admitted and put under treatment in the form of antiviral, antibiotics, and high dose of injectable steroids. The patient started improving within 5 days of starting treatment and complete recovery of facial nerve took place in 3 months (**Fig. 6.5**).

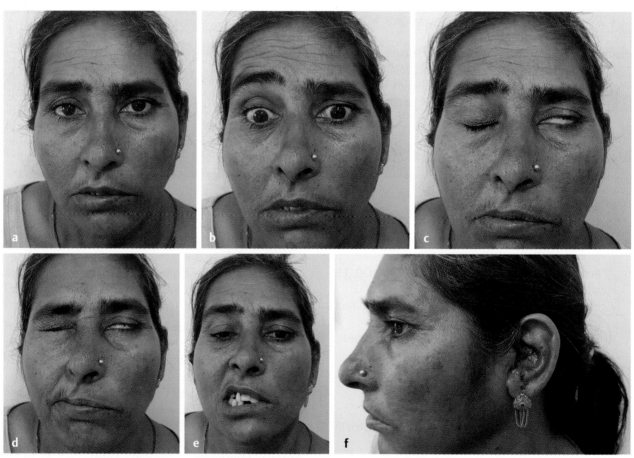

Fig. 6.3 **(a)** Left sided facial nerve palsy, grade VI (House-Brackmann's scale [HBS]), with loss of normal facial tone at rest, **(b)** inability to wrinkle forehead and lift the eyebrow, and **(c)** inability to close eye on light closure **(d)** inability to close eye on forceful closure with Bell's phenomenon visible. **(e)** Inability to lift angle of mouth. **(f)** Vesicles involving left auricle.

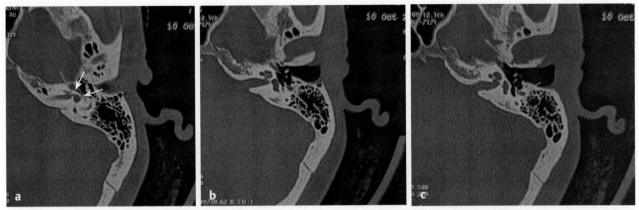

Fig. 6.4 High-resolution computed tomography (HRCT) of temporal bone showing normal facial nerve from IAM till stylomastoid foramen, **(a)** showing the LS (*orange arrow*), first genu (*white arrow*), and TS (*yellow arrow*), **(b)** the second genu (*orange arrow*), and **(c)** the MS (*orange arrow*).

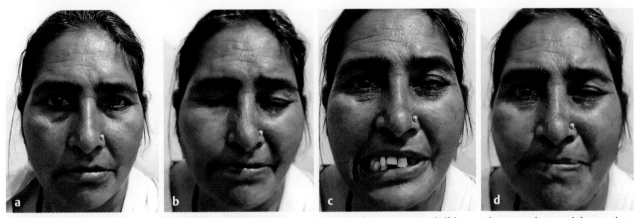

Fig. 6.5 After 3 months of treatment (left side): **(a)** face at rest, normal tone regained, **(b)** complete eye closure, **(c)** complete lifting of angle of mouth, and **(d)** appearance of nasolabial fold.

Case 2

A 32-years-old male presented with left-sided facial weakness and left-sided hearing loss and tinnitus since 10 days which was sudden in onset and progressive. There was history of fever, sore throat, and vesicular eruptions over left pinna 12 days back for which he had taken treatment in the form of tab acyclovir 800 mg four times a day for 7 days. On examination, there was left-sided lower motor neuron grade III FP (HBC) (**Fig. 6.6a–c**). There was no other focal or systemic neurological deficit. The vesicles on left pinna were in healing phase along with bilaterally intact tympanic membrane (**Fig. 6.7**). He gave a history of chicken-pox infection in childhood. As he was tested positive for COVID-19, so he was kept in isolation while getting treatment for COVID-19. Diagnosis made was RHS, with reactivation of VZV in left facial nerve along with sudden-onset hearing loss. Investigations performed were pure tone audiometry (PTA), MRI of brain and skull base, and HRCT of temporal bone. The PTA revealed profound sensorineural hearing loss on the right side and severe sensorineural hearing loss on the left side. MRI study showed no abnormality with bilateral normal IAM and VIIth–VIIIth nerve complexes (**Fig. 6.8**). HRCT also revealed essentially normal study with facial canal dimensions within normal limits (**Fig. 6.9**). His routine blood investigations were well within normal limits with marginally increased CRP levels. IgG and IgM titers for HSV were negative.

Medical treatment started in the form of intravenous (IV) Dexamethasone 8 mg twice daily, IV Xanthinol Nicotinate 1 g twice daily, and IV Neurobion Forte once daily with an antibiotic cover for lesion on pinna. He was also administered 0.5 mL intratympanic triamcinolone acetonide 40 mg/mL bilaterally on days 1, 3, and 5 under local anesthesia. However, the patient showed only a 5 dB improvement in the left hearing thresholds after the first injection and no improvement after the second and third injections. Speech discrimination score after all three intratympanic injections was 70% with the use of hearing aid bilaterally. His facial paresis improved completely to grade I on day 10 (**Fig. 6.6d–f**) with improvement in tinnitus as well. The steroids were tapered off in 3 weeks and he was advised use of hearing aids.

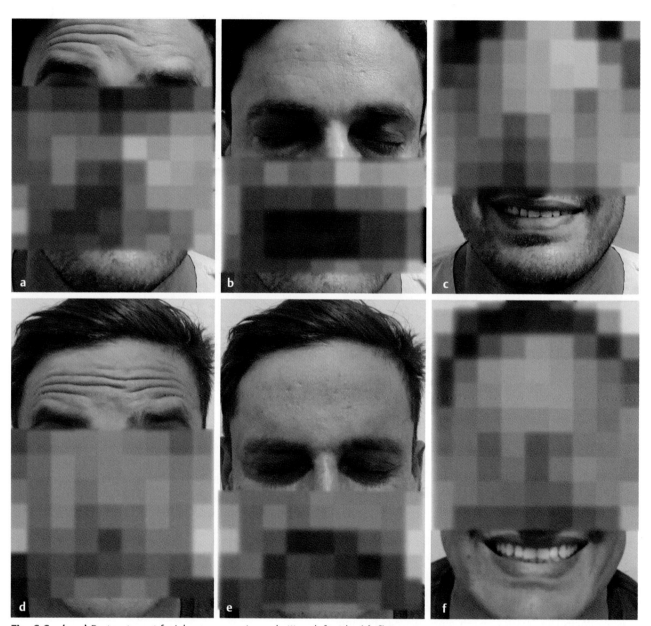

Fig. 6.6 **(a–c)** Pretreatment facial nerve paresis grade III on left side. **(d–f)** Post-treatment recovery up to grade I.

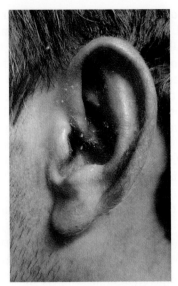

Fig. 6.7   Vesicular eruptions over left pinna.

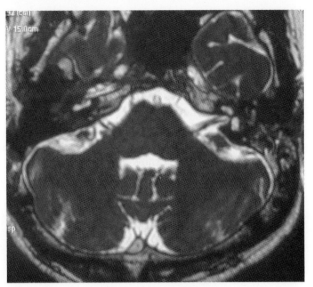

Fig. 6.8   Normal study of facial nerve in internal auditory meatus (IAM) and labyrinthine segment (LS).

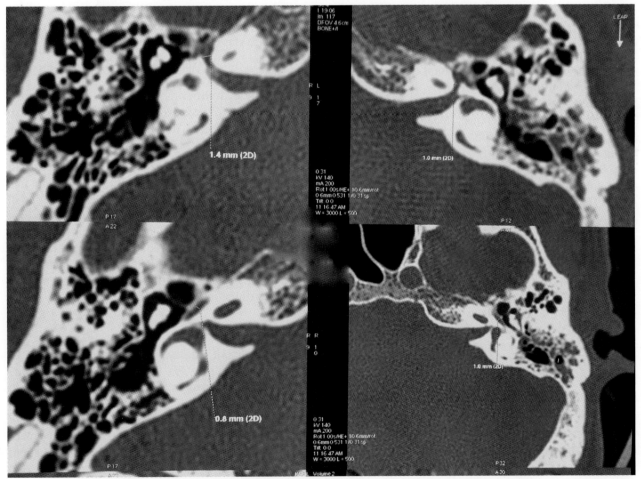

Fig. 6.9   Comparison of facial canal on both sides on high-resolution computed tomography (HRCT) of temporal bones showing essentially normal study with facial canal dimensions within normal limits on both sides.

Case 3

A 51-year-old patient presented with sudden-onset, left-sided facial palsy since 6 months, without any associated symptoms pointing toward some specific cause for the palsy. On examination, there was complete grade VI FP involving left side with Bell's phenomenon noted (**Fig. 6.11**). Examination showed normal nose, ears, oral cavity, and nervous system. MRI (**Fig. 6.12**) and HRCT of temporal bone (**Fig. 6.13**) showed normal facial nerve course and dimensions from IAM to stylomastoid foramen, other than the dehiscence of facial nerve at and just distal to geniculate ganglion on left side (**Fig. 6.13c**). The patient had already received conservative treatment in the form of oral prednisolone 1 mg/kg body weight in tapering dosage in the starting 1 month of palsy. No antiviral drug was prescribed in the past.

As 6 months had already passed, and grade VI FP persisted, surgical management became the treatment of choice.

Surgical Steps

On otomicroscopy, the tympanic membrane was found intact (**Fig. 6.14a**). Through post aural approach, skin incision was made, posteroinferiorly based musculoperiosteal flap was raised, skin of bony EAC lifted in three-fourths of circumference. Meatotomy incision made just lateral to the bony annulus and canal skin retracted anteriorly in self-retaining mastoid retractor (**Fig. 6.14b–d**). Canaloplasty was performed till tympanic annulus became visible in its total circumference (**Fig. 6.15a, b**).

Tympanic membrane lifted in its posterior quadrant. Middle ear and ossicular chain were found normal (**Fig. 6.15c, d**).

With 2 mm and 3-mm diamond burrs, lateral wall of epitympanum was drilled in an inside-out manner (**Fig. 6.16**). The incus, malleus, stapes, and horizontal part of facial nerve visualized (**Fig. 6.17**). After separating the incudostapedial and incudomalleolar joint with a right angle pick, the incus was taken out (**Fig. 6.18**). Further, head of malleus was nipped and removed (**Fig. 6.19**). Inside-out atticotomy continued till lateral wall of anterior, superior, and posterior attic drilled away and complete attic was exposed (**Fig. 6.20**).

Facial canal visualized in its tympanic portion up to the first genu. The nerve found dehiscent and inflamed at the first genu and anterior most part of TS (**Fig. 6.21**).

Drilling of suprafacial and supralabyrinthine cells was started and bony chips removed from around to expose facial nerve at the first genu (**Fig. 6.22**). With 2-mm diamond burr, the cells surrounding the first genu and LS drilled away and exposure of the LS achieved in 270-degree circumference (**Fig. 6.23**) as the edema and inflammation could be seen reaching up to labyrinthine portion as well. Decompression was achieved till medial end of the LS (**Figs. 6.24–6.26**). To decompress and expose the LS completely, the thick block of bone superior to the first genu and anterior part of TS, and anterior to ampulla of both superior and lateral semicircular canal needs to be drilled with a diamond drill (**Fig. 6.25**). This step is to be performed carefully, so as to avoid injuring ampulla of lateral semicircular canal (LSC) and superior semicircular canal (SSC) (**Figs. 6.24** and **6.25**).

The decompression of facial nerve in its TS was also achieved by drilling away the thin shell of bone, first with the diamond burr (**Fig. 6.27**) followed by removal with a curette and tympanic membrane elevator (**Fig. 6.28**). The decompression is to be achieved almost 4 to 5 mm beyond the level of inflammation of facial nerve, which in this case was up to the second genu (**Fig. 6.28**).

After decompression, the sheath of facial nerve (epineurium) was opened up with ophthalmic keratome (**Fig. 6.29**) from the first genu up to the second genu (**Fig. 6.30**). As labyrinthine portion does not have an epineurium sheath, never try to move blade or any sharp instrument on the LS (**Fig. 6.31**).

The posterosuperior canal wall reconstructed with the tragal cartilage graft with perichondrium on side facing the neotympanum (**Fig. 6.32**). Reconstruction of ossicular chain by placing reshaped head of malleus over head of stapes as a columella graft was performed and round window reflex checked. Finally, temporalis fascia graft was placed medial to true tympanic membrane (TM) to support the posterior quadrant of TM over the neoposterosuperior canal wall (**Fig. 6.33**).

Postsurgery Status

After 24 hours of surgery, the patient had grade VI FP persisting on left side (**Fig. 6.34**). After 3 months of surgery, the improvement in facial nerve functioning could be achieved up to grade V (**Fig. 6.35**). After 6 months of surgery, the improvement reached up to grade IV (**Fig. 6.36**). After 1 year of surgery, the improvement could be achieved up to grade I (**Fig. 6.37**). The patient was put on regular physiotherapy sessions to avoid synkinesis.

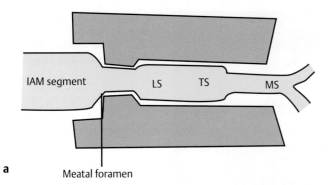

a   Meatal foramen

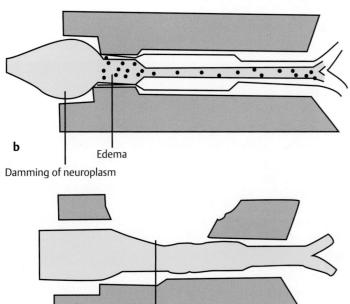

b
Damming of neuroplasm   Edema

c   Drilling away the bone around LS and MF

Fig. 6.10 **(a)** The different segments of facial nerve and anatomical location of meatal foramen (MF). **(b)** Edema of labyrinthine segment (LS) blocking the axoplasmic flow at the meatal foramen leading to the swelling of meatal segment of facial canal (damming of neuroplasm). **(c)** Decompression of the LS by drilling away bone of fallopian canal (FC) relieves this edema of the LS and meatal segment.

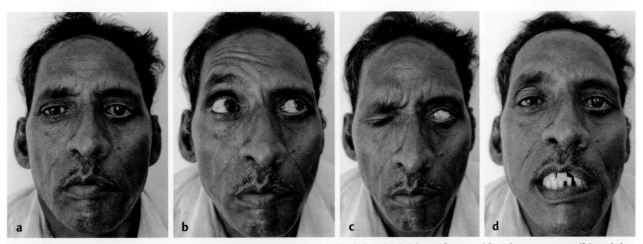

Fig. 6.11 Clinical images showing grade VI (HBS) facial palsy on the left side, **(a)** loss of normal facial tone at rest, **(b)** inability to wrinkle the forehead and lifting of eyebrow, **(c)** inability to close eye on forceful closure with Bell's phenomenon visible, **(d)** inability to lift angle of mouth. HBS, House Brakmann's scale.

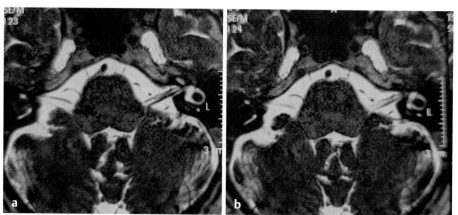

Fig. 6.12 (a, b) Magnetic resonance imaging (MRI) showing normal facial nerve course in meatal segment and labyrinthine segment (LS).

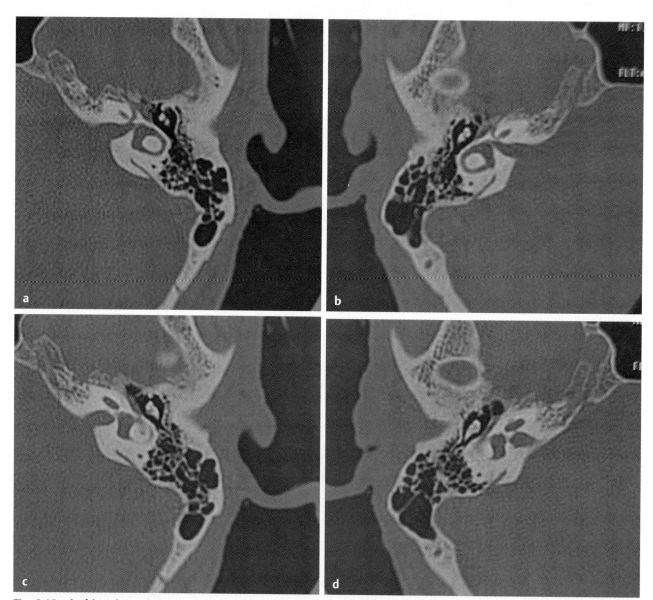

Fig. 6.13 (a, b) High-resolution computed tomography (HRCT) images showing normal course and dimensions of facial nerve in the internal auditory meatus (IAM), labyrinthine segment (LS), and first genu segment on both left and right sides. There is dehiscence noted in the first genu area on left side (*orange arrow*). **(c, d)** normal course and dimensions of facial nerve in its TS on both sides. *(Continued)*

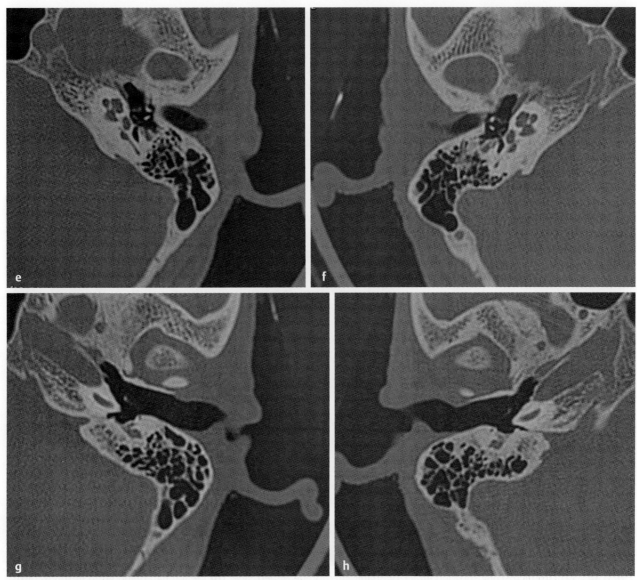

Fig. 6.13 *(Continued)* **(e, f)** Normal course and dimensions of facial nerve at the second genuon both sides. **(g, h)** normal course and dimensions of facial nerve in mastoid segment (MS) on both sides.

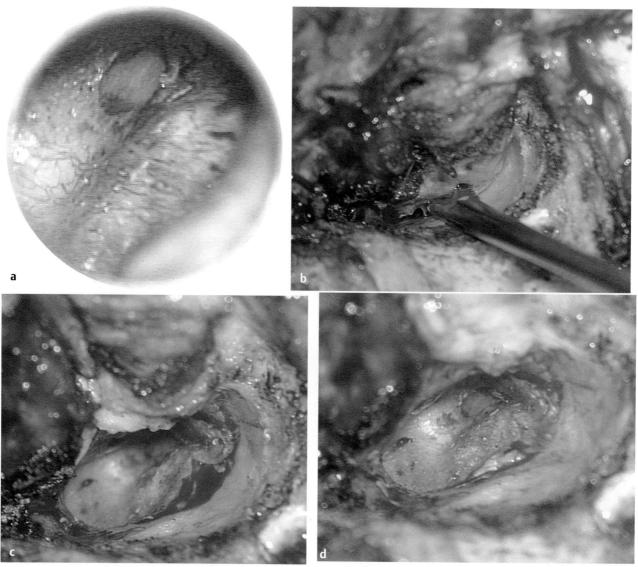

Fig. 6.14 **(a)** Otomicroscopy showing intact tympanic membrane on left side. **(b)** Meatal flap being lifted in three-fourths of its circumference. Meatotomy incision is given just lateral to the tympanic annulus. **(c, d)** After lifting of meatal flap it is retracted anteriorly in self-retaining mastoid retractor. The intact TM is visible.

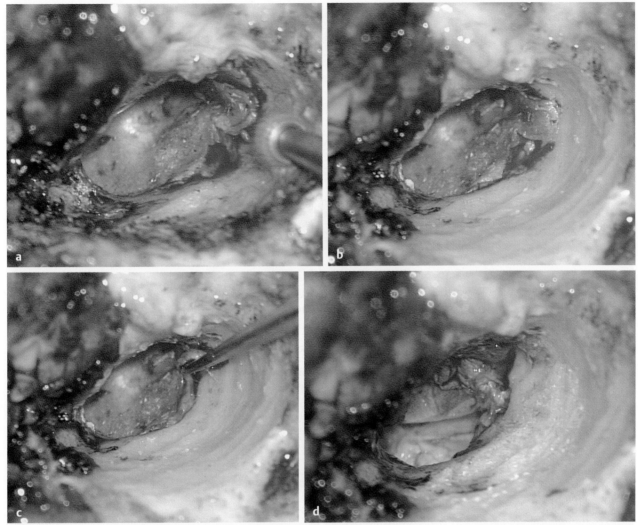

Fig. 6.15 **(a, b)** Canaloplasty performed from lateral to medial direction with size 4- and 3-mm diamond burrs respectively and bony overhangs removed. **(c, d)** Tympanic membrane lifted in its posterior quadrant and middle ear visualized.

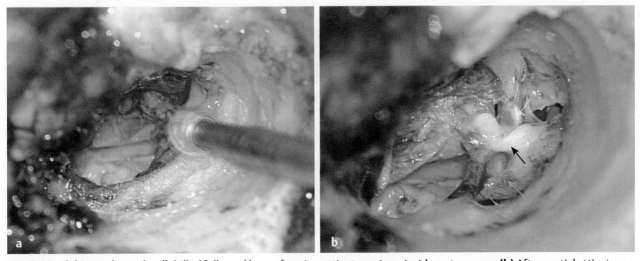

Fig. 6.16 **(a)** Lateral scutal wall drilled followed by performing atticotomy in an inside-out manner. **(b)** After partial atticotomy, head and neck of malleus (*black arrow*), anterior malleolar ligament (*yellow arrow*), long process of incus (*blue arrow*), and chorda tympani (*red arrow*) are visualized.

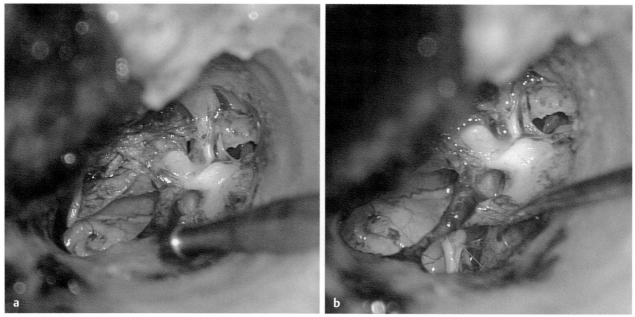

Fig. 6.17   (a, b) Further drilling exposes stapes (*green arrow*) and horizontal segment (TS) of facial nerve (pointed by a sickle knife).

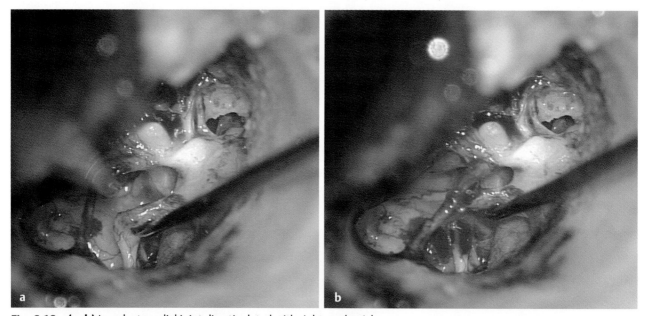

Fig. 6.18   (a, b) Incudostapedial joint disarticulated with right angle pick.

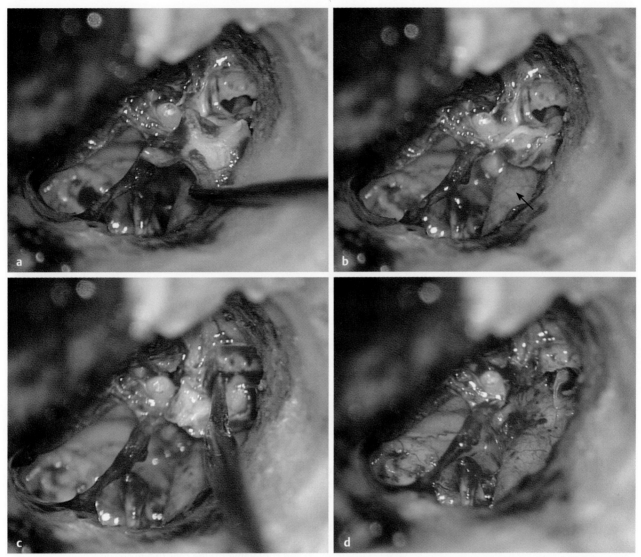

Fig. 6.19 **(a, b)** After disarticulating incudomalleolar joint, incus is being taken out. Tympanic segment (TS) of facial nerve visualized (*black arrow*). **(c, d)** Head of malleus excised after cutting with malleus head cutter.

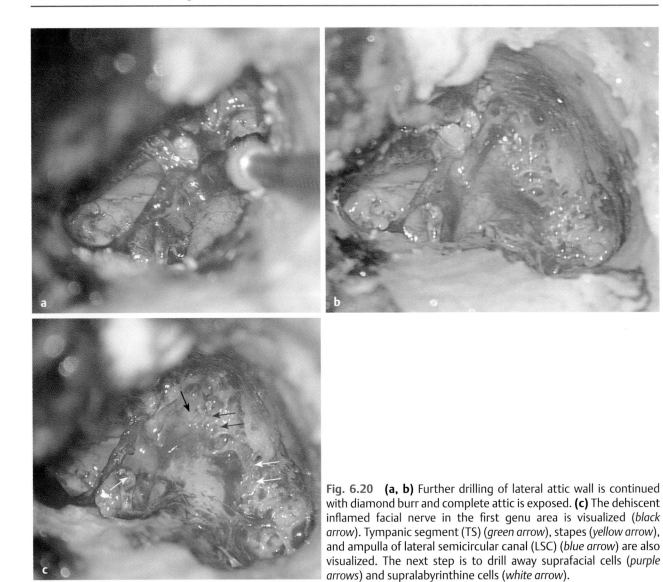

Fig. 6.20 **(a, b)** Further drilling of lateral attic wall is continued with diamond burr and complete attic is exposed. **(c)** The dehiscent inflamed facial nerve in the first genu area is visualized (*black arrow*). Tympanic segment (TS) (*green arrow*), stapes (*yellow arrow*), and ampulla of lateral semicircular canal (LSC) (*blue arrow*) are also visualized. The next step is to drill away suprafacial cells (*purple arrows*) and supralabyrinthine cells (*white arrow*).

Fig. 6.21 **(a)** Drilling of supra facial and supra labyrinthine cells in progress. **(b)** Dehiscent facial nerve at first genu area is clearly visualized (*yellow arrows*).

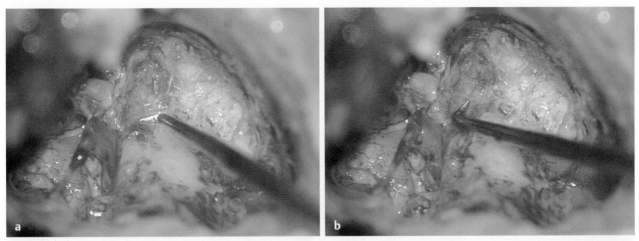

Fig. 6.22 **(a)** Very thin bony shell present over anterior part of tympanic segment (TS) being pointed with the right angle pick. **(b)** Proximal to which bony cover is missing on facial nerve (dehiscent facial nerve in first genu area).

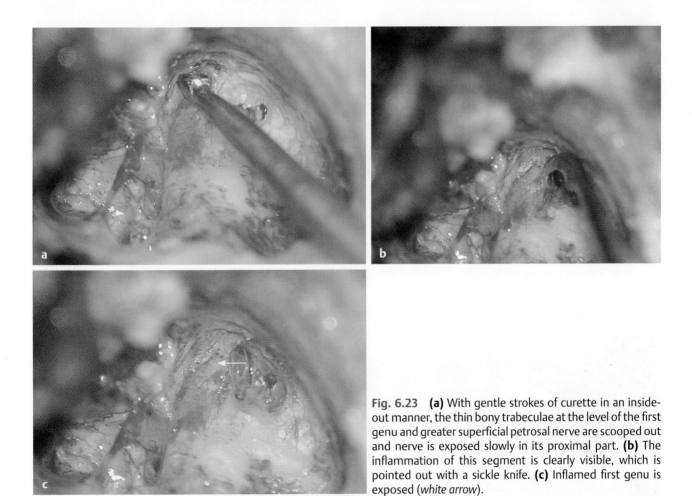

Fig. 6.23 **(a)** With gentle strokes of curette in an inside-out manner, the thin bony trabeculae at the level of the first genu and greater superficial petrosal nerve are scooped out and nerve is exposed slowly in its proximal part. **(b)** The inflammation of this segment is clearly visible, which is pointed out with a sickle knife. **(c)** Inflamed first genu is exposed (*white arrow*).

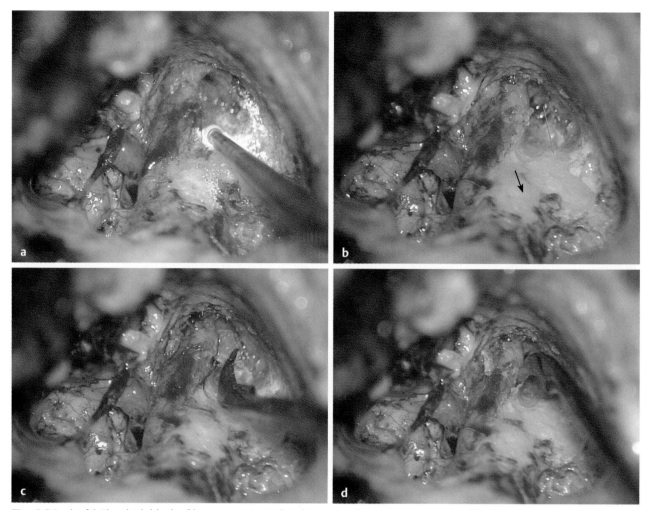

Fig. 6.24 **(a, b)** The thick block of bone superior to facial nerve and anterior to ampulla of both superior semicircular **canal** (SSC) (a landmark for exposing labyrinthine segment [LS]) and lateral semicircular canal (LSC) (a landmark for exposing tympanic segment [TS]) is removed with a diamond burr, size always biggest for that given area. This step is to be performed carefully so as to avoid injuring ampulla of LSC (*black arrow*) and SSC (*green arrow*). **(c, d)** Final thin shell of bone is removed with a sickle knife or TM) elevator.

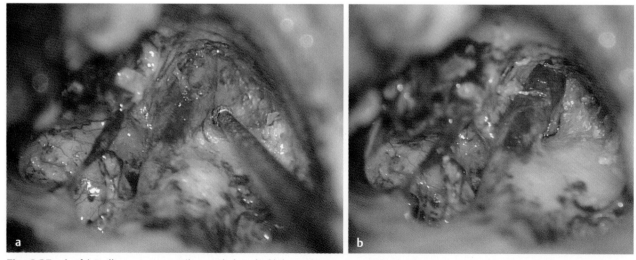

Fig. 6.25 **(a, b)** Drilling to expose the medial end of labyrinthine segment (LS). The nerve seems inflamed till the medial end of LS proximally.

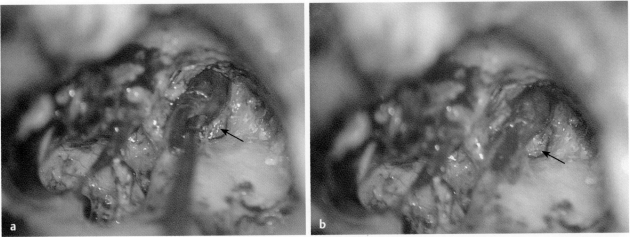

Fig. 6.26 **(a)** Labyrinthine segment (LS) exposed in 270 degrees till its medial end (*black arrow*). **(b)** Medial end of LS (meatal foramen, *black arrow*) visualized.

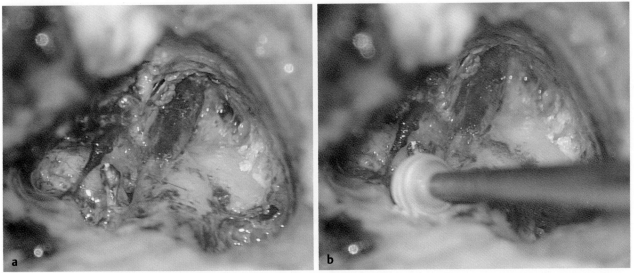

Fig. 6.27 **(a)** On distal side, inflammation of nerve is involving the tympanic segment (TS) (*green arrow*) so **(b)** drilling of bone around the TS in progress.

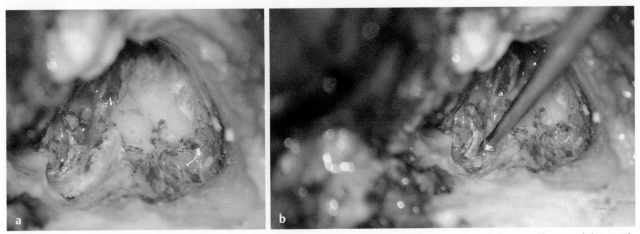

Fig. 6.28 **(a, b)** Exposure of the tympanic segment (TS) in its whole length is in progress first with diamond burr and then with a curette to scoop out the last thin bony shell over the nerve. *(Continued)*

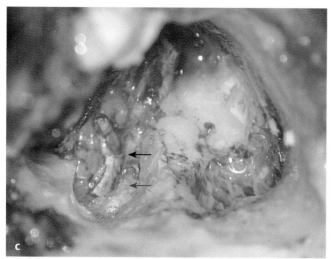

Fig. 6.28 *(Continued)* **(c)** Inflammation noticed up to mid part of the TS, so decompression of nerve achieved till the second genu (at least 4–5 mm of healthy nerve beyond inflammation). The inflammed and healthy nerves are depicted by *black* and *red arrows*, respectively.

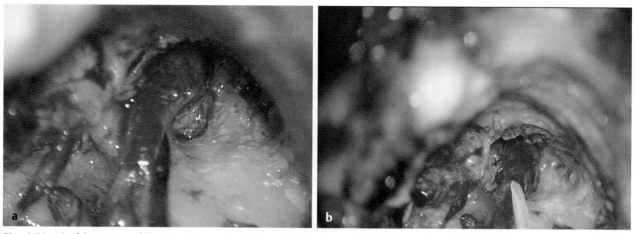

Fig. 6.29 **(a, b)** Incision of the sheath over the inflamed first genu portion in progress with ophthalmic keratome.

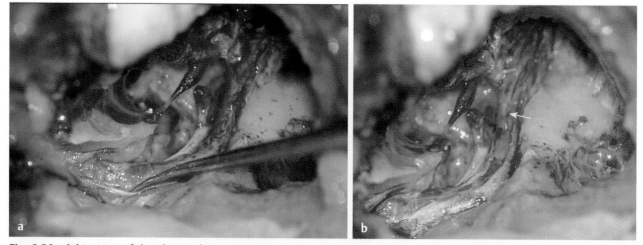

Fig. 6.30 **(a)** Incision of sheath over the second genu in progress. **(b)** Decompressed nerve with incised epineurium visualized from the first genu up to the second genu. The difference in colour of nerve in its inflamed part (yellow arrow) and healthy part (blue arrow) can be visualized.

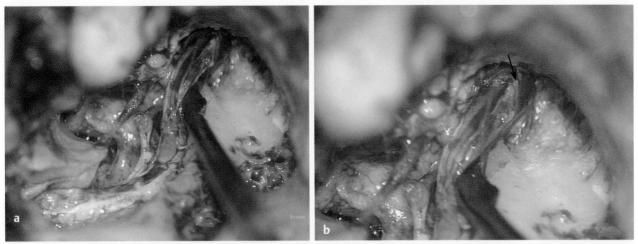

Fig. 6.31 **(a, b)** Decompressed facial nerve visualized from the second genu up to the **labyrinthine segment** (LS) but the incising of epineurial sheath is up to the geniculate ganglion only (*black arrow*).

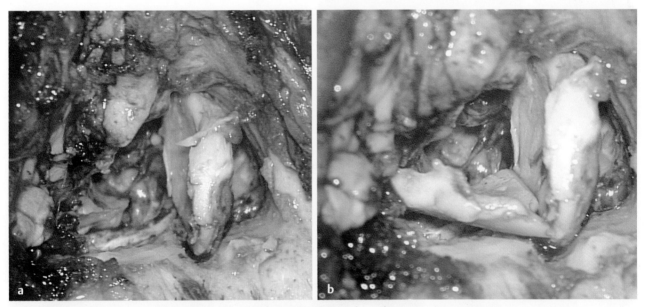

Fig. 6.32 **(a, b)** Posterosuperior canal wall reconstructed with tragal cartilage.

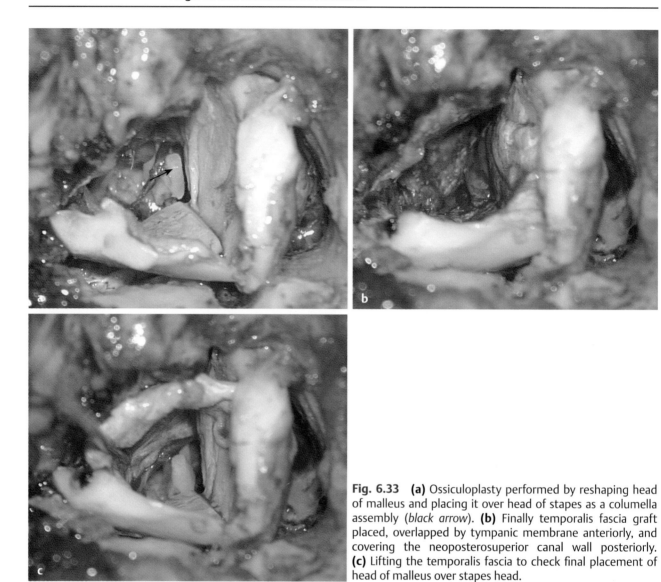

Fig. 6.33 **(a)** Ossiculoplasty performed by reshaping head of malleus and placing it over head of stapes as a columella assembly (*black arrow*). **(b)** Finally temporalis fascia graft placed, overlapped by tympanic membrane anteriorly, and covering the neoposterosuperior canal wall posteriorly. **(c)** Lifting the temporalis fascia to check final placement of head of malleus over stapes head.

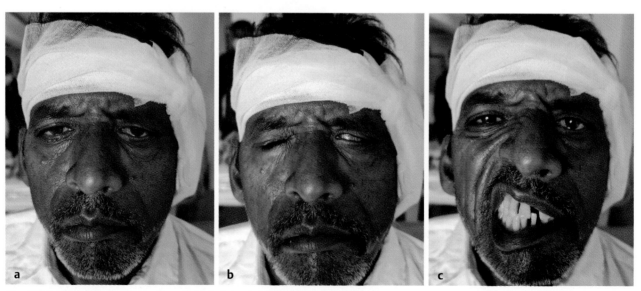

Fig. 6.34 **(a–c)** Persistence of grade VI facial palsy 24 hours post surgery.

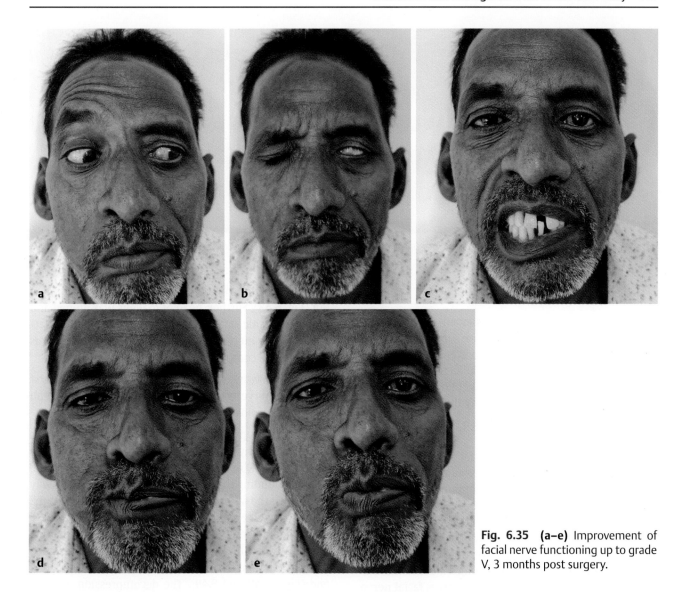

Fig. 6.35   (a–e) Improvement of facial nerve functioning up to grade V, 3 months post surgery.

Fig. 6.36   (a–d) Improvement of facial nerve function up to grade IV, 6 months post surgery.

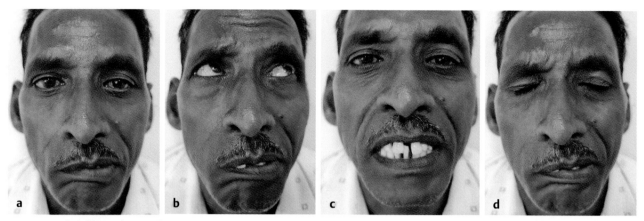

Fig. 6.37 **(a–d)** Facial nerve function recovery up to grade I with mild ocular oral synkinesis on left side 1 year post surgery.

Case 4

A 32-year-old patient came with sudden-onset grade VI facial palsy left side (**Fig. 6.38**) since 4 months. He was also suffering from essential hypertension since few years along with renal ailment. Radiological investigations like HRCT of temporal bone and MRI (**Figs. 6.39** and **6.40**) did not show any abnormality in facial nerve and no lesion was found to be affecting facial nerve. Vesicles were seen on left pinna (**Fig. 6.41**).

He was already on treatment for severe hypertension, Diabetes mallitus and kidney ailment. High dose steroids could not be given due to immunocompromised state of the patient. Low dose steroids along with treatment for kidney disease and hyperglycemia were given for 1 month. Tarsorrhaphy was performed on left side to avoid damage to cornea. No recovery in FP was observed after 1 month of medical therapy (which meant 5 months post onset of FP), so surgery to decompress facial nerve was planned.

Surgical Steps

On otomicroscopy, the tympanic membrane was found intact (**Fig. 6.42**). Through post aural approach, skin incision was made, posteroinferiorly based musculoperiosteal flap raised, skin of cartilaginous and bony EAC lifted in three-fourths of circumference, and retracted anteriorly in self-retaining mastoid retractor. Meatotomy incision was made just lateral to the bony annulus and skin lifted anteriorly. Canaloplasty was performed till tympanic annulus became visible in its total circumference.

Tympanic membrane was lifted in its posterior quadrant. Middle ear and ossicular chain were found normal. With a 2-mm diamond burr, lateral wall of epitympanum was drilled in an inside-out manner. The incus, malleus, stapes, and TS of facial nerve were visualized. After separating the incudostapedial (IS) and incudomalleolar

(IM) joint with a right angle pick, the incus was taken out (**Fig. 6.43**). Further, head of malleus was nipped and removed. Inside-out atticotomy was continued till, lateral wall of anterior, superior, and posterior attic was removed and complete attic exposed (**Fig. 6.44**).

Facial nerve was visualized in its TS up to the first genu. The nerve was found dehiscent at the first genu and anterior-most part of TS (**Fig. 6.45**).

Drilling of suprafacial and supralabyrinthine cells was started and bony chips removed from around to expose the first genu (**Fig. 6.46**). With 2-mm diamond burr, the cells surrounding the first genu and LS were drilled away along with the fallopian canal bone and exposure of the LS in 270-degree circumference was achieved (**Fig. 6.47**). As the edema and inflammation could be seen reaching up to labyrinthine portion, the LS was decompressed in its whole length and circumference upto its medial end (**Figs. 6.48** and **6.49**). The decompression of facial nerve in its TS was also achieved by drilling away the thin fallopian bone, first with the diamond burr followed by removing with a curette and tympanic membrane elevator (**Fig. 6.50**). On distal side, the decompression is achieved up to the second genu (almost 4–5 mm beyond the level of inflammation of facial nerve which in this case was up to mid part of the TS) (**Fig. 6.51**).

After decompression, the sheath of facial nerve (epineurium) was opened up with a keratome knife, from the second genu up to the first genu (**Figs. 6.51** and **6.52**).

Reconstruction of ossicular chain by placing reshaped head of malleus over head of stapes as a columella graft was performed (**Figs. 6.53** and **6.54**) and round window reflex checked. The posterosuperior canal wall reconstruction was done with the tragal cartilage graft with perichondrium on side facing outside. Finally, temporalis fascia graft was placed medial to the tympanic membrane to support the posterior part of membrane over the neoposterosuperior canal wall (**Figs. 6.55** and **6.56**).

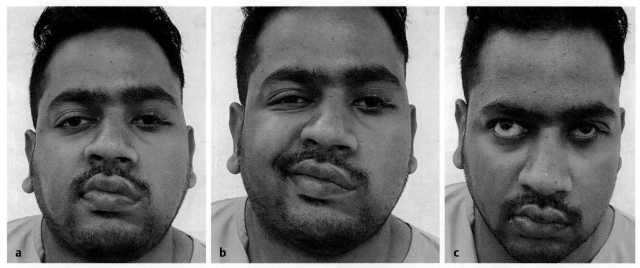

Fig. 6.38   (a–c) Grade VI facial palsy on left side. Tarsorrhaphy on the left side already performed.

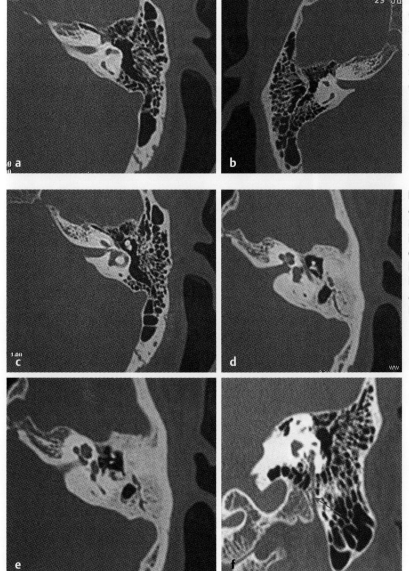

Fig. 6.39 High-resolution computed tomography (HRCT) of temporal bone images showing facial nerve in the internal acoustic meatus (IAM), labyrinthine segment (LS), and first genu: **(a)** left side **(b)** right side. Both sides showing normal course and dimensions of facial nerve.

Fig. 6.39 (c–e) HRCT of temporal bone axial cuts of left side showing facial nerve in HS, second genu, and mastoid segment (MS) in normal location and dimensions **(f)** HRCT of temporal bone coronal cut showing whole length of MS (*red arrow*). HRCT Temporal bone axial cuts showing normal dimensions and anatomy of facial nerve in its meatal part, LS, first genu a) left side b) right side.

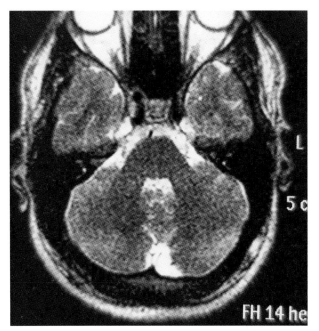

Fig. 6.40 Magnetic resonance imaging (MRI) showing normal cisternal and internal acoustic meatus (IAM) segment of facial nerve on both sides.

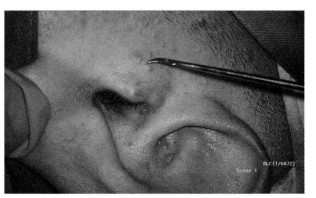

Fig. 6.41   Vesicles in left pinna.

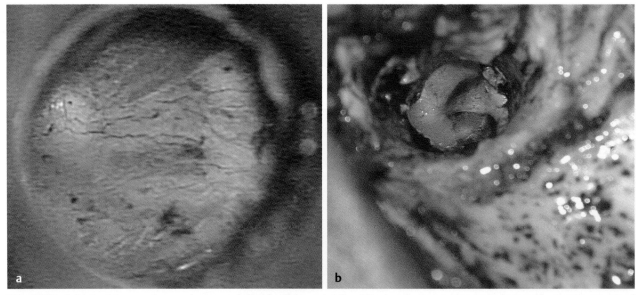

Fig. 6.42 **(a)** Intact tympanic membrane on left side, **(b)** meatal flap lifted and retracted anteriorly in self-retaining mastoid retractor.

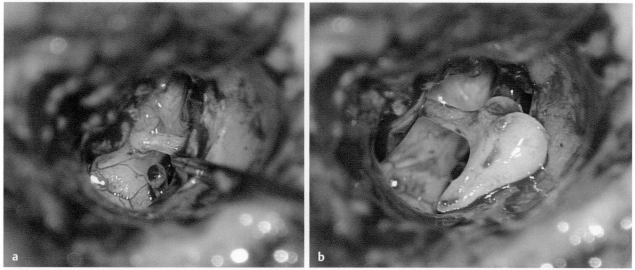

Fig. 6.43 **(a)** After lifting tympanic membrane in its posterior quadrant, incudostapedial (IS) and incudomalleolar (IM) joint disarticulated and **(b)** incus taken out.

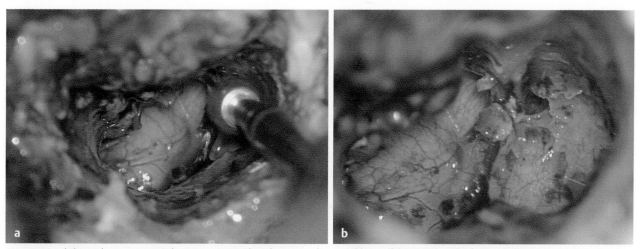

Fig. 6.44 **(a)** Inside-out mastoidectomy started with 3-mm diamond burr. **(b)** Lateral wall of attic drilled out.

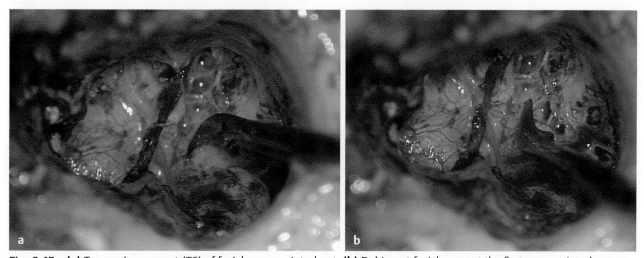

Fig. 6.45 **(a)** Tympanic segment (TS) of facial nerve pointed out. **(b)** Dehiscent facial nerve at the first genu pointed out.

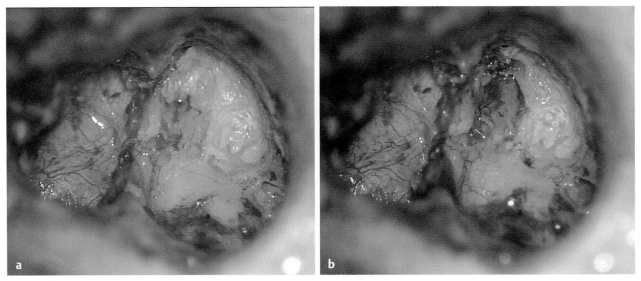

Fig. 6.46 **(a, b)** Drilling of suprafacial and supralabyrinthine cells to expose the tympanic segment (TS) and labyrinthine segment (LS) of facial nerve in progress.

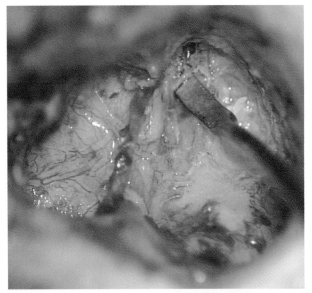

Fig. 6.47 After drilling with diamond burr, the thin shell of bone over the first genu is lifted with tympanic membrane (TM) elevator.

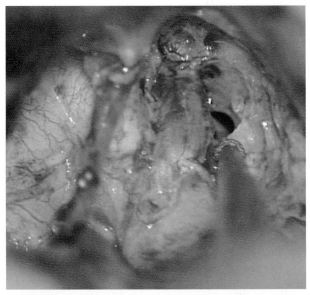

Fig. 6.48 Drilling of block of bone superior to the tympanic segment (TS) and first genu and anterior to ampulla of both lateral semicircular canal (LSC) and superior semicircular canal (SSC).

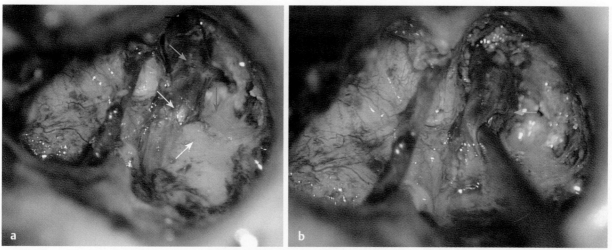

Fig. 6.49   (a) Decompression of anterior half of the tympanic segment (TS) (*yellow arrow*), first genu (*green arrow*), greater superficial petrosal nerve (GSPN) (*black arrow*), *White arrow* is lateral semicircular canal (LSC) ampulla, and orange arrow is superior semicircular canal (SSC). **(b)** Decompression of labyrinthine segment (LS) (*blue arrow*) achieved.

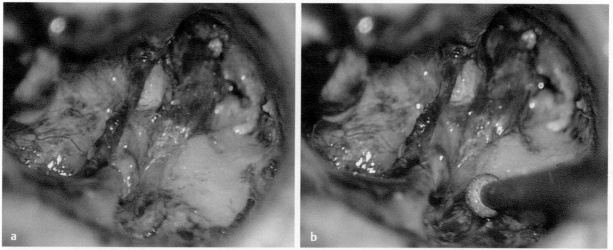

Fig. 6.50   (a, b) Decompression of 4 to 5 mm of healthy nerve beyond the level of inflammation and exposure of complete tympanic segment (TS) in progress.

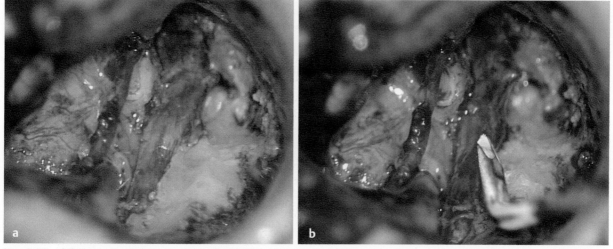

Fig. 6.51   (a) Decompression up to TS in distal direction achieved. **(b)** Incising the nerve sheath with keratome in progress.

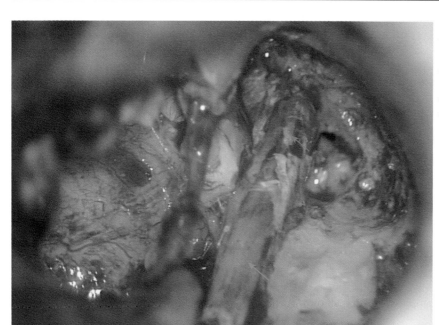

Fig. 6.52 Decompression of the tympanic segment (TS), first genu, and labyrinthine segment (LS) with incised epineurium achieved. The difference in inflamed part of facial nerve (*orange arrow*) and healthy facial nerve (*blue arrow*) can be appreciated.

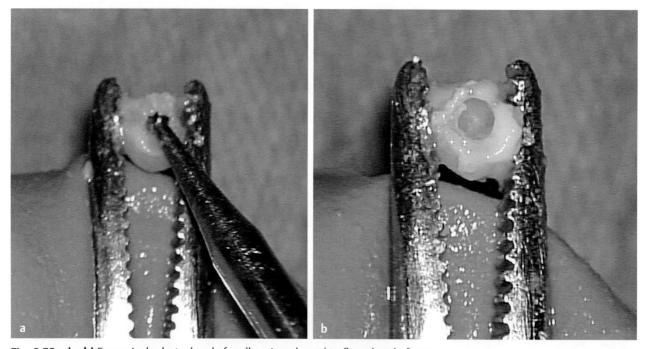

Fig. 6.53 **(a, b)** For ossiculoplasty, head of malleus is reshaped to fit on head of stapes.

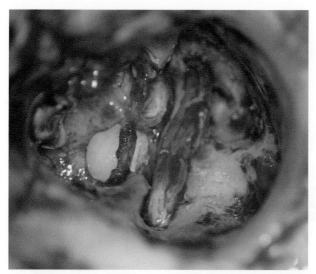

Fig. 6.54 Reshaped head of malleus on head of stapes for columella assembly.

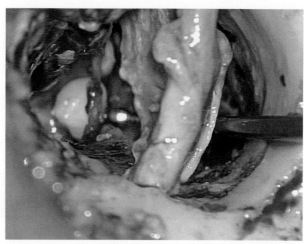

Fig. 6.55 Posterosuperior canal wall reconstruction with tragal cartilage. For patency, Few millimeters space is left medial to the cartilage graft, which is shown by passing a probe.

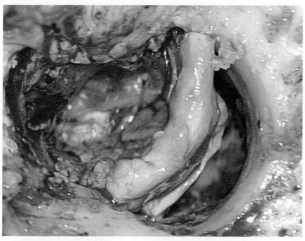

Fig. 6.56 Temporalis fascia graft in place.

Postsurgery Status

After 24 hours of surgery, the patient continued with grade VI FP on left side (**Fig. 6.57**). After 3 months of surgery, the improvement in facial nerve functioning could reach up to grade IV (**Fig. 6.58**). After 6 months of surgery, the improvement was up to grade III (**Fig. 6.59**). After 1 year of surgery, the improvement could be achieved up to grade II (**Fig. 6.60**). The patient was put on regular physiotherapy sessions to avoid formation of synkinesis.

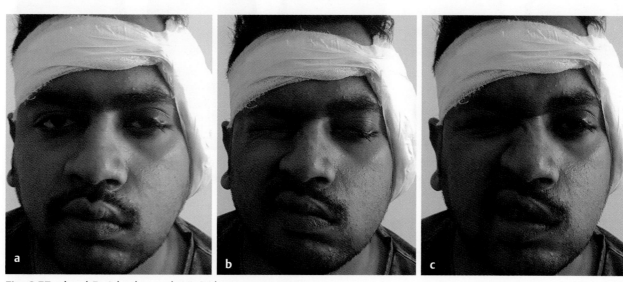

Fig. 6.57 **(a–c)** Facial palsy grade VI, 24 hours post surgery.

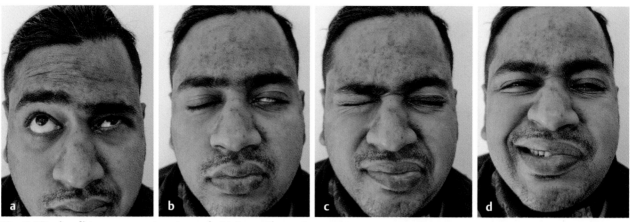

Fig. 6.58 **(a–d)** Improvement up to grade IV, 3 months post surgery.

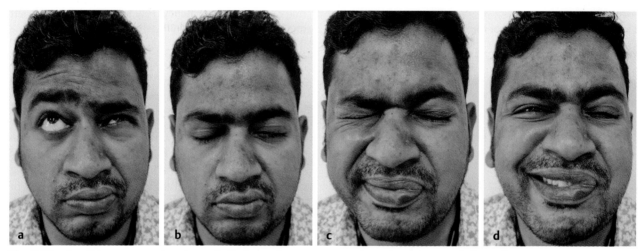

Fig. 6.59 **(a–d)** Improvement up to grade III, 6 months post surgery. Least improvement in frontal area.

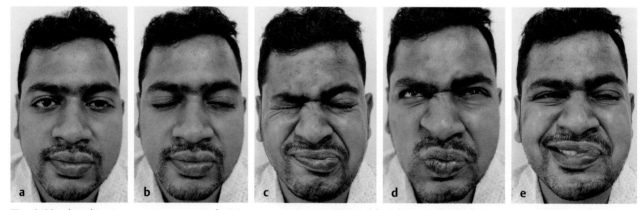

Fig. 6.60 **(a–e)** Improvement up to grade II 1 year post surgery. Normal facial tone achieved at rest. Complete eye closure on light and forceful closure. Nasolabial fold has reappeared though not complete. Smile improved but not complete.

Case 5

Transzygomatic anterior attic technique: This technique has been designed by the author along with her collegue Dr. K. P. Morwani, specifically to, deal with the lesion around labyrinthine segment and first genu area and scores over all other transtemporal techniques.

It has been described in detail in Chapter 12 titled "Management of Post-traumatic Facial Nerve Palsy."

As already explained in this chapter, in BP, pathogenesis lies mostly in the LS, so transzygomatic anterior attic technique in one of the cases of BP, which persisted for more than 5 months, has been described here.

Surgical Steps

Through post aural approach, skin with subcutaneous flap is raised, and posteroinferiorly based musculoperiosteal flap lifted. Then, after meatal flap, tympanic flap is lifted from 3 o'clock to 9 o'clock position and retracted inferiorly along with handle of malleus after cutting at the neck of malleus. Incus is taken out after disarticulating IS and IM joint.

Now the surgeon shifts and sits in front of the patient, and performs rest of the steps via transzygomatic, anterior attic technique. The drilling to reach the LS is started at the root of zygomatic process of temporal bone with a cutting burr and drilling progressed from lateral to medial side. The cells drilled on the way are zygomatic cells, supratubal cells, lateral wall of anterior and superior attic, and suprafacial and supralabyrinthine cells (**Figs. 6.61** and **6.62**).

As it is an anterior attic approach, the LS lies closest to the surgeon. So, the first segment to be decompressed is first genu and LS itself and then can be extended distally up to stylomastoid foramen according to the requirement of the case (**Figs. 6.63–6.68**).

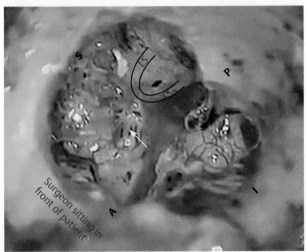

Fig. 6.61 Left ear of patient. Surgeon sitting in front of the patient and the anterior (A), posterior (P), superior (S) and inferior (I) positions are marked. Processus cochleariform (*white arrow*) and stapes (*green arrow*) are visualized. The *black curved lines* depict the location of the tympanic segment (TS), first genu, and labyrinthine segment (LS) of facial nerve.

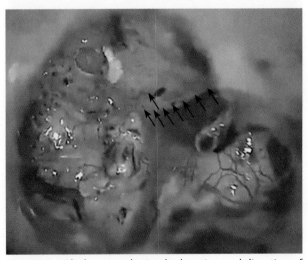

Fig. 6.62 *Black arrows* depict the location and direction of facial nerve (from TS to LS).

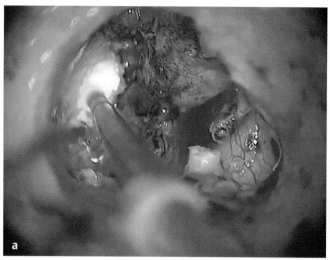 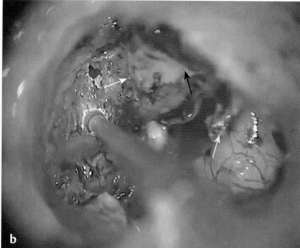

Fig. 6.63 **(a, b)** The drilling of supratubal and suprafacial cells is so easy in this technique as there are least chances of injuring the stapes (*yellow arrow*) and ampulla of the lateral semicircular canal (LSC) (*black arrow*) and superior semicircular canal (SCC) (*white arrow*), which lie much posterior and away from the area of drilling.

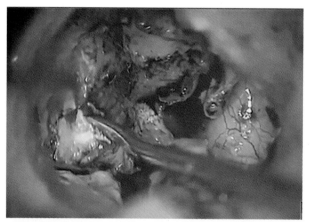 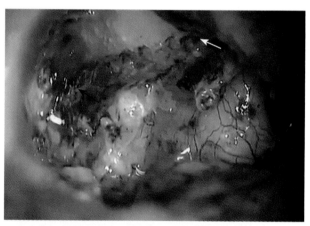

Fig. 6.64 Lifting the final thin shell of bone with a tympanic membrane (TM) elevator.

Fig. 6.65 Decompression from the first genu (*black arrow*) to the second genu (*white arrow*) visualized.

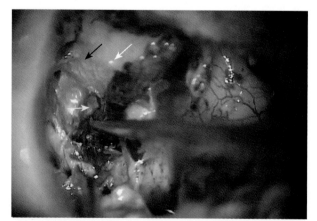 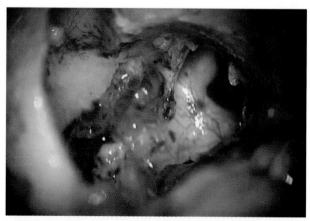

Fig. 6.66 Decompression of the labyrinthine segment (LS) visualized (*yellow arrow*). Ampulla of the superior semicircular canal (SSC) (*black arrow*) and ampulla of lateral semicircular canal (LSC) (*white arrow*) are visualized.

Fig. 6.67 Decompression with normal nerve visualized 4 to 5 mm beyond the site of inflammation on distal side (*red arrow*).

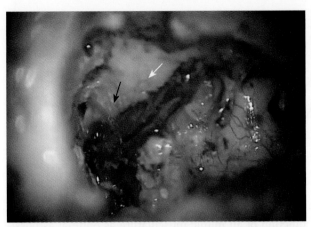

Fig. 6.68 Incision of the sheath of decompressed facial nerve performed. Ampulla of LSC is white arrow and ampulla of SSC is black arrow.

Conclusion

AFP is an emergency situation which should be managed at the earliest. The list of differential diagnosis is broad; however, the most common cause is idiopathic BP. A comprehensive history and physical examination are essential for making the right diagnosis. Management depends on the specific diagnosis; however, corticosteroids and antiviral medications are the mainstay of treatment. Most of the cases of AFP recover completely with medical management only. A small percentage of patients requires surgical management. Waiting period for self-recovery is up to 3 to 4 months and lack of recovery after 4 months should prompt further diagnostic workup and consideration for surgical management. Timely management and surgical intervention can save patient from permanent cosmetic deformity and complications like incomplete closure of eyelids leading to cornea injury, epiphora, crocodile tear syndrome (gustatolacrimal reflex), inadequate function of the mouth, nasal obstruction, dysgeusia or ageusia, dysesthesia, and sequels like synkinesis.

Bibliography

1. Teresa MO. Medical management of acute facial paralysis. Otolaryngol Clin North Am 2018;51(6): 1051–1075
2. WebMD Editorial Contributors; Best Exercises for Bell's Palsy By. Medically Reviewed by Dan Brennan; 2020 (https://www.webmd.com/brain/best-exercises-bells-palsy)
3. Karina C (Original Editor); Karina C, Bell J, Walker W, van der Stockt T, Jackson K, Knott C (Top Contributors). Neuromuscular Reeducation in Facial Palsy (https://www.physio-pedia.com/Neuromuscular_Reeducation_in_Facial_ Palsy)

7 Management of Flaccid Facial Palsy of Short and Intermediate Duration with Proximal Stump Available

■ Introduction

This chapter includes cases of complete (grade VI) facial palsy of short duration (less than 3 weeks) and intermediate duration (from 3 weeks to 2 years with viable facial mimetic musculature) and where the proximal and the distal stump of traumatized facial nerve are viable and available for repair. In such cases, the facial mimic muscles are expected to be viable and receptive to regeneration.

The short-term palsy cases include iatrogenic facial nerve palsy recognized in intraoperative or within 3 weeks of postoperative period, post-traumatic facial palsy whereas the intermediate duration facial palsy includes iatrogenic, post traumatic facial nerve palsy, any tumor in viscinity causing compression on facial nerve and tumor involving facial nerve in its different segments, with duration up to 2 years.

The management of such cases starts with a thorough history and clinical examination of ear, nose, and throat (ENT), neurological, ophthalmological, and facial nerve (the details have already been discussed in Chapter 4 "Preoperative Evaluation and Diagnosis").

The medical history should focus on the onset and characteristics of the paralysis (acute, chronic, paresis slowly worsening to paralysis), associated symptoms, and whether some recovery of facial functioning has started or not. Any medical or surgical treatment in the past should also be inquired. Assessment of the cause as well as the site of pathology also needs to be done before starting any treatment.

Management in totality includes medical and surgical treatment, and surgical intervention includes decompression, primary nerve repair, or interposition cable nerve grafting as per the requirement of the case. The surgical repair of the nerve is followed by training the patient in the postoperative period for symmetrical facial movements with good tone of functioning muscles, and avoiding complications like synkinesis, dyskinesis, hyperkinesis, or mass movements.

The aim of surgical reconstruction is to restore the function of all mimic musculature as optimal as possible, which means restoration of frontal frowning, wrinkling of forehead while lifting the eyebrow, closure of the eye, a symmetric nasolabial fold, and the ability to smile symmetrically.

Before any surgical intervention, the patient should be educated about the possible results after surgery. Both the patient and the surgeon should appreciate that once facial nerve is damaged, complete normal facial nerve functioning can never be achieved. The voluntary movement will improve dramatically, but the involuntary controls will remain deficient.

■ Selection of the Optimal Surgical Concept

Once surgical intervention is the treatment of choice, we must focus on factors deciding timing and technique of surgery in that specific situation.

As already discussed in Chapter 5, the two most important factors other than etiology which decide the timing and selection of the rehabilitation technique are duration of palsy and presence or absence of proximal stump of facial nerve for anastomosis shown in Flowchart 5.1 in Chapter 5. Using these parameters, the possible surgical techniques for short and intermediate duration flaccid facial palsy with proximal stump available can be summed up into the following different categories:

- Facial nerve decompression.
- Primary repair of facial nerve through end-to-end anastomosis.
- Facial nerve repair with interposition cable grafting.

All three techniques have already been described in detail in Chapter 3 "Facial Nerve Unit, Structure, Lesions and Repair".

These surgical techniques can be further divided depending upon the segment of facial nerve involved (intracranial, intra temporal or extra temporal segment or multiple segments) and further categorization can be done, depending upon the cause of palsy (post traumatic, infective, iatrogenic or tumor involvment). The acute infective situations have been discussed in details in chapter 6 "Management of Acute Facial Palsy".

Intracranial Facial Nerve Reconstruction

Usually it is the tumor involvment or compression to the facial nerve by tumor in viscinity or the iatrogenic trauma itself that leads to facial nerve palsy in intracranial route. The facial nerve gets traumatized (the trauma can be from simple compression or strectch trauma to complete transaction of nerve) in its intracranial route during lateral skull base surgery while removing tumor from posterior or middle cranial fossa. These lesions are usually large acoustic schwannomas, meningiomas, and other tumors. Other than that, resection of facial nerve schwannoma involving its intracranial with or without extension into its intratemporal and/or extratemporal segment can be the cause for facial palsy. Most of the times, in such situations, the proximal viable stump is available for repair of facial nerve either through direct end-to-end anastomosis or interposition graft suturing/glue. In case, the proximal stump is too small or not available for repair, motor nerve transfer or substitution (XII–VII or V–VII coaptation) becomes the procedure of choice and is discussed in Chapter 8 "Short and Intermediate Duration Flaccid Facial Palsy with Proximal Stump Unavailable."

In case the proximal stump is sufficiently long and viable, and distal segment is closeby (gap <5 mm) direct end to end anastomosis should be attempted, during primary surgery only. In case the gap between the proximal and the distal segment is more than 5 mm even after rerouting, interposition cable grafting is to be performed, for which two types of anastomoses are possible. It can be either intracranial to intracranial graft technique in case the distal stump is close by (great auricular nerve as cable graft suffices) or intracranial to extracranial graft technique in case the gap is long and distal segment is in extracranial region (long sural nerve graft preferred). Whenever we use interposition graft, there are always going to be two neurorrhaphy sites. The first category includes intradural anastomosis wherein the proximal neurorrhaphy site is at the brainstem and the distal site is in the internal auditory meatus (IAM) the second category includes transdural anastomosis, wherein the proximal site is in the cerebellopontine angle (CPA) or the IAM and the distal site is either intratemporal or extratemporal that remained after excision of the lesion (**Fig. 7.1**).

The procedure is either through combined middle fossa and transmastoid approach or posterior fossa approach. In posterior fossa approach, the central or proximal stump is identified at its origin and sutured or glued to one end of the cable graft. If the distal stump is extracranial, the cable graft is placed along the inferior aspect of posterior fossa, passed through a perforation in the dura, and is led to the distal segment which is in the extracranial part beyond the stylomastoid foramen (SMF). The second end is sutured to the distal end of the facial nerve. At least two to three sutures should be applied on each anastomotic site.

The repair can be performed in the same stage as primary surgery or in the second stage but within a month of primary surgery to avoid fibrosis and collagenization of endoneurium surrounding the facial nerve fibers.

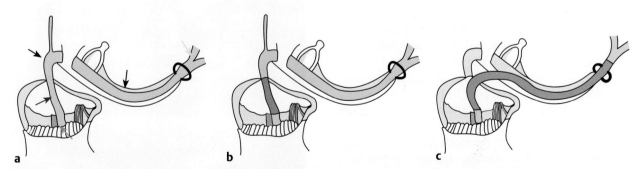

Fig. 7.1 **(a)** The diagrammatic depiction of facial nerve course from cerebellopontine angle (*green arrow*) (intracranial course) till pes ansarinus (extra temporal course). **(b)** Intracranial to intracranial graft technique in case the distal stump is close by (in internal auditory meatus). Great auricular nerve (GAN) is used as cable graft. **(c)** Intracranial to extracranial graft technique in case the distal stump is in the intratemporal or extratemporal portion (sural nerve is used as cable graft). Facial nerve is in *yellow color*, cable graft is in *orange color*, cerebellopontine angle is shown by *green arrow*, internal auditory meatus (IAM) is in *red arrow*, intratemporal is in *black arrow*, and extratemporal is in *yellow arrow*.

The procedure remains the same for facial palsy recognized in post operative period, (short or intermediate duration).

Intratemporal Facial Nerve Reconstruction

Intra temporal facial nerve decompression or repair depends upon the cause which can be:

- Post infective facial palsy (explained in details in chapters 6 and 11)
- Post traumatic facial palsy(explained in details in Chapter 12)
- Iatrogenic facial palsy(explained in details Chapter 13)
- Post tumor excision facial palsy(explained in details Chapter 17).

Post-traumatic Facial Nerve Palsy

In post-traumatic immediate complete (grade VI) facial nerve palsy cases, high-resolution computed tomography (HRCT) of temporal bone plays an important role in deciding the right management. If the injury has led to nerve compression only (CT scan shows longitudinal fracture line reaching up to fallopian canal), conservative management is the treatment of choice, followed by exploration and decompression at the site of injury, in case the facial palsy does not show any improvement within 3 months. But if the CT scan shows transverse fracture line transecting the facial nerve or bony fragment impinging into the facial nerve, the surgical repair should be performed as early as possible because delay can cause incomplete or defective recovery. When explored, most cases demonstrate damage due to impingement by bony fragment, contusion, stretch trauma, intraneural hematoma, surrounding fibrosis, or crush injury rather than complete transection. Following are certain points of consideration:

- Cases of microfracture or impacted bony fragment in dehiscent facial nerve will require decompression. Decompression will be for few millimeters on either side of the site of injury and if decompressed nerve is edematous or inflamed, decompression will be extended further till the healthy, non-edematous, and noninflamed nerve is reached in both directions. Incision of nerve sheath is performed when there is gross edema of the nerve or intraneural hematoma. Incision of sheath is avoided if there is presence of infection around.
- Cases with damage to nerve sheath or minimal thickness of nerve fibers will also require decompression of the facial nerve along with incision of nerve sheath in both directions. Exposed and decompressed nerve need to be protected by placing boomerang-shaped cartilage (**Fig. 7.2**) lateral to it, in that area, to avoid fibrosis and adhesions. There should be space between the cartilage and exposed facial nerve, so as to avoid pressure of cartilage on the nerve.
- Partial-thickness cable grafting: Cases with damage to almost 50% facial nerve fibers will require excision of damaged nerve fibers with partial-thickness nerve grafting; greater auricular nerve remains the nerve of choice. The author gives a minimum of two sutures on either side whenever it is technically possible to suture. When this is not possible, the author uses tissue glue. Suture line should be protected to avoid fibrosis and adhesion. The technique is similar as described earlier in the chapter.
- End-to-end anastomosis: Cases with either damage to more than 50% of nerve thickness or complete transection of facial nerve fibers will require end-to-end anastomosis between the proximal and distal stump of facial nerve provided after trimming the damaged fibers the gap between the two ends is less than 5 mm. If the gap is more than 5 mm, rerouting of the distal stump can be done to bring the two ends in close proximity for a tension-free end-to-end suturing.

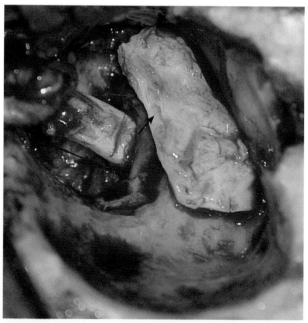

Fig. 7.2 Showing case of left ear canal wall down mastoidectomy showing ossiculoplasty performed with cartilage strip and facial nerve decompressed in TS segment. A cartilage graft placed lateral to the decompressed TS with gap of at least 5 mm in between (*arrow*).

- Full-thickness cable grafting: When there is more than 5 mm gap between the two cut ends of the facial nerve, even after rerouting, excision of damaged part of the nerve with full-thickness nerve grafting between the healthy ends of the nerve with protection of suture line is performed. One of the sensory nerves, namely, great auricular or sural nerve, is used as interposition graft between the two cut ends of the facial nerve. The donor nerve is cut on both sides. Edges of the graft should be cut sharp and bevel shaped. Length of the graft should be at least 10% longer than the defect so as to avoid tension on the suture line. It is then reversed at inset (rotating the donor nerve graft so that its distal end is sutured to the proximal end of the facial nerve). This maximizes the number of useful tubules through which the new nerve will grow and minimizes the possibility of new nerve fibers growing out ineffectively through small branches that have been cut (Dr. Henstroms reconstructive procedure protocols for nerve grafting for facial paralysis). This theory has been challenged lately.
- The ends of the injured facial nerve are identified. Both ends are cut sharply, any fibrosis, neuroma or lacerated fibers are trimmed away. The two ends of the facial nerve should be freed up for few millimeters on both sides before placing the cable graft to facilitate the suturing. If possible, place a square piece of dry gelfoam underneath the two ends for providing a stable platform. Suturing of both ends of the nerve is preferred whenever technically possible with monofilament of size 8'0 and minimal two sutures on either side with protection of suture line to avoid fibrosis and adhesions. Suturing a fresh injury can be from epineurium to epineurium and if it is an old injury with development of fibrosis at both ends, suturing is performed from perineurium to perineurium after trimming off the fibrotic tissue. For that, after excising fibrotic tissue, the epineurium at the cut end is stripped back (on both facial nerve stump and cable graft ends) for a few millimeters and perineurium and endoneurium are exposed. The two anastomotic sites are then approximated and matched without tension in a bony canal or soft tissue bed and suture applied entering through perineurium and out of endoneurium of facial nerve stump to through endoneurium and out of perineurium on the cable graft side. The same is repeated on the second anastomotic site. This helps in well-matched approximation of ends which allows maximum number of axons to pass through

the nerve graft. In technically difficult situations, use of surgical glue gives comparable results. Axons regenerate at approximately 1 mm per day after an initial period of 2 to 4 weeks of no growth through the cable graft which acts as a bridge/conduit for the nerve fibers to grow across and it takes almost 1 year for the facial nerve recovery to start showing.

Case 1: Post-traumatic, Immediate, Complete Facial Nerve Palsy (Grade VI) (Left Side)

The patient had developed immediate complete facial nerve palsy left side post head injury (**Fig. 7.3**) in a roadside accident. He was treated under neurosurgical care where he was put on ventilator for 15 days. He presented to the ENT surgeon after 3 weeks. Clinical examination showed grade VI facial palsy (House-Brackmann's scale [HBS]) on the left side.

HRCT of temporal bone showed longitudinal fracture of the left temporal bone, passing through the squamous temporal bone and attic and reaching up to fallopian canal at the first genu and labyrinthine part (**Fig. 7.4**). The temporal bone had got fragmented at the first genu area and might be the cause of facial injury in that portion of facial nerve. Pure tone audiometry showed mild conductive hearing loss with associated mild sensorineural hearing loss in high frequencies on left side.

Surgical Steps (Left Side)
Post aural incision was made. Posteroinferiorly based musculoperiosteal flap was lifted. Meatal flap was mobilized and retracted anteriorly. Fracture line was visualized running across the squamous temporal bone and the posterior canal wall (**Fig. 7.5**). Tympanic membrane (TM) was found intact (**Fig. 7.5**). Canaloplasty was performed (**Fig. 7.6**) and posterior half of the TM lifted. Ossicular chain was found intact (**Fig. 7.7a**). The incus was dislocated and removed (**Fig. 7.7b**). Head of the malleus was also excised (**Fig. 7.7c, d**). Inside-out tympano-mastoidectomy was performed to open up the anterior and superior attic area. Fibrotic and hypertrophic mucosa was found filling the attic region (**Fig. 7.8**). The fracture line was found extending to medial wall of anterior attic reaching up to the first genu (**Fig. 7.9**). After clearing the hypertrophic mucosa and fibrotic tissue, drilling of suprafacial and supratubal cells was performed with diamond burr (**Fig. 7.10**).

After clearance of all fibrotic and hypertrophic tissue, skeletonization of fallopian canal was performed. The bone over the first genu and tympanic segment (TS) was first thinned with diamond burr and then lifted with TM elevator and right-angle pick (**Fig. 7.11**). The facial nerve was found inflamed and edematous in proximal part of TS, first genu, and greater superficial petrosal nerve (GSPN) (**Fig. 7.12**). The nerve sheath is incised in the TS, first genu, and labyrinthine segment (LS) to expose the normal healthy nerve segment on both sides of the site of injury (**Figs. 7.13–7.15**).

For ossiculoplasty, the incus was reshaped and used as interposition graft between the stapes head and handle of malleus (**Fig. 7.16**). Tragal cartilage graft was reshaped and used to reconstruct the posterosuperior

canal wall (**Fig. 7.17**). Temporalis fascia graft was placed between the posterior margin of TM and posterior canal wall (**Fig. 7.18**). External canal wall skin was replaced back.

Postoperative facial nerve recovery after 1, 3, and 6 months, 1 year and 18 months are shown in **Figs. 7.19–7.23**.

Postoperative endoscopic view shows intact TM with ossiculoplasty and reconstructed posterosuperior canal wall reflecting through the membrane (**Fig. 7.24**). Postoperative pure tone audiometry (PTA) showed no further increase in air bone gap.

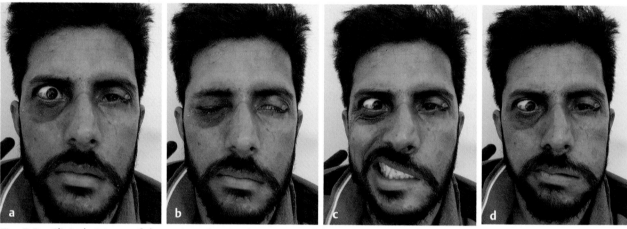

Fig. 7.3 Clinical pictures of the patient showing hematoma of the right eye (raccoon eye) and grade VI (House-Brackmann's scale [HBS]) facial nerve palsy on the left side. Temporary tarsorrhaphy has already been performed on left side by the ophthalmologist.

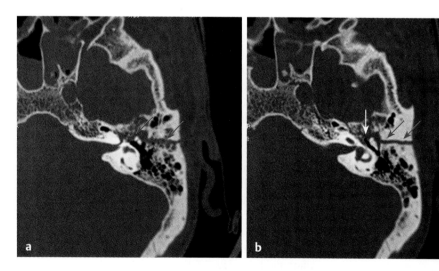

Fig. 7.4 (a, b) High-resolution computed tomography (HRCT) of temporal bone showing longitudinal fracture of the left temporal bone, passing through the squamous temporal bone, attic wall, and fallopian canal at the first genu and labyrinthine segment (LS) (*red arrows*). Fragmentation of temporal bone is visible in the first genu area (*white arrow*).

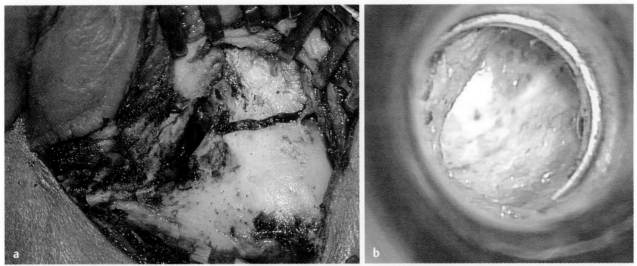

Fig. 7.5   Left ear: **(a)** After post aural incision and lifting of musculoperiosteal flap posteroinferiorly and tympanomeatal flap anteriorly, the mastoid cortex is exposed. The fracture line crossing the squamous temporal bone and posterior canal wall is visible. **(b)** Intact tympanic membrane.

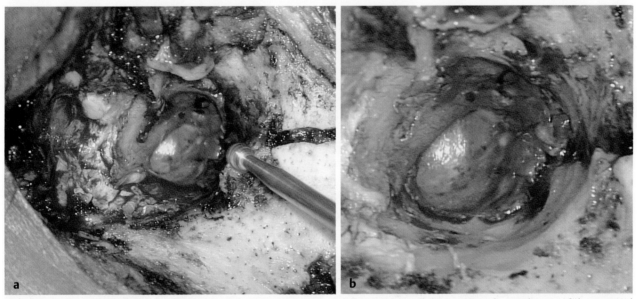

Fig. 7.6   **(a)** Canaloplasty in progress. **(b)** Tympanic membrane annulus visible in all dimensions after widening of the external auditory canal (EAC).

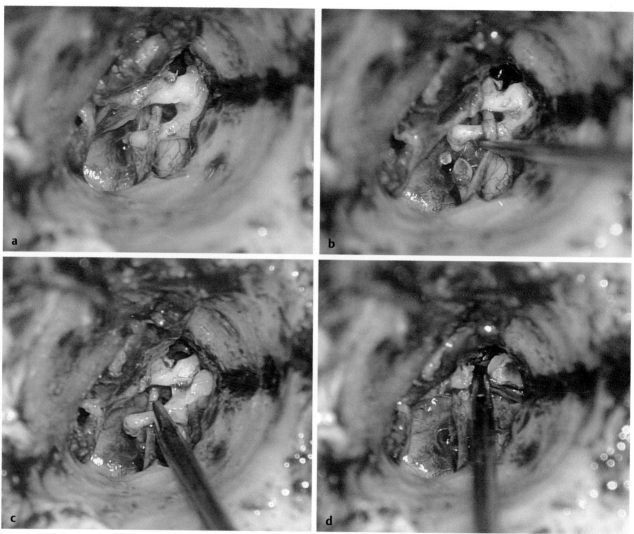

Fig. 7.7 **(a)** Tympanic membrane lifted in its posterior quadrant. Intact ossicular chain visualized. **(b)** Incus dissociated from stapes head and being lifted to be taken out. **(c)** Incus being taken out. **(d)** Head of malleus cut and removed with the help of malleus head nibbler.

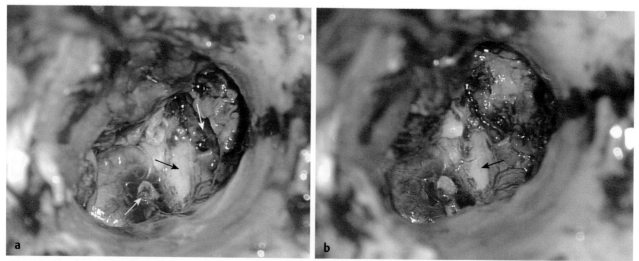

Fig. 7.8 **(a, b)** Inside-out atticotomy in process after removing incus and head of malleus. Excessive mucosal hypertrophy and fibrosis visualized in anterior and middle attic (*white arrow*). Tympanic segment (TS) of facial nerve visualized (*black arrow*). Stapes head visualized (*yellow arrow*).

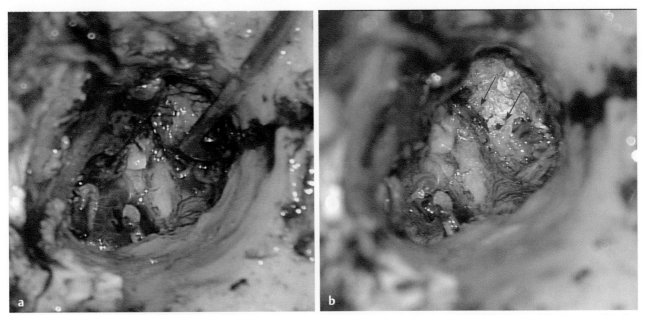

Fig. 7.9 **(a)** Flag knife showing extension of fracture line up to the medial wall of attic and reaching up to fallopian canal in the region of the first genu. **(b)** After clearance of hypertrophic mucosa, the cells in suprafacial and supratubal area to be cleared to reach the first genu and labyrinthine portion (*red arrows*).

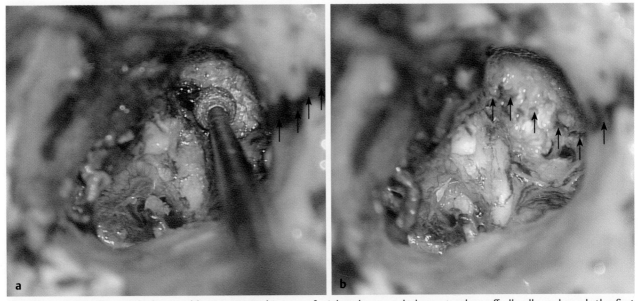

Fig. 7.10 **(a)** Drilling with diamond burr is started in suprafacial and supratubal area to clear off all cells and reach the first genu and labyrinthine segment (LS). **(b)** Drilling continued further to skeletonize the facial canal. Continuity in fracture line can be seen up to the first genu (*multiple black arrows*).

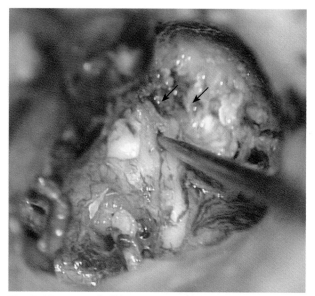

Fig. 7.11 Bony shell being removed from the first genu of the facial nerve. The extent of fracture line can be visualized reaching up to the first genu (*black arrows*).

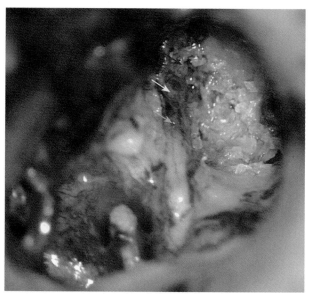

Fig. 7.12 Edema involving anterior part of the tympanic segment (TS) (*blue arrow*), first genu (*yellow arrow*), and greater superficial petrosal nerve (GSPN) (*red arrow*).

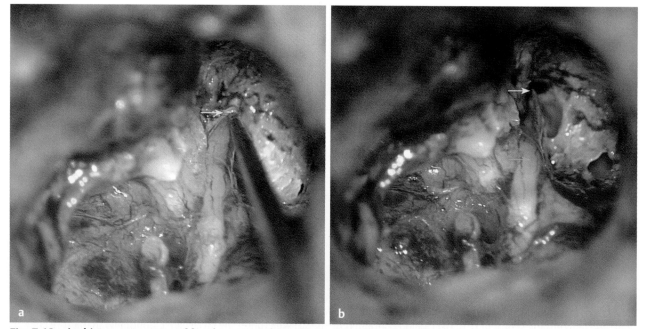

Fig. 7.13 **(a, b)** Decompression of facial nerve is achieved by incising the nerve sheath over the tympanic segment (TS) (*blue arrow*) and the first genu (*yellow arrow*). As there is no epineurium covering over labyrinthine segment (LS) no sharp instrument is to be rubbed over the LS.

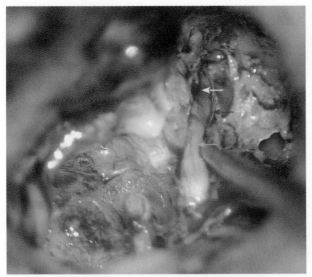

Fig. 7.14 Exposure of the labyrinthine segment (LS) in progress. Decompression of the LS, first genu, and tympanic segment (TS) achieved. The first genu (*yellow arrow*) is found inflamed and inflammation is extending to both the LS (*red arrow*) and TS (*blue arrow*) on either side.

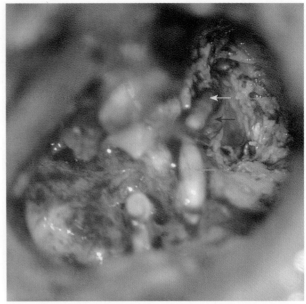

Fig. 7.15 The tympanic segment (TS) (*blue arrow*), first genu (*yellow arrow*), and labyrinthine segment (LS) (*red arrow*) are decompressed.

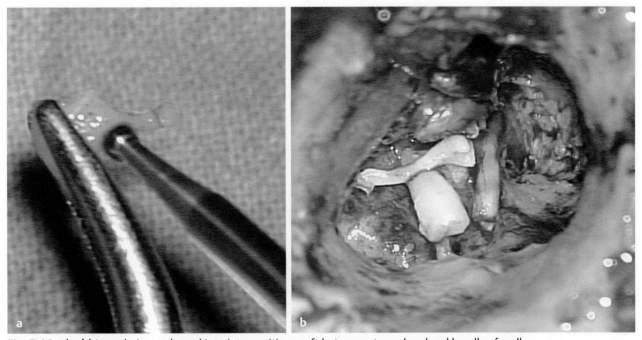

Fig. 7.16 **(a, b)** Incus being reshaped into interposition graft between stapes head and handle of malleus.

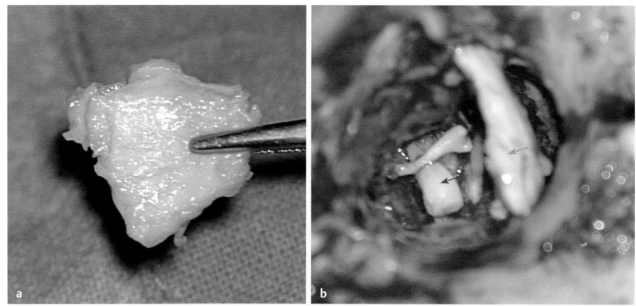

Fig. 7.17 **(a)** Tragal cartilage graft harvested. **(b)** Incus already placed between head of stapes and handle of malleus (*red arrow*). Decompressed nerve is visible. Tragal cartilage graft placed to reconstruct the posterosuperior canal wall (*blue arrow*).

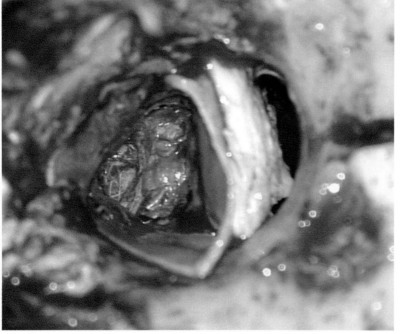

Fig. 7.18 Temporalis fascia graft placed and tympanic membrane reflected back.

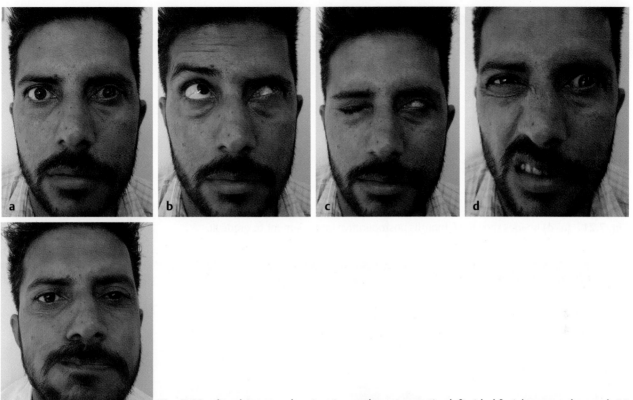

Fig. 7.19 (a–e) Images showing 1 month postoperative left sided facial nerve palsy grade VI persisting with asymmetry of the face at rest.

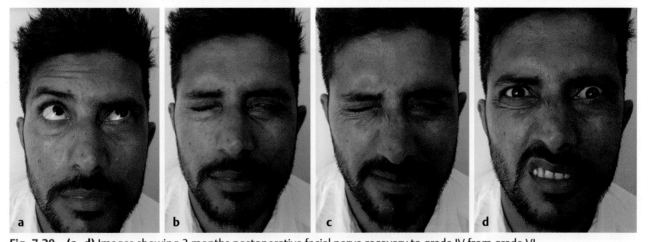

Fig. 7.20 (a–d) Images showing 3 months postoperative facial nerve recovery to grade IV from grade VI.

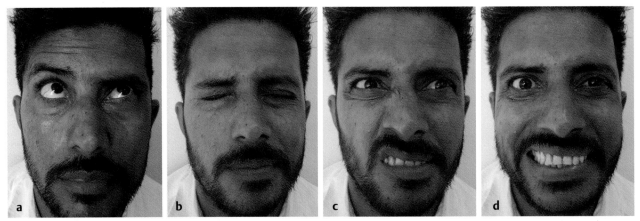

Fig. 7.21 (a–d) Images showing 6 months postoperative improvement to grade III.

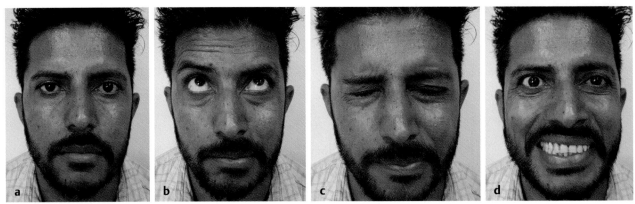

Fig. 7.22 (a–d) Images showing 1 year postoperative recovery up to grade II and complete symmetry at rest.

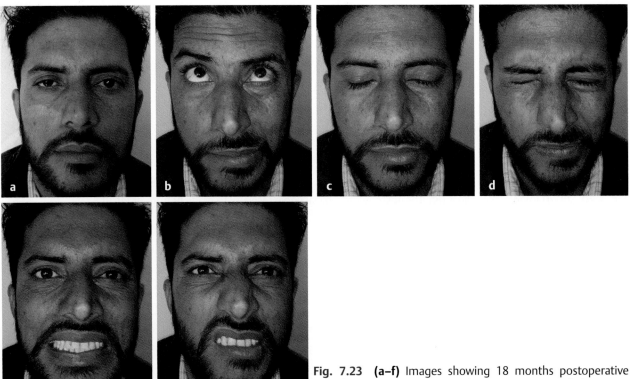

Fig. 7.23 (a–f) Images showing 18 months postoperative complete symmetry at rest and recovery up to grade I.

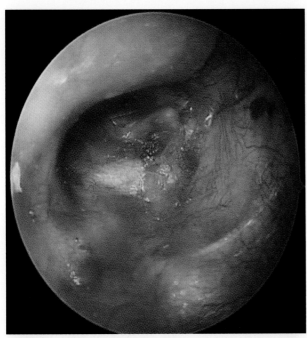

Fig. 7.24 Endoscopic image showing completely healed tympanic membrane with reconstruction of posterosuperior canal wall and ossiculoplasty chain.

Iatrogenic Facial Nerve Palsy (discussed in details in chapter 13 " Management of Iatrogenic Facial Nerve Plasy". The injury can be identified either intraoperatively or in post operative period.

Intraoperative Iatrogenic Trauma

If the surgeon is sure of facial nerve injury during surgery, end-to-end repair or repair through cable grafting in the same stage is the best treatment. In end-to-end repair, the cut ends are approximated to each other and anastomosis performed either through suturing or application of fibrin glue, but the anastomosis or coaptation should be without tension. If any stretch is felt in the suture line or the sutures cut through the perineurium, then a cable graft should be used to fill the gap. If the injury has happened in the intratemporal region, where nerve has a bed in the form of fallopian canal, the cut ends with cable graft are placed in bony canal and coapted to each other. Whereas if the injury has happened in the intracranial segment or the intratemporal region with already destroyed bony canal due to primary disease (e.g., glomus tumor), pedicled musculoperiosteal flap is used as base to give support and vascularity to the grafted facial nerve. In the initial phase of recovery, the facial nerve draws its vascularity from the surrounding tissue only.

Case 2: Intraoperative Iatrogenic Injury to Facial Nerve During a Case of Surgery for Glomus Jugulare Tumor (Left Side)

Surgical Steps (Left Side)

While performing anterior transposition of facial nerve during glomus jugulare surgery, the nerve got stretched and then disrupted in its mastoid segment (MS) (**Figs. 7.25–7.31**). Immediate intraoperative end-to-end repair of facial nerve was performed after trimming away the torn ends and releasing the nerve sufficiently on both sides (**Figs. 7.33 and 7.34**). Fallopian canal was found partially eroded by disease and the rest drilled away as part of surgical procedure. So, the pedicled musculoperiosteal flap from sternocleidomastoid muscle was placed underneath the repaired nerve for support as well as vascularization (**Fig. 7.35**). Pedicled musculoperiosteal flap from temporalis muscle was used to obliterate the mastoid cavity and cover the facial nerve from lateral side (**Fig. 7.35**).

After 2 years of surgery, the recovery of facial nerve could be reached up to grade II (HBS) (**Fig. 7.36**) which includes obvious but not disfiguring difference between the sides; there is noticeable but not severe synkinesis, eye can be completely closed with effort, and slight asymmetry at the angle of mouth has persisted.

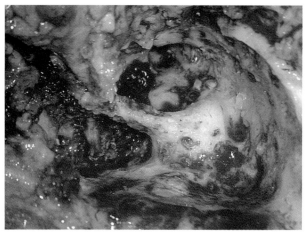

Fig. 7.25 Left ear after subtotal petrosectomy, for anterior transposition of facial nerve is in progress. Skeletonization of fallopian canal in lower half of MS already performed.

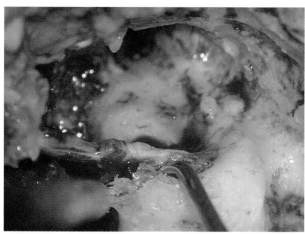

Fig. 7.26 After drilling away the facial canal bone, the facial nerve is being lifted in its MS.

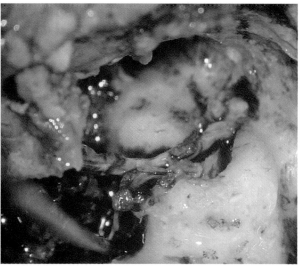

Fig. 7.27 Facial nerve lifted up to the first genu.

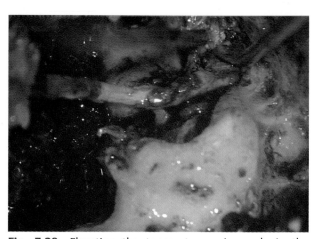

Fig. 7.28 Elevating the tensor tympani muscle in the anterior quadrant to create space to lift the nerve up to the labyrinthine segment (LS) for complete anterior transposition of the nerve.

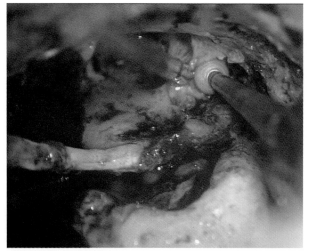

Fig. 7.29 Drilling the bone in the anterior attic area to expose the first genu.

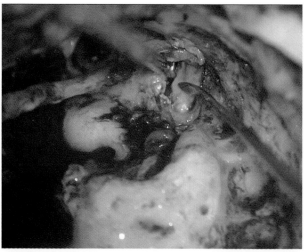

Fig. 7.30 Facial nerve lifted till the labyrinthine segment (LS).

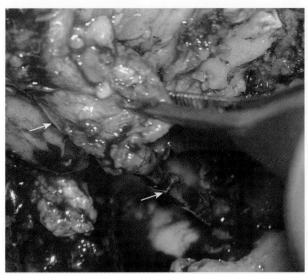

Fig. 7.31 Separating the facial nerve at stylomastoid foramen area (*white arrow*). The nerve got stretched at this point (*yellow arrow*).

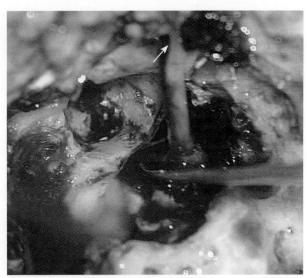

Fig. 7.32 Disruption in continuity of facial nerve at its exit from SMF can be visualized (*white arrow*)

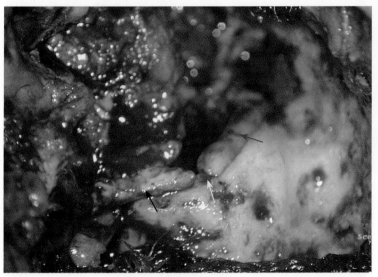

Fig. 7.33 For repair, the distal stump of the nerve is released till its bifurcation (pes ansarinus) and both proximal and distal stumps of the facial nerve are trimmed sharply and placed on bony bed approximating each other (*yellow arrow*) the proximal stump is marked red and distal stump is marked black.

Iatrogenic Grade VI Facial Nerve Palsy (Intact Facial Nerve) Recognized in Postoperative Period

Immediate, complete (grade VI) facial nerve palsy noticed within 24 hours of surgery will need surgical intervention unless the first surgeon is very sure of not damaging the nerve and has video recording of the procedure which is not showing any significant damage to the facial nerve. If review of the video recording confirms minimal handling of the facial nerve, the patient can be reassured of early recovery of the facial nerve function. Occasionally, the patient is given the choice of facial nerve decompression in such a situation to hasten the recovery and avoid negligible mismatching of fibers as the author believes that decompression will help in reducing the edema of nerve fibers and its consequences. Longer duration of recovery is noticed in cases of damage to the facial nerve sheath leading to fibrosis around facial nerve fibers. In case no video recording is available or the surgeon is not sure whether injury took place or not, the author strongly recommends re-exploration of the cases with grade VI palsy at the earliest in the presence of experienced surgeon or in an institute well versed with experience of managing various degrees of facial nerve injury.

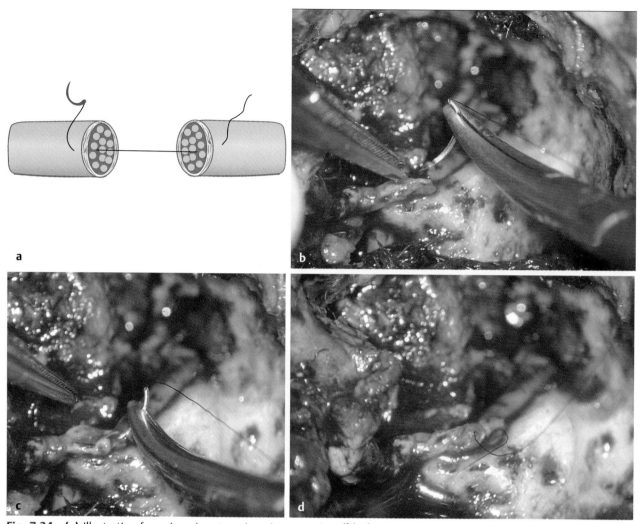

Fig. 7.34 **(a)** Illustration for epineurium to epineurium suturing. **(b)** The same step is being shown in live surgery. **(c)** The suture is being passed through epineurium of proximal stump to epineurium of distal stump. **(d)** The 8-0 monofilament nylon suture passed through both ends is tied.

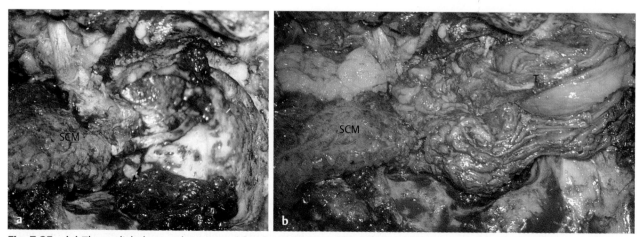

Fig. 7.35 **(a)** The pedicled musculoperiosteal flap from sternocleidomastoid muscle (SCM) is placed underneath the repaired nerve for support as well as vascularization. **(b)** Pedicled musculoperiosteal flap from temporalis muscle (T) is used to obliterate the mastoid cavity and cover the facial nerve from lateral side.

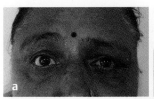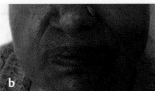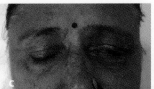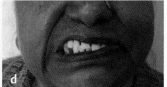

Fig. 7.36   Post surgery after 2 years **(a)** Face at rest showing normal tone but slight asymmetry on the left side. **(b)** Nasolabial fold has appeared on the left side along with mild oculo-oral synkinesis. **(c)** Eye closing on light closure. **(d)** Slight asymmetry at the angle of mouth on smiling.

The principle for surgical technique remains the same as in post-traumatic cases, although in iatrogenic cases, there are more chances of different forms of neuroma formation depending on the extent of injury and time taken to reach the surgeon.

Result again depends on the time of surgical intervention post onset of palsy and the extent of damage to the facial nerve. The best results are achieved when surgical intervention takes place within 30 days. Still excellent result can be achieved if performed within 3 months, fairly good results till 6 months, after which the recovery is incomplete or defective due to collagenization of endoneurial sheath at the cut ends. In collagenization, there starts progressive shrinkage in axon diameter over 3 months followed by gradual thickening of the collagen in the endoneurial layer surrounding the nerve fibers. Early repair promotes axons to grow into the collapsing tubules in time, thus expanding them and avoiding collagenization.

Case 3: Residual Cholesteatoma with Iatrogenic Facial Nerve Palsy (Grade VI) of 2 Months Duration (Left Side)

The patient presented with profuse foul-smelling ear discharge with complete facial palsy left side of 1 month duration which developed immediately after first ear surgery which the patient went through 1 month back. Facial palsy was assessed as grade VI according to HBS. There were no operative notes by the first surgeon explaining the details of surgery performed and any injury inflicted on the facial nerve during the first surgery. Post surgery, medical treatment in the form of steroids and antibiotics were prescribed by the first surgeon.

On his first visit, the patient was assessed for the residual ear disease and the status of facial nerve on the left side.

HRCT of temporal bone was performed which showed soft tissue shadow in the middle ear, with facial nerve found dehiscent from TS till geniculate ganglion (**Fig. 7.37a**). The intensity of soft tissue in the middle ear was different from that of the facial nerve. The second genu and MS on the distal side and the first genu and LS on the proximal side had intact bone over them. A large defect was noted in the tegmen antri with slight herniation of brain tissue (**Fig. 7.37b**).

As there were no surgical details available regarding the extent of injury to the facial nerve in the first surgery and HRCT of temporal bone did not confirm the extent of injury, the patient was put on antibiotic treatment depending upon culture sensitivity testing of the purulent discharge performed on the first visit along with local toilet of ear with vinegar (2% acetic acid) and normal saline (1:1) for few weeks. The patient was also given steroids. As facial nerve function did not improve after 1 month of conservative treatment, the patient was taken up for surgery after 2 months of the first surgery.

Preoperative pictures showed grade VI facial nerve palsy on the left side (**Fig. 7.38**).

Otomicroscopy was suggestive of plastered TM (**Fig. 7.39a**). Scar of previous surgery was visualized in post aural area (**Fig. 7.39b**).

Surgical Steps (Left Side)
After post aural incision and harvesting of temporal fascia graft, musculoperiosteal flap is mobilized posteroinferiorly, cavity skin is elevated, mobilized laterally and held in position with mastoid retractor (**Fig. 7.40**).

Inside-out drilling is started along the bony margin of cavity, bone dust harvested, and margin and part of cavity saucerized and polished (**Fig. 7.41**). Skin lying on the superior part of the cavity is mobilized toward the annulus and TM. Dehiscence of tegmen is visualized. The granulation tissue is found adherent to the dura which is mobilized and dissected from the dura and exposed dura is bipolarized (**Fig. 7.42**).

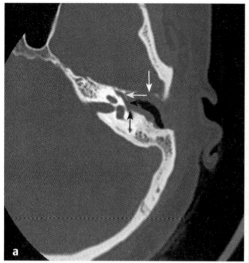
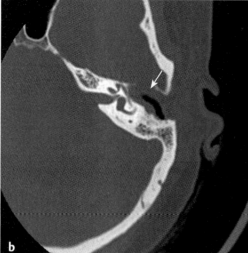

Fig. 7.37 **(a, b)** High resolution computed tomography (HRCT) temporal bone axial cuts left side showing soft tissue shadow in the middle ear with dehiscent tympanic segment (TS) of the facial nerve in its posterior part up to the second genu (*black arrow*). Bony fallopian canal is intact at the first genu area and the anterior part of TS (*yellow arrow*). Defect in tegmen antri is shown (*white arrow*).

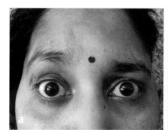
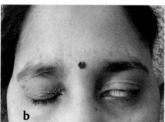
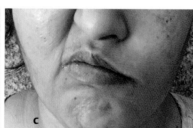
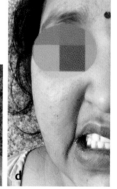

Fig. 7.38 **(a–d)** Preoperative pictures of the patient depicting grade VI facial nerve palsy (House-Brackmann's scale [HBS]) on the left side.

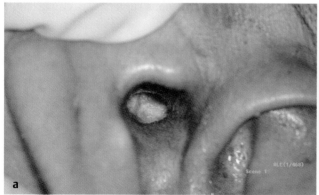
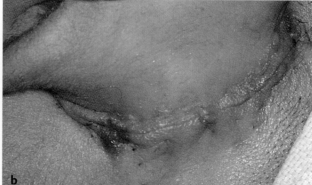

Fig. 7.39 Left ear **(a)** Plastered tympanic membrane visualized. **(b)** Scar of previous surgery in post aural area visualized.

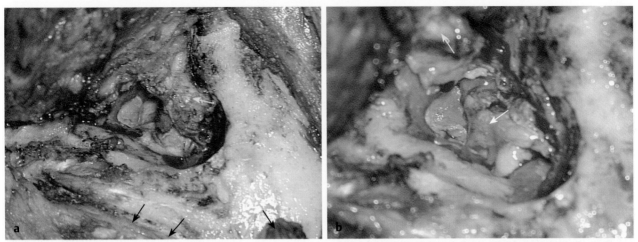

Fig. 7.40 **(a)** Musculoperiosteal incision made along the margin of the cavity and between post aural and superficial temporal muscle and mobilized posteroinferiorly (*black arrow*). Cavity skin being elevated (*yellow arrow*). **(b)** Canal skin and part of cavity skin mobilized laterally and held in mastoid retractor (*yellow arrow*). Sloughing of fascia from previous surgery is visualized (*white arrow*).

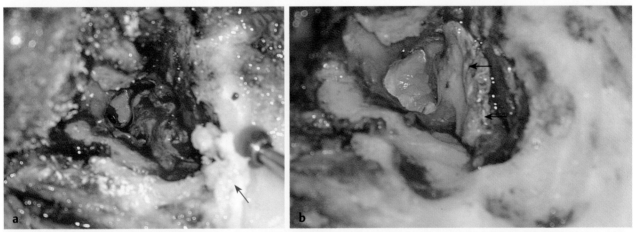

Fig. 7.41 **(a)** Drilling of the margins of the cavity of the mastoid bone started with harvesting and collection of bone dust (*red arrow*). **(b)** After drilling of the margins of the cavity, margins of false epithelium and residual cholesteatoma are reached (*black arrows*).

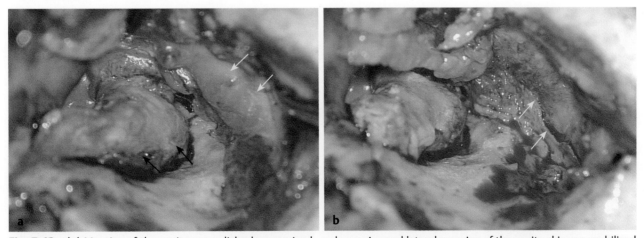

Fig. 7.42 **(a)** Margins of the cavity are polished, saucerized, and superior and lateral margins of the cavity skin are mobilized toward the annulus (*black arrows*). The false epithelium still covering the tegmen area and a big tegmen defect with herniation of brain visualized (*yellow arrows*) underneath the false epithelium. **(b)** Margins of tegmen defect visualized after clearing the granulation tissue and lifting the epithelial layer (*yellow arrows*).

The dehiscent horizontal portion of facial nerve is visualized (**Fig. 7.43**). Before starting work on the facial nerve, the granulation tissue and residual cells in mastoid cavity and antrum are cleared and the cavity polished (**Fig. 7.44**).

Plastered TM is elevated from the exposed horizontal part of the facial nerve (**Fig. 7.45**). The adhesions between the plastered TM and facial nerve are dissected sharply with scissors and sickle knife. Lowering and thinning of the facial ridge is performed with diamond burr (**Fig. 7.46a, b**). The thinning of facial ridge is performed to expose the posterior limit of the plastered TM. The plastered TM is mobilized from promontory gradually in continuity (**Fig. 7.46c**). Occasionally, the plastered TM may be elevated along with mucosa overlying the promontory (**Fig. 7.46d, e**). It is better to remove a bit

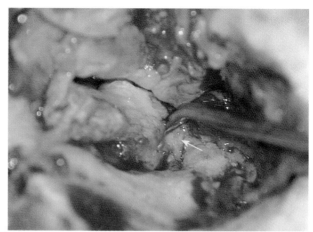

Fig. 7.43 Cavity skin along with plastered tympanic membrane (TM) mobilized further from dehiscent horizontal portion (TS) of the facial nerve (*yellow arrow*).

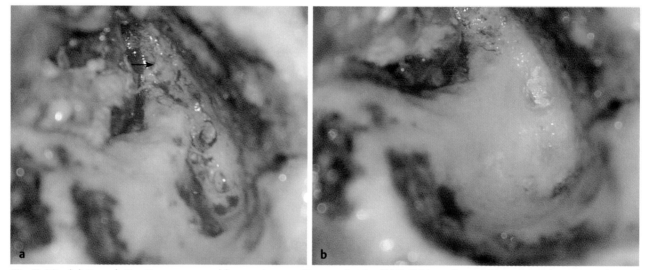

Fig. 7.44 **(a)** Granulation tissue removed from antrum, aditus, and attic. **(b)** Polishing of mastoid cavity and antrum achieved with diamond burr.

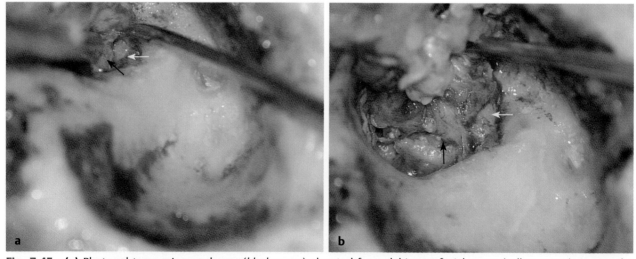

Fig. 7.45 **(a)** Plastered tympanic membrane (*black arrow*) elevated from dehiscent facial nerve (*yellow arrow*). Notice the polished cavity. **(b)** Tympanic membrane plastered over the promontory (*black arrow*) and dehiscent facial nerve (*yellow arrow*).

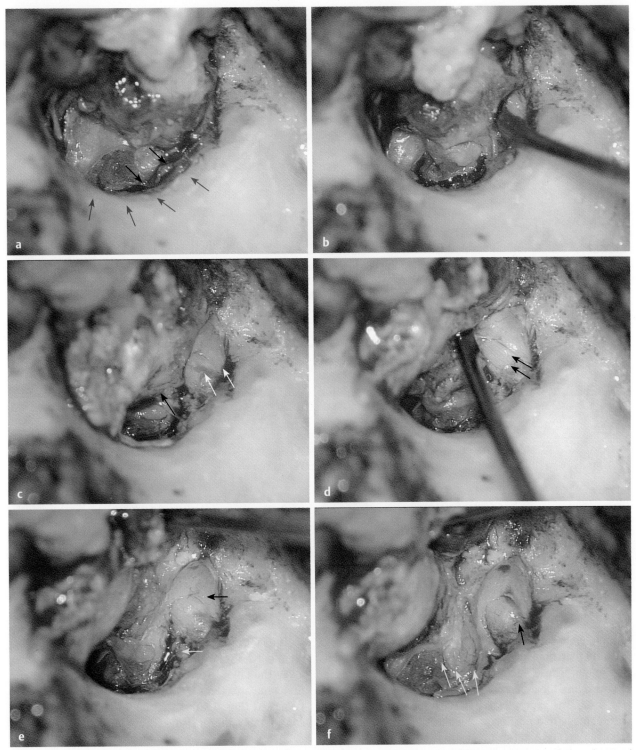

Fig. 7.46 **(a)** Lowering and thinning of the facial ridge (*red arrows*) exposes the posterior-most margin of the plastered tympanic membrane in sinus tympani (*black arrows*). **(b)** Plastered tympanic membrane is separated from the dehiscent facial nerve with sharp sickle knife. **(c)** Elevation of tympanic membrane from posteroinferior part (*black arrow*). Dehiscent facial nerve in the tympanic segment (TS) visualized (*white arrows*). **(d)** Tympanic membrane further elevated from the promontory and the exposed facial nerve. The sheath of the nerve is missing in the posterior part of the exposed nerve (*black arrows*). **(e)** TS seems to be damaged in its posterior part with edema and formation of neuroma-in-continuity (*black arrow*). The second genu area seems to be compressed or damaged (*yellow arrow*). **(f)** Notice the exposed facial nerve with small area devoid of sheath (*black arrow*). Adhesions between the tympanic membrane and promontory mucosa are visualized (*yellow arrows*). *(Continued)*

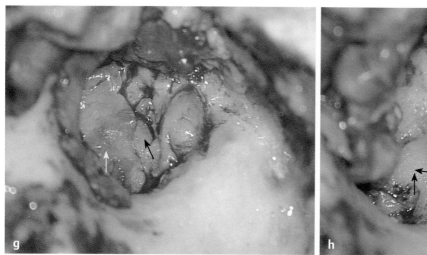
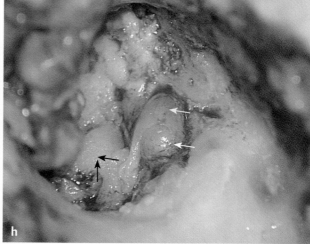

Fig. 7.46 *(Continued)* **(g)** After excising the false epithelium, the residual plastered tympanic membrane is visible in inferior part (*yellow arrow*). Promontory devoid of mucosa is also visible (*black arrow*). **(h)** Plastered tympanic membrane elevated from the promontory, dehiscent edematous facial nerve exposed (*white arrow*), and preserved facial nerve sheath (*yellow arrow*). Bare bone of promontry visualized (*black arrows*).

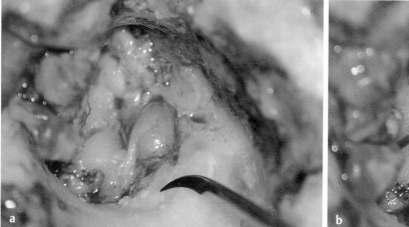
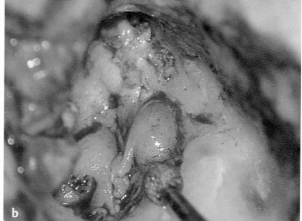

Fig. 7.47 **(a)** Bone over the second genu to be drilled for its decompression (for releasing the compressed or damaged nerve). **(b)** Bone over the second genu being drilled with diamond burr.

of middle ear (ME) mucosa with TM epithelium if both are adherent than to leave the TM epithelium behind that might cause recurrent cholesteatoma. Plastered TM overlying the dehiscent facial nerve is then elevated (**Fig. 7.47**). The exposed facial nerve is found edematous with damage to a portion of the sheath of the exposed facial nerve (**Fig. 7.46f–h**).

The facial nerve is decompressed for few millimeters on either side of exposed edematous nerve after drilling away the fallopian canal bone in the second genu and first genu area (**Figs. 7.48** and **7.49**). Facial nerve sheath is incised (**Fig. 7.50**). Facial nerve edema is regressed considerably after incising sheath (**Fig. 7.51**).

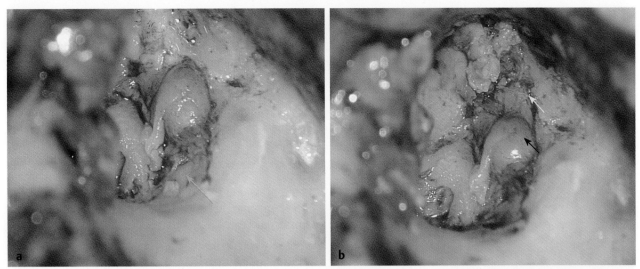

Fig. 7.48 **(a)** Facial nerve which seemed compressed or damaged at the second genu (*blue arrow*) is exposed. **(b)** Facial nerve with neuroma in continuity in TS (*black arrow*) exposed completely. Decompression of the facial nerve segment proximal to site of neuroma achieved with exposure up to first genu. About 3 to 4 mm of healthy facial nerve (*yellow arrow*) proximal to injured part (*black arrow*) has been decompressed.

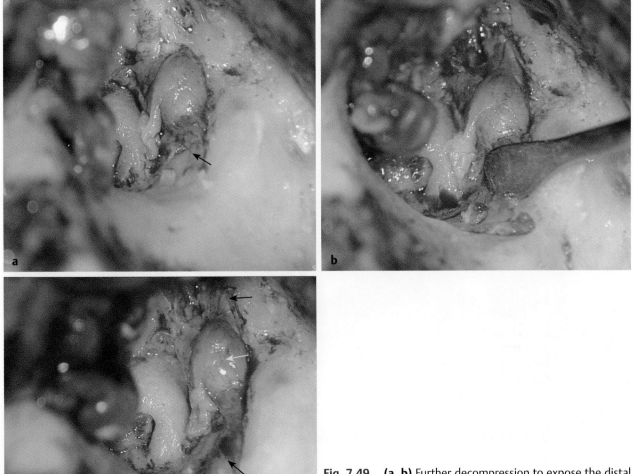

Fig. 7.49 **(a, b)** Further decompression to expose the distal compressed part of facial nerve (second genu) (*black arrow*) by removing the bony shell lateral to it is in progress. **(c)** The healthy facial nerve (*black arrows*) can be differentiated from the inflamed facial nerve with fusiform neuroma-in-continuity (*yellow arrow*) on both sides.

After incising the sheath, fibrotic band compressing on the facial nerve at the injury site is removed (**Fig. 7.51**). The neuroma at the injury site is exposed completely but not excised, as it is involving less than 30% thickness of the facial nerve (**Fig. 7.52**).

In view of large tegmen defect, repair of the defect is performed through mini middle cranial fossa approach with squamous temporal bone graft. Temporalis muscle is elevated to expose squamous part of the temporal bone. 3 × 3 × 2 cm sized craniotomy is performed (**Fig. 7.53**). The bone piece is elevated from the dura and harvested (**Fig. 7.53**). The dura is elevated around the tegmen defect in complete circumference (**Fig. 7.54**). Fascia graft bigger than the size of defect is placed over the bipolarized dura from the mastoid side and tucked inside the defect in all directions (**Fig. 7.54**). Squamous temporal bone graft placed between the fascia graft and the bony margins of the defect from the middle cranial fossa side (**Fig. 7.54**).

For ossiculoplasty, the tragal cartilage is reshaped into a boomerang-shaped cartilage graft to be used as columella graft between the foot plate and anteroinferior part of the bony annulus (**Fig. 7.55**). Another piece of cartilage is placed lateral to decompressed facial nerve in the attic to avoid adhesion and fibrosis (**Fig. 7.55**). The fascia graft is placed to reconstruct the TM and cover the mastoid cavity (**Fig. 7.56**).

Postoperative facial nerve recovery after 3 months, 6 months, and 1 year can be seen in **Figs. 7.57** and **7.58**. Improved meatal opening and widened canal are depicted in **Fig. 7.59**.

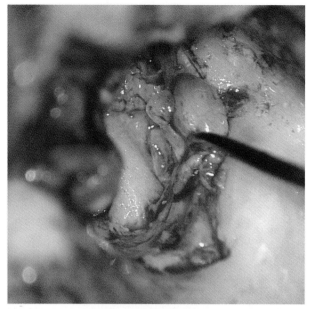

Fig. 7.50   Sheath of facial nerve being incised.

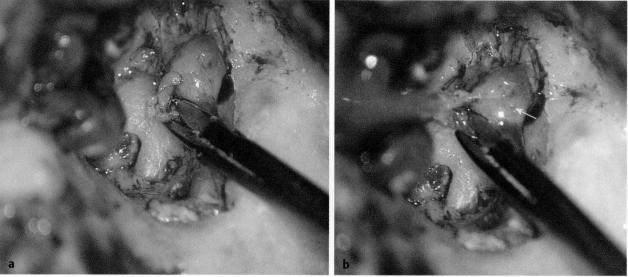

Fig. 7.51   **(a, b)** Facial nerve sheath along with fibrotic bands is being excised gently. Fusiform neuroma-in-continuity (*yellow arrow*) noticed beneath the fibrotic layer. It is involving only the partial thickness of the facial nerve, so-named fusiform neuroma, and is not excised, although the fibrotic bands around it are removed completely.

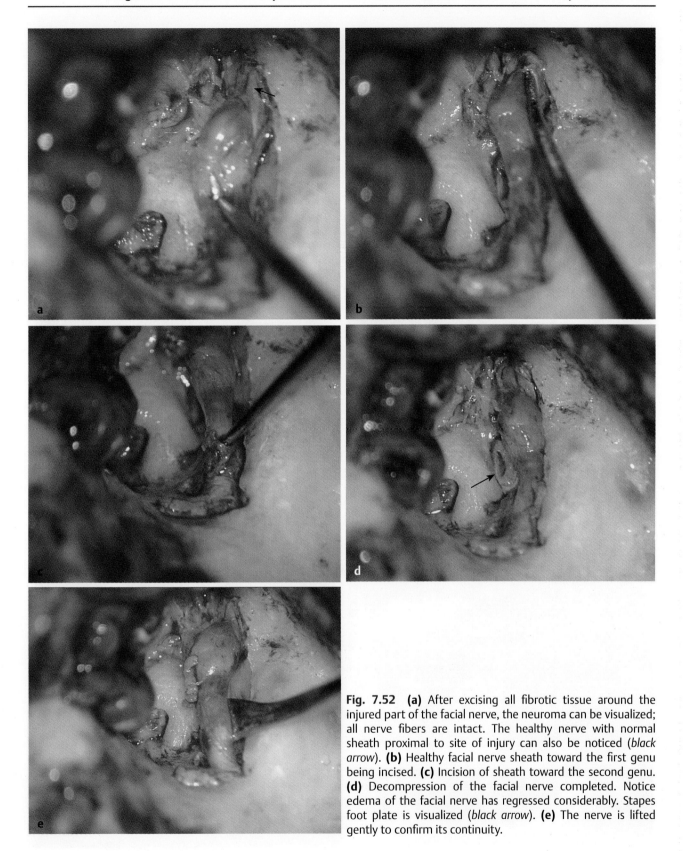

Fig. 7.52 **(a)** After excising all fibrotic tissue around the injured part of the facial nerve, the neuroma can be visualized; all nerve fibers are intact. The healthy nerve with normal sheath proximal to site of injury can also be noticed (*black arrow*). **(b)** Healthy facial nerve sheath toward the first genu being incised. **(c)** Incision of sheath toward the second genu. **(d)** Decompression of the facial nerve completed. Notice edema of the facial nerve has regressed considerably. Stapes foot plate is visualized (*black arrow*). **(e)** The nerve is lifted gently to confirm its continuity.

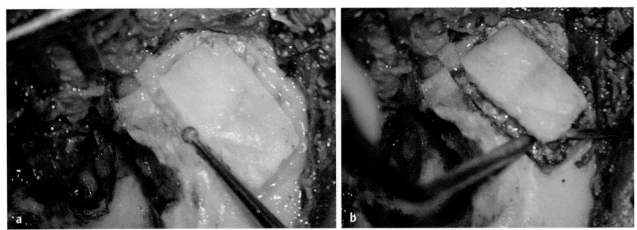

Fig. 7.53 **(a)** After marking of craniotomy in squamous temporal bone by lifting temporalis muscle, drilling is started to harvest a 3 × 2 cms sized bone graft with cutting burr and switched to diamond burr when reaching closer to the dura. **(b)** Bone piece is elevated from the dura with the help of blunt dissector.

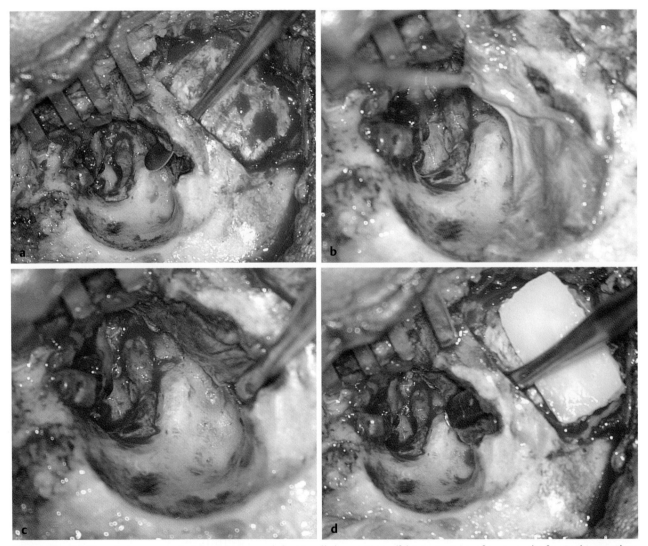

Fig. 7.54 **(a)** Dura being separated from tegmen defect in all dimensions. **(b)** Large piece of temporalis fascia, bigger than defect, being placed over the defect from the mastoid side. **(c)** Fascia being tucked beyond the defect in all directions. **(d)** The fascia is pressed with brain to create space for placing the bone graft. *(Continued)*

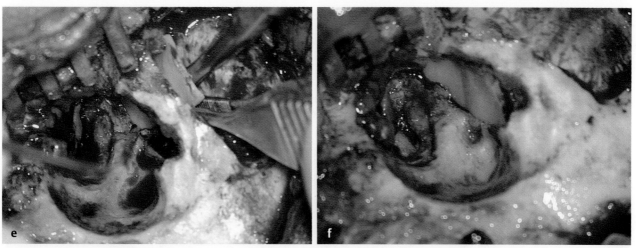

Fig. 7.54 *(Continued)* **(e)** Bone piece being placed from middle cranial fossa side between the fascia graft and tegmen bone to repair the tegmen defect. **(f)** Tegmen defect repaired with bone piece.

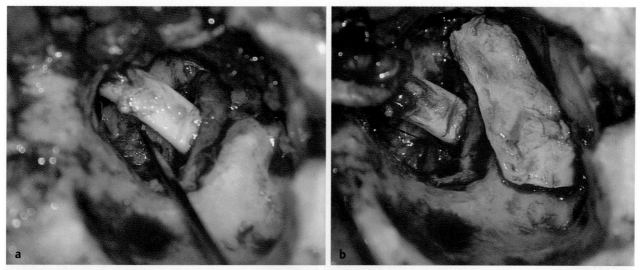

Fig. 7.55 **(a)** Boomerang-shaped cartilage placed from the foot plate to the anteroinferior bony sulcus. Instrument demonstrating the middle ear space preserved. **(b)** Piece of cartilage placed lateral to the decompressed facial nerve in the attic.

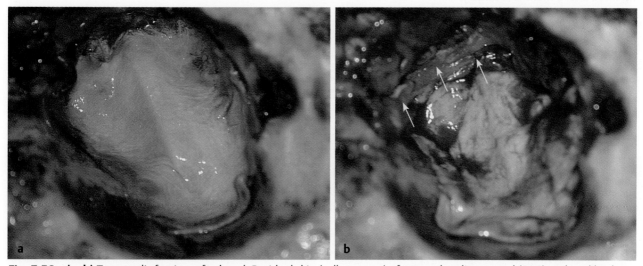

Fig. 7.56 **(a, b)** Temporalis fascia graft placed. Residual skin (*yellow arrow*) of external auditory canal (EAC) replaced back.

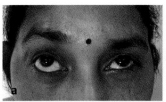 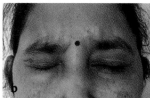 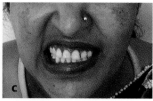 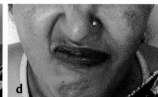

Fig. 7.57   (a–d) Left-sided facial nerve function returning to grade II after 6 months.

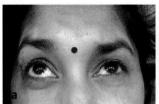 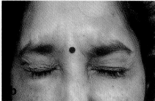 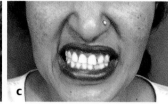 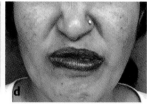

Fig. 7.58   (a–d) Recovery of the facial nerve up to grade I (House-Brackmann's scale [HBS]) 1 year post surgery. Appearance of forehead wrinkling, complete eye closure on light and forceful effort, symmetrical nasolabial fold on both sides, and lifting of the angle of mouth. Mild synkinetic movement of left oral commissure on tight eye closure (oculo-oral) and slight narrowing of palpebral fissure on lifting of the angle of mouth (oral-ocular).

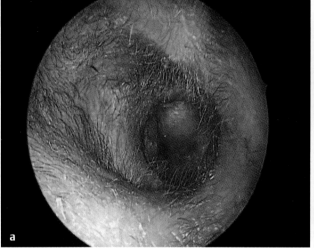 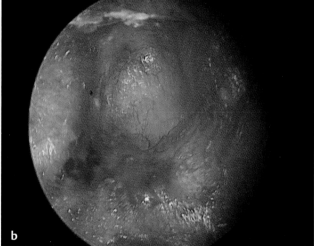

Fig. 7.59   (a, b) Adequate meatal opening, smooth circular widened canal, well-healed neotympanum, and small cavity achieved after 6 months of surgery.

Case 6: Residual Cholesteatoma with Iatrogenic Grade VI Facial Palsy (Right Ear)

The following is an interesting case where the previous surgeon while performing inside-out mastoidectomy traumatized the facial nerve in its TS on the right side.

Surgical Steps (Right Side)
While performing revision surgery, after lifting the tympanomeatal flap gently in posterior and superior quadrant, the damaged TS of the facial nerve could be visualized (**Fig. 7.60**). Almost 50% of fibers were found

transacted. After decompression on both sides of the site of injury for up to 3 to 4 mm, the extent of injury was assessed. (**Fig. 7.61**). The traumatized fibers were found lacerated which were trimmed and cut ends were approximated to each other. As there was a gap of >5 mm between the cut fibers, decision taken was to place a cable graft between the transected fibers on both sides, keeping the continuity of the rest of the fibers intact (partial-thickness grafting) (**Figs. 7.62–7.67**). Interposition cable grafting has already been explained in detail in Chapter 3 "Facial Nerve Unit, Structure, Lesions, and Repair."

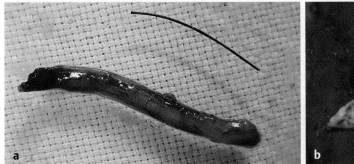 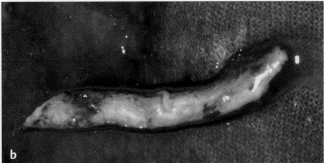

Fig. 7.60 (a, b) Great auricular nerve graft bigger than the size of gap between cut ends of facial nerve has been harvested. The edges of graft are cut sharp and bevel shaped.

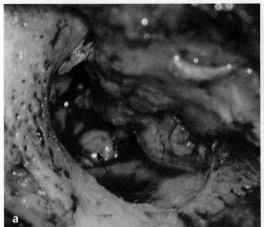 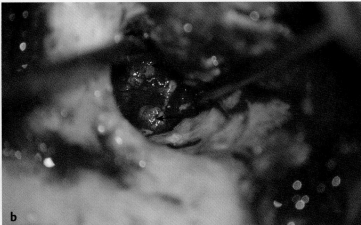

Fig. 7.61 The right ear inside out atticotomy performed. **(a)** The damaged fibers in the distal part of the tympanic segment (TS) visualized while lifting the tympanomeatal flap (*arrow*). **(b)** Partial-thickness sectioning of the facial nerve observed in the TS. The lacerated fibers of the proximal part (*black arrow*) and distal part (*black arrow*) of the TS are visible. *(Continued)*

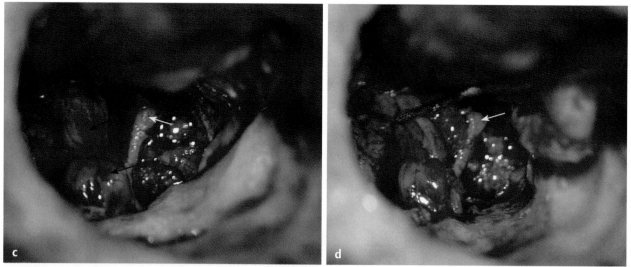

Fig. 7.61 *(Continued)* **(c)** Further lifting of the tympanomeatal flap showed absence of incus and malleus and only stapes (*yellow arrow*) was found intact. the transected fibers are approximated with each other at the site of injury (*black arrows*). **(d)** The amount of lacerated fibers to be trimmed on the proximal segment pointed out by sickle knife.

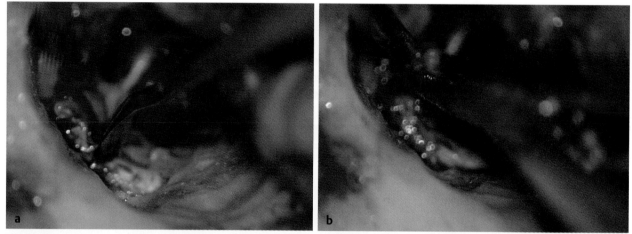

Fig. 7.62 **(a)** Amount of lacerated fibers to be trimmed in the distal segment is pointed out by the instrument. **(b)** The lacerated fibers on both sides are being excised with a sharp iris scissors.

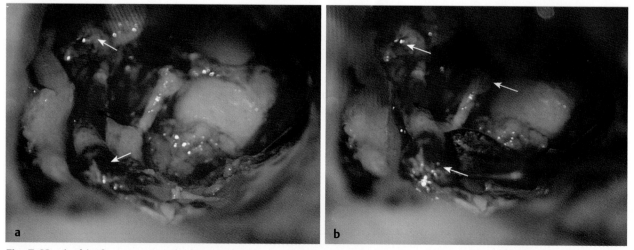

Fig. 7.63 **(a, b)** After trimming the lacerated edges, a gap of >10 mm between cut ends (*white arrows*) is noticed. The intact thickness of facial nerve in its tympanic segment is visible (*black arrow*). Stapes is shown by the *yellow arrow*.

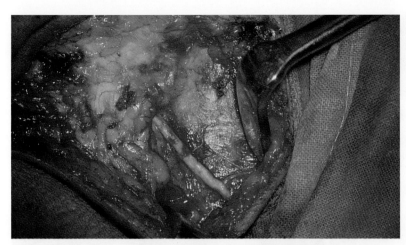

Fig. 7.64 Great auricular nerve to be harvested exposed in the neck.

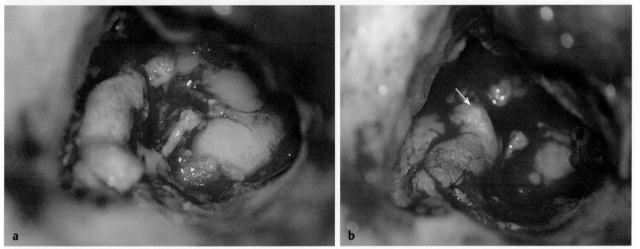

Fig. 7.65   (a, b) Cable graft placed between the two cut ends of sectioned portion of the facial nerve and anastomosed to both the stumps with sutures on distal site (*red arrow*) and glue on proximal site (*white arrow*).

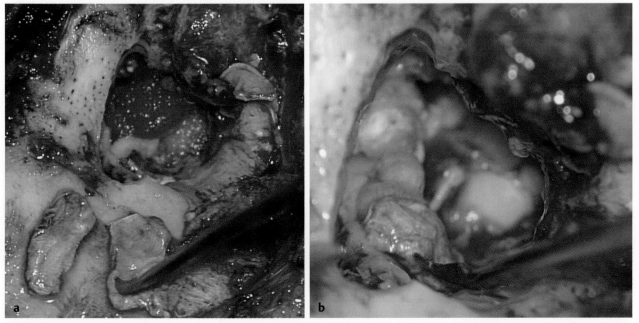

Fig. 7.66   (a) Two pieces of periosteal graft harvested. **(b)** Both anastomotic sites are covered with periosteal graft to protect and keep the anastomosis stable.

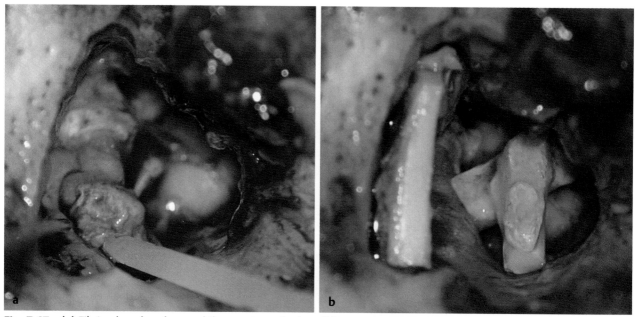

Fig. 7.67 **(a)** Fibrin glue placed around the anastomotic sites. **(b)** Reconstruction of posterosuperior canal wall is performed with tragal cartilage and ossicular chain with tragal cartilage strip between stapes head and anteroinferior bony annulus. Additional cartilage strip is placed over the first strip to create enough height to avoid adhesion with repaired facial nerve.

Case 7: Cholesteatoma with Iatrogenic Grade VI Facial Nerve Palsy (Right Side)

This is a case of iatrogenic grade VI facial nerve palsy right side of 2 months duration developed immediately after cholesteatoma surgery (**Fig. 7.68**) performed in the past. On his visit to present surgeon, the patient persisted with grade VI facial palsy along with foul smelling ear discharge and profound hearing loss on the same side.

HRCT of temporal bone was performed, which demonstrated thickening of the TM, erosion of horizontal fallopian canal, with soft tissue shadow seen in the middle ear, antrum, and mastoid cavity (**Fig. 7.69**). Erosion of the tegmen with herniation of brain in cavity is also visualized (**Fig. 7.70**).

Otomicroscopy also revealed thickened TM (**Fig. 7.71**).

Surgical Steps (Right Ear)
All the routine steps till canal wall down mastoidectomy were performed. Further, the area of tegmen defect with meningoencephlocoele was exposed (**Figs. 7.72** and **7.73**).

The tegmen was polished around the herniated brain to expose it in complete circumference (**Fig. 7.74a**). The herniated nonfunctional part of the meningoencephlocoele was then reduced with the help of bipolar cauterization (**Fig. 7.74b**). After complete reduction of herniated brain with meninges, inside-out mastoidectomy was

completed (**Fig. 7.75**). The cholesteatoma sac was mobilized from the mastoid cavity, antrum, and attic and debulked up to the TS of the facial nerve, followed by polishing of the residual cells from the medial wall of the mastoid cavity and antrum. Residual matrix was visualized over the fallopian canal around the TS and foot plate area from where it was extending toward the sinus tympani. Further thinning of the facial ridge along with drilling of pyramid was performed to exteriorize the sac completely. The sac was elevated from the foot plate. Cholesteatoma sac was cleared from the sinus tympani and foot plate area and damaged TS of the facial nerve exposed (**Fig. 7.76**). More than 80% of the fibers in the TS were found damaged (**Figs. 7.77** and **7.78**). Fallopian canal was decompressed on both sides of the damaged TS.

The damaged TS and the first genu were exposed. Injury caused by moving burr in the previous surgery had led to formation of dumbbell-shaped neuroma in the region of the TS and first genu. The neuroma involving the first genu was preceded by thin fibrotic segment of the nerve in place of the TS and it continued into a small-sized neuroma distal to it making it a dumbbell-shaped neuroma (**Fig. 7.78**). As this neuroma led to complete blockage of nerve impulse, the proximal and distal parts of neuroma were excised along with the fibrotic TS in between (**Fig. 7.79**). A few millimeters of unhealthy and fibrotic part of the nerve beyond neuroma on both sides was also excised (*orange lines* in **Fig. 7.78a**). This was followed by nerve grafting.

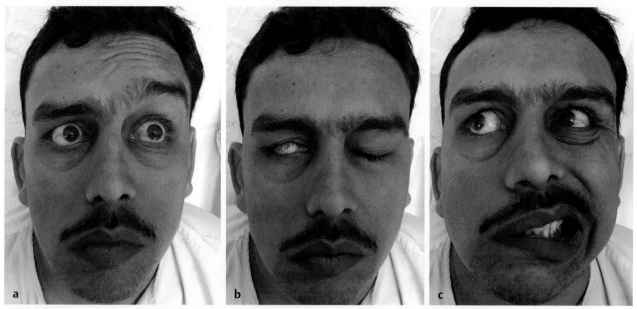

Fig. 7.68   (a–c) Preoperative images of the patient depicting grade VI facial nerve palsy on the right side.

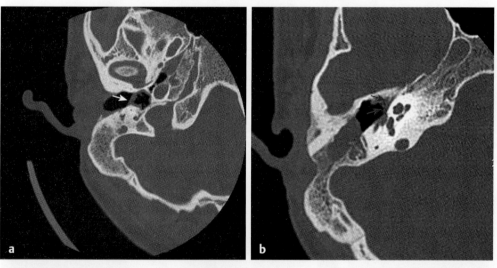

Fig. 7.69 (a) High-resolution computed tomography (HRCT) of the temporal bone axial cut right side demonstrating lateralized thickened tympanic membrane (*white arrow*). **(b)** Dehiscent tympanic segment (TS) of facial nerve (*red arrows*).

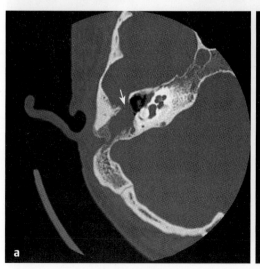

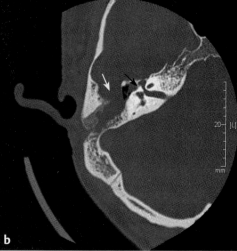

Fig. 7.70 (a) High-resolution computed tomography (HRCT) of the temporal bone axial cut right side demonstrating the tegmen defect with herniation of brain (*arrow*). **(b)** Image demonstrating soft tissue shadow just proximal to the horizontal facial nerve at the level of the first genu (*black arrows*).

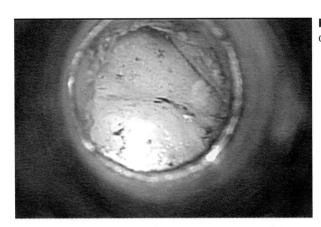

Fig. 7.71 Thickened tympanic membrane right side visualized on otomicroscopy.

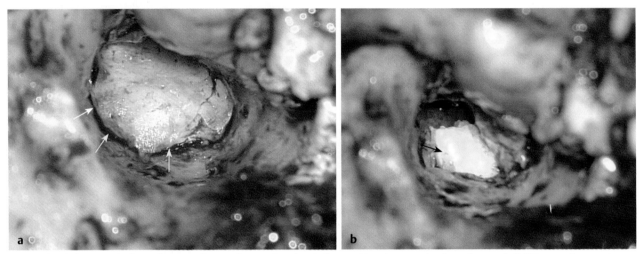

Fig. 7.72 **(a)** Intact thickened tympanic membrane visualized after performing canaloplasty (*arrows*). **(b)** Tympanic membrane elevated. Cholesteatoma sac visualized in the middle ear (*black arrow*).

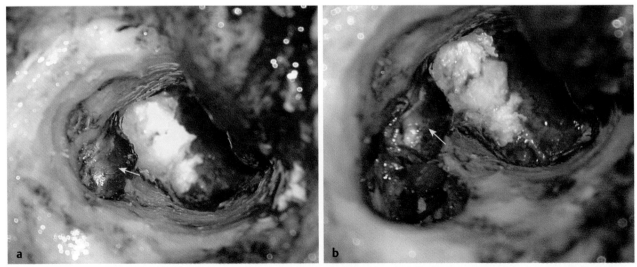

Fig. 7.73 **(a, b)** Inside-out mastoidectomy performed. Outer atticoantral wall drilled out and tegmen defect with herniation of brain visualized (*yellow arrow*).

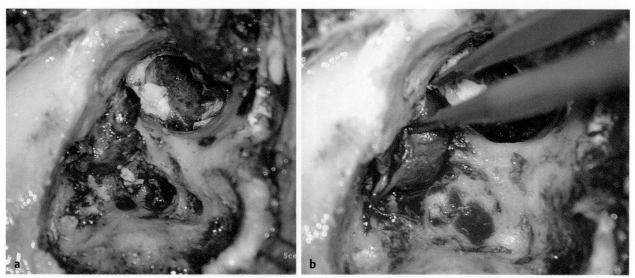

Fig. 7.74 **(a)** Exposure of the mastoid tip cells and polishing of the sinus plate. **(b)** Reduction of herniated tissue with the help of bipolar cautery.

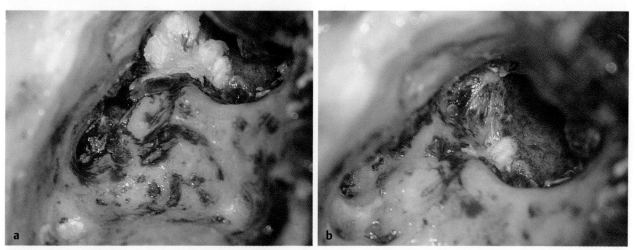

Fig. 7.75 **(a)** Complete reduction of the herniated tissue which has exposed the cholesteatoma matrix and the sac in the anterior attic extending to the mesotympanum and sinus tympani. **(b)** Cholesteatoma sac mobilized from aditus and attic and debulked. Sac left over the fallopian canal and foot plate area.

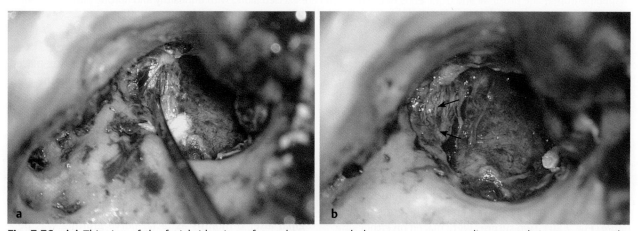

Fig. 7.76 **(a)** Thinning of the facial ridge is performed to expose cholesteatoma sac extending toward sinus tympani. The thinned out, traumatized TS pointed out with instrument. **(b)** Cholesteatoma sac cleared from the sinus tympani and foot plate area and damaged horizontal portion of the facial nerve exposed. More than 80% of the fibers in the tympanic segment (TS) found damaged (*arrows*).

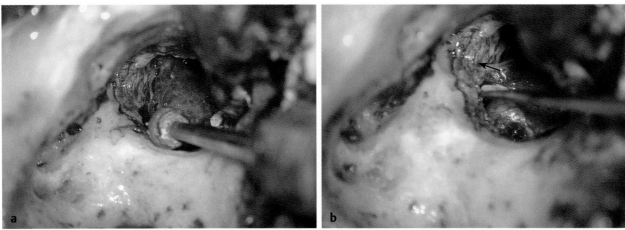

Fig. 7.77 **(a)** Decompression of the facial nerve distal to the site of injury (TS) including second genu is being performed with diamond burr. **(b)** Bone chip around the damaged horizontal portion of the facial nerve is being removed and the complete tympanic segment (TS) is exposed. Residual damaged fibers of the TS visible (*black arrow*).

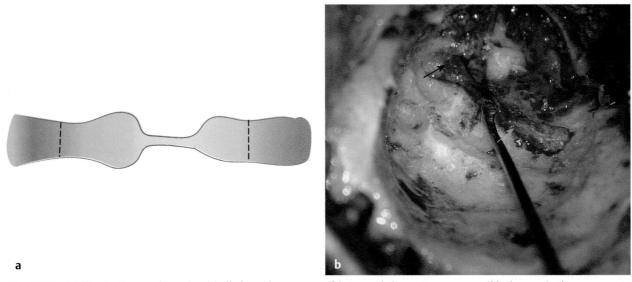

Fig. 7.78 **(a)** Illustration to show dumbbell-shaped neuroma. **(b)** Beyond the main neuroma (*black arrow*), the nerve gets changed into a thin fibrotic segment (*red arrow*) which continues into a small-sized neuroma (*blue arrow*) making it dumbbell-shaped neuroma. The proximal and distal ends of the neuroma are excised along with unhealthy and fibrotic part of the nerve beyond the neuroma on both sides (depicted by *orange lines* in the illustration) followed by nerve grafting.

The greater auricular nerve was harvested and all the loose areolar tissue around the nerve was excised. The polarity of the nerve was reversed, i.e., proximal end of the graft to be sutured to the distal end of the facial nerve and vice-versa. The edges of the graft were cut sharply in bevel shaped manner, so also the edges of the facial nerve after complete excision of dumbbell neuroma. This was done to have maximum axons for approximation (**Fig. 7.79**). 8-0 monofilament sutures were used for suturing the cut ends of the graft and the nerve (**Fig. 7.80**). Two sutures were placed on either side and the suture line was further reinforced with tissue glue (**Fig. 7.81**). Small periosteal grafts were placed to cover both the suture lines (**Fig. 7.82**).

After repair, a circular piece of cartilage was placed lateral to the grafted nerve to avoid plastering the graft to neotympanum. This avoids fibrosis and ischemia of the nerve and also displacement of cable graft. No ossiculoplasty performed as patient had profound sensorineural hearing loss post first surgery on left side.

Figs. 7.83 and **7.84** show postoperative results of the facial nerve function after 6 months and 1 year, respectively. Improvement in facial nerve palsy is marginal after 6 months as facial nerve grafting was performed. After 1 year the improvement is up to grade III which is the maximum recovery possible after facial nerve grafting.

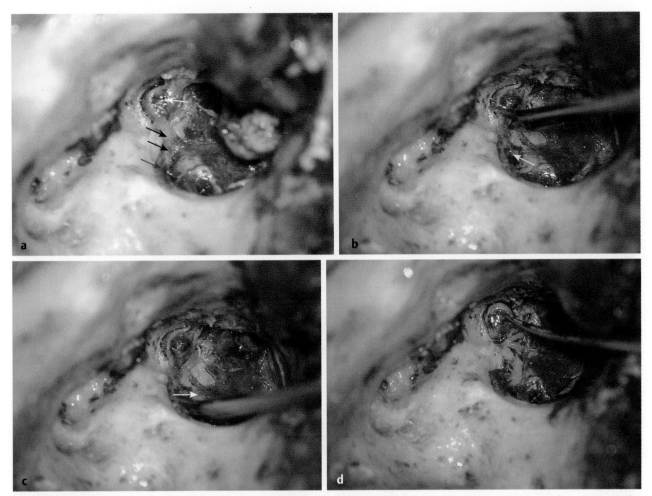

Fig. 7.79 **(a)** Thinned out facial nerve fibers of the tympanic segment (TS) (*black arrows*) with formation of neuroma at the first genu area (*white arrow*) and small neuroma in posterior part of the TS (*red arrow*) visualized. **(b)** Foot plate area (*yellow arrow*) visualized. Proximal end of the thinned out portion of the facial nerve is being cut. **(c)** The distal end of the neuroma is being cut. **(d)** Healthy distal stump of facial nerve pointed out (*white arrow*). Neuroma involving the first genu to be excised being pointed out.

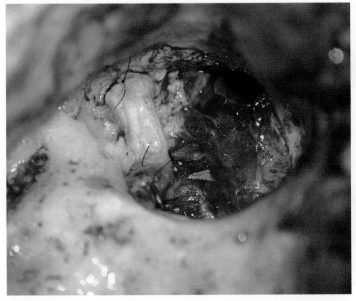

Fig. 7.80 Great auricular nerve (GAN) as interposition graft is sutured to two cut ends of the facial nerve after excision of the neuroma.

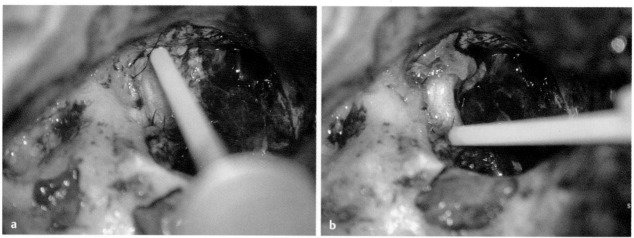

Fig. 7.81 **(a)** Suture line reinforced with tissue glue at the proximal end. **(b)** Suture line reinforced with tissue glue at the distal end. Small perichondrium pieces have been prepared to cover the proximal and the distal neurorrhaphy site.

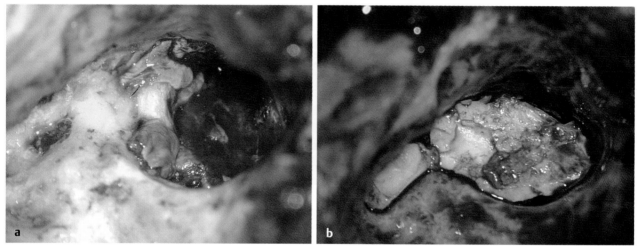

Fig. 7.82 **(a)** Both the suture lines draped with the pieces of perichondrial graft. **(b)** A big piece of tragal cartilage placed lateral to grafted facial nerve and piece of cartilage placed in the attic.

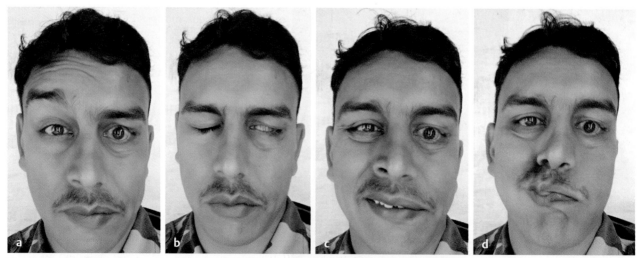

Fig. 7.83 **(a–d)** Marginal improvement in facial nerve palsy to grade V (right side) after 6 months.

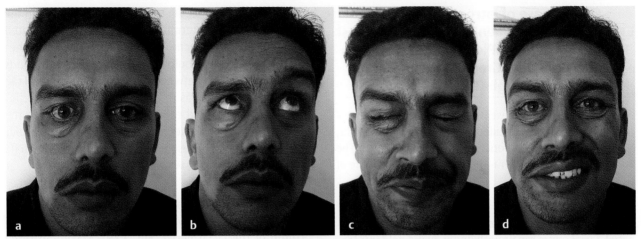

Fig. 7.84 **(a)** Face at rest looking close to normal. **(b–d)** Recovery of facial nerve function on the right side to grade III (House-Brackmann's scale [HBS]) after 1 year.

Facial Palsy Post Tumor Excision

This topic has been dealt in detail in Chapter 15 "Management of Facial Nerve Schwanomma".

Extratemporal Facial Nerve Reconstruction

In extratemporal region, the most common causes for facial nerve palsy are post-traumatic (mostly due to act of violence or accident), invasion of nerve by malignancy itself or iatrogenic trauma to facial nerve while removal of either benign or malignant tumor. Iatrogenic injury can also happen while excising the first branchial cleft cyst and sinus tracts in very young children where facial nerve is always at risk.

First branchial cleft cysts occur just in front (of) or below the ear at the angle of the jawline. The external sinus tract opening can be above the jawline (type I) or below the jawline in the upper neck above the level of the hyoid bone (type II). If there is an internal opening, it will be in the ear canal such situation of iatrogecic facial nerve injury while excising first branchial cleft sinushas been described in details in Chapter 16 " Management of Facial Nerve in Extra temporal segmen".

Close observation is required in case of post-traumatic facial palsy. If it has been blunt injury with nerve still intact, the patient is put on medical treatment, although synkinesis may result from axonotmesis. But once it becomes evident that the nerve has got traumatized or has been sacrificed, a good assessment is required to see whether the nerve is partially involved or transacted, the surgical procedure for both situations being different. In any case, the surgery should be performed as early as possible, before any fibrosis or collagenization takes place. In case the repair gets delayed, the nerve ends tend to retract, leading to a gap in between, making direct nerve suturing impossible. Also, fibrosis around retracted cut ends makes their identification from surrounding fibrosis in soft tissue almost impossible. Nerve monitoring is only useful in case the continuity in nerve is maintained. Once the nerve is completely transected, even nerve monitor would not be able to help in locating the distal stump of the nerve for reconstruction. So early repair is very important in injury involving extratemporal segment.

In case of tumor, the reconstruction of the facial nerve should be done intraoperatively at the same stage with primary surgery to get the best results.

Free the nerve in both proximal and distal direction from the site of injury for at least 3 to 4 mm so as to have a good length for repair on both sides; however, excessive exposure can devascularize the nerve.

The epineurium around the cut ends need to be separated from perineurium so as to perform suturing from perineurium to endoneurium on one side and endoneurium to perineurium on the other side using an 8-0 monofilament. Even if the suturing is performed from epineurium to epineurium, it gives equally good results provided the nerve fibers of both sides are well approximated. Not more than four sutures are to be applied. Use the least number of sutures to achieve accurate coaptation. The suture should not be under undue tension. The rule of thumb is "breakage or cut through" of 8-0 monofilament shows that the suturing is under tension. In that case we should choose to put interposition cable graft in place of direct suturing.

Accurate, tension-free anastomosis with minimal sutures performed within 1 year is the way to best results. Delayed repair can be carried out till 3 years of injury, after which the facial muscles get atrophied and primary repair of nerve may not help in facial reanimation.

Case 8: Case of Iatrogenic Injury to Extratemporal Segment of Facial Nerve Post Parotid Surgery for Pleomorphic Adenoma with Complete Grade VI Facial Palsy (Right Side)

A 58-year-old patient presented with grade VI facial palsy immediately post parotidectomy surgery (**Fig. 7.85**) with a big fistula in parotid region since 1 month. The fistula was located in infra-auricular region at the site of pes ansarinus (**Fig. 7.86**).

Surgical Plan
As it was obvious that the facial nerve had got transacted, facial nerve repair with upper eyelid gold implantion surgery was planned, as the recovery of facial nerve functioning may take as long as 3 to 5 years and immediateclosure of eye can be achieved with gold implantation in the upper eyelid.

Surgical Steps (Right Side) (Figs. 7.86–7.92)
Modified Blair's incision made exactly at the previous incision site (**Fig. 7.86**). The skin flap was lifted around the fistula. A lot of tissue necrosis and slough was found occupying the area of parotid at the pes ansarinus (the site of bifurcation of facial nerve into its terminal branches). On exploration at the previous surgical site with careful dissection, the proximal stump of the completely transacted facial nerve could be located at the

level of pes ansarinus. On further dissection through the necrotic tissue, the terminal branches could be located one by one. Two branches from upper and two branches from lower division could be located with lacerated ends (**Fig. 7.87**). The gap between the proximal stump and the terminal branches was more than 2 cm, so an interposition cable graft had to be placed and sutured to the cut ends of the facial nerve. For that the great auricular nerve with its branches (anterior and posterior, with its further two branches) was harvested (**Fig. 7.88a**).

Once the area was cleared of slough and necrotic tissue, the cable graft shifted to the site (**Fig. 7.88b**). One end of the cable graft was sutured to the main proximal stump of the facial nerve (**Fig. 7.89**). Maximum three sutures applied. Two branches of great auricular nerve sutured one by one to the cut ends of the upper division of the facial nerve, seemingly zygomatic and buccal branches (**Fig. 7.90**). After that, the third branch of GAN was sutured to the lower two branches, seemingly mandibular and cervical branches (**Fig. 7.91**). After completing the anastomosis (**Fig. 7.92**), the nerve was covered laterally by parotid tissue by suturing the cut ends of the gland.

As it is going to take a minimum of 2 to 5 years for the nerve to regenerate through the GAN graft, upper eyelid gold implant was placed in the same stage to achieve the closure of upper eyelid (**Fig. 7.93**).

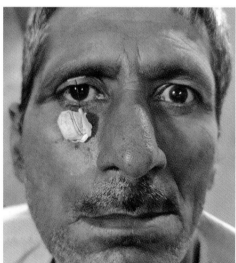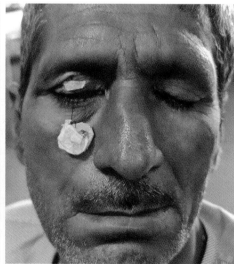

Fig. 7.85 Facial nerve palsy grade VI right side with weights hanging from upper eyelid. The weight of 2.15 mg attached to the upper eyelid was found sufficient enough for complete eye closure.

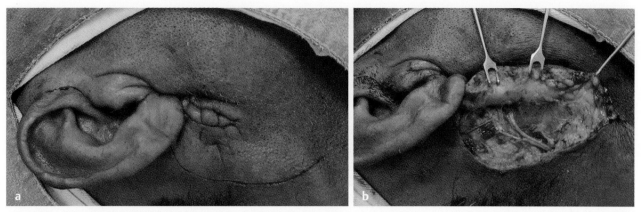

Fig. 7.86 **(a)** Incision site of previous surgery with fistula in infra-auricular region (pes ansarinus). **(b)** GAN with its branches exposed in the neck to be harvested later on.

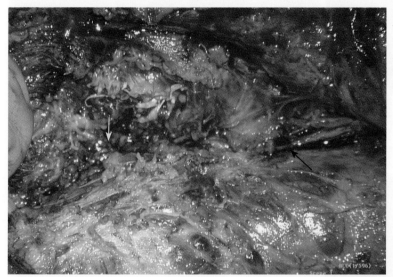

Fig. 7.87 After lifting the skin and subcutaneous flap, careful dissection could expose the proximal stump of the facial nerve (*yellow arrows*) at pes ansarinus and two branches each from upper (*green arrows*) and lower (*black arrows*) divisions of the facial nerve.

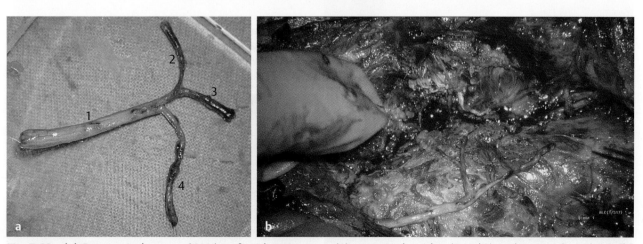

Fig. 7.88 **(a)** Great auricular nerve (GAN) graft with main stump (1), posterior branches (2 and 3), and anterior branch (4). **(b)** GAN graft placed at the operative site.

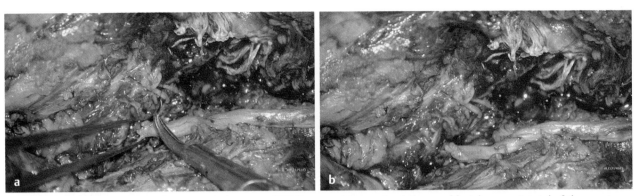

Fig. 7.89   (a, b) Main stump of great auricular nerve (GAN) sutured to proximal stump of facial nerve. A total of three sutures were applied.

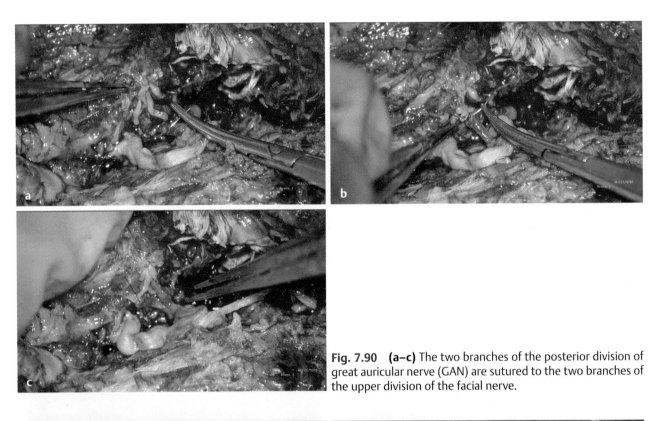

Fig. 7.90   (a–c) The two branches of the posterior division of great auricular nerve (GAN) are sutured to the two branches of the upper division of the facial nerve.

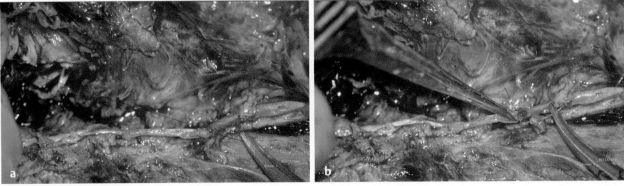

Fig. 7.91   (a, b) The anterior branch of great auricular nerve (GAN) sutured to the two branches of the lower division of the facial nerve.

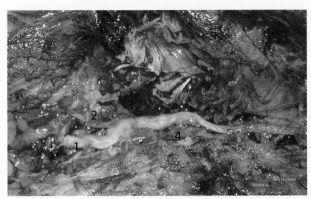

Fig. 7.92 The final anastomosis of all branches of the facial nerve to the great auricular nerve (GAN) graft. Number 1 is main trunk of GAN, number 2and 3 are 1st and 2nd posterior branches respectively, and number 4 is anterior branch of GAN.

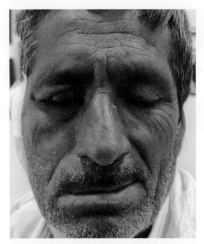

Fig. 7.93 Complete closure of right eyelid achieved after placing gold implant of weight 2.15 gm in upper eyelid.

Bibliography

1. Solares CA, Chan J, Koltai PJ. Anatomical variations of the facial nerve in first branchial cleft anomalies. Arch Otolaryngol Head Neck Surg 2003;129(3):351–355

2. Miller PD, Corcoran M, Hobsley M. Surgical excision of first cleft branchial fistulae. Br J Surg 1984;71(9): 696–697

3. Mehta RP. Surgical treatment of facial paralysis. Clin Exp Otorhinolaryngol 2009;2(1):1–5

8 Management of Flaccid Facial Palsy of Short and Intermediate Duration with Proximal Stump Unavailable

■ Introduction

This chapter details the situation and cases where the duration of facial palsy is less than 2 years, which means that the facial muscles are still viable and capable of functioning (facial mimetic muscle fibrillations positive on electromyography), but ipsilateral proximal stump of facial nerve is unavailable. As the source to transmit nerve impulses in the ipsilateral facial nerve is absent, a motor nerve transfer is required to provide the neural input. Nerve transfer uses functioning motor nerve close to the target muscles to transmit the nerve impulses to residual distal stump of facial nerve to provide source for faster and complete recovery though spontaneous activity of face cannot be achieved.

The nerve transfers are best suited for providing input to the facial nerve following removal of tumors arising from facial nerve itself like extensive facial nerve schwannomas or following surgeries on other skull base tumors like acoustic schwannomas leading to iatrogenic trauma to proximal part of facial nerve. Also, skull base lesions lying close to the facial nerve, impinging and stretching it, leading to its ischemia and nonfunctioning are the cases where proximal stump may not be available for repair and nerve transfer is the right technique provided the palsy is not of long duration.

The development of techniques for facial nerve rerouting in various lateral skull base procedures like infratemporal fossa approach (anterior transposition of facial nerve) and transcochlear approach (posterior transposition of facial nerve) have enabled performing surgeries without the need to interrupt the nerve (discussed in details in chapter 16 titled ' Management of Facial Nerve in Lateral Skull Base Surgery'). Still, surgeries performed for deep-seated tumors in lateral skull base can lead to interruption of the facial nerve and nonavailability of its proximal stump. In such cases, the repair must be performed immediately to get the best results, by means of motor nerve transfer.

Other situations can be extensive skull base osteomyelitis or tubercular mastoiditis where the disease has led to avascular necrosis of facial nerve in its intracranial and intratemporal segment, making the proximal stump of facial nerve nonviable or unavailable.

The two most commonly used motor nerves for nerve transfer are the masseter nerve (CN V) and hypoglossal nerve (CN XII).

■ Motor Nerve Transfer

Indications

- Duration of palsy is less than 2 years with facial muscles capable of useful function after reinnervation.
- Proximal, ipsilateral facial nerve stump is unavailable for grafting, which means the ipsilateral nerve impulse is absent.
- The distal stump of facial nerve is present.
- Masseter nerve (CN V) or hypoglossal nerve (CN XII) is intact.

Contraindications

- Cases of congenital absence of facial nerve (Moebius syndrome) with nonviable facial muscles.
- Tumors with multiple cranial nerve involvement like neurofibromatosis (type II).
- Malignancy in parotid gland invading the peripheral branches of facial nerve, which means the distal stump of facial nerve is nonviable.
- Concomitant, ipsilateral lower cranial nerve dysfunction (CNs IX, X, and XI) palsies.

Motor nerve transfers are relatively easy to do and require nerve regeneration mostly over a single neurorrhaphy (single anastomosis), unless there is a big gap between the ends of both functioning motor nerve and facial nerve in which case a cable graft is used as conduit between the two ends. Also, as the diameter and thickness match perfectly with the facial nerve trunk, nerve transfer provides powerful reinnervation, and good muscle tone and mobility, closest to normal.

The results are equally rewarding in a way that normal appearance and excellent tone at rest can be achieved in most of the patients. The voluntary, intentional facial movements improve dramatically, although the true spontaneous reflexive facial function or emotional expression cannot be achieved. Recovery usually starts at around 6 months and continues to improve up to 2 years, but can go as late as up to 5 years.

Outcomes are variable; best recovery is in mid face, to a lesser degree in lower part of face, and the least is in the upper face. The most probable explanation is that the axonal pathways toward forehead are fewer as compared to mid face.

The disadvantages include the loss of function of donor nerve and more chances of synkinesis or mass facial movement if donor nerve is used in full thickness. So, in cases of nerve transfer, patients are trained to reprogram how to move their face. That is, if it is facio-masseteric anastomosis, the patients in order to move their face need to think about biting down (the normal function of the masseter muscle). Similarly, if the hypoglossal nerve is used, then the patients need to think about moving their tongue in order to get facial movement. Over the time, the two actions can be dissociated with practice.

Out of the two motor nerves (CN V and CN XII) used for cooptation with distal facial nerve stump, hypoglossal nerve (CN XII) has been the preferred one since long, but lately the masseter nerve (CN V) is becoming the nerve of choice for the reasons described further in this chapter.

Facio-hypoglossal Anastomosis

Anatomy of Hypoglossal Nerve (CN XII)

It arises from brainstem as small rootlets, travels with CNs X and XI in the neck, and passes between internal jugular vein (IJV) and internal carotid artery (ICA) over carotid sheath. At the level of angle of mandible, it emerges from behind the posterior belly of digastric, runs lateral to hyoglossus muscle, medial to stylohyoid muscle and lingual nerve, and enters the tongue.

Classical End-to-End Facio-hypoglossal Anastomosis

For classical end-to-end facio-hypoglossal anastomosis, the entire thickness of hypoglossal nerve distal to ansa cervicalis is transected and anastomosed in an end-to-end manner to the main trunk of the facial nerve (**Fig. 8.1**). The disadvantage is the postsurgery paralysis and atrophy of the ipsilateral tongue due to its denervation leading to speech and swallowing impairment (Conley and Baker, 1979).

Physiotherapy

As the recovery of motor functions is taking place, the patient is trained to manipulate the tongue for facial movements. The two moments can be dissociated over a period of few months. The details of physiotherapy and adjuvant therapies have been discussed in detail

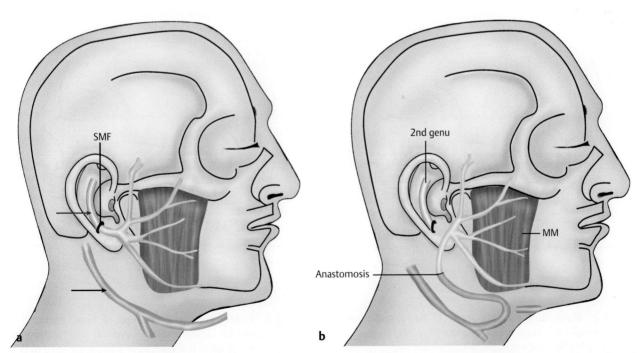

Fig. 8.1 **(a)** Illustration showing right sided facial nerve (*red arrow*) in its intra and extra temporal course and hypoglossal nerve (*black arrow*)in neck. **(b)** Illustration showing end-to-end anastomosis between full-thickness hypoglossal nerve (CN XII) stump and facial nerve (CN VII) stump. Level of stylomastoid foramen (SMF), second genu and masseter muscle (MM) have been marked.

in Chapter 10 "Management of Nerve Regeneration Complications."

The patient is also taught to suppress the normal side, while the recovery is taking place on the affected side.

The classical end-to-end hypoglossal–facial nerve anastomosis using the entire proximal hypoglossal nerve is now being replaced with hemi end-to-end facio-hypoglossal–jump nerve anastomosis.

Hemi End-to-End Facio-hypoglossal–Jump Nerve Anastomosis

This technique is an improvisation on the classical technique designed to preserve the functioning of hypoglossal nerve. It involves partial sectioning of hypoglossal nerve rather than complete transection, thus avoiding tongue atrophy. An end-to-side anastomosis is performed between the partially sectioned surface of hypoglossal nerve and cable graft which acts as a jump graft and sutured on the other side with distal stump of facial nerve in an end-to-end manner (**Fig. 8.2**). Hyperkinesia, often seen after the classical technique, is avoided in this technique because less nerve fibers regenerate to the periphery. The hypoglossal nerve is incised partially in its approximately 30% thickness. A needle can be passed through the nerve at 30% thickness to avoid incising more than that. The nerve opens up in a wedge-shape

manner making it possible to house the graft on the proximal surface of the wedge for the end-to-side nerve anastomosis.

The advantage over classical end-to-end anastomosis is that functioning of ipsilateral hypoglossal nerve can be preserved. The disadvantage remains that the nerve fibers have to grow through the whole length of cable graft, so the recovery takes a longer time, and due to two anastomotic or neurorrhaphy sites, recovery may not be up to grade I (maximum improvement expected is up to grade II or III (HBS)).

As it is not possible to approximate intact hypoglossal nerve and facial nerve stump without using interposition cable graft, a further modification to this technique is hemi end-to-end facio-hypoglossal anastomosis.

Hemi End-to-End Facio-hypoglossal Anastomosis

To avoid the use of cable graft, extra length of facial nerve is attained by mobilizing the mastoid segment (MS) of the facial nerve as far as the second genu, and transecting it there rather than at its exit at stylomastoid foramen (SMF). In this way, a much longer distal stump of the facial nerve is created which can now be directly sutured to partial-thickness cut surface of the hypoglossal nerve in an end-to-side anastomosis, without using any cable graft in between (**Fig. 8.3**). The length of

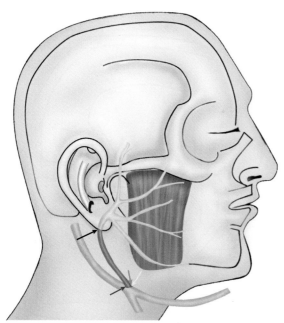

Fig. 8.2 Illustration showing steps of hemi end-to-end facio-hypoglossal jump graft anastomosis technique. 'V' shaped cut in 30% thickness of CN XII is visible (*red arrow*). CN VII sectioned at its exit from SM foramen. Illustration showing great auricular nerve (GAN) free cable graft being used for end to side anastomosis with CN XII (*green arow*) and end to end anastomosis with CN VII (*black arrow*).

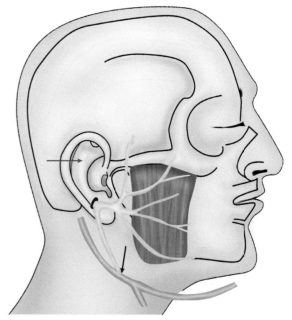

Fig. 8.3 Illustration showing steps of hemi end-to-end facio-hypoglossal anastomosis. Level of transection of CN VII at second genu is shown by red arrow and end to side anastomosis between CN VII and CN XII without the use of interposition graft is shown by *black arrow*.

the mastoid part of facial nerve is approximately 15 to 18 mm and length from its exit at SMF to its bifurcation is around 16 to 20 mm, so total length attained becomes around 35 mm. The length of hypoglossal nerve from close to IJV to its turn toward tongue is around 31.6 mm. So, the length which could have been attained by rotating full-thickness hypoglossal nerve has been compensated by the longer distal stump of facial nerve transacted at the second genu. The use of interposition graft is thus avoided, and nerve fibers regenerate through one neurorrhaphy site only, making it easy for the nerve to regenerate faster and up to grade I (HBS).

Procedure

Steps involved in hemi end-to-end facio-hypoglossal anastomosis are:

- Additional cortical mastoidectomy is performed.
- Facial nerve is followed proximally from the SMF and traced up to the second genu.
- Complete transection of facial nerve at the second genu, and distal stump released till its bifurcation in parotid gland.

This procedure may not be possible in facial nerve tumors like schwannoma where the mastoid segment is involved by tumor till its exit at SMF and has already been excised.

Cases

Classical Facio-hypoglossal End-to-End Anastomosis

Steps involved in classical facio-hypoglossal end-to-end anastomosis are:

- Just after its exit from SMF, the facial nerve is exposed and then mobilized by dissecting and freeing it from the parotid tissue till its bifurcation (pes ansarinus). This step is performed to create maximum length of facial nerve for coaptation.
- The facial nerve is then transected close to its exit at the SMF.
- The horizontal portion of the hypoglossal nerve is identified just inferior to the posterior belly of the digastric and the greater cornu of the hyoid bone.
- The hypoglossal nerve is further exposed posteriorly by dividing the lingual veins.
- The sternomastoid branch of the occipital artery is identified and divided to further free up the vertical portion of the hypoglossal nerve up to the anterior aspect of the IJV.
- The hypoglossal nerve is exposed anteriorly, pulled back a bit, and divided toward its distal-most part to secure an adequate length of nerve.
- Further length of hypoglossal nerve can be achieved by releasing and bringing it up from under the posterior belly of digastric muscle.

- The cut end of hypoglossal nerve is approximated to the distal facial nerve stump over a bed of underlying muscles.
- End-to-end suturing of hypoglossal and facial nerves is achieved with 8-0 monofilament nylon. At least three sutures need to be placed to secure anastomosis. Always perform a tension-free suturing to have the optimal results.

Case 1: Skull Base Osteomyelitis with Facial Palsy Grade VI (Left Side)

A 57-year-old patient presented with excruciating pain in chronically discharging left ear for 3 months along with progressively increasing facial palsy left side (presently grade VI HBS) since 2 months. She was a known case of diabetes and on antidiabetic treatment since long. She had already taken treatment in the form of antibiotics based on culture sensitivity report of ear discharge. As the condition did not improve after medical treatment and facial nerve palsy (grade VI HBS persisted, surgical intervention was planned. Pure tone audiometry showed moderate conductive hearing loss left side.

High-resolution computed tomography (HRCT) of temporal bone depicted extent of osteomyelitic lesion along with involvement of facial nerve in the left temporal bone (**Fig. 8.4**).

Preoperative clinical assessment showed grade VI HBS facial palsy on the left side (**Fig. 8.5**).

Surgical Planning

Tympanoplasty with cortical mastoidectomy with planning certain procedure pertaining to facial nerve.

Surgical Steps

Permeatal microscopic examination showed multiple polyps filling external auditory canal (EAC) and middle ear (ME) (**Fig. 8.6**). On lifting the tympanomeatal flap, polypi found filling the ME (**Fig. 8.7**). ME exploration with cortical mastoidectomy was performed. Excessive granulation tissue with polypi were found filling the mastoid cavity and the ME along with complete blockage of patency between the mastoid air cell system and ME (**Fig. 8.8**). All polypi, granulation tissue, and hypertrophic mucosa from mastoid cavity and ME were excised. Incus and malleus found entrapped in granulation tissue were removed. The mucosa of promontory was inseparable from the granulation tissue, so it was excised as well, making the promontory bone bare in posterior part (**Fig. 8.9**). Facial nerve was found dehiscent in its mastoid segment (MS) up to its exit at SMF (**Fig. 8.10**). The exposed facial nerve seemed hyperemic and necrotic in different segments. Further decompression of facial nerve performed to reach normal facial

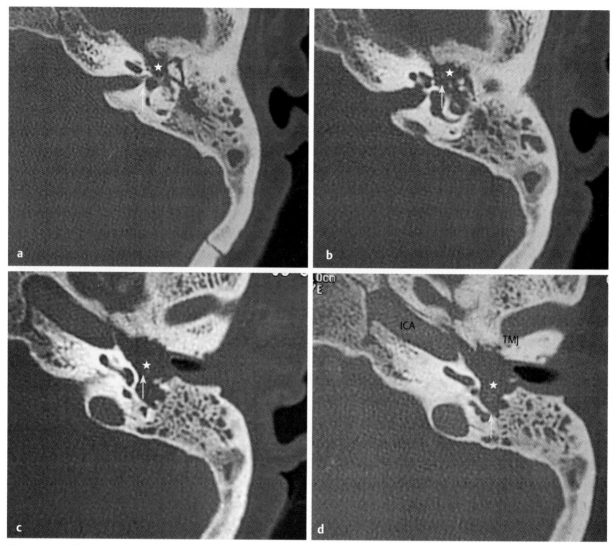

Fig. 8.4 High-resolution computed tomography (HRCT) temporal bone axial cuts of the left side showing soft tissue shadow (*white asterisk*) filling mastoid cavity, antrum, attic, middle ear, and medial part of external auditory canal (EAC). Anteriorly, the soft tissue shadow is seen involving labyrinthine segment (LS) of facial nerve and reaching up to internal carotid artery (ICA) and temporomandibular joint (TM). The fallopian canal (*yellow arrow*) is eroded from **(a)** the LS to **(b)** the first genu, **(c)** tympanic segment (TS), and **(d)** second genu and whole length of mastoid segment (MS).

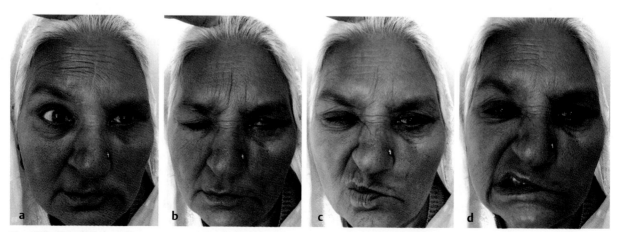

Fig. 8.5 **(a–d)** Preoperative pictures of the patient showing grade VI (HBS) facial palsy on the left side.

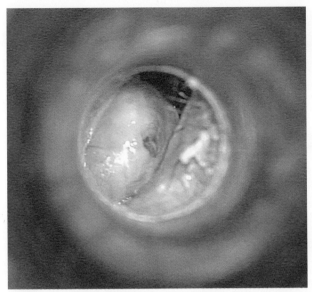

Fig. 8.6 Otomicroscopy showing big polyp filling external auditory canal (EAC) left ear.

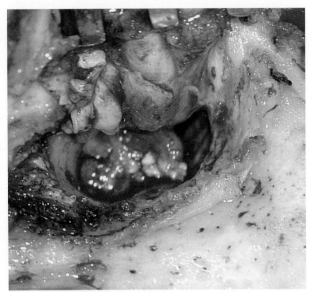

Fig. 8.7 On lifting and retracting the tympanomeatal flap, multiple polypi filling the middle ear (ME) are visualized.

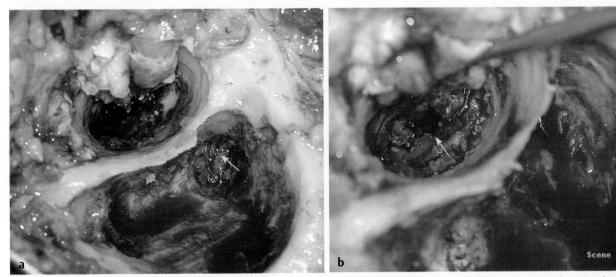

Fig. 8.8 **(a)** Canal wall up mastoidectomy performed to clear all granulations (*yellow arrow*) filling antrum and mastoid cavity and achieve patency between middle ear and mastoid. **(b)** Multiple polypi with hypertrophic mucosa filling the middle ear (*yellow arrow*) are visualized.

nerve on both sides (**Fig. 8.10**). Normal nerve could not be reached up to the labyrinthine segment (LS), which also seemed ischemic and necrosed. Further exploration of facial nerve proximal to the LS was stopped there only. On distal side, there was ischemic necrosis of facial nerve extending till SMF so exploration stopped there

only. After confirming the complete clearance of disease occupying the ME (including the disease around and reaching up to ICA and temporomandibular joint [TMJ]), attic, antrum, and mastoid cavity, reconstruction of ossicular chain was performed by placing tragal cartilage graft between stapes and bony annulus along with

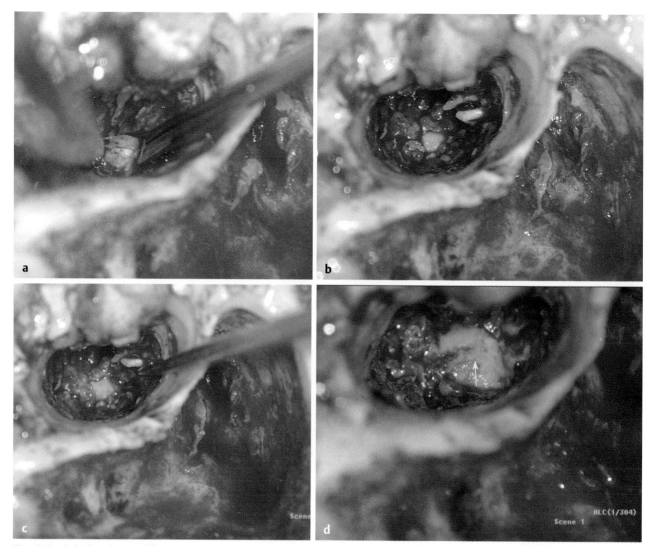

Fig. 8.9 **(a)** All polypi and hypertrophic mucosa filling the middle ear (ME) being excised with microscissors. **(b)** Raw area on promontory visualized after clearance of hypertrophic tissue. Ossicles seem entrapped in granulations. **(c)** Incus and malleus removed as they are found entrapped in granulations. **(d)** The mucosa of promontory was inseparable from the granulations, so removed along with the granulations. The bare bone of promontory in posterior part can be visualized (*yellow arrow*).

repair of tympanic membrane with temporalis fascia. As the whole intratemporal course of facial nerve found necrosed and nonviable, the repair of facial nerve was not possible. Any procedure for facial reanimation was planned for second stage after settling down of infection and inflammation depending upon availability of neural input.

Postsurgery Results

After 6 months of surgery, the osteomyelitis got cured, patients hearing improved with reduction in air bone gap upto 10dB and the neo tympanum was well taken up but complete facial nerve palsy grade VI persisted (**Fig. 8.11**).

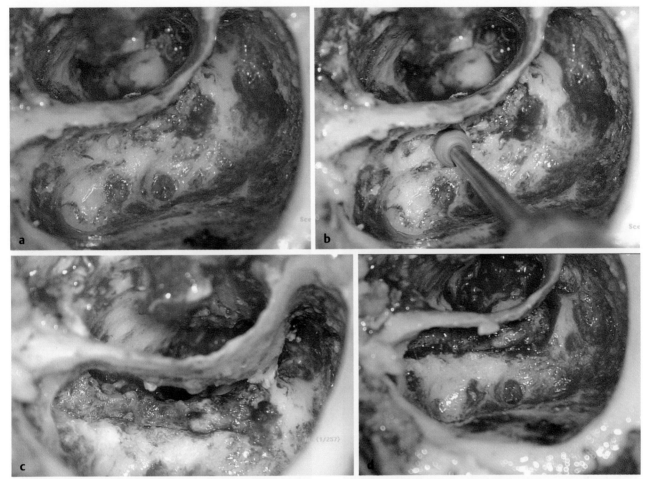

Fig. 8.10 (a–d) Decompression of intratemporal segment of facial nerve in progress. There is complete ischemic necrosis of intratemporal facial nerve and it seems non-viable and non-functional.

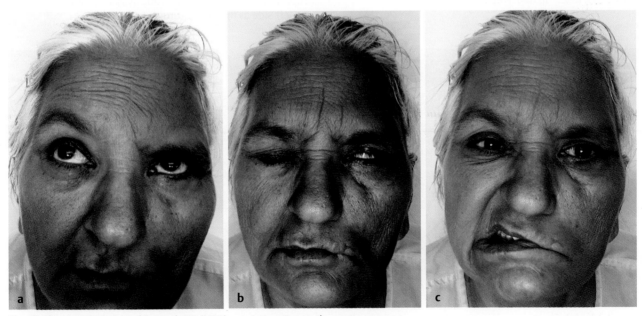

Fig. 8.11 (a–c) Facial palsy grade VI (HBS) persisting 6 months post surgery.

Second Stage Surgery: Classical End-to-End Facio-hypoglossal Anastomosis (Left Side)

As the osteomyelitis had caused complete avascular necrosis of facial nerve up to labyrinthine part, the proximal stump was nonviable up to the LS. As the hearing was well preserved on ipsilateral side in this patient, translabyrinthine approach to reach proximal healthy part could not be the procedure of choice. To preserve the hearing on ipsilateral side, motor nerve transfer procedure in the form of facio-hypoglossal anastomosis was chosen for facial reanimation.

Surgical Steps

The second stage surgical steps are as follows:

- The neotympanum found intact after first surgery, which showed the healing of the ME and mastoid (**Fig. 8.12**).
- Modified Blair's incision made. Skin with superficial muscular aponeurotic system (SMAS) flap was lifted (**Fig. 8.13**). The great auricular nerve (GAN) graft was harvested.
- Facial nerve exposed at its exit at SMF and released up to its bifurcation in parotid gland (**Fig. 8.14**).

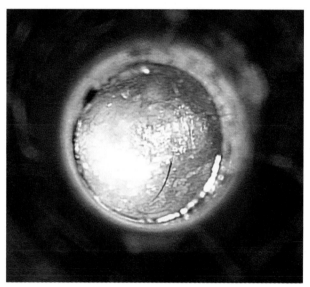

Fig.8.12 6 months post first surgery otomicroscopy showing intact well taken up neotympanum.

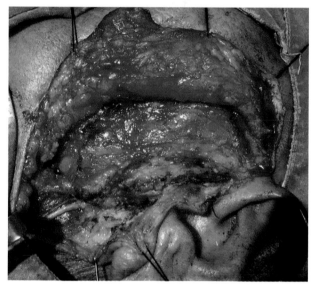

Fig. 8.13 Modified Blair's incision made and skin with superficial muscular aponeurotic system (SMAS) flap lifted on left side as in parotid surgery.

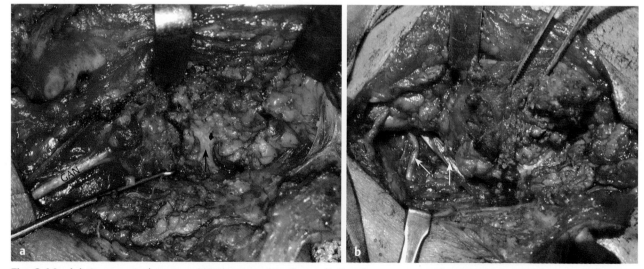

Fig. 8.14 **(a)** Great auricular nerve (GAN) exposed in the neck. Facial nerve exposed at its exit from stylomastoid foramen (SMF) (*black arrow*). **(b)** Hypoglossal nerve exposed in the neck (*yellow arrow*). Posterior belly of digastric muscle visible (*white arrow*).

- Hypoglossal nerve exposed in the neck. The horizontal portion of the hypoglossal nerve is identified just inferior to the posterior belly of the digastric and the greater cornu of the hyoid bone (**Fig. 8.14**).
- The hypoglossal nerve was further exposed posteriorly till the anterior aspect of the IJV after ligating lingual vein and branch of the occipital artery.
- The hypoglossal nerve was divided toward its distal-most part to secure an adequate length of nerve (**Fig. 8.15**).
- The facial nerve was then transected close to its exit from the SMF (**Fig. 8.15**).
- Both cut ends were placed on a piece of gelfoam and approximated to each other in a very precise manner (**Fig. 8.15**).

- Suturing (end to end) of approximated ends of facial and hypoglossal nerve is performed with 8-0 monofilament nylon. At least three to four sutures are placed for stable assembly (**Fig. 8.16**).
- The anastomotic site was covered with a piece of gelfoam and posterior margin of parotid resutured to sternocleidomastoid muscle and preauricular soft tissue (**Fig. 8.17**).

Postsurgery Results

After 1 year of surgery, the recovery of facial nerve function was up to grade I HBS (**Fig. 8.18**), but there was atrophy of left-sided tongue (**Fig. 8.18**). The patient felt difficulty in swallowing for the first few months which improved over 6 months. The tongue paresis also improved over time.

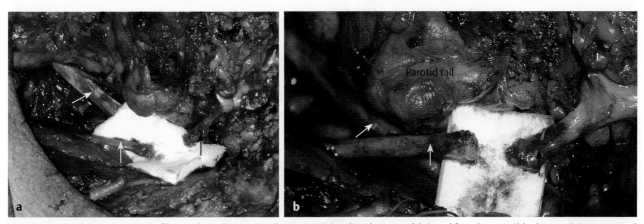

Fig. 8.15   (a, b) Transaction of hypoglossal nerve (*yellow arrow*) (as distal as possible) and facial nerve (*black arrow*) (as proximal as possible) performed. Both cut ends brought together and placed on a piece of gelfoam. Posterior belly of digastric (*white arrow*) and tail of parotid also visualized.

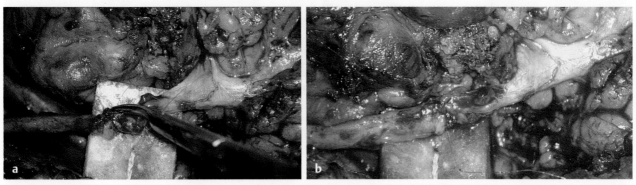

Fig. 8.16   (a) End-to-end suturing with 8-0 monofilament nylon from epineurium to epineurium through both cut ends of CN XII and CN VII stumps in progress. **(b)** first suture in progress. *(Continued)*

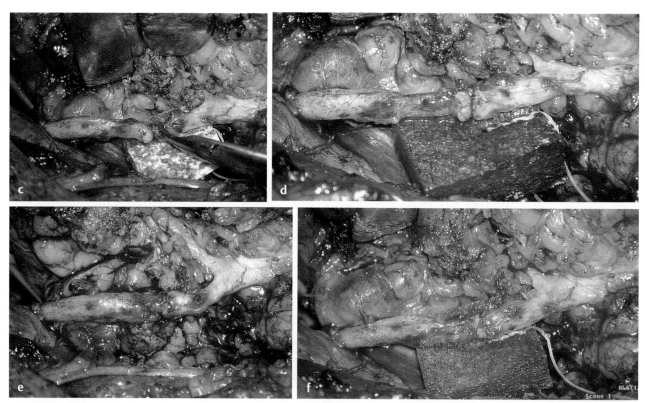

Fig. 8.16 *(Continued)* **(c, d)** Second suture being applied. **(e, f)** third suture also applied and perfect approximation of both cut ends is achieved.

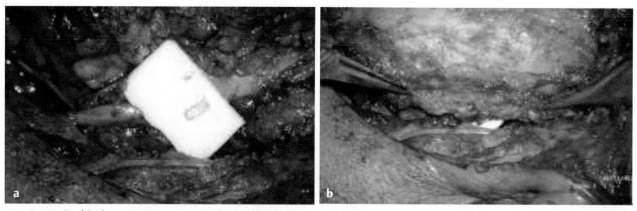

Fig. 8.17 **(a, b)** The anastomotic site is covered with a piece of gelfoam and posterior margin of parotid to be sutured to sternocleidomastoid muscle.

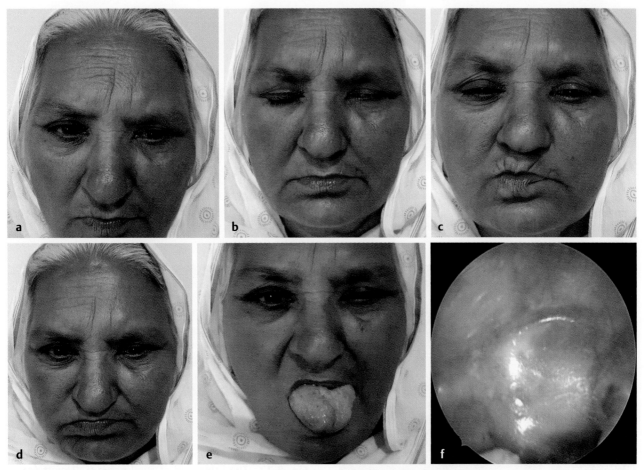

Fig. 8.18 **(a–d)** Facial nerve recovery to grade I after 1 year of surgery. **(e)** Left-sided tongue atrophy and mild paresis, although the patient has learned to swallow with the help of self-training and physiotherapy. **(f)** Healthy intact neotympanum.

Case 2: Patient with Facial Nerve Neuroma Involving the Nerve from Cerebellopontine Angle (CPA) to the SMF (Right Side)

Surgery was performed in two parts. First part of surgery included complete excision of facial nerve neuroma from the CP angle to the SMF. As the proximal stump of facial nerve was not available, motor nerve transfer became the procedure of choice for facial reanimation. The second part of surgery was performed in the same stage for facial reanimation, in the form of motor nerve transfer (hemi end-to-end facio-hypoglossal jump nerve anastomosis).

Second Stage Surgical Procedure (Right Side)

After harvesting the sural nerve (SN) for cable grafting (as longer cable graft was needed) and exposing facial nerve at the SMF and hypoglossal nerve in the neck, the following steps were performed:

- The facial nerve stump was prepared by identifying it after its exit from SMF and exposed further till its bifurcation in terminal branches in parotid gland and transected at the SMF (**Fig. 8.19**).
- SN with sharp cut bevel-shaped ends was prepared to be used as interposition cable grafting (**Fig. 8.20**).
- The cable graft (SN) was sutured on one end with the distal stump of facial nerve in end-to-end manner (**Fig. 8.21**).
- The second end of cable graft was approximated to the hypoglossal nerve at a site where wedge was to be created (**Fig. 8.22**).
- A partial section (30% incision) of hypoglossal nerve was performed with a very sharp microscissors. This allowed the defect to splay open and create a wedge-shaped wider surface area for anastomosis (**Fig. 8.22**).
- The other end of cable graft was sutured to the hypoglossal nerve in end-to-side manner (with the proximal surface of V-shaped wedge created) with 8-0 monofilament nylon (**Figs. 8.23** and **8.24**).

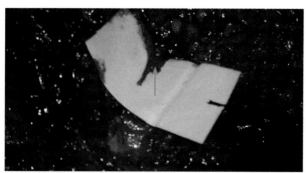

Fig. 8.19 Right side of face showing, cut end of CN VII after its exit from SMF which has already been drilled away. The stump of facial nerve is created with exposure till its division into terminal branches in parotid gland (*green arrow*).

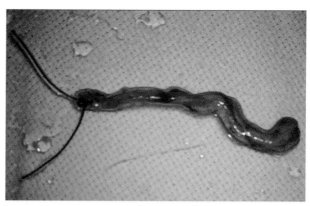

Fig. 8.20 Harvested sural nerve graft.

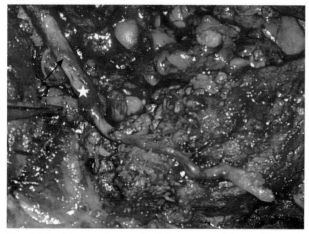

Fig. 8.21 The sural nerve (SN) (*green arrow*) free cable graft is sutured in an end-to-end manner (*white asterisk*) with the distal stump of facial nerve (*black arrow*).

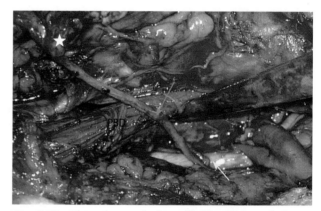

Fig. 8.22 The other end of sural nerve (SN) graft (*green arrow*) placed close to hypoglossal nerve (*yellow arrow*) appearing from underneath the posterior belly of digastric (PBD). The cut end of cable graft is placed at a point on hypoglossal nerve, where partial-thickness cut is to be given.

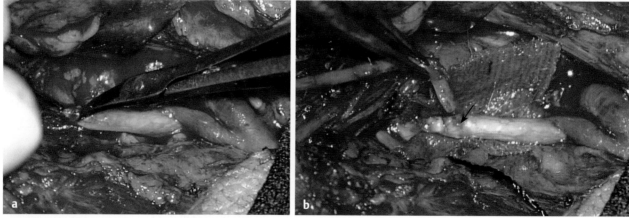

Fig. 8.23 **(a)** A partial cut (up to 30% thickness) is being given in hypoglossal nerve (HN). **(b)** The "V"-shaped cut and wedge-shaped opening up of CN XII at incision site (*black arrow*).

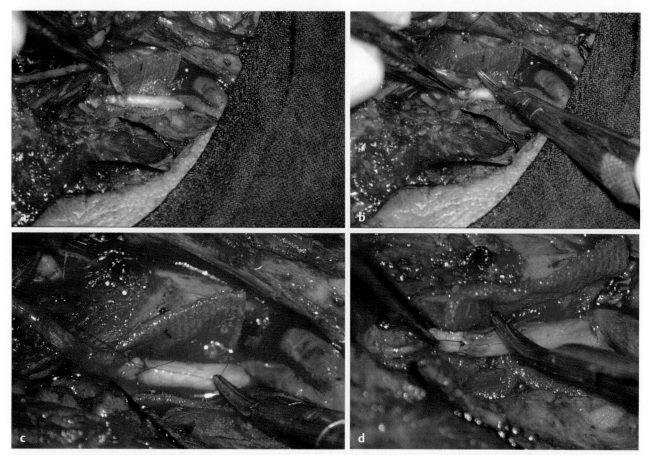

Fig. 8.24 **(a, b)** The second cut end of cable graft being approximated to the proximal surface of the V-shaped cut and first suture applied with 8-0 monofilament. Suture is passed from epineurium to perineurium on facial nerve stump side and then passed from perineurium to epineurium on cut surface of hypoglossal nerve in an end-to-side manner. **(c)** Suturing in progress for end-to-side anastomosis between cut end of cable graft and the proximal surface of V-shaped wedge on hypoglossal nerve. **(d)** Second suture being placed. *(Continued)*

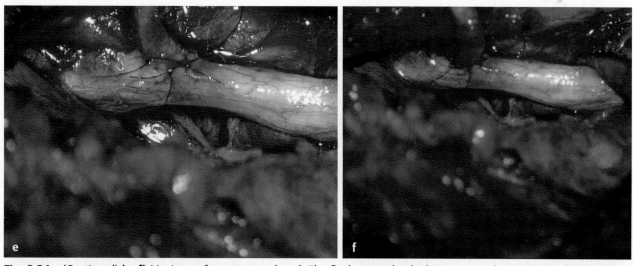

Fig. 8.24 *(Continued)* **(e, f)** Maximum four sutures placed. The final neurorrhaphy between sural nerve (SN) cable graft and hypoglossal nerve is visualized.

Facio-masseteric Anastomosis

The masseter nerve lately has become the preferred choice for motor nerve transfer procedures due to its comparable size, easy dissection as in the same surgical field, early recovery due to close proximity, and minimal compromise in masticatory function (as there are alternative muscles for mastication available), although the length may not be sufficient in certain situations.

Use of masseter nerve can be in the form of direct end-to-end anastomosis with facial nerve stump if the length of both nerves is sufficient and there is no gap between the two cut ends after approximating. In case there is a gap of more than 5 mm between approximated cut ends (due to shorter length of the facial nerve stumpin cases of facial nerve tumors involving the MS up to (SMF), interposition cable graft (**Fig. 8.25**) has to be used in between, which delays the recovery by few months and facial nerve recovery cannot be better than grade II or grade III HBS.

Advantages Over Facio-hypoglossal Anastomosis

- Anatomical location is in the same surgical field, so more proximity and relative ease of dissection.
- There is optimal motor neural output leading to similar nerve recovery with low morbidity.
- Unlike facio-hypoglossal anastomosis, where the patient has difficulty in the first stage of deglutition and articulation post surgery for a long time, this anastomosis does not cause any restriction of function. The donor deficit is very minimal and not clinically relevant as there are other muscles for mastication available.
- It is better nerve for producing spontaneous effortless smile as it is the natural function of masseter muscle which is supplied by masseter nerve.
- There is early reinnervation and improved symmetry.
- Its use is not contraindicated in patients with lower cranial nerve deficits or palsies or in patients susceptible to develop multiple cranial nerve deficits (neurofibromatosis type II).

Disadvantages Over Facio-hypoglossal Anastomosis

- It is quite close to temporal and zygomatic branches of the facial nerve which can get injured while locating the masseter nerve.
- Unless the surgeon is well versed with the surgical anatomy of masseter nerve, it may take long and at times difficult to locate the nerve, as the tendinous fibers of masseter muscle are glistening white in appearance and may look like nerve and create confusion.

Physiotherapy

Physiotherapy includes various techniques, for example, bite and smile, decrease bite and increase facial function, and getting an independent facial function. The detailed techniques of physiotherapy and adjuvant therapy have been explained in Chapter 10"Management of Nerve Regeneration Complications."

Anatomy of Masseter Nerve

Masseter nerve originates from anterior division of mandibular branch of trigeminal nerve (CN V). It leaves the mandibular nerve shortly after its entrance to the infratemporal fossa. The nerve passes over the lateral pterygoid muscle and leaves the infratemporal fossa through the sigmoid notch, accompanied by the masseteric artery. Distance from the notch to the entrance of the muscle is around 32 mm. It is located in the plane between the middle and deep lobes of masseter muscle and enters from its medial surface.

Surface Marking for Masseter Nerve

The masseteric nerve is proving to be the most viable nerve for motor nerve transfer. The only limitation is that surgeons are not well versed with the surgical anatomy of the nerve, so they usually do not opt for it as a first choice. To make the surgery simple, surface anatomy with few landmarks has been specified, which allows surgeons to quickly and accurately identify the nerve intra-operatively.

- It is approximately 3.06 cm anterior to tragus.
- It is approximately 1.16 cm inferior to inferior margin of zygomatic arch.
- It lies around 1.5 cm deep to the SMAS.
- It bisects the subzygomatic triangle, which is described in details below.
- It is in close proximity to zygomatic branch of facial nerve, forming an angle of around 50 degrees with it while descending.
- In its proximal part, it is often identified deep to and between two branches of zygomatic division of facial nerve, one traveling toward lower eyelid and other to the zygomatic muscle.

Subzygomatic triangle is an important landmark to locate masseter nerve (**Fig. 8.26**).

The boundaries of the triangle are as follows:

- Superior side formed by zygomatic arch inferior margin.

- Posterior side formed by vertical line through TM joint anterior margin.
- Anteroinferior side formed by zygomatic branch of facial nerve.

The masseter nerve bisects this triangle.

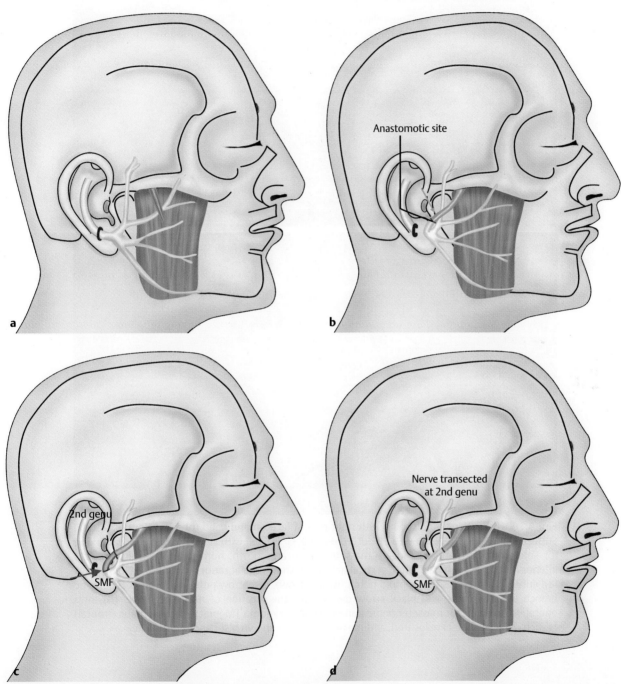

Fig. 8.25   Illustrations showing **(a)** exposure of facial nerve (*yellow coloured*) from SMF till its terminal branches and exposure of masseter nerve (*orange coloured*). **(b)** showing end to end anastomosis between cut end of masseter nerve and distal stump of facial nerve at SMF, **(c)** showing GAN interposition graft (*dark orange coloured*) between cut ends of masseter nerve and facial nerve in an end to end manner (anastomotic site shown with *red lines*), **(d)** showing extra length of facial nerve achieved by transecting it at the level of 2nd genu rather than at SMF and end to end anastomosis performed between cut ends of both nerves.

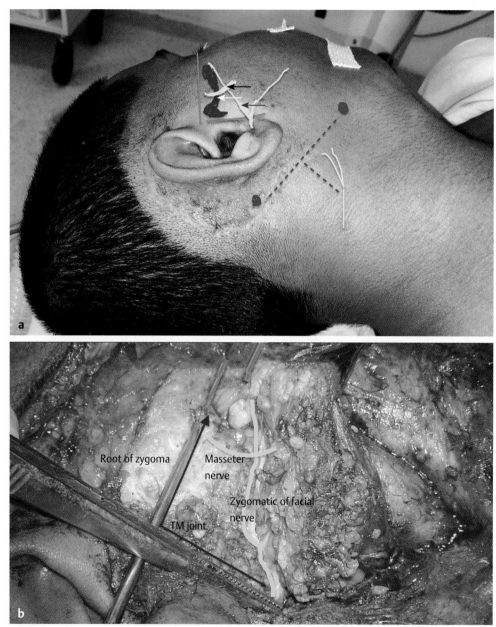

Fig. 8.26 **(a)** Patient lying supine with right side of face up and head rotated to opposite side. Surface marking for GAN shown with dotted red line, GAN itself with yellow lines. Surface marking for subzygomatic triangle to locate masseter nerve are shown. horizontal green line depicts inferior margin of zygomatic arch, vertical green line shows the anterior margin of TM joint, thick red curved line depicts the sigmoid notch (white arrow), red arrow pointing towards zygomatic branch of facial nerve and black arrow demarcates the location of masseter nerve. **(b)** Intra operative markings for masseter nerve namely, root of zygoma TM joint, and zygomatic (frontal) branch of facial nerve, are located, and masseter nerve is shown bisecting the triangle.

Case 3: Case of Post Gamma Knife Treated Facial Nerve Schwannoma Tumor with Complete Grade VI Facial Palsy (Right Side)

This is a case of a 15-years-old patient who had received gamma knife treatment for facial nerve schwannoma 18 months back at some center. He presented with recurrence of tumor with grade VI facial palsy for 9 months.

Surgical Planning

Surgical management was planned in two stages. First stage included complete excision of tumor along with affected part of facial nerve through infra temporal fossa Type A approach (the details of first stage surgery has been described in details in chapter 15 " Facial Nerve Schwanomma").

While excising the tumor, surgical exploration showed ischemic and fibrotic changes in facial nerve in whole of its intratemporal part (*arrows*) and meatal segment (porus of internal auditory meatus [IAM]). As the

viability of proximal stump of facial nerve after excising the affected part was doubtful, second stage surgery in the form of facio-masseteric anastomosis was performed after 2 months of primary surgery.

Fig. 8.27 shows right-sided facial nerve palsy grade VI HBS when taken up for surgery (facio masseteric anastomosis).

Surgical Steps (Fig 8.28-8.43)

First surgery was performed through Infra temporal fossa Type A approach. All fibrotic tissue surrounding the intratemporal segment and meatal segment of facial nerve (post gamma knife treatment) was excised. As the facial nerve was found ischemic and necrotic from porus of internal auditory meatus till its exit at the SMF; hence the whole affected segment was excised. As the viability of proximal stump was doubtful, motor nerve transfer technique was chosen for facial reanimation and masseter nerve was used for anastomosis with distal stump of facial nerve at the SMF.

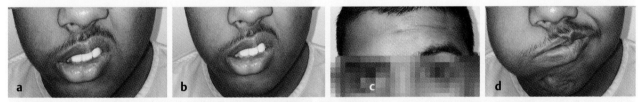

Fig. 8.27   (a, b, c, d) Preoperative pictures of the patient's face showing grade VI facial palsy on right side.

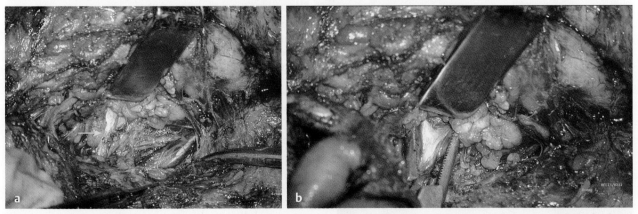

Fig. 8.28   (a) For identification of facial nerve, the posterior belly of digastric muscle (*green arrow*) has been exposed. The facial nerve (*yellow arrow*) is identified at its exit from stylomastoid foramen, 1 cm superior and parallel to superior border of posterior belly of digastric muscle. **(b)** Facial nerve exposed up to its bifurcation in parotid tissue by lifting and cutting the parotid tissue lateral to the nerve. For that, the artery forceps is inserted in the plane lateral to facial nerve, lifted and spread and the parotid tissue lateral to it is cut and separated.

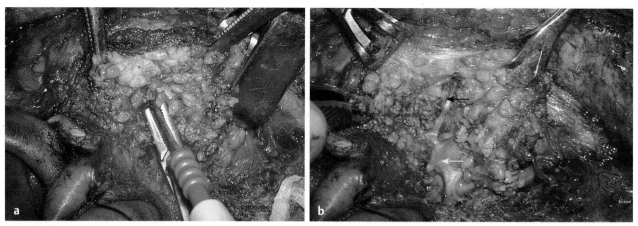

Fig. 8.29 **(a)** Insertion, lifting, spreading, and cutting the tissue lateral to facial nerve while tracing and exposing zygomatic branch. **(b)** Identifying and exposing the upper division of facial nerve (*yellow arrow*) and completely exposing the zygomatic branch (*black arrow*).

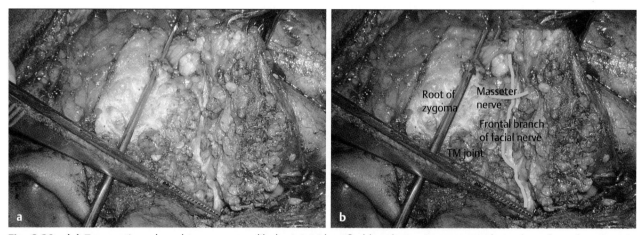

Fig. 8.30 **(a)** Zygomatic arch and temporomandibular joint identified by placing instrument along them for subzygomatic triangle. **(b)** Borders of subzygomatic triangle. The three sides of triangle are: inferior border of root of zygoma, line drawn along the anterior border of temporomandibular joint (depicted by two *red lines*), and zygomatic branch of facial nerve (*yellow line* showing nerve beneath). Location of masseter nerve (which bisects this triangle) is marked with curved *yellow line*.

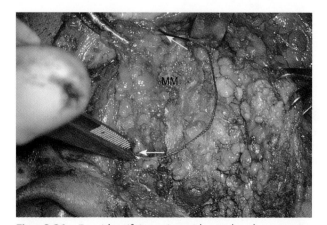

Fig. 8.31 For identifying sigmoid notch, the anterior margin of condylar process (*white arrow*) and posterior margin of coronoid process (*yellow arrow*) are marked. Sigmoid notch is marked with silk suture. Masseter muscle (MM) is identified. The masseter nerve crosses the sigmoid notch after crossing medial to the zygomatic arch.

Surgical steps for facio-masseteric anastomosis:

- Preauricular modified Blair's incision was made.
- Skin with SMAS flap was lifted.
- Parotid gland and masseter muscle exposed.
- The great auricular nerve identified in the neck.
- Facial nerve was identified at its exit at the SMF and dissected from surrounding parotid tissue till its division into two terminal branches.
- *Different markers for identifying facial nerve at SMF are:*
  - ➤ Tragal pointer: The anterior part of tragus points anterior, inferior, and deep to superficial surface of the preauricular area. Its anterior end takes a bluntly pointed shape on its medial aspect and is called "pointer." The facial nerve at its exit at the SMF lies approximately 1 cm inferior and deeper to tragal pointer.

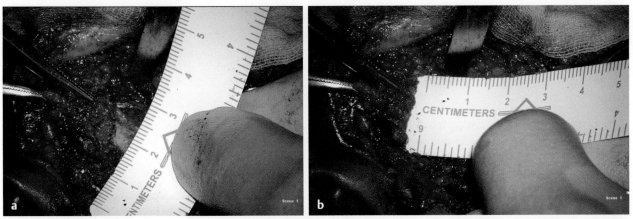

Fig. 8.32 Scale being used to measure right distanceto locate masseter nerve. it is around **(a)** 3.06 cms from tragus and **(b)** 1.16 cms from inferior margin of root of zygoma as depicted in pictures.

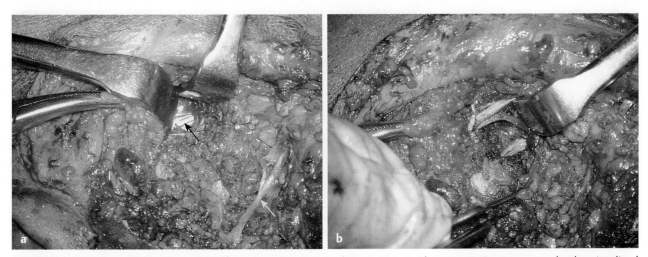

Fig. 8.33 **(a)** Transmuscular dissection through masseter muscle in progress. The zygomatic nerve can also be visualized (*yellow arrow*). The glistening white fibers of muscle tendon are visible (*black arrow*). **(b)** Superficial part of masseter muscle separated; deeper part of masseter muscle being dissected. The white fibers of tendon of muscle look like masseter nerve, but they are flatter and broader than the nerve.

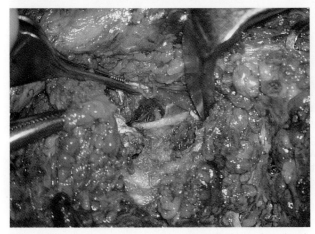

Fig. 8.34 The masseter nerve identified in the depth of masseter muscle. Maximum length of masseter nerve exposed till its entry from the medial side of muscle.

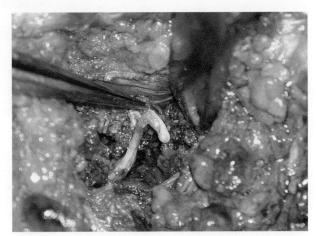

Fig. 8.35 After exposing the complete length, the masseter nerve is transected at its entry into masseter muscle. The cut end of nerve is lifted and brought to the surface.

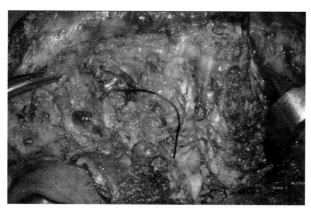

Fig. 8.36 A piece of thread is used to measure the gap between the cut end of masseter nerve and facial nerve stump at the stylomastoid foramen (SMF).

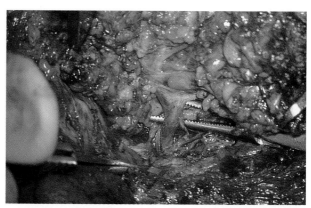

Fig. 8.37 The artery forceps lifting the facial nerve at its exit from the stylomastoid foramen (SMF). The nerve is to be cut as proximal as possible at its exit from SMF.

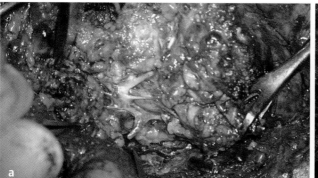

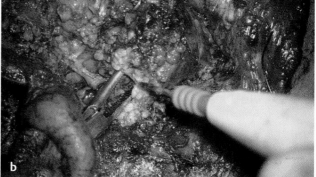

Fig. 8.38 **(a)** Facial nerve stump prepared by transecting the nerve at the stylomastoid foramen (SMF). The temporozygomatic branch is already exposed. **(b)** Parotid tissue lateral to lower division of facial nerve is lifted and cut to expose the lower trunk. This step is performed to create longest possible stump of facial nerve for tension free anastomosis.

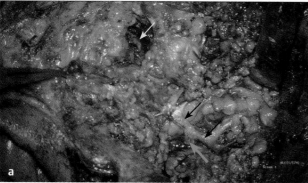

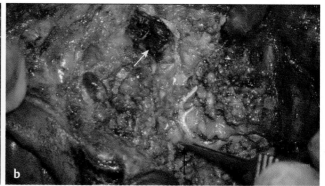

Fig. 8.39 **(a)** Facial nerve stump (*thick blue arrow*) with both upper and lower division exposed (*thin black arrows*). The masseter nerve is also visible in the vicinity (*yellow arrow*). **(b)** There is a gap of almost 1.5 cm between lower end of masseter nerve (*yellow arrow*) and facial nerve stump (*thick blue arrow*). As this was a case of facial nerve neuroma where first stage surgery involved total excision of neuroma extending from internal acoustic meatus (IAM) to stylomastoid foramen (SMF), the mastoid portion up to the second genu is not available to increase the length of facial nerve stump.

> Tympanomastoid suture: It is palpable as a hard ridge deep to the cartilaginous part of EAC. The facial nerve emerges few millimeters deep to its outer edge. Its mean distance from facial nerve trunk is 3.5 mm (2.5–4.5 mm).

> Posterior belly of digastric muscle: It is the most easily identifiable and consistent landmark for facial nerve dissection. After lateral retraction of sternocleidomastoid muscle, the posterior belly of digastric muscle can be identified as it

inserts on mastoid ridge. The facial nerve trunk lies approximately 1 cm above and parallel to the upper border of the digastric muscle near its insertion (**Fig. 8.28a** and **b**).

- After identifying and locating the facial nerve at its exit till its bifurcation, the nerve was followed along the course of temporozygomatic trunk the superior terminal branch of facial nerve (**Fig. 8.29**).
- The sigmoid or mandibular notch, between condylar and coronoid process of mandible, was then identified (**Fig. 8.31**).

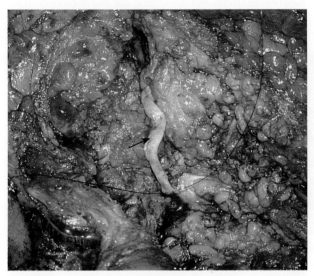

Fig. 8.40 Great auricular nerve (GAN) (*black arrow*) is used as cable graft between the two motor nerves.

- After making a transverse incision in the parotid capsule, a blunt dissection was carried through the parotid tissue up to the surface of the masseter muscle, keeping in plane with the temporozygomatic branch of facial nerve, so as to avoid transecting it accidentally. The whole length of zygomatic branch was exposed as it makes the third side of subzygomatic triangle which is used to locate the masseter nerve (**Fig. 8.30**). Also by exposing zygomatic branch, the iatrogenic trauma to zygomatic branch is avoided.
- The masseter nerve location was demarcated with a scale measuring approximately 3.06 cm anterior to anterior border of tragus, 1.16 cm inferior to inferior border of zygomatic arch, and approximately 1.5 cm deep to the SMAS (**Fig 8.32**). The nerve is to be located in the plane between the middle and deep lobes of masseter muscle entering from medial deeper surface of masseter. Keeping all these measurements/parameters in mind, the masseter muscle was dissected in the direction of masseter nerve till the medial surface of masseter muscle reached (**Fig. 8.33**). The distance from the origin of masseter nerve to its ramification in masseter muscle is around 3.2 to 3.5 cm, which means almost 3 cm length of branch-free segment of nerve can be dissected for direct end-to-end anastomosis.
- Transmuscular identification of masseter nerve is important as the tendon of masseter muscle have glistening white fibers which almost look like the

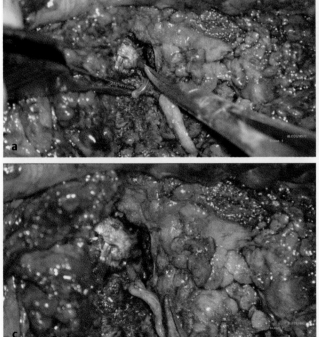

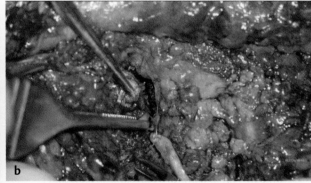

Fig. 8.41 **(a)** End-to-end anastomosis between cut ends of masseter nerve and GAN cable graft. For placing sutures, the epineurium is stripped back, suture passed entering from perineurium, out through endoneurium on masseter nerve side. **(b)** The same suture is passed through endoneurium and out from perineurium on cable graft side. **(c)** Three sutures are applied.

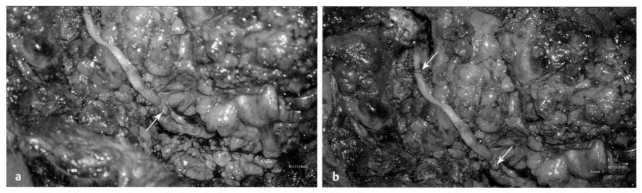

Fig. 8.42 **(a)** Suture being applied in similar way, between distal facial nerve stump and the second cut end of cable graft for end-to-end anastomosis (*white arrow*). **(b)** Final sutures between facial nerve stump and cable graft lower end (*white arrows*).

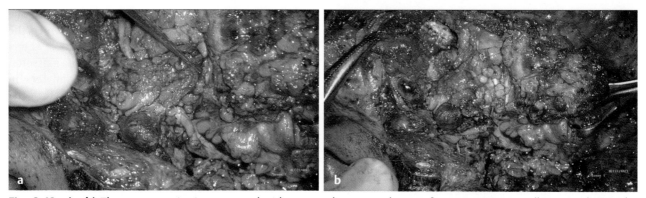

Fig. 8.43 **(a, b)** The anastomotic sites wrapped with surrounding parotid tissue for protection as well as vascularity. The parotid tissue sutured together.

masseter nerve (**Fig. 8.34**). That is why knowing the anatomy and surface marking of the nerve are very important.

- The nerve was transected at its distal-most end at its entry into masseter muscle and reflected laterally into the wound (**Fig. 8.35**).
- At this stage, the facial nerve stump was prepared by transecting it at the SMF (**Figs. 8.36** and **8.37**).
- In situations where the length of the masseter nerve is not sufficient, extra length can be achieved by transecting the facial nerve at the second genu rather than at the SMF. The extra length of MS added to the distal stump of facial nerve makes end-to-end anastomosis possible (**Fig. 8.26d**).
- In cases of facial nerve neuroma resection, where the tumor might be involving facial nerve up to the SMF as in this case, the facial nerve stump may not be long enough to be directly coapted with the masseter nerve. In that situation, great auricular cable nerve graft is interposed between masseter and facial nerves, as was performed in this case.

After creating stump of facial nerve at the SMF, the two divisions of facial nerve in parotid gland were identified and exposed, so as to create the maximum length of facial nerve stump for neurorrhaphy (**Figs. 8.38** and

8.39). The motor branch to posterior belly of digastric and stylohyoid muscle were transected to release few extra millimeters of facial nerve. In this case, as there was a big gap between the cut ends of masseter nerve and facial nerve stump, an interposition grafting with GAN graft (**Figs. 8.40, 8.41,** and **8.42**) was performed to avoid stretching of the nerves and tension at suture line. With cable graft in between the two nerves, there were two neurorrhaphies, so recovery was expected to be delayed and improvement in facial nerve functioning expected, maximumup to grade III or II HBS. Finally, the parotid tissue was replaced back to cover the anastomotic sites for support and vascularity and was sutured back to the soft tissue in preauricular region on the face and sternocleidomastoid muscle in the neck (**Fig. 8.43**).

- As facial nerve recovery takes almost 2 years to recover to optimal functioning after facio-masseteric anastomosis, the exposed cornea of the ipsilateral eye may develop complications due to inability to close eyelid. Static procedure in the form of upper eyelid gold implant was performed in the same stage to achieve immediate eyelid closure, details of which are described in Chapter 9 "Management of long duration flaccid facial palsy".

Postsurgery Results

Immediate postoperative pictures show complete facial palsy with closure of upper eyelid achieved due to gold implantation (**Fig. 8.44**). One year postoperative pictures show facial nerve improvement up to grade III (**Fig. 8.45**). After 2 years of surgery, gold implant could be taken out as right upper eyelid could close on its own. Facial nerve recovery up to grade II was achieved after 2 years of facio-masseteric anastomosis (**Fig. 8.46**).

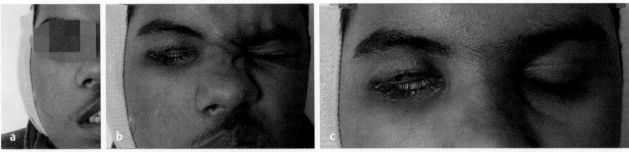

Fig. 8.44   **(a–c)** Immediate postoperative pictures showing grade VI facial palsy right side with closure of upper eyelid. Suture marks for gold implantation upper eyelid (which was performed in the same sitting) can be noticed on right side.

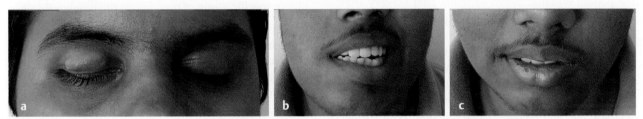

Fig. 8.45   **(a–c)** Improvement in facial nerve functioning up to grade III after 1 year of surgery. Good closure of eyelid along with lifting of angle of mouth and appearance of nasolabial fold is visible.

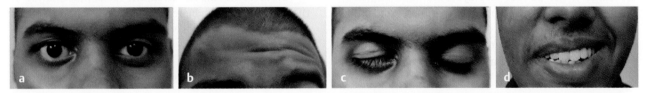

Fig. 8.46   **(a–d)** Pictures showing facial nerve recovery up to grade II after removal of gold implant 2 years post surgery.

Case 4: An Operated Case of Facial Nerve Neuroma with Facial Palsy Grade VI (Right Side)

The primary surgery performed was excision of facial nerve schwannoma involving facial nerve in its entire meatal and intratemporal segment. As the proximal stump of facial nerve was not available for facial nerve repair, motor nerve transfer in the form of facio-masseteric anastomosis was performed as second stage surgery for facial reanimation. In this case, as the length of facial nerve stump was sufficiently long enough, end-to-end anastomosis could be achieved between the cut end of masseter nerve and distal stump of facial nerve without any stretch or tension on suture line (**Fig. 8.47**).

Postoperative Care and Physiotherapy Training

The patient was discharged 48 hours after surgery after removal of dressing. First follow-up was 10 days after surgery when the sutures were removed. After 6 weeks of surgery, on the first rehabilitative visit, the patient was taught to activate the reinnervated facial muscles through teeth clenching, which means bite and smile together. Slowly over time, the patient was taught to decrease bite and increase facial function. With regular physiotherapy training, facial muscles showed signs of recovery within 2 to 9 months. Around 18 months after the surgery, the patient displayed dramatic improvement of voluntary control on facial symmetry and smile and remarkable reduction of disability, and finally the patient had an independent facial function. However, the patient was unable to achieve an effortless spontaneous smile.

Cross-Face Nerve Grafting (CFNG)

CFNG with nerve transfer is another technique in cases where it is short duration facial palsy with proximal stump unavailable (motor end plates of facial muscles are viable and likely to respond to new axonal ingrowth).

CFNG, first introduced by Scaramella, uses the peripheral branches of the contralateral, intact facial nerve (mostly buccal) to innervate corresponding areas of the paralyzed side of face to produce spontaneous and voluntary facial movements. It can be done in one stage, where both ends are sutured in single stage through interposition SN graft. Or the procedure can be performed in two stages, where in stage one, one end of SN is sutured to the branches of facial nerve on healthy side and the whole length of SN is passed through a subcutaneous tunnel created from across the upper lip to bring it to opposite side. In the second stage, the distal end of SN graft is sutured to the corresponding branches supplying specific group of muscles on the paralyzed side.

Use of CFNG as sole procedure is limited to cases with less than 6 months duration of nerve palsy, as in cross-face facial nerve grafting, due to long distance interposition graft, there is already delay in recovery, along with the continuing atrophy of denervated facial muscles. So, in already long duration palsy (though less than 2 years), further delay may cause irreversible muscle atrophy leading to incomplete recovery.

To overcome this situation, the facial musculature of the affected side can be reanimated additionally by a so-called "babysitter" procedure, described by Terzis and Konofaos in cases where the denervation time is longer than 6 months but less than 2 years before surgery. Parallel to the cross-face surgery, in the same sitting, the

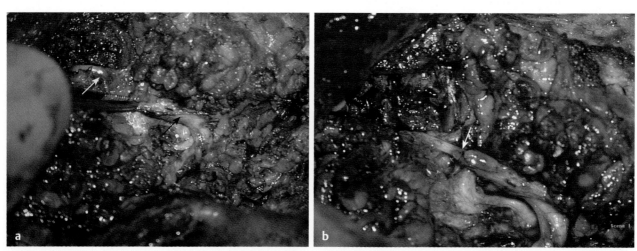

Fig. 8.47 Right side, facio-masseteric anastomosis in progress. **(a)** Cut end of masseter nerve (*yellow arrow*) and facial nerve (*black arrow*) are visible in the operative field. **(b)** Direct end-to-end anastomosis performed between the cut ends of both nerves with 8-0 monofilament nylon. Three sutures placed from perineurium to perineurium (*white arrow*).

facial musculature is reanimated by a facio-hypoglossal jump anastomosis or facio-masseteric end-to-end suturing to provide more rapid neural output. Static procedure in the form of upper eyelid gold implant can also be performed simultaneously for immediate eye closure.

Disadvantages

- CFNG carries the risk of disrupting the nonparalyzed donor facial nerve, although every effort is made to choose nondominant buccal branches.
- Additional surgery on the normal side of the face may not be acceptable to the patient.
- This procedure takes a longer time for recovery as the distance for reinnervation is very long.

◼ Conclusion

Motor nerve transfer procedures have the potential to restore close to normal innervation to the mimetic facial musculature. The success of nerve transfer depends on proper patient and technique selection and performing the procedure at the earliest to have optimal recovery through reinnervation. The ideal time recommended for surgery is, during the first 12 months of paralysis. Long-term facial palsy of more than 2 years duration is usually not the right situation for nerve transfer. Although both motor nerves, namely, CN V and CN XII, are good substitutes for providing neural input to facial nerve, the masseteric nerve has few advantages over hypoglossal nerve. Several modifications to the facio-hypoglossal anastomosis have been done with better results and least morbidity to speech and swallowing. The CFNG technique which seems appealing to plastic surgeons and can achieve a true spontaneous smile, has limitations in terms of axonal load, unnecessary surgery and handling of facial nerve on contralateral healthy side, added babysitter procedure to achieve early results,

unpredictable outcomes, and delayed recovery time due to use of long cable interposition graft. New developments are ongoing and many new ways are being developed to use these donor nerves for better and early facial nerve regeneration.

References

1. House JW. Facial nerve grading systems. Laryngoscope 1983;93(8):1056–1069
2. May M. Anatomy for the clinician. New York, NY: Thieme Medical Publishers; 2000
3. Terzis JK, Konofaos P. Nerve transfers in facial palsy. Facial Plast Surg 2008;24(2):177–193
4. Scaramella LF. Anastomosis between the two facial nerves. Laryngoscope 1975;85(8):1359–1366
5. Lee EI, Hurvitz KA, Evans GR, Wirth GA. Cross-facial nerve graft: past and present. J Plast Reconstr Aesthet Surg 2008;61(3):250–256
6. Terzis JK, Tzafetta K. The "babysitter" procedure: minihypoglossal to facial nerve transfer and cross-facial nerve grafting. Plast Reconstr Surg 2009;123(3):865–876
7. Galli SK, Valauri F, Komisar A. Facial reanimation by cross-facial nerve grafting: report of five cases. Ear Nose Throat J 2002;81(1):25–29
8. Conley J, Baker DC. Hypoglossal-facial nerve anastomosis for reinnervation of the paralyzed face. Plast Reconstr Surg 1979;63(1):63–72
9. Rochkind S, Shafi M, Alon M, Salame K, Fliss DM. Facial nerve reconstruction using a split hypoglossal nerve with preservation of tongue function. J Reconstr Microsurg 2008;24(7):469–474
10. Lee Peng G, Azizzadeh B. Cross-facial nerve grafting for facial reanimation.
11. Borschel GH, Kawamura DH, Kasukurthi R, et al. The motor nerve to the masseter muscle: An anatomic and histomorphometric study to facilitate its use in facial reanimation. Plastic Reconstructive and Aesthetic Surg
12. Collar RM, Byne PJ, Boahene KDO. The Subzygomatic Triangle: Rapid, Minimally Invasive Identification of the Masseteric Nerve for Facial Reanimation.

9 Management of Long Duration Flaccid Facial Palsy

Introduction

Facial expressions play a very important role in our day-to-day life, where we require using them for communication, social interaction, and showing our feelings. These complex but coordinated movements and expressions of face are achieved by the facial mimetic muscles supplied by the facial nerve. Facial nerve denervation for a long time can lead to fibrosis and atrophy of these facial mimetic muscles and degeneration of motor end plates making them nonviable permanently.

In long-term facial palsy (>2 years with EMG negative or >3 years) where the facial muscles have seemingly become nonviable and motor end plates are thought to have atrophied, primary corrective procedures like decompression, end-to-end repair, nerve grafting, or nerve transfer are not the procedures of choice (though we still perform these procedures as primary surgery along with added procedures). Even procedures like motor nerve transfer are not of any use in such situations, as facial muscles themselves have become nonviable. In such cases, the facial reanimation is planned with certain other procedures which can be both dynamic and static depending upon the region of the face to be reanimated. The aim of facial reanimation is to restore facial symmetry at rest as well as replace functioning of the atrophied facial muscles by dynamic transposition of some other functioning muscle so as to have spontaneous and coordinated reconstruction of facial expression and movements.

Management of long-term facial palsy can be divided into two categories:

1. Long-term facial nerve palsy with proximal or distal portion of facial nerve available

The literature suggests that facial nerve palsy of more than 2 years duration will not improve after facial nerve repair procedures like decompression, suturing, grafting, or nerve transfer due to irreversible atrophy and fibrosis of the mimetic muscles caused by long-term denervation. So, procedures like dynamic muscle transplants or elongation along with static and adjuvant procedures are more apt for providing optimal results. Electromyography (EMG) test plays an important role in

facial palsy of >2 years of duration, as it can accurately show the viability of facial muscles for reinnervation.

It is a very interesting observation in the author's cases though, that revision surgery through repair of facial nerve for long-standing facial nerve palsy could produce rewarding results even after a gap of >3 years.

So the author's philosophy is that in all primary or revision cases of iatrogenic or post-traumatic facial palsy or revision middle ear surgery, with facial palsy of long-term duration, re-exploration and primary repair in the form of decompression, end-to-end repair, or cable grafting should always be performed along with static procedures like upper eyelid implant and fascia lata slings. Because in the author's experience, especially in revision cases, the re-exploration at the anastomotic sites has shown that the two ends of the nerve were pulled apart from each other either because of infection, tension, or faulty repair. In such cases, the author performs facial nerve reconstruction along with static reanimation procedures. These additional procedures should be performed in the same sitting for immediate facial reanimation results till the repaired facial nerve starts functioning.

The patients in such cases are clearly explained that the outcome may not be excellent due to long-term denervation of facial muscles.

The viability of muscle fibers, sustaining even after a long period extending beyond 3 years, has been explained in the literature, that in spite of complete facial nerve denervation, the muscle fibers can get reinnervation from nerves in the vicinity, like fifth cranial nerve through branches of communication.

2. Long-term facial nerve palsy with proximal or distal portion of facial nerve unavailable, or the facial nerve not developed (Moebius syndrome) or mimic muscles atrophied due to long-term facial nerve palsy (duration of 2–3 years with EMG showing facial muscles atrophy or >3 years with or without EMG)

These cases are not going to improve by performing primary surgeries on facial nerve like nerve repair, grafting, or nerve transfer because of the nonavailability of proximal or distal stump of facial nerve and long-term denervation of the facial muscles leading to atrophy of muscle fibers and motor end plates. The choice of surgery is either dynamic or static procedures for facial reanimation. The nerve transfer like cranial nerves (CN) V–VII anastomosis can also be used, although not as primary surgery, but as a "babysitter" procedure along with dynamic procedure named "free micro neurovascular muscle transfer (FMMT)." Dynamic reconstruction and static procedures for facial reanimation are used separately or as combination of multiple procedures or used along with primary nerve repair. As different procedures are designed for different parts of the face, thorough examination of the whole face is conducted by dividing it into three anatomical regions. An independent analysis of upper, mid, and lower face is done and rehabilitation of each of these interconnected regions is planned according to the dysfunction in different parts. All these procedures require thorough education and counseling of the patient prior to surgery regarding the limited movements restored or achieved through these procedures.

For treatment purpose, the face can be divided into upper face (forehead, eyes), midface including nose , and lower face (oral) region. The region of the eye can be further divided into eyebrow, upper eyelid, ocular surface, and lower eyelid.

For forehead and eyes region, usually static procedures are performed, whereas in midface and oral region both dynamic and static procedures are performed in combination. Along with them, adjuvant therapy also forms part of the protocol.

The different procedures are:

Static Procedures

The different static procedures for different zones of the face can be performed separately or in combination and these include:

- Brow lift.
- Eye:
  - Temporary tarsorrhaphy.
  - Upper eyelid implants, palpebral spring.
  - Lower eyelid procedures like canthopexy and wedge resection.
- Face-lift.
- Static slings.

Dynamic Reconstruction Procedures

These include the following:

- FMMT with masseter nerve transfer in single-stage or cross-face nerve graft in two-stage surgery.
- Muscle transposition or dynamic transplant:
  - Temporalis muscle.

- Masseter muscle.
- Lengthening temporalis myoplasty (Labbe's technique).
- Anterior belly of digastric muscle transplant.

Adjuvant Procedures

These include:

- Physiotherapy.
- Botulinum toxoid injections.

These have been discussed in detail in Chapter 10 "Management of Nerve Regeneration Complications."

■ Static Corrections for Asymmetry

Static correction aims to correct facial asymmetry at rest only. The static procedures do not reproduce the dynamic movement of the face, although the advantages are that they provide eye closure, corneal protection, improve the nasal airway, and prevent drooling from oral cavity.

Indications

- Long-term facial nerve palsy without viable facial muscles.
- Cases of malignancy of parotid invading whole thickness of facial nerve and/or its peripheral branches.
- Extensive crushing trauma of the face, damaging the peripheral branches of facial nerve.
- Tumor removal causing damage to the extratemporal part of facial nerve along with its peripheral branches.
- In cases where dynamic procedures have failed.
- As an additional procedure with primary facial nerve repair for early recovery.
- Patients unfit for major surgical procedure.

Through static procedures, the goal of treatment is to restore symmetry in all three facial zones, namely, upper, middle, and lower face, by modifying either the affected side, the normal side of the face, or both.

Upper Face

Management of the upper third of the face involves the restoration of brow symmetry and protection of the eye.

Eyebrow

The frontalis-orbicularis oculi antagonistic muscle complex acts as a secondary elevator of eyelid. Whereas the orbital portion of the orbicularis oculi along with the procerus and corrugator muscles form the depressor of the eyebrow. This way they act together to close the eyelids. All these muscles are supplied by temporal branch of facial nerve. Any dysfunction of eyebrow elevator muscles can produce brow ptosis. This ptosis is more in the lateral part of eyebrow due to less fibers of frontalis muscle and more retro-orbicularis oculi fat pad. The lowering of brow along with loss of muscle tone can cause redundant skin (especially in old people) between eyebrow and the eyelid to hang on eyelid margin leading to cosmetic deformity and vision compromise due to obstruction of the upper visual field, especially in elderly patients.

Surgical Repair

Open brow approaches or the endoscopic correction has been developed for achieving brow elevation. Endoscopic approach is slightly better as there is negligible scar, less sensory loss, and faster recovery. The results can be enhanced by using botulinum injections to suppress hyperactive muscles on the contralateral side of the brow.

Procedure

Incision is placed just along the superior line of hair follicles (**Fig. 9.1**). An ellipse of the skin and frontalis muscle is excised and resuturing is done. A bit of overcorrection is needed to bring symmetry with the normally active healthy side.

Upper Eyelid

Upper eyelid is responsible for most of lubrication, protection, and clearance of ocular surface of the eye. If the eyelid is drooping low as in ptosis, it can protect eye but obscure the vision and if eyelid is not closing and remains retracted, the vision is good, but the protection of ocular surface is gone leading to excessive tearing, foreign body sensation, keratitis, vision loss, etc.

The muscles responsible for retraction of upper eyelid are levator palpebrae superioris supplied by oculomotor nerve and Horner superior tarsal muscle supplied by branches of sympathetic nervous system. Eyelid closure is due to the contraction of palpebral part of orbicularis oculi muscle (anatomy described in Chapter 2 "Facial Nerve Anatomy") supplied by facial nerve. In patients with long-standing facial nerve palsy, the upper eyelid rests in an elevated position due to paralysis of orbicularis oculi muscle leading to unopposed action of elevators. Varying degrees of lagophthalmos (inability to close the eyelids) is noticed with loss of both reflexive involuntary blinking and voluntary eye closure.

Inability to close the eye also leads to abnormal functioning of lacrimal pump mechanism, which is the function of lacrimal part of orbicularis oculi muscle. There is abnormal distribution of tears on the affected side leading to tear overflow or epiphora.

To examine upper eyelid closure, the patient is asked to first lightly close the eye and then tightly close the eye with full force. The patient is asked to resist manual opening by the clinician. The patient should be examined both in sitting and supine position for eyelid closure so as to rule out the aid of gravity. Also, the degree of Bell's phenomenon (reflexive upward rotation of the eyeball with the closure of eyelid) should be noticed.

Surgical Repair

The primary goal in addressing the eye in facial paralysis is the preservation of vision and avoidance of exposure keratopathy. This can be achieved by the following procedures.

Temporary Lateral Tarsorrhaphy

It is a temporary procedure performed till there is planning for some definitive surgical procedure or in case there is chance of self-recovery. It is performed by the ophthalmologists to protect the cornea during this short duration till the corrective procedures take over. It narrows the palpebral fissure by approximating parts of the eyelids, which helps in eyelid closure (suturing of free outer edge of the upper and lower eyelids together).

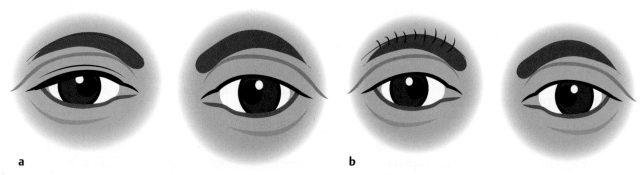

a   b

Fig. 9.1 **(a)** Illustration showing incision site right eyebrow (*red mark*) with lax and drooping right upper eyelid. **(b)** Illustration showing corrected right upper eyelid and eyebrow after surgery.

Procedure: Surgical apposition of lateral part of both upper and lower eyelids is performed with nonabsorbable sutures in a mattress fashion. The suture enters partial thickness (skin and orbicularis oculi) through upper eyelid, beginning 5 mm above the eyelid margin and exiting at the gray line of the eyelid margin. The suture continues as a margin-to-mid eyelid suture passing through the lower eyelid (exiting through the orbicularis oculi and skin 5 mm below the eyelid margin). The suture ends can be tied over bolsters made of rubber tubing. The suture is tied like a shoe lace, with a bow to facilitate tying and untying in future (**Fig. 9.2**).

Upper Eyelid Implants
These implants work on the principle that the eye opens due to the action of levator palpebrae superioris muscle supplied by the oculomotor nerve (CN III), whereas the eye closes due to the action of orbicularis oculi, which is supplied by facial nerve (CN VII). As the levator relaxes, the orbicularis contracts and vice versa. In the paralyzed eyelid, due to facial nerve palsy, the closure does not happen. The predetermined weight of gold/platinum chain placed in upper eyelid helps to substitute the action of paralyzed orbicularis oculi and the eye closes completely (gravity-dependent closure). The different materials used for loading the upper eyelid have kept changing over time. The ones which are still in use are gold or platinum implants and palpebral springs etc. Gold weights are most commonly used due to their malleable and inert quality.

These procedures are generally easy to do and performed under local anesthesia only. The procedure can be reversed easily. Good symptomatic relief from corneal exposure is achieved and cosmetic improvement is also there. Surgical success of upper eyelid procedures is defined as at least 50% reduction in lagophthalmos and induction of less than 2 mm of ptosis.

The disadvantage is possibility of its extrusion in later years as depicted in **Fig. 9.3**.

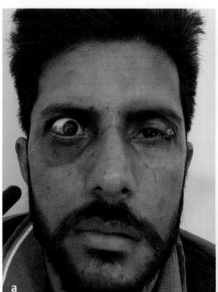
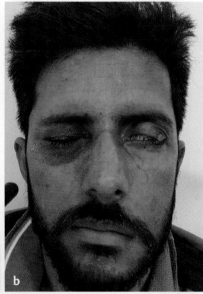

Fig. 9.2 (a, b) Tarsorapphy performed on eyelids (left side).

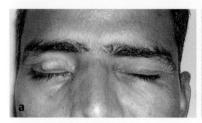
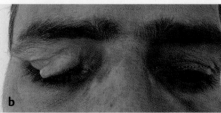

Fig. 9.3 (a, b) The lateral end of implant is showing signs of extrusion after 6 years of surgery.

Procedure: Select the appropriate gold weight preoperatively by taping a series of weights (used in chemistry lab) to the upper eyelid (**Fig. 9.4**) till the patient is able to achieve complete eyelid closure. The implants are designed as per individual needs. In the author's cases so far, mostly the weight required were between 1.5 to 2 g.

Implant is made up of 24 carat gold. Length of implant is middle two-thirds of the length of upper eyelid measured from medial to lateral canthus. The breadth of implant measures 5 mm at the medial end and 4 mm at the lateral end, as a fractionally greater weight is required to close the medial end.

The right curvature is acquired by placing a flexometalic strip on the contour of upper eyelid. The edges of the implant are rounded and smoothened. There are three holes in the implant for fixation to surrounding soft tissue and partial thickness of tarsal plate.

Case 1: Operated Case of Extensive Facial Nerve Schwannoma Involving the Intracranial and Intratemporal Segments with Grade VI Facial Palsy (Right Side)

Excision of facial nerve schwannoma was performed in first stage 6 months back. This is the second-stage surgery where the patient is taken up for facial reanimation. Preoperative pictures show grade VI facial palsy on the right side (**Fig. 9.5**). Facio-masseteric anastomosis with static reanimation procedures in the form of gold implant surgery is performed together in the same sitting. Gold implant is for immediate protection of eye till the nerve fibers regenerate through facio-masseteric anastomosis. Facio-masseteric anastomosis has already been described in Chapter 8 titled "Short Duration Flaccid Facial Palsy with Proximal Stump Unavailable."

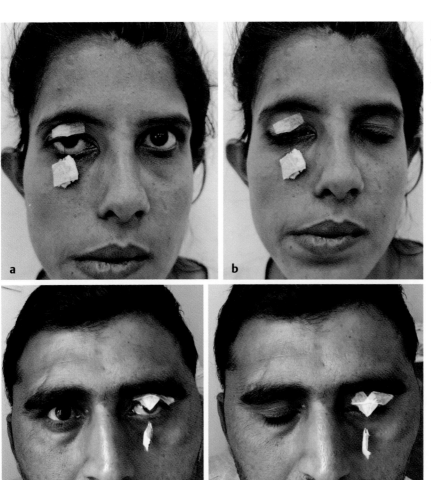

Fig. 9.4 (a–d) Appropriate gold weight is being selected preoperatively by taping a series of weights (1.5g in **Fig. 9.4a, b** and 1.95g in **Fig. 9.4c, d**) to the upper eyelid.

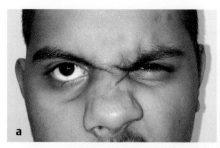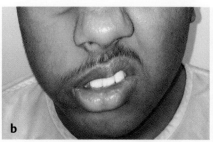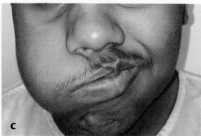

Fig. 9.5 **(a–c)** Preoperative pictures of patient face showing grade VI facial nerve palsy on right side.

Surgical Steps (Figs. 9.6–9.10)

- Surgery is performed under local anesthesia.
- A corneal protector is fixed with 6-0 ethilon to protect the cornea.
- Vernier caliper is used to measure the distance between the eyelid margin and the incision line.
- The incision line is marked about 6 mm from the inferior eyelid margin (**Fig. 9.6**).
- Two percent xylocaine with adrenaline (1 in 100,000) is injected into the upper eyelid.
- A 2-cm incision is made with a scalpel in the middle two-thirds of the eyelid through the skin and subcutaneous tissue in the marked line (**Fig. 9.7**).
- The incision is enlarged through the skin and subcutaneous tissue with the help of microscissors.
- The fibers of the orbicularis oculi muscle are incised (along the direction of muscle fibers) by going vertically down and medially toward tarsal plate and the tarsal plate is exposed (**Fig. 9.8**).
- A pocket is created on both sides of incision for placing the implant between the orbicularis oculi and the tarsal plate. This pocket extends medially and laterally further from the incision site. The tarsal plate is exposed up to the orbital septum. The lower end of pocket should remain 3 mm above the lash line so that the final placement of implant should be 3 mm above the eyelid margin. It is to avoid the implant reaching too close to the roots of the eyelashes.
- The gold weight should be centered over the medial limbus of the iris.
- While placing the implant, it should lie directly on the tarsal plate and the broader side of the implant should be on the medial side (**Fig. 9.9**).
- The gold implant is fixed by passing 6-0 ethilon sutures through the holes in the implant and soft tissue lateral to it. The suture can be anchored through partial thickness of the tarsal plate. Complete thickness should be avoided as the plate contains glands and there can be chances of infection once the glands are damaged. The suture is additionally run around the implant to suture it superiorly as well as inferiorly and achieve maximum anchorage (**Fig. 9.10**).
- The underside of the eyelid is inspected to ensure that the conjunctiva has not been breached.
- The fibers of orbicularis oculi muscle are then sutured back with interrupted 5-0 vicryl sutures.
- The skin incision is sutured with 6-0 fast absorbable sutures.

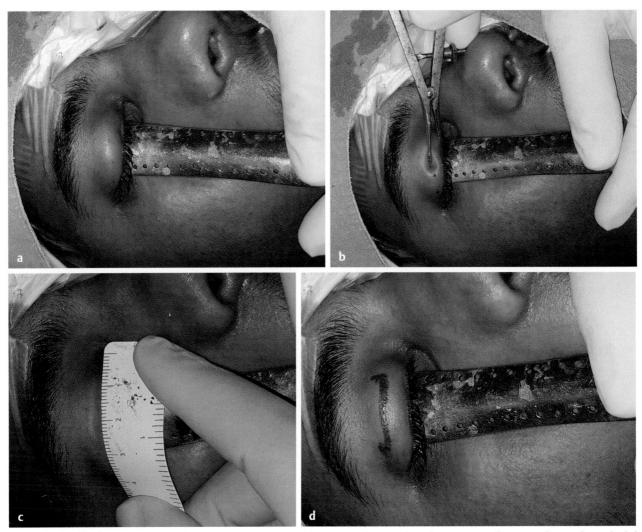

Fig. 9.6 **(a)** Corneal protector in place to protect the eye. **(b)** Vernier caliper is placed to measure distance of 6mm from the lid margin for giving incision. **(c)** 2 cms long incision marking is measured in the mid of upper eyelid (middle 2/3rd of upper eyelid), 6 mm from the lid margin. **(d)** The incision line is marked with a marker.

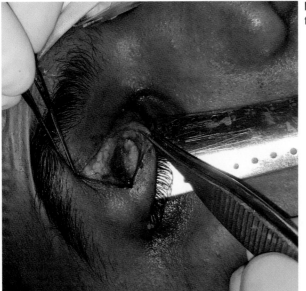

Fig. 9.7   2 cm long skin incision given in the middle 2/3rd of lid through skin and subcutaneous tissue over the marked line.

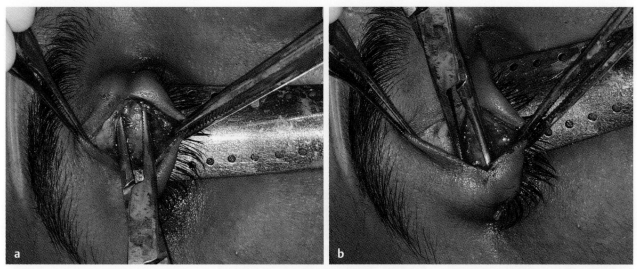

Fig. 9.8 **(a, b)** Incising and separating the fibres of the orbicularis oculi muscle (along the direction of muscle fibres) till the tarsal plate is reached and exposed. A pocket on either side of incision is being created for the implant to be placed between the orbicularis oculi and the tarsal plate.

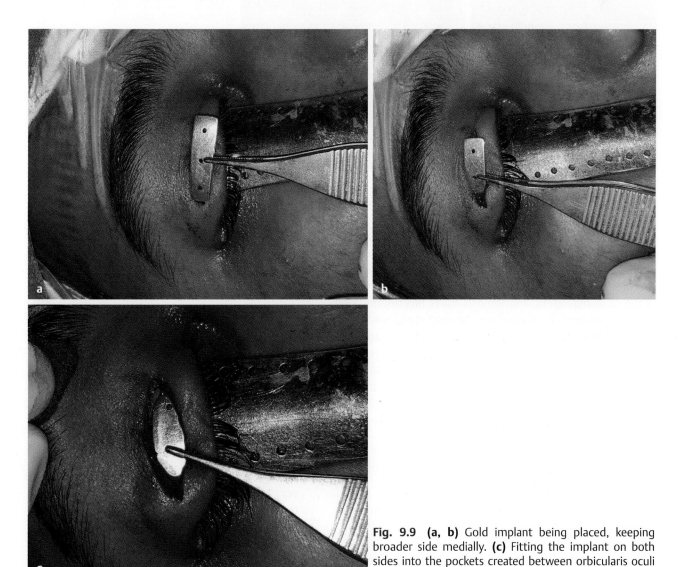

Fig. 9.9 **(a, b)** Gold implant being placed, keeping broader side medially. **(c)** Fitting the implant on both sides into the pockets created between orbicularis oculi and tarsal plate on both sides of incision.

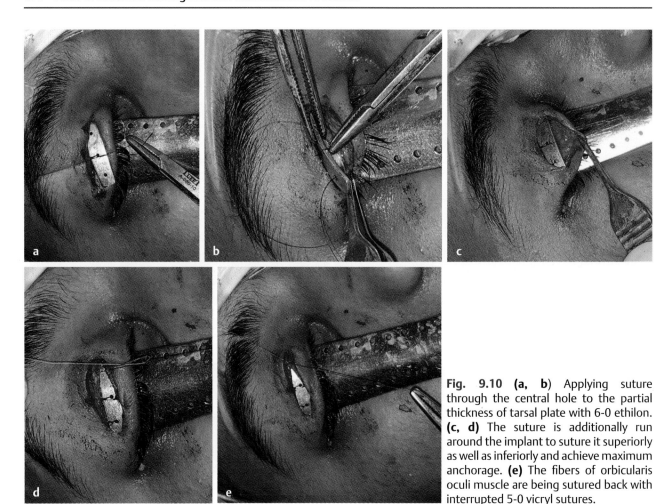

Fig. 9.10 (a, b) Applying suture through the central hole to the partial thickness of tarsal plate with 6-0 ethilon. **(c, d)** The suture is additionally run around the implant to suture it superiorly as well as inferiorly and achieve maximum anchorage. **(e)** The fibers of orbicularis oculi muscle are being sutured back with interrupted 5-0 vicryl sutures.

Postoperative Outcome

Immediate and 3 months postoperative results (as depicted in **Fig. 9.11**) showed grade VI facial palsy of the right side persisting but the closure of upper eyelid is achieved with gold implant. After 1 year of surgery, as the facio-masseteric anastomosis starts functioning, and facial recovery is taking place, the right eyelid could be closed voluntarily with angle of mouth lifting and the patient regaining smile. The patient was instructed to learn to smile with action of biting. Over the next 6 months, the patient learned to dissociate both actions and now he can smile without the action of bite. After 18 months, the gold implant could be removed, with upper eyelid closing on its own (**Fig. 9.11g, h**).

Advantages

This is the simplest, most reliable, and reproducible of all the procedures performed for upper eyelid loading. The implant is easily available commercially and can be performed under local anesthesia. It has lowest rejection rate and lowest complication rate as far as cosmetic deformity is concerned. It can be easily revised or

reversed, once the eyelid moment is recovered in certain cases post repair of facial nerve (**Fig. 9.11g**).

Disadvantages

- There can be inadequate upper eyelid closure if the weight of gold implant is less than required and overclosure of upper eyelid if the weight of gold implant is more than required.
- Extrusion of gold implant can also take place. The causes can be many which include surgical errors like not placing the implant in the right plane, not applying proper sutures (extra run around the implant for stability), sutures giving way (**Fig. 9.3**), constant irritation over eyelid skin leading to lot of rubbing by the patient leading to extrusion, and finally, if the choice of patient is not right like in very old patients with skin of upper eyelid being too loose and thin. The implant can be too prominent at times and its shape reflects through the skin of upper eyelid. At times the contour of the implant may not match the contour of the upper eyelid leading to extrusion of the implant.

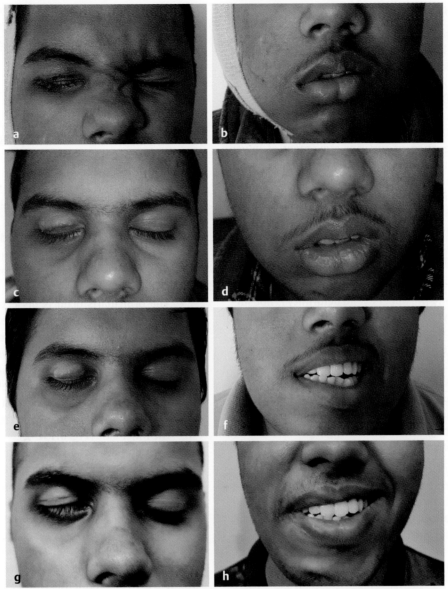

Fig. 9.11 **(a, b)** Immediate postsurgery (facio-masseteric anastomosis and upper eyelid gold implant) pictures showing right side grade VI palsy persisting but upper eyelid closure is achieved. **(c, d)** Pictures showing facial palsy of the right side persisting with eye closure achieved 3 months post surgery. **(e, f)** Pictures showing complete closure of upper eyelid, with gold implant in place, and facial nerve recovery of up to grade III after 1 year of surgery. **(g)** Pictures showing closure of right upper eyelid after removal of gold implant and **(h)** the patient regaining smile 18 months post surgery.

Lower Eyelid Surgery (Figs. 9.12–9.14)

This is performed for correction of paralytic ectropion. The lower eyelid provides a stable platform against which the upper eyelid rests during sleep leading to complete seal of ocular surface during sleep and intentional closure. Depression of lower eyelid is by the capsulopalpebral fascia supplied by oculomotor nerve and the inferior tarsal muscle supplied by sympathetic nervous system. Elevation or superior movement of lower eyelid is by contraction of orbicularis oculi which is supplied by facial nerve. In long-standing facial nerve palsy, there is unrestricted depression or retraction along with ectropion of lower eyelid (outward turning of lower eyelid caused by gravitational pull of atonic cheek) due to paralysis of orbicularis oculi muscle leading to incomplete closure of eye, epiphora, exposure keratitis, and cosmetic deformity.

Correcting only the upper eyelid deformity is not sufficient to achieve complete closure of the eyelids, tear drainage, and the distribution system. Lower eyelid retraction and ectropion also need to be corrected by certain surgical procedures to lift it and improve its position, reduce watering, and complete the closure of the eye. Surgical outcomes are considered favorable when the lower eyelid rests at the limbus, while acceptable when the lower eyelid margin rests within 1 mm above or below the lower limbus.

Before surgery, the position of the lower eyelid should be assessed, noting the extent and location of retraction of lower eyelid and extent of widening of the eyelid aperture. Lateral ectropion can be surgically addressed by a lateral tarsal strip procedure or a lateral transorbital canthopexy, while laxity in the medial portion of the lower eyelid can be corrected by performing a medial canthopexy.

Case 2: Operated Case of Chronic Otitis Media with Iatrogenic Facial Palsy (mostly involving upper part of face) of Thirteen Years Duration (Right Side)

This being long-term facial palsy, with EMG showing silent graph, primary repair is not the procedure of choice. The upper eyelid closure is achieved by gold implant in the first stage. The lower eyelid laxity and retraction is corrected by lateral canthoplexy procedure, in which lateral tarsal strip is elevated and sutured to the periosteum inside the lateral orbital rim. This simple procedure tightens the lower eyelid by around 6 mm.

Preoperative picture shows inability to close upper eyelid and laxity of lower eyelid more in lateral part (**Fig. 9.12a**). Upper eyelid gold implant surgery was first performed and the closure of upper eyelid could be

achieved. The lateral ectropion and retraction of lower eyelid persisted (**Fig. 9.12b**) for which the second surgery in the form of lateral canthoplexy was performed after 3 months of the first surgery.

Surgical Procedure (Fig. 9.13)

- The incision is marked in lateral part of the eye (lateral canthus) and another mark is placed, which decides how much tightening is required (**Fig. 9.13a**).
- Local anesthesia is instilled in the lateral canthus area involving lateral end of both lower and upper eyelids deep up to orbital rim.
- A horizontal incision is made starting at the junction of upper and lower eyelids, through skin, orbicularis oculi, and down to orbital rim (**Fig. 9.13b**).
- The orbicularis oculi is dissected and the orbital rim exposed by using cotton peanuts.
- After holding the lateral edge of tarsal plate, it is stripped by creating plane between the tarsal plate and orbicularis oculi on outer side. The upper edge is trimmed off to remove eyelid margin in that limited area. The exposed extra part of tarsal plate is trimmed after clearing it from conjunctiva on the inner side (**Fig. 9.13c–g**).
- Tarsal plate is sutured to the orbital rim with double armed 5-0 prolene. Initially, suture passed with help of one needle from anterior to posterior at the upper free margin of tarsal plate and then with second needle from anterior to posterior at the lower border of tarsal plate to have a total control of the eyelid (**Fig. 9.13h**). The superior string of suture is tied to periosteum of superior part of orbital rim from inside outwards and in the same manner, inferior string of suture is tied to slightly inferior part of orbital rim, and then the two sutures are pulled along the natural curve of the lower eyelid toward the orbital rim in a way that it puts lateral canthus in the accurate position (**Fig. 9.13i–l**). At least three knots are to be tied. Now before trimming off the sutures, each prolene needle is passed posteriorly and trimmed at the exit point (**Fig. 9.13l**). The excess skin is trimmed off (**Fig. 9.13m**).
- Orbicularis oculi is sutured back with 6-0 vikoryl suture to cover the prolene knots.
- Tarsal plates are sutured. Skin is also sutured back (**Fig. 9.13n**).

Complete closure of the upper and lower eyelids with correction of ectropion of lower eyelid could be achieved post surgery, and results 3 months post surgery is shown in **Fig. 9.14**.

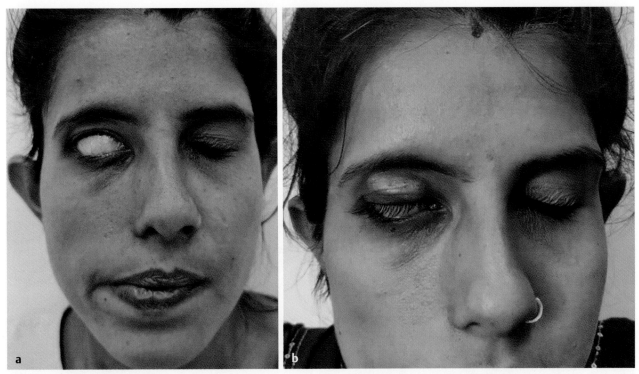

Fig. 9.12 **(a)** Picture showing paralysis of both upper and lower eyelids before surgery. **(b)** Picture showing upper eyelid closure after upper eyelid gold implant surgery. The lower eyelid is retracted with ectropion in lateral part leading to incomplete closure of the eye.

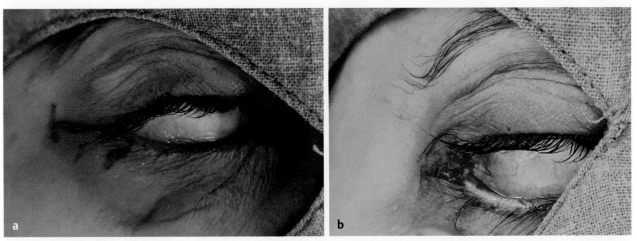

Fig. 9.13 **(a)** Incision marks in lateral part of the eye (lateral canthus). **(b)** Incision made at the junction of the upper and lower eyelids, through skin, orbicularis oculi, and down to orbital rim. (*Continued*)

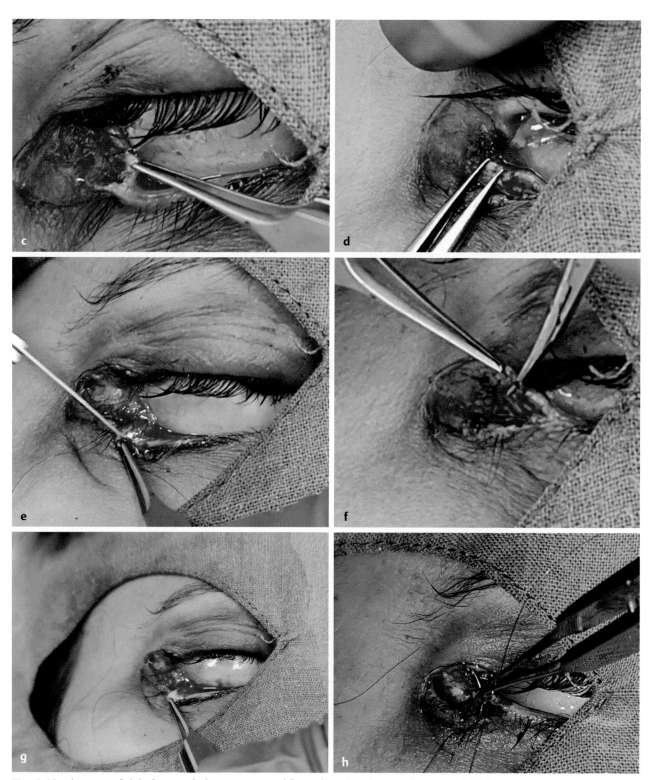

Fig. 9.13 (*Continued*) **(c)** The tarsal plate is separated from the orbicularis oculi muscle. **(d)** The length of tarsal plate to be trimmed to achieve optimal tightening is measured with vernier caliper. **(e)** Separation of tarsal plate from conjunctiva. **(f)** The excess tarsal plate trimmed. **(g)** After trimming the excess tarsal plate, the suture is applied. **(h)** The suture is passed through upper and lower part of tarsal plate with the help of 5-0 prolene suture with needle at its both ends. (*Continued*)

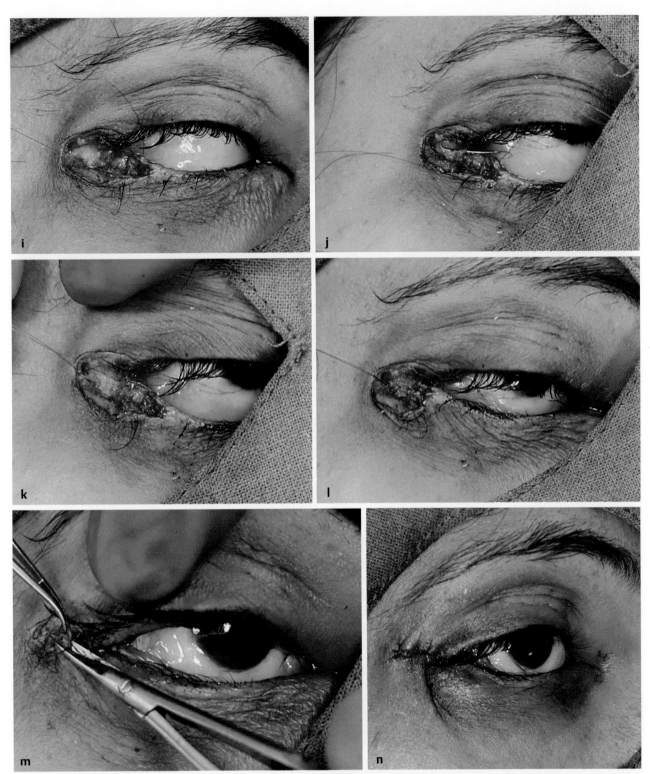

Fig. 9.13 (*Continued*) **(i)** The double armed suture passed through the upper and lower part of tarsal plate lateral margin. **(j)** The superior string of suture is tied to periosteum of superior part of orbital rim from inside outwards and in the same manner, inferior string of suture is tied to slightly inferior part of orbital rim. **(k)** The two sutures are pulled along the natural curve of the lower eyelid toward the orbital rim. **(l)** Both ends of prolene suture are tied to each other and each prolene needle is passed further posteriorly and trimmed at the exit point. **(m)** The excess skin is trimmed off. **(n)** Final skin sutures in place.

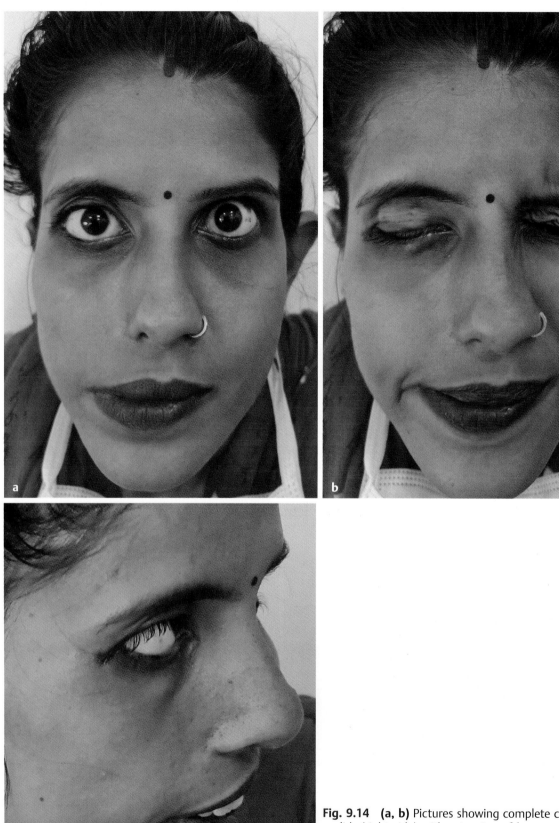

Fig. 9.14   (a, b) Pictures showing complete closure of both eyelids (right side) with ectropion of lower eyelid corrected 3 months post surgery. **(c)** Picture showing completely healed surgical site.

Ocular Surface

Due to malposition of both upper and lower eyelids, there is lagophthalmos and incomplete blink reflex in the affected eye leading to damage to the ocular surface of eye in the form of drying and damage to corneal surface leading to abrasion, ulceration, or in extreme stages perforation of cornea leading to endophthalmitis and loss of eye.

Timely correction of functioning of eyelids can prevent all complications and prevent the cosmetic deformity of the face. To avoid damage to cornea, till the procedures take place, lubrication of ocular surface can be achieved with artificial tears in the day time and artificial tear ointments at night.

Midface

In midface, long-term facial palsy leads to loss of facial muscles functioning resulting in laxity and drooping of the affected side of the face, especially in aged patients. It leads to impaired facial expressions, facial deformity, and difficulty in speech, smile, and eating. It may also lead to obstruction of nasal airway.

Treatment of the midface deformities aims to alleviate this obstruction of the nasal airway and to counteract the forces of gravity on the malar soft tissues. It includes suspension of parts of the face by a sling or face-lift.

Other Static Procedures

Most techniques for static facial reconstruction involve suspension of parts of the face by a sling. Static facial slings are commonly used to suspend the oral commissure, which results in improved facial symmetry and oral competence. Surgical exposure for the placement of a static sling can be obtained via a preauricular rhytidectomy incision and incisions at the vermilion border of the upper lip, lower lip, and oral commissure. A cheek-temple flap is elevated medially to the level of the nasolabial fold and orbicularis oris muscle, which is dissected circumferentially from the surrounding skin and mucosa. Temporalis fascia, tensor fascia lata, or tendon can be harvested if autogenous tissue is desired; autogenous tissue is preferred over polytetrafluoroethylene for immediate reconstruction in patients with a history of radiation therapy. The grafts selected are sutured laterally to the temporal fascia or zygoma and medially to the corner of the lip, and tension is adjusted to achieve the ideal amount of elevation.

Multiple-vector suspension is a procedure in which the lateral canthus, melolabial crease, and lower lip are suspended with nonabsorbable sutures and/or polytetrafluoroethylene through several small stab incisions. Slings can also be used to suspend a collapsed nostril by pulling the lateral alar base to the ascending maxillary buttress. Subperiosteal midfacial suspension—including a suborbicularis oculi fat lift (SOOF) via a temporal, lower eyelid, and buccal approach—allows for suspension of stretched and atrophied facial muscles for improved static facial symmetry.

Cheek

Paralysis of the midface becomes quite obvious and needs addressal. Face-lift surgeries help in reducing the disfigurement of the face and also prevent nasal valve stenosis (**Fig. 9.15**). Different threads create different effects (such as firming or lifting), for example, long bidirectional slings (barbed suture lift), or long unidirectional threads (contour threads). These threads can be used in conjunction with traditional open face-lift surgery or endoscopic techniques.

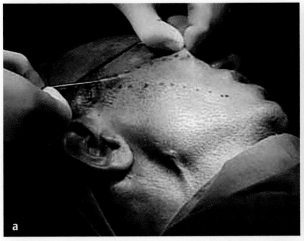
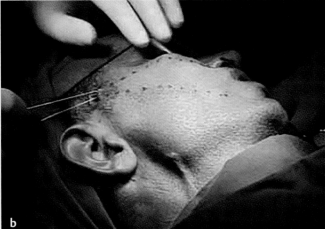

Fig. 9.15   (a, b) Face-lift procedure with barbed suture lift.

Nose

Same procedure as described above or a percutaneously placed fascia lata sling to suspend the nasolabial fold is performed. This also improves the nasal valve collapse.

Lower Face

Disability in the lower face resulting from facial paralysis consists mainly of oral incompetence leading to loss of smile, poor articulation, drooling, and difficulty in chewing food. Static slings, suspended from the zygomatic arch or deep temporal fascia to support the oral commissure and upper lip, lead to the elevation of these structures.

Static Slings

Slight overcorrection is better than undercorrection as the tissue gets lax after few months and overcorrection at rest adds to the symmetry when the patient is smiling.

Case 3: Operated Case of Extensive Facial Nerve Schwannoma Involving the Intracranial and Intratemporal Segments with Grade VI Facial Palsy (Right Side)

The excision of facial nerve schwannoma was performed in the first stage, 6 months back. This is the second stage surgery where the patient is taken up for facial reanimation. Preoperative pictures show grade VI facial palsy of the right side with inability to close upper eyelid and lift the angle of mouth (**Fig. 9.16a, b**). Facio-masseteric anastomosis is performed in the second stage. Static reanimation procedures like upper eyelid gold implant and fascia lata sling surgery are performed together in the third stage almost 2 months after the second surgery,

as the patient was not ready for the static implants in the second stage. Static procedures are performed for immediate protection of the eye till the nerve fibers regenerate through facio-masseteric anastomosis. Facio-masseteric anastomosis has already been described in Chapter 8 "Management of Short and Intermediate Duration Flaccid Facial Palsy with Proximal Stump Unavailable."

Surgical Procedure (Fig. 9.17)

- A long fascia lata sling is harvested from the thigh. One side of this sling is divided into three slips.
- The harvested sling is placed on the affected side between the angle of mouth and the temporal region to measure the size (**Fig. 9.17a, b**).
- Then a tunnel is created under the subcutaneous tissue on that side from orbicularis oris to temporalis muscle tendon.
- The modiolus (a chiasma of facial muscles held together by fibrous tissue, located lateral and slightly superior to angle of the mouth on each side, which is important in moving the mouth and creating facial expression) is identified.
- Three vertical stab incisions are made in the midline of the upper and lower lips and modiolus and one stab incision is made in the temporal region above zygomatic arch (**Fig. 9.17c**).
- The sling is passed through the tunnel and taken out on surface through the stab incisions on both sides (**Fig. 9.17c–e**). Out of three slips on one side of fascial sling, the upper slip is passed through the stab incision on the upper lip and sutured around the orbicularis oris with a nonabsorbable suture (4-0 prolene). The lower slip is secured to the lower lip, a bit tighter than that of the upper lip and the final slip is anchored to the orbicularis oris at the modiolus.

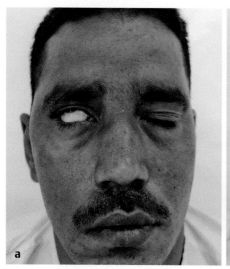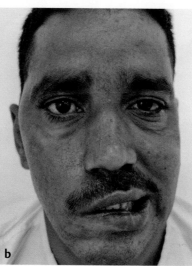

Fig. 9.16 (a, b) Preoperative pictures (before the second stage surgery) showing grade VI facial palsy of the right side.

- The proximal end of fascial sling is sutured under tension to deep temporalis fascia (**Fig. 9.17f**).

After 9 months of facio-masseteric surgery and 7 months of static procedures, facial symmetry at rest along with closure of upper eyelid could be achieved along with voluntary lifting of angle of mouth on the right side (**Fig. 9.18**).

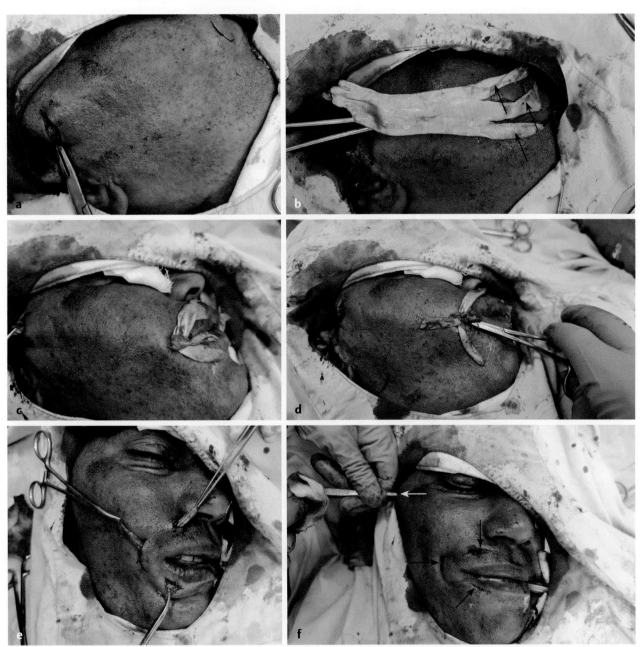

Fig. 9.17 **(a)** Picture showing stab incision made in temporal region superior to zygomatic arch for taking out the proximal end of fascia lata sling and suturing to deep temporal fascia. **(b)** The harvested fascia lata broad strip is placed in its final location on the right side of the face (between the angle of mouth and the temporal region) to measure the exact size required. The distal end of fascial sling is divided into three slips (*arrows*). **(c)** After giving stab incision over modiolus, tunnel is created on the face beneath the subcutaneous tissue, between the two stab incisions and the fascial sling is passed through it. **(d)** All three slips on the distal end of fascia sling are taken out from the stab incision in the region of oral commissure. **(e)** Two more vertical stab incisions in the midpoint between angle of mouth and midpoint of upper and lower lip are made. The upper slip of the fascia lata sling is passed through the upper incision and sutured around the orbicularis oris with a nonabsorbable suture (4-0 prolene). The lower slip is sutured to the orbicularis oris fibers in lower lip, a bit tighter than that of the upper lip and the third final slip is anchored to the modiolus (*black arrows*). **(f)** Final lifting of angle of mouth on right side after suturing the proximal end of the fascia lata sling under tension to deep temporalis fascia (*yellow arrow*).

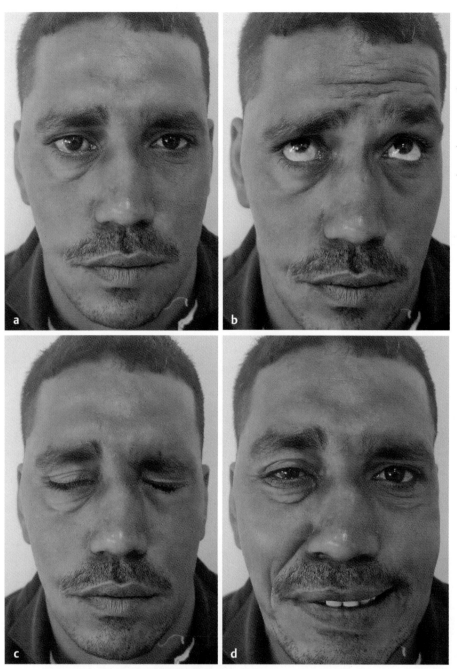

Fig. 9.18 Recovery of face, post surgery: **(a)** After 9 months of facio-masseteric anastomosis and static procedures, facial symmetry at rest can be visualized. **(b)** Wrinkling of forehead not appeared **(c)** Upper eyelid closing perfectly after gold implant and **(d)** Angle of mouth regaining voluntary movement on the right side (due to facial nerve recovery leading to regeneration of facial muscles).

Case 4: A Case of Adenocystic Carcinoma Parotid with Grade VI Facial Palsy (Left Side)

First surgery in the form of total parotidectomy was performed followed by complete course of radiotherapy and chemotherapy. Although the facial nerve could be preserved, as the disease had already invaded the extratemporal part of facial nerve. After taking complete course of radiotherapy and chemotherapy, the second stage surgery including of static procedures in the form of gold implant in the upper eyelid and fascia lata sling surgery for midface were performed.

Fig. 9.19 depicts the images of face after the first surgery and radiotherapy and chemotherapy course. The images show grade VI facial palsy left side. **Fig. 9.20** shows images 7 days post upper eyelid gold implant and facial sling surgery showing closure of upper eyelid and facial symmetry at rest. **Fig. 9.21** showing pictures of the face 3 months post second surgery. There is further improvement in the face at rest and complete closure of the eye and with lifting of drooping angle of mouth, the face looks symmetrical at rest.

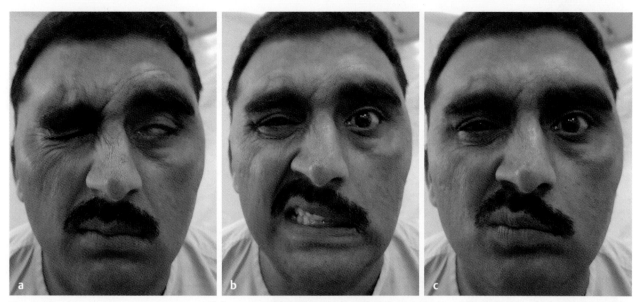

Fig. 9.19 **(a–c)** Preoperative pictures of the patient showing grade VI facial nerve palsy of the left side. Slight closure of the left eye can be visualized (due to incomplete involvement of facial nerve by the tumor).

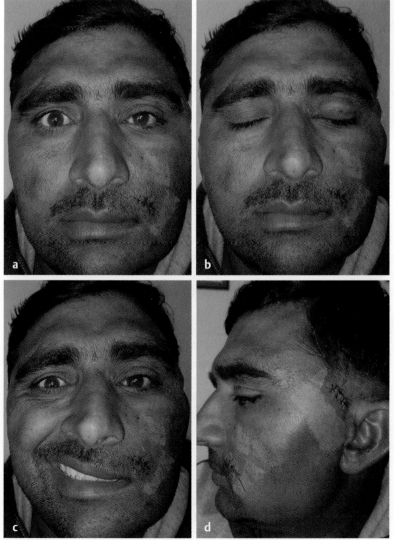

Fig. 9.20 **(a)** Immediate postsurgery result after static procedures shows facial symmetry at rest due to fascia lata sling. **(b)** Complete eye closure could be achieved with upper eyelid gold implant. **(c)** Absence of voluntary lifting of angle of mouth. **(d)** The suture lines in nasolabial fold and temporal region for suturing and holding fascia lata sling are visible (*red arrows*).

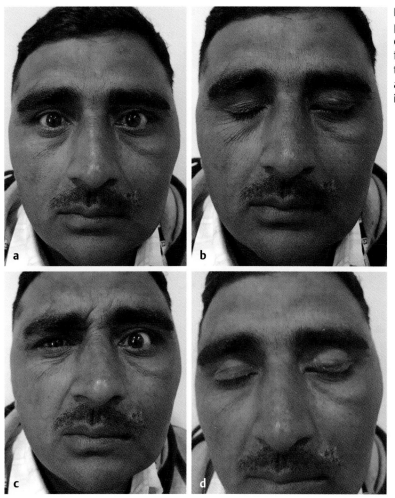

Fig. 9.21 (a–d) Pictures of the face 3 months post second surgery and radiotherapy and chemotherapy, with further improvement in facial symmetry at rest, complete closure of the eye, and voluntary lifting of angle of mouth achieved to some extent due to improvement in facial nerve functioning.

■ Dynamic Reconstruction

In dynamic reconstruction, a functional muscle is used to replace the functioning of atrophied and nonviable facial mimetic muscles. The functioning muscle usage can be in the form of locoregional muscle transposition or lengthening orFMMT. Locoregional muscle lying close to the facial muscles like temporalis or masseter muscle are the choice for replication of function. A specific muscle tendon unit (MTU) is chosen for replacing the function of the original facial muscle.

Biomechanics of Muscle Transfer

When a skeletal functional muscle is used to replicate the action of facial mimetic muscles, the minimal prerequisite is that the muscle should maintain a normal action of contraction as it is going to overtake the function of mimetic muscles.

Myofibrils, the contractile elements of skeletal muscles, are composed of actin and myosin proteins which generate the mechanical force to create muscle contraction. But if we put too much tension on these rotated, transpositioned fibers, it can disturb the actin–myosin interaction leading to reduced contraction of muscle fibers. So, muscle is to be transferred in a way that it is not in a stretched form at rest and should maintain its pretransfer resting tension. To select the muscle, few important prerequisites are:

- The selected MTU should be causing minimal donor site morbidity.
- The selected MTU should have good contractility and its vector of contraction should be almost similar to that of the original set of muscles.
- A soft tissue bed in the form of buccal pad of fat should be there around the transferred MTU for its free movement.
- The muscles around the oral commissure and modiolus should be flexible and strong enough to give support to the tension generated by transpositioned muscle tendon sutured to them.
- Innervation to transposed muscles should be intact.

- The insertion or suture point for transpositioned muscle is assessed prior to surgery by asking the patient for full smile and calculating by observing on the contralateral normal side. There are three types of smile out of which the lateral smile can be achieved easily by muscle transposition and the temporalis muscle transposition is considered the best because its vector of contraction is in upwards and lateral direction. Both the canine smile and the full smile are difficult to reproduce because trying to attain this level of smile results in oral incompetence which may further need correction.

Regional Muscle Transfer

The temporalis or the masseter muscle is used for dynamic reanimation, alone or in combination with upper eyelid implant for eye closure restoration in cases of long-term denervation and atrophy of facial muscles or absence of suitable mimetic muscles.

Retrograde Temporal Muscle Transplant

Sir Harold Gilles (1934) originally described the temporalis muscle flap with fascia lata graft to reach the oral commissure. The temporalis muscle is innervated by the trigeminal nerve. The muscle can be used to provide static support to the oral commissure and trigeminal-innervated dynamic movement.

Surgical Steps

Separate the temporal muscle from temporal fossa, and turn it down in front of or deeper to zygomatic arch to reach orbicularis oris. Additional fascia lata graft may be required. This technique gives static symmetry as well as voluntary activity based on trigeminal nerve. Care is taken not to injure the very thin facial nerve branches entering the orbicularis oris muscle (**Fig. 9.22**).

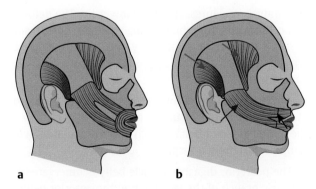

a   b

Fig. 9.22 (a) The middle part of temporalis muscle (*red arrow*) is rotated, leaving behind the anterior and posterior parts (*blue arrows*) and its cut end is bifurcated into two slips which are sutured to orbicularis oris in its superior and inferior parts close to modiolus directly or through **(b)** additional fascia lata graft (*black arrow*).

The disadvantage is that it gives a depression at the original site of temporalis muscle and an abnormal prominence in the region of cheek bone. So as a modification is done in which, only the middle part of muscle is rotated, leaving behind the anterior and posterior parts (**Fig. 9.22**). The cut end is bifurcated into two slips which are sutured to orbicularis oris in its superior and inferior parts close to modiolus. Fascia lata extension flap can be added to lengthen the MTU if it falls short. But the disadvantage is that it reduces the tensile force of the MTU.

Further modification came with the lengthening of the temporalis muscle (temporalis myoplasty) by Labbe which eliminates the use of fascia lata extension flap.

Temporalis Myoplasty

Temporalis myoplasty involves detaching the insertion of the temporalis muscle to the coronoid process of the mandible and transposing and inserting it around the orbicularis oris muscle. In spite of temporalis myoplasty providing good static control, it has a drawback in the form of not being able to recreate a spontaneous, dynamic smile as its activation requires clenching of the teeth. This technique is also not useful in cases of congenital facial palsy syndromes associated with other cranial nerve anomalies including CN V (trigeminal nerve). Severe temporalis atrophy, found in the edentulous patient, is another contraindication.

Surgical Steps (Fig. 9.23)

Posterior half of temporalis muscle is dissected in anterograde direction from its origin in the temporal fossa and reached up to zygomatic arch. The zygomatic arch is then detached using two osteotomies and the tendinous part of the temporalis is released further. Then it is detached from the coronoid process, and tunneled through the buccal fat pad to reach the mouth. The detaching of temporalis tendon from its insertion on the coronoid process is performed from the incision in nasolabial fold. Here the muscle is split into three slips, each sutured to orbicularis oris in the upper lip, modiolus, and lower lip. Temporalis myoplasty has been modified by many surgeons. Surgeons have modified the procedure to allow a more limited incision directly over the temporalis and without a need for zygomatic osteotomies.

Masseter Muscle Transplant

All or part of the masseter can be used as a local muscle flap for facial reanimation.

Surgical Steps (Fig. 9.24)

The anterior half of the muscle's insertion is detached from the lower mandibular border, transposed anteriorly, divided into three slips, and inserted into the

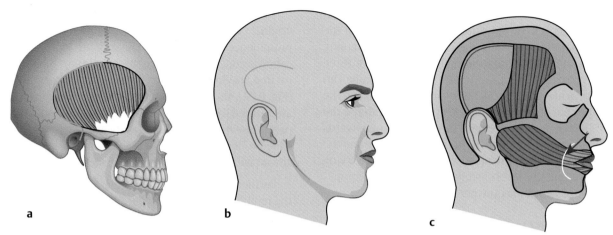

Fig. 9.23 (a–c) Illustration showing incision line in temporal region (*red line*). Temporalis muscle is exposed and posterior half of muscle dissected. The separation of the temporalis tendon from coronoid process is performed from the incision in nasolabial fold (*red arrow*). The tendon of temporalis muscle has been slid inferiorly through a tunnel to reach modiolus and its three slips are sutured to orbicularis oris in upper lip, modiolus, and lower lip.

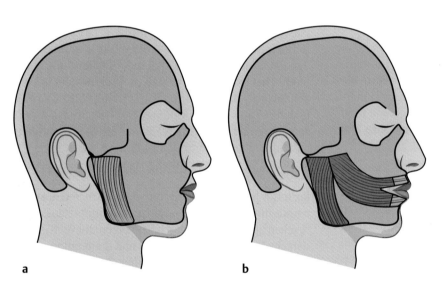

Fig. 9.24 (a, b) Anterior part of the masseter muscle has been detached from the lower mandibular border transposed anteriorly, divided into slips, and inserted into the dermis of upper lip, modiolus, and lower lip.

dermis of upper lip, modiolus, and lower lip (**Fig. 9.24**). This procedure gives motion to the lower half of the face and usually achieves good static control. This is usually performed in cases where the masseter muscle is already exposed in primary surgery (radical parotidectomy). Both temporalis and masseter muscles can also be transplanted together, temporalis for the upper lip and nasolabial fold and masseter for the corner of mouth and lower lip.

Anterior Belly of Digastric Muscle Transplantation (ABDMT)

Lower lip palsy is caused by the paralysis of marginal mandibular nerve. Cosmetic as well as functional deformity in the form of inability to depress, lateralize the lower lip, and evert the vermilion border is caused

by paralysis of depressors of the lower lip. The deformity becomes obvious while talking when the normal side has lip corner moving inferiorly and away from teeth, whereas on the paralyzed side lip corner remains in elevated form.

ABDMT is indicated for restoration of the depressor of the corner of the mouth in cases of isolated palsy of the marginal mandibular branch or in combination with temporalis muscle transplant.

The posterior digastric muscle belly is innervated by digastric branch of the facial nerve; the anterior belly is innervated by the nerve to mylohyoid, a branch from the inferior alveolar nerve of the mandibular division of the trigeminal nerve (V_3). So, anterior belly can be used as a nerve source for contraction of rest of the muscle when transplanted.

Surgical Procedure (Fig. 9.25)

Incision in submandibular region is made and subplatysmal flap is raised. Digastric muscle is identified. The intermediate tendon of digastric is released from the fibrous sling attached to greater cornu and body of hyoid. A part of posterior belly of digastric is also included with the intermediate tendon. This flap is mobilized from underlying mylohyoid muscle and the submandibular gland. The neurovascular bundle is left intact.

A 2-cm incision is made in vermilion border of lower lip on the affected side close to the commissure. A tunnel is created between the lower lip incision and the submandibular region to accommodate the sling of digastric muscle. The sling is then lifted and passed through the tunnel to reach out of incision on vermilion border. The tendon with small part of posterior belly is then divided into three parts which are one by one sutured to different parts of orbicularis oris muscle. The lateral-most slip is attached near the commissure, the medial one at the mid of the lower lip, and the intermediate one in between the previous two. Suturing is done just above the vermilion border (**Fig. 9.25**).

Free Microneurovascular Muscle Transfer (FMMT)

Free muscle transfer is another technique which is used for long-term facial nerve palsy leading to nonviability of facial musculature. This technique provides new, vascularized muscle that can pull in various directions and can replicate a spontaneous, dynamic smile. This is best utilized in patients with congenital facial nerve palsy (Moebius syndrome), where the nerve and the mimetic musculature do not exist, which is why this technique is mostly practiced by plastic surgeons. The other clear-cut indications for free muscle transfer are radical parotidectomy where malignancy itself led to perineural infiltration of terminal branches of facial nerve and post-traumatic damage to the distal branches of facial nerve. The most frequent muscles used are the gracilis and the pectoralis minor muscle. It can be performed as a one- or two-stage surgery. There are two ways of performing this procedure.

In one-stage surgery, the nerve used to transmit nerve impulse is masseter nerve which is anastomosed end to end with obturator nerve which is the nerve to the free gracilis muscle, whereas in two-stage surgery, free muscle transfer with cross-face nerve grafting (CFNG) is the technique. If masseter nerve has been used to innervate the neural bundle of free muscle graft, the smile achieved is bite activated volitional smile, whereas if the free muscle is innervated by the contralateral facial nerve branches, it produces spontaneous smile on the affected side.

Two-Stage Surgery

First Stage
The sural nerve is harvested (procedure explained in Chapter 3 "Facial Nerve Unit, Structure, Lesions, and Repair"). Donor nerve branches (buccal or zygomatic branch of the facial nerve of contralateral healthy side) are assessed through modified Blair's incision. A sub-superficial muscular aponeurotic system (SMAS) flap is lifted off the parotidomasseteric fascia and required branch of facial nerve is identified at the anterior border of parotid, with very fine meticulous dissection performed in the direction of facial nerve branches. A nerve stimulator can be used at this stage to identify the branches and choose the right one by stimulating the required branch and its supply to specific muscle. After identification, the branch is cut sharply and in an elliptical manner to have maximum surface area for coaptation with sural nerve.

Sural nerve as CFNG is anastomosed on one end to this functioning buccal branch of the facial nerve from the normal, nonparalyzed side. A tunnel is created across the face through a labial mucosal incision above the upper lip and the sural nerve graft is passed through this tunnel to the opposite (affected) side. A fascia passer is used to inlay the sural nerve in this tunnel. Then either "bank" the distal end of the nerve graft in the upper

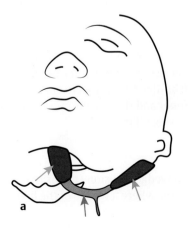 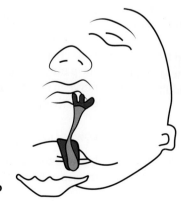

Fig. 9.25 (a, b) Illustrations showing anterior belly digastric muscle (*blue arrow*) rotation with the tendon (*orange arrow*) and small part of posterior belly of digastric (*green arrow*) divided into three parts sutured to respective parts of lower lip on the left side.

buccal sulcus at the level of the root of the upper canine tooth or the free end of the sural nerve can be sutured to the tragus or mark it with a permanent, colored suture to facilitate its identification at the second stage.

Second Stage
It is performed after 9 months of the first surgery, when it is anticipated that the nerve fibers from the normal side have regenerated through the cable graft and reached the affected side. This can also be confirmed by "Tinel's sign." When the nerve is lightly tapped, the patient feels an electric tingling sensation in the region where nerve is regenerating. It is similar to the feeling of uncomfortable tingling or discomfort similar to what one feels when his or her foot falls asleep or recovering from the effect of local anesthesia.

A muscle flap to replicate the pull of the zygomaticus major is harvested. The gracilis muscle with neurovascular pedicle which contains obturator nerve and adductor vessel branch of profunda femoris vessels is most commonly used as it is thin (only a segment of muscle is used) and perfectly replicates the facial muscle. The advantage is that it causes minimal donor site morbidity, leaves no functional deficit, and has a relatively long motor nerve. It has strong contractility also. For more favorable position of free muscle flap and shorter distance for neural regeneration, the ipsilateral muscle flap is harvested if we are using masseter nerve for innervating the flap and contralateral muscle flap is harvested if CFNG is used.

Surgical Procedure
A 7-cm longitudinal incision up to subcutaneous tissue is made in the medial side of the thigh, posterior to the pubic tubercle, below the inguinal crease. The adductor compartment fascia is dissected and gracilis muscle identified. The pedicle comes around the central part of the muscle. The neurovascular bundle containing obturator nerve identified as it runs superficial to adductor magnus muscle around 8 cm inferior to inguinal crease and vascular pedicle in the form of arterial branch of profunda femoris, associated with its two venae comitans, running inferior to the nerve is prepared. Now, the gracilis free muscle flap with its neurovascular bundle is mobilized in a sliced manner, taking out only the posterior segment and leaving behind the anterior segment. The muscle flap once delivered can be trimmed to exact weight and size depending upon the age of the patient (in pediatric patient it is around 10 g and in adults it is around 15 g).

The affected side is opened with modified Blair's incision. A skin with subcutaneous flap is lifted keeping superficial to temporoparietal fascia when moving superior to zygomatic arch and skin; subcutaneous tissue with SMAS flap is lifted keeping lateral to parotidomasseteric fascia when moving inferior to zygomatic arch. The flap is lifted over the whole lateral surface of parotid gland up to the anterior border of the masseter muscle to create the right size of pocket for gracilis muscle flap positioning. The facial vein is now located as it moves upwards keeping anterior to anterior border of masseter muscle. The facial artery is also identified along with vein. It courses superiorly and anteriorly from the inframandibular region toward the oral commissure. The facial artery is just cut proximal to its bifurcation. The buccal pad of fat is reduced to locate the artery properly and also to reduce bulkiness and bogginess on the face postoperatively. The artery once ligated can be moved posteriorly for microvascular anastomosis. The skin flap is finally lifted up to nasolabial fold to expose the modiolus, orbicularis oris in lower lip, and upper lip. Now anchoring sutures with 2-O vikoryl sutures are placed through the modiolus, lower lip, and upper lip. The suture through the upper lip creates the nasolabial fold. To create anchorage to the gracilis muscle flap, the exact distance is measured between the oral commissure and the root of the helix. This much length of the free gracilis graft is required. The harvested free muscle graft is now placed under the skin flap already created. Its distal end is sutured to the orbicularis oris near the modiolus, just lateral to the oral commissure to replicate the smile as on the contralateral side. To lock the muscle in position, almost five interlocking sutures are first placed along the cut edge of the muscle. Now the main anchoring sutures are passed through the muscle, proximal to these interlocking sutures. The proximal end of muscle is sutured onto the body of the zygoma or onto the deep temporal fascia. Microvascular anastomosis is performed between the vascular pedicle of the muscle flap and facial vessels if available or the superficial temporal vessels. The obturator nerve is sutured end to end with the distal stump of sural nerve graft through which the regeneration of contralateral buccal nerve has taken place. If the muscle graft seems bulky then the buccal or subcutaneous fat can be trimmed or resected to achieve a normal facial contour (**Fig. 9.26**).

Single-Stage Surgery

If we plan for single-stage surgery, the better alternative is to create nerve transfer using the masseter nerve on the paralyzed side. It can be directly sutured to obturator nerve in end-to-end manner and the gracilis muscle can get activated in the same stage (**Fig. 9.26**).

Lower Lip Surgery

Lip wedge excision: A lip wedge excision is considered in case of lower lip paralysis, where a wedge of the lip is

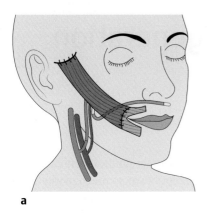
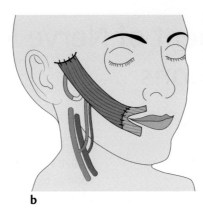

Fig. 9.26 (a, b) Illustration showing one-stage surgery with end-to-end anastomosis between masseter nerve (*orange arrow*) and obturator nerve in place of cross-face sural nerve graft.

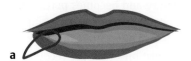
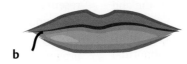

Fig. 9.27 (a, b) Illustration showing wedge resection of the lower lip on the right side for paralyzed lower lip.

removed, and the remaining tissue is sewn together to lift and tighten the corner of the mouth (**Fig. 9.27**).

Conclusion

The goals of treatment for long-term facial palsy include facial symmetry at rest, corneal protection, eye closure, oral competence, and restoration of voluntary and spontaneous facial movements. Multiple static and dynamic procedures can be performed depending on different areas of the face to achieve these goals. The results of dynamic procedures are better than those of static procedures. For optimal reanimation of the face, usually multiple surgeries are required with combination of both types of procedures. The patients should always be properly counseled regarding the post surgery results which may not replicate the normal facial movements and the recovery may take a very long time.

Bibliography

1. Volk GF, Pantel M, Guntinas-Lichius O. Modern concepts in facial nerve reconstruction. Head Face Med 2010;6:25
2. Collar RM, Byrne PJ, Boahene KD. Cross-facial nerve grafting. Operative Techniques in Otolaryngology-Head and Neck Surgery 2012;23(4):258–261
3. Sainsbury D, Borschel G, Zuker R. Surgical reanimation techniques for facial palsy/paralysis. In: Fagan J, ed. Open Access Atlas of Otolaryngology, Head & Neck Operative Surgery; 2017
4. Faris C, Heiser A, Hadlock T, Jowett N. Free gracilis muscle transfer for smile reanimation after treatment for advanced parotid malignancy. Head Neck 2018; 40(3): 561–568
5. Greene JJ, Fullerton Z, Jowett N, Hadlock T. The Tinel Sign and Myelinated Axons in the Cross-Face Nerve Graft: Predictors of Smile Reanimation Outcome for Free Gracilis Muscle Transfer? Facial Plast Surg Aesthet Med 2022; 24(4): 255–259

10 Management of Nerve Regeneration Complications

■ Introduction

While the facial nerve is regenerating after repair or injury, there could be abnormal facial movements due to defective healing. It is a part of nerve regeneration process and may lead to various involuntary static and dynamic alteration of facial expression. Even when we are expecting complete recovery of facial nerve functioning to grade I, there still can be additional abnormal involuntary movements of facial muscles on the same or the contralateral side of the face. This is what is referred to as facial synkinesis. It is one of the most distressing complications associated with recovery from facial paralysis. It can create functional derangements with important activities like closing eyes, smiling, and eating leading to cosmetic disfigurement causing psychological trauma to the patient.

The facial synkinesis can be defined as the abnormal involuntary facial movement which takes place along with voluntary reflex activity of a different set of facial muscles, which do not normally act together, on the same or the contralateral side of the face. It can develop during recovery from post-traumatic or iatrogenic injury to facial nerve, post facial nerve repair, or as a sequelae

of Bell's palsy or Ramsay Hunt's syndrome. It can be so mild as to be barely perceptible or so much marked and incapacitating that it can lead to mass movement of all parts of the involved side of the face, making the patient unable to move each part separately. It usually is a representation of faulty recovery and becomes perceptible at around 3 to 4 months post injury or repair, when the recovery of nerve fibers has already started and can keep progressing up to 2 years post onset till the recovery is complete.

The different manifestations of facial synkinesis can be in the form of:

- Synkinesis: These are synchronous and involuntary movements of facial muscles on the ipsilateral side while the patient is performing another voluntary movement. These synkinetic movements can be in the form of:
  - ➢ Ocular–oral synkinesis (commonest presentation) (**Fig. 10.1**): Voluntary eye contraction such as raising the eyebrow, blinking, or eye closure elicits an involuntary mouth movement, like lifting of angle of mouth on the affected side of the face.

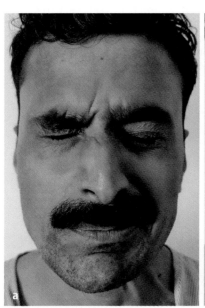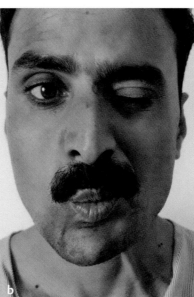

Fig. 10.1 Case of incomplete recovery of Bell's palsy left side. **(a)** Ocular-oral synkinesis left side, leading to lifting of angle of mouth while closing the eye tightly and a deeper nasolabial fold on affected side of the face, causing the cheek to appear bulky. **(b)** The neck muscle tightened while patient tries to smile or whistle.

➢ Oral–ocular synkinesis (**Fig. 10.2**): Volitional mouth movement such as smiling, eating, or lip puckering elicits involuntary eye contraction (partial or complete closure of eyelid) on the affected side of the face.

➢ Other types of facial synkinesis include chin–oral synkinesis, platysma synkinesis, ocular–chin synkinesis, ocular–nasal synkinesis, and chin–ocular synkinesis.

Common signs of synkinesis are as follow:

- The angle of mouth and cheek lifts when a person closes his or her eyes (**Fig. 10.1a**).
- A deeper nasolabial fold on affected side of the face, causing the cheek to appear bulky (**Fig. 10.1a**).
- The neck muscle tightens when a person tries to laugh, smile or whistle (**Fig. 10.1b**).
- The eyes narrow when an individual smiles (**Fig. 10.2**).
- Facial twitching in the cheek and chin.
- Facial muscles become tight, leading to facial pain and headaches.
- Hyperkinesia: It consists of static and dynamic asymmetry of the face due to hypertonia, that is, abnormal and much stronger mimic movement than normal like periocular synkinesis leading to narrowed palpebral fissure width (**Fig. 10.2**), more than normal prominence of nasolabial fold and corner of the mouth pulled laterally in upward or downward direction, or stiffness in the neck due to platysmal synkinesis. Hyperkinesia develops due to compensatory hyperactivity of the muscles of facial expression on the nonparalyzed side when the patient is putting effort to regain maximum facial movements on the affected paralyzed side. As there is weak antagonism of the affected side muscles, it leads to hyperactivity of muscles on the contralateral side (**Fig. 10.3**).

- Auto paralytic syndrome: This is a special form of synkinesis characterized by synkinetic activity of antagonistic muscles. It can be characteristically seen in the frontalis muscle while recovering from palsy. Due to synkinetic reinnervation of antagonistic muscles, the frontalis muscle may not show movement during active frowning; although the nEMG shows muscle activity. This happens due to the simultaneous pathological activation of the frontalis muscle and its antagonist, the orbicularis oculi muscle.

- Spasms: This facial movement dysfunction can be spontaneous or secondary to involuntary contraction of facial muscles on the paralyzed side. These are characterized by rapid and rhythmic contractions like a "tick" or can present as sustained muscle contraction. These spasms can present on the face as facial twitching in the cheek and chin or facial muscles becoming tight, leading to facial pain and headaches. In the neck, it may present as tightening of the neck muscle while a person tries to laugh or smile.

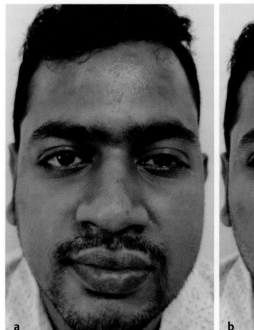 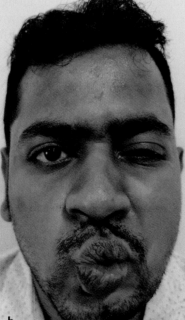 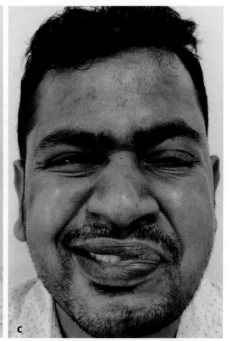

Fig. 10.2   (a–c) Oral–ocular synkinesis on the left side leading to narrowing of palpebral fissure while smiling or puckering of the lips.

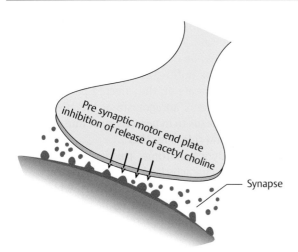

Fig. 10.3 Injection of botulinum toxin type A causing inhibition of the release of acetylcholine from the presynaptic motor end plates into the synapse.

Pathophysiological Basis of Facial Synkinesis

There are many theories postulated for explaining the development of synkinesis while recovering from facial nerve injury out of which the four most appropriate ones are:

- Aberrant regeneration: After injury or repair, the axons while regrowing from the facial nucleus till their entry into myoneural junction may get connected to different axons or incorrect peripheral muscle groups. Although the commonest site of misconnection is at the injury site, but it can happen at three levels, namely, the facial nerve nucleus in pons (neuronal stripping), the axons getting connected with other axons on the way, and the connections at myoneural junction.
- Nuclear hyperexcitability theory: It explains that at the myoneural junction, the postsynaptic cell, when it does not get neural input from the degenerated nerve fiber (axon), creates additional neurotransmitter receptors for receiving different nerve terminals. This leads to newer connections developing with neighboring axons, which were previously not connected to these myoneural junctions.
- Ephaptic transmission: At the injury site, the myelin sheath covering, after regeneration, becomes quite thin and weak leading to poor insulation of axons. This causes electrical cross-connection between different axons leading to synkinesis.
- Maladaptive cortical plasticity: According to this theory, other than faulty regeneration at periphery or on the way, the cortical reorganization also

happens in the primary sensorimotor area and the supplementary motor area in the brain.

Keeping all these theories in mind, it can be said that synkinesis may be a multifactorial process, and more than one factor may be responsible for it.

Nerve Regeneration Evaluation

Evaluation of synkinesis is most of the times a subjective measurement through clinical examination over time. As the knowledge and presence of synkinesis got registered, new or modified facial grading scales have been developed to measure it in an objective manner.

Clinical Examination

Synkinesis being a clinical diagnosis, it is mandatory on the part of the clinician to properly assess the patient's face on the basis of the presenting symptoms along with physical examination of the facial nerve. The clinician must keep in mind that *the final aesthetic changes on the face is a combined effect of the absence of movement or synkinetic movement on the paralyzed side* and/or the compensatory hyperactivity of the facial muscles on the nonparalyzed side. It is *the final response that the complete facial musculature produces after the loss of balance between the paralyzed and nonparalyzed sides.*

Facial muscles should be carefully assessed at rest and during different stages of facial movements. The seven standard facial movements are wrinkling forehead by lifting eyebrows, eye closure on light and full effort, nose wrinkling, smile, lower lip depression, and puckering of lips, which are documented with digital photography and video so that the grading and synkinesis can be measured. Along with the standard views, the face is examined for the trigger actions which lead to synkinesis, the commonest being forceful eye closure or a puckering movement of the lips.

Measuring Synkinesis through Facial Grading Scales

The most common scale, which is used for evaluation of facial palsy and its recovery, is House-Brackmann's classification, but it does not have a rating for recording the presence and measurement of synkinesis. It is because this system was only developed to classify acute facial palsy. Assessment of postrecovery defective healing was never a part of this classification system.

- A modification of House-Brackmann's classification is available that includes synkinesis in its measuring scale (explained in Chapter 4).

- Another grading system which accurately measures synkinesis including the assessment of defective healing is Sunnybrook facial grading system (SFGS) which, besides assessing the functional evaluation, also helps in measuring quality of life after facial reconstruction surgery (explained in Chapter 4).
- Even better are objective observer-independent measurement tools like video-based semiquantitative measurement systems. Objective measures of synkinesis using computerized video analysis show promise although no objective techniques are currently widely used.
- The Synkinesis Assessment Questionnaire consists of nine questions and has been shown to be both valid and reliable as a dedicated measurement of synkinesis; it can be accurately correlated with the synkinesis component of the SFGS.

■ Management/Interventions

Once the facial nerve palsy has started recovering, numerous facial rehabilitation techniques are incorporated for prevention of impending synkinesis or treatment of synkinesis once it has started developing or has completely developed. The management can be in two forms which can be performed separately or in combination:

- Physiotherapy intervention.
- Nonphysiotherapy intervention.

Physiotherapy Interventions

The following physiotherapy interventions have been shown to be effective in reducing or minimizing synkinesis.

Facial Neuromuscular Retraining (NMR)

It is a set of training sessions to teach the patient the coordination of appropriate facial muscle movements. These regimes can train a patient with synkinesis to limit abnormal movement patterns that may otherwise progress to "auto-paralysis" of different facial muscle groups. The exercises are to be started after the wound has completely healed.

During NMR, the abnormally contracting facial muscles are identified. Then, a multistep process is used to help the patient retrain the muscles at the neurological (brain) level. Certain massage techniques are also incorporated along with NMR to provide optimal results. The set of exercises used in NMR vary depending upon the cause and the surgical treatment given.

For Motor Nerve or Muscle Transfer Cases

The patient is taught to train the transferred nerve or muscle for its new function.

Physiotherapy in Facio-masseteric Anastomosis

The patient is taught to bite (action of masseter muscle) and smile (action of facial nerve). The patient has to slowly dissociate the two actions by decreasing function of bite and increasing facial function that is smile and closing eye and finally get an independent facial function.

Physiotherapy in Facio-hypoglossal Anastomosis

The patient is taught to move the tongue to get facial function. The direction of tongue thrust is toward palate while trying to achieve action of facial nerve. The patient starts normalizing the strength of the tongue and links the direction and the strength of the tongue to facial movements and finally gets independent facial function.

Physiotherapy for Cases of Hyperkinesis or Spasms

A physical therapy program is incorporated which is a combination of manual stretching and massage exercises. It is aimed to reduce the facial tissue tightness and hyperactivity by using the proper muscles to smile, frown, and make other facial expressions.

Most of the synkinesis exercises can be performed at home after initial training by a physiotherapist. A therapist ensures that the patients fully understand the technique to be able to perform each exercise on their own. The treatment plans are customized depending on requirement of the patient.

Mime Therapy

Mime is a form of performance art which uses nonverbal expression to convey a story. The aim of mime therapy is to train the patient to improve symmetry of the face at rest and during movement and simultaneously training to prevent synkinesis formation through the art of mime. Mime therapy should be started only after the reinnervation signs have started appearing clinically.

The various components of mime therapy include:

- The patient assessed for synkinesis using a standard grading system and then explained the cause, treatment, and prognosis of the ailment. Photography and videography sessions are conducted while the patient is at rest and while performing seven standard facial movements.
- Face and neck self-massage along with stretching exercises of muscles on the affected side is taught.
- Breathing and relaxation exercises are performed.
- Exercises to enhance coordination between both sides of the face and to reduce synkinesis or hyperkinesis are done.

- Exercises to achieve better facial nerve functioning like eye and lip closure are performed.
- Letter and word exercises to increase the patient's awareness of lip movements and mouth position for various sounds (to pronounce AA, EE, and OO) are taught.
- Facial expression exercises (related to different moods) are taught to develop an awareness of the connection between the use of specific muscles to achieve facial expressions.

A session of 45 minutes to 1 hour once a week for at least 10 to 12 weeks is the regime. Once the patients learn them, they can perform these exercises at home also. All these exercises are to be practiced at different speed and force and each exercise is to be repeated five times in one session. Mime therapy should be started once the synkinesis has started setting in (around 3 months after onset of facial palsy). Mirrors can be used as a feedback tool.

Biofeedback Therapy

EMG biofeedback is a perfect tool for retraining muscles and reducing synkinesis movement along with mirror therapy.

"Facial Re-education"

It is sometimes used to help minimize the effects of synkinesis after Bell's palsy. It involves teaching the patient how to perform various facial exercises, such as keeping the face up when speaking and chewing food with the eyes open. Facial re-education also involves wearing sunglasses to prevent squinting and massaging the intraoral buccal area. These sessions where patient works on slow and symmetric movements of the face to improve facial muscle coordination are held for at least 4 to 6 months.

Electrostimulation

This increases activity of already overactive muscles, so should not be used as part of neuromuscular training. While the NMR focuses on muscle recoordination rather than stimulation, the electrostimulation does the opposite; hence, it is to be avoided in cases of synkinesis. So, electrostimulation or muscle-strengthening exercises are to be completely avoided as part of the treatment or only can be tried in earliest days of palsy, when the nerve fibers have yet not started regenerating.

Nonphysiotherapy Interventions

Nonsurgical

Other than physiotherapy, the most effective modality which can effectively restrict the synkinesis though temporarily is botulinum toxin injection, which is used to paralyze or weaken hyperactive muscles. Injections are usually given on the affected side to weaken the involuntary movement seen with synkinesis. Additionally, injections can be given to the unaffected side in order to achieve symmetry.

Surgical

Surgical procedures are almost obsolete nowadays. This modality is used very rarely, and reserved for severe synkinesis which has not responded to physiotherapy and/or Botox. The surgeries include selective neurolysis, selective myectomy, selective neurectomy, and even cross-facial nerve grafting. As these surgical procedures are irreversible and radical in nature, the author does not practice them for treating synkinesis.

Botulinum Toxin Type A Injection

It is an effective temporary treatment to relax the hyperactive muscles of the face. The injections can effectively reduce the dyskinesis and synkinesis. The effects of botulinum toxin are reversible so can be injected in different sets of muscles at different stages. First, it is injected into muscles on the affected side. While the affected side is recovering, the contralateral healthy side starts showing hyperactive movements due to overuse. In such situations, botulinum toxin can also be applied on the unaffected side to reduce these overactive muscle movements (usually the depressor anguli oris muscle and orbicularis oculi muscle).

BTX-A (botulinum toxin type A): It is a protein derived from bacteria *Clostridium botulinum*, which is an anaerobic, gram-positive, rod-shaped organism. *Clostridium botulinum* produces eight exotoxins, out of which type A, a high molecular weight protein, is the one used for treating the hyperactive muscles. It is named as botulinum toxin type A. Its mechanism of action starts at the neuromuscular junction, where it, by binding to the presynaptic cholinergic nerve terminals, leads to inhibition of the release of acetylcholine from the presynaptic motor end plates into the synapse (**Fig. 10.4**). Through this procedure it causes paralytic effect, which prevents the muscular contraction. This procedure is called chemodenervation. The paralytic effect on muscle fibers is dose dependent.

Preparation and Injection

Botulinum toxin (Botox) is provided in vials of 50 or 100 Units (U) in a frozen lyophilized form (at −5° C). One unit equals to 0.25 ng of toxin. Its toxic dose is 40 U/kg in human beings and above 200 U it causes systemic paralysis. Do not shake while reconstituting the dose as it destroys the toxin. It is best to use the reconstituted dose on the same day. The vial can be kept in freezer

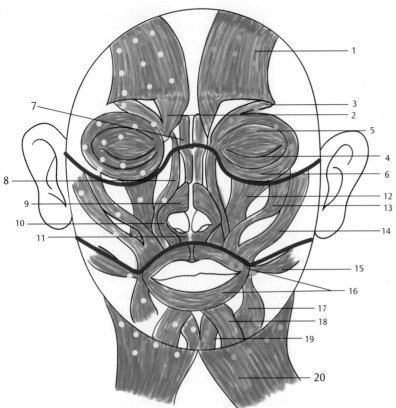

Fig. 10.4 The face has been divided into three zones by two red lines. The numbers show the facial muscles. Yellow bullet points are for injection of Botox on the affected side muscles (*right side*) and green bullet points are for injecting Botox on the normal side overactive muscles (*left side*). The facial mimetic muscles are shown as follows: (1) Frontalis medial and lateral; (2) depressor supracilii; (3) corrugator supercili; (4) orbicularis oculi: pretarsal portion; (5) orbicularis oculi: preseptal portion; (6) orbicularis oculi: orbital portion; (7) procerus; (8) levator labii superioris alaeque nasi; (9) compressor nasi; (10) dilator nasi; (11) depressor septi; (12) levator labii superioris; (13) zygomaticus minor; (14) zygomatic major; (15) risorius; (16) orbicularis oris; (17) depressor anguli oris; (18) depressor labii; (19) mentalis; and (20) platysma.

at –20° C, if we want to use the residual botulinum toxin in vial after days or weeks of opening the vial, although the efficacy may reduce.

After injection, the paralytic effect is noticed within 12 to 16 hours, although the maximum effect becomes visible after 5 to 6 days. The effect remains up to 12 weeks usually, but some muscles take time to recover and the effect stays for up to 6 months. Injection can be repeated to create the effect again, but it must be kept in mind that repetitive use can lead to muscle atrophy. So, the Botox injection should be done in conjunction with physiotherapy, mime therapy, and biofeedback mechanism.

Evaluation, Dose, and Location

Once the diagnosis of synkinesis is established, the location and severity of spasm is measured on a scale from 1 (mild) to 4 (severe). Photographs and video recording before and after injections are very helpful in measuring the effect.

Counseling of the patient is mandatory as this being a temporary relief and the patient needs to be educated about other alternatives also. The risks need to be informed before starting the sessions.

An individualized injection plan is formed, and specific points and dose per point is defined. The main objective is to balance the facial expression and not paralyze the face. Depending on the number of sites, the total dose is calculated and prepared. Each site receives around 2 to 7 U of botulinum toxin. Few sites require more dose than others depending upon severity of synkinesis and strength of the muscle involved.

The injection is given on the affected side to reduce or treat synkinesis and on the unaffected side to reduce hyperkinesis. The final aim is facial symmetry both at rest and activity. Accurate injection technique and dosage are a very important aspect of this therapy. The exact origin and insertion of the mimetic muscle which is to be injected should be marked. The injection site, along with depth and angle of the needle while injecting, should be accurate to have optimal results.

Regarding dosage, it depends on the severity of synkinesis or hyperkinesis, as well as the strength of the muscle involved. In the initial sessions of therapy, less than recommended dosage is injected followed by customized optimal dosage according to the requirement in the following sessions.

The injection sites are marked are shown in **Fig. 10.4**. The skin is cleaned with spirit, avoiding contact with exposed eye. The reconstituted toxin is filled in tuberculin syringe and with a 30-gauge needle, the Botox toxin is directly injected into the desired muscle. The smaller muscles require to be injected at one or two sites whereas bigger muscles like frontalis, orbicularis oris, orbicularis oculi, and platysma require injection at multiple sites.

Upper Face

While injecting botulinum toxin in the upper part of the face, a natural appearance is to be achieved by making a balance between the elevator and depressor muscle groups: the elevator being frontalis and depressors being corrugator supercilii, procerus, depressor supercilii, and orbicularis oculi.

- Frontalis muscle: Injection given at multiple sites.
- Corrugator supercilii: There are two points of injections, one at the origin and the other at the insertion of muscle.
- Procerus: Single injection is sufficient.
- Depressor supercilii: Single injection is sufficient.
- Orbicularis oculi:
    - ➤ Upper eyelid: The site chosen is either the mid of eyelid close to the eyelid margin, or at more than one site, and the Botox toxin is injected directly into the pretarsal muscles in a dose of around 5 U. Care is to be taken not to accidentally inject into levator palpebrae superioris because the muscle being extremely sensitive to the toxin can lead to temporary ptosis (drooping of upper eyelid) which is to be avoided. The theory behind choosing mid point for injection is that the lateral and medial parts of muscles keep functioning, so the hyperactivity is avoided but normal eyelid closure is not disturbed.
    - ➤ Lower eyelid: It requires lesser dose of toxin (3–4 U) as its role in closing the eye is less than the upper eyelid. At mid point of lower eyelid or at multiple sites, close to the margin, the toxin is injected in pretarsal orbicularis oculi. Avoid its diffusion through orbital septum into deeper structures like inferior oblique and inferior rectus muscle as their paralysis can lead to temporary vertical diplopia.
    - ➤ Additional few units of toxins can be used to inject posterior to the lateral temporal rim of the orbit to further enhance the paralytic effect on orbicularis muscle in cases of severe spasm.

Mid and Lower Parts of the Face

- Nasalis: One or two injections near the superior third of the lateral nasal wall.
- Levator labii alaeque nasi: Single injection in the naso-facial groove at the superior point of the nasal ala.
- Levator labii superioris: Single injection lateral to the bony nasal prominence.
- Zygomaticus major: First point 2 cm from the oral commissure on a diagonal line to the malar prominence; second point on the malar prominence.

- Zygomaticus minor: Single injection, 1 cm above the zygomaticus major.
- Orbicularis oris: Injection at or 2 mm above the vermilion border.

The cheek becomes flaccid after these injections and can lead to self-bite by the patient unknowingly, so the dose should accurate. Orbicularis oris is to be injected with very low doses as its paralysis can lead to loss of good water seal leading to drooling of saliva.

- Risorius: Single injection, 2 cm medially to the anterior border of the masseter.
- Depressor labii inferioris: Single injection, 1.5 cm from lower lip border, 1 cm from the midline.
- Depressor anguli oris: Single injection, immediately above the angle of the mandible and 1 cm lateral to the oral commissure.
- Mentalis: Its spasm can lead to deep dimpling of chin; single injection on the chin prominence, close to the midline, at a distance of more than 2 cm from the lower lip.
- Platysma: 1.5 to 2 cm apart along the mandible margin and platysma bands.

During all these times and post injection, the patient's input is very important. The patient can guide us all through and after the procedure for the exact site of twitching or tightness of muscles.

First follow-up visit is after 10 to 15 days of initial treatment.

Adverse effects depend upon the injection site and can be in the form of ptosis, diplopia, lagophthalmos, oral incompetence, speech abnormalities, diplopia, worsening of paralysis, and dysphonia. They wean off slowly over time, but the clinician should try to be accurate in injecting botulinum A so as to avoid all these adverse effects.

Synkinesis is a situation which cannot be prevented; however, there are certain things that patients can do to minimize its effect on the face. These include facial re-education techniques, physiotherapy techniques, mime therapy, and biofeedback mechanism. Along with that chemodenervation with botulinum toxoid is a very effective alternative.

Bibliography

1. Chua CN, Quhill F, Jones E, Voon LW, Ahad M, Rowson N. Treatment of aberrant facial nerve regeneration with botulinum toxin A. Orbit 2004;23(4):213–218
2. Dall'Angelo A, Mandrini S, Sala V, et al. Platysma synkinesis in facial palsy and botulinum toxin type A. Laryngoscope 2014;124(11):2513–2517

3. Patel PN, Owen SR, Norton CP, et al. Outcomes of buccinator treatment with botulinum toxin in facial synkinesis. JAMA Facial Plast Surg 2018;20(3):196–201

4. Shinn JR, Nwabueze NN, Patel P, Norton C, Ries WR, Stephan SJ. Contemporary review and case report of Botulinum resistance in facial synkinesis. Laryngoscope 2019;129(10):2269–2273

5. Cooper L, Lui M, Nduka C. Botulinum toxin treatment for facial palsy: a systematic review. J Plast Reconstr Aesthet Surg 2017;70(6):833–841

6. Shinn JR, Nwabueze NN, Du L, et al. Treatment patterns and outcomes in Botulinum therapy for patients with facial synkinesis. JAMA Facial Plast Surg 2019;21(3):244–251

7. Raslan A, Guntinas-Lichius O, Volk GF. Altered facial muscle innervation pattern in patients with post-paretic facial synkinesis. Laryngoscope 2020;130(5): E320–E326

8. Moran CJ, Neely JG. Patterns of facial nerve synkinesis. Laryngoscope 1996;106(12 Pt 1):1491–1496

9. Choi D, Raisman G. After facial nerve damage, regenerating axons become aberrant throughout the length of the nerve and not only at the site of the lesion: an experimental study. Br J Neurosurg 2004;18(1): 45–48

10. Yamada H, Hato N, Murakami S, et al. Facial synkinesis after experimental compression of the facial nerve comparing intratemporal and extratemporal lesions. Laryngoscope 2010;120(5):1022–1027

11. Sadjadpour K. Postfacial palsy phenomena: faulty nerve regeneration or ephaptic transmission? Brain Res 1975;95(2-3):403–406

12. Husseman J, Mehta RP. Management of synkinesis. Facial Plast Surg 2008;24(2):242–249

13. Wang Y, Wang W-W, Hua X-Y, Liu H-Q, Ding W. Patterns of cortical reorganization in facial synkinesis: a task functional magnetic resonance imaging study. Neural Regen Res 2018;13(9):1637–1642

14. Beurskens CH, Oosterhof J, Nijhuis-van der Sanden MW. Frequency and location of synkineses in patients with peripheral facial nerve paresis. Otol Neurotol 2010;31(4):671–675

15. Fujiwara K, Furuta Y, Nakamaru Y, Fukuda S. Comparison of facial synkinesis at 6 and 12 months after the onset of peripheral facial nerve palsy. Auris Nasus Larynx 2015;42(4):271–274

16. Pourmomeny AA, Asadi S. Management of synkinesis and asymmetry in facial nerve palsy: a review article. Iran J Otorhinolaryngol 2014;26(77):251–256

17. House JW, Brackmann DE. Facial nerve grading system. Otolaryngol Head Neck Surg 1985;93(2):146–147

18. Ross BG, Fradet G, Nedzelski JM. Development of a sensitive clinical facial grading system. Otolaryngol Head Neck Surg 1996;114(3):380–386 fckL

19. Neely JG, Cherian NG, Dickerson CB, Nedzelski JM. Sunnybrook facial grading system: reliability and criteria for grading. Laryngoscope 2010;120(5): 1038–1045

20. Fattah AY, Gurusinghe ADR, Gavilan J, et al; Sir Charles Bell Society. Facial nerve grading instruments: systematic review of the literature and suggestion for uniformity. Plast Reconstr Surg 2015;135(2):569–579

21. Mehta RP, WernickRobinson M, Hadlock TA. Validation of the Synkinesis Assessment Questionnaire. Laryngoscope 2007;117(5):923–926

22. Brach JS, VanSwearingen JM, Lenert J, Johnson PC. Facial neuromuscular retraining for oral synkinesis. Plast Reconstr Surg 1997;99(7):1922–1931, discussion 1932–1933

23. Manikandan N. Effect of facial neuromuscular re-education on facial symmetry in patients with Bell's palsy: a randomized controlled trial. Clin Rehabil 2007;21(4):338–343

24. Ross B, Nedzelski JM, McLean JA. Efficacy of feedback training in long-standing facial nerve paresis. Laryngoscope 1991;101(7 Pt 1):744–750

25. Balliet R, Shinn JB, Bach-y-Rita P. Facial paralysis rehabilitation: retraining selective muscle control. Int Rehabil Med 1982;4(2):67–74

26. de Maio M, Bento RF. Botulinum toxin in facial palsy: an effective treatment for contralateral hyperkinesis. Plast Reconstr Surg 2007;120(4):917–927

27. Filipo R, Spahiu I, Covelli E, Nicastri M, Bertoli GA. Botulinum toxin in the treatment of facial synkinesis and hyperkinesis. Laryngoscope 2012;122(2):266–270

28. Markey JD, Loyo M. Latest advances in the management of facial synkinesis. Curr Opin Otolaryngol Head Neck Surg 2017;25(4):265–272

29. Bran GM, Lohuis PJ. Selective neurolysis in post-paralytic facial nerve syndrome (PFS). Aesthetic Plast Surg 2014;38(4):742–744

30. Guerrissi JO. Selective myectomy for postparetic facial synkinesis. Plast Reconstr Surg 1991;87(3):459–466

31. van Veen MM, Dusseldorp JR, Hadlock TA. Long-term outcome of selective neurectomy for refractory periocular synkinesis. Laryngoscope 2018;128(10): 2291–2295

32. Zhang B, Yang C, Wang W, Li W. Repair of ocular-oral synkinesis of postfacial paralysis using cross-facial nerve grafting. J Reconstr Microsurg 2010;26(6): 375–380

33. Beurskens CHG, Devriese PP, Heiningen I, Oostendorp RAB. The use of mime therapy as a rehabilitation method for patients with facial nerve paresis. Int J Ther Rehabil 2004;11(5):206–210

34. Wang Y, Wang W-W, Hua X-Y, Liu H-Q, Ding W. Patterns of cortical reorganization in facial synkinesis: a task functional magnetic resonance imaging study. Neural Regen Res 2018;13(9):1637–1642. The above-mentioned study conducted in 2018 using MRI concluded this fact.

35. Finsterer J. Management of peripheral facial nerve palsy. Eur Arch Otorhinolaryngol 2008;265(7):743–752

36. Armstrong MWJ, Mountain RE, Murray JAM. Treatment of facial synkinesis and facial asymmetry with botulinum toxin type A following facial nerve palsy. Clin Otolaryngol Allied Sci 1996;21(1):15–20

37. Salles AG, da Costa EF, Ferreira MC, do Nascimento Remigio AF, Moraes LB, Gemperli R. Epidemiologic overview of synkinesis in 353 patients with longstanding facial paralysis under treatment with Botulinum toxin for 11 years. Plast Reconstr Surg 2015;136(6):1289–1298

38. Heydenrych I. The treatment of facial asymmetry with Botulinum toxin: current concepts, guidelines, and future trends. Indian J Plast Surg 2020;53(2): 219–229

39. Sadiq SA, Khwaja S, Saeed SR. Botulinum toxin to improve lower facial symmetry in facial nerve palsy. Eye (Lond) 2012;26(11):1431–1436

40. Macgregor FC. Facial disfigurement: problems and management of social interaction and implications for mental health. Aesthetic Plast Surg 1990;14(4): 249–257

41. de Carvalho VF, Vieira APS, Paggiaro AO, Salles AG, Gemperli R. Evaluation of the body image of patients with facial palsy before and after the application of botulinum toxin. Int J Dermatol 2019;58(10): 1175–1183

42. de Maio M. Use of botulinum toxin in facial paralysis. J Cosmet Laser Ther 2003;5(3–4):216–217

43. Frevert J. Pharmaceutical, biological, and clinical properties of botulinum neurotoxin type A products. Drugs R D 2015;15(1):1–9

44. Cabin JA, Massry GG, Azizzadeh B. Botulinum toxin in the management of facial paralysis. Curr Opin Otolaryngol Head Neck Surg 2015;23(4):272–280

45. Benichou L, Labbe D, Le Louarn C, Guerreschi P. Facial palsy sequel and botulinum toxin. Ann Chir Plast Esthet 2015;60(5):377–392

46. Maria CM, Kim J. Individualized management of facial synkinesis based on facial function. Acta Otolaryngol 2017;137(9):1010–1015

47. Mehdizadeh OB, Diels J, White WM. Botulinum toxin in the treatment of facial paralysis. Facial Plast Surg Clin North Am 2016;24(1):11–20

48. Zarins U. Anatomy of facial expression. In: Anatomy of Facial Expression. 3rd ed. Seattle, WA, USA: Exonicus, Inc.; 2018:48

11 Facial Nerve in Cholesteatoma and Infections

Introduction

Facial nerve involvement in any infective pathology is not common, but once it gets involved, the right cause should be diagnosed, and the treatment should be started at the earliest. The common inflammatory causes for facial palsy include various viral as well as bacterial pathologies out of which idiopathic facial palsy (Bell's palsy) and many other viral pathologies have been described in detail in Chapter 6 titled "Evaluation and Management of Acute Facial Palsy." This chapter focuses on bacterial infections including acute suppurative otitis media (ASOM), chronic suppurative otitis media (CSOM), malignant otitis externa (MOE), and granulomatous diseases like tubercular otitis media (TOM) leading to facial palsy.

As the clinical picture of all patients with acute facial palsy is identical, most often they are wrongly diagnosed and treated as Bell's palsy. That makes it mandatory to evaluate each patient based on the symptoms and clinical manifestations and treat accordingly.

Late and inadequate treatment is a common cause of deterioration in facial palsy and development of other otogenic complications like acute mastoiditis, otogenic meningitis, and cerebral and cerebellar abscesses.

Acute Suppurative Otitis Media (ASOM)

The advent of so many antibiotics over time has reduced the incidence of facial nerve involvement in acute otitis media; nevertheless, facial paralysis, as an otogenic complication, can originate from acute otitis media and secretory otitis media and may present as the first symptom of ASOM.

Pathophysiology

The involvement of facial nerve in acute middle ear infections is either due to direct extension of infection to the facial nerve through existing dehiscence in bony canal or through naturally present canaliculi connecting middle ear and mastoid air cells to the fallopian canal which includes perivascular spaces, spaces around muscles like stapedius muscle, and nerves like chorda tympani. Congenital dehiscence of the fallopian canal results due to failure of the ossification progression along the length or around the circumference of the facial canal. The inflammatory changes in the nerve lead to swelling of endoneurium inside the unyielding perineurium leading to nerve anorexia and finally causing degeneration of nerve.

Clinical Presentation

The classical presentation of this disease, which is usually seen in pediatric age group, is an episode of upper respiratory tract infection followed by ear pain, hearing loss, and sudden onset of facial palsy or paresis. The presence of an opaque or red congested and bulging tympanic membrane (TM) is confirmatory of diagnosis.

Treatment

These cases are primarily treated with medical management, which should be started as early as possible. It includes therapeutic dose of intravenous antibiotics followed by oral antibiotics for at least 14 days. Associated surgical procedures include:

- **Myringotomy:** In cases with opaque or red bulging TM, where exudate has collected in middle ear, myringotomy is to be performed along with medical therapy for drainage of exudate and collecting sample for culture sensitivity.
- **Mastoid surgery:** The mastoid surgery is selected for those few patients where the computed tomography (CT) scan is showing coalescent mastoiditis or the facial palsy is unresponsive to medical treatment, or presence of subperiosteal abscess, meningitis, or Gradenigo's syndrome (petrositis with cranial nerves VI and VII involvement).

The surgery includes cortical mastoidectomy, clearance of the infected exudate, bone, and soft tissue, and achieving aeration in middle ear and mastoid air cells. The facial nerve mostly does not require decompression; just releasing the pressure due to exudate on dehiscent facial nerve is good enough most of the times. In case the facial nerve has to be decompressed (depending upon the extent of damage), the nerve sheath is not opened to avoid infection traversing to nerve fibers. The sheath is breached only in very few cases where the pus is seen extending into the fallopian canal.

Chronic Suppurative Otitis Media (CSOM)

Facial palsy is a rare but significant complication of CSOM with or without cholesteatoma disease. Although the incidence of this complication has decreased over time with use of antibiotics, but once it happens, urgent addressal is required. The treatment includes medical therapy in the form of specific antibiotics and steroids, and surgical intervention in the form of mastoid exploration with or without facial nerve decompression.

Chronic Suppurative Otitis Media without Cholesteatoma

Pathophysiology

Several years of pathological process in CSOM causes changes in mucosa of middle ear, manifested by edema, submucous fibrosis, and infiltration with chronic inflammation cells. Progressive spreading of these inflammation changes causes osteitis, which provokes invasion and bone destruction of inner ear, durae, or facial canal and development of facial palsy. In chronic infections, especially in cases of cholesteatoma, the facial nerve involvement is by extraneural compression. Usually it is less than grade VI, which means that the infections rarely involve the nerve directly and completely. Prompt treatment usually results in a good outcome, but if treatment is delayed the prognosis can be difficult to predict.

Clinical Presentation

The patient presented with chronically discharging ear with slow-onset facial weakness on left side which progressed to grade IV House-Brackmann scale (HBS) (**Fig. 11.1**).

Pure tone audiometry shows mild to moderate conductive hearing loss.

High-resolution computed tomography (HRCT) of temporal bone shows presence of soft tissue in middle ear and mastoid, and presence of dehiscence in some segment of the facial nerve.

Treatment (Figs. 11.2–11.5)

The treatment remains surgical intervention in the form of clearance of mastoid disease, reconstruction of TM, excising adhesions and fibrous tissue between TM and middle ear mucosa and dehiscent or exposed facial nerve, and protection of facial nerve by putting some tissue like a boomerang-shaped cartilage bridge to avoid further fibrosis between TM and facial nerve. Medical therapy in the form of antibiotics based on culture sensitivity report and steroids forms an important part of treatment. 6 months post surgery the facial nerve functioning improved to grade I HBS (**Fig. 11.6**).

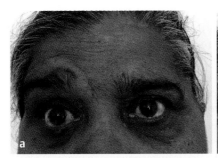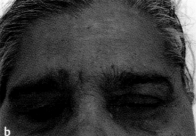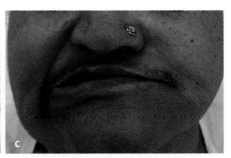

Fig. 11.1   (a–c) Left-sided facial palsy of grade IV.

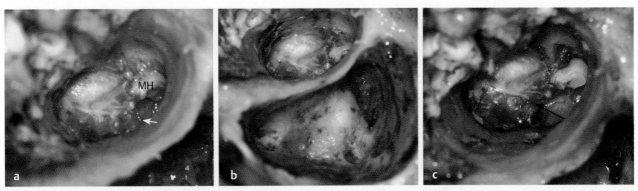

Fig. 11.2 **(a)** Perforation in posterosuperior quadrant with tympanosclerosis in anterior quadrant of tympanic membrane (TM) and adhesions between TM and middle ear mucosa in the left ear. Mucosal folds around horizontal part of fallopian canal also visualized (*arrow*). Malleus head (MH) is exposed. **(b)** Cortical mastoidectomy with clearance of granulation tissue and patency achieved between antrum and middle ear. **(c)** As the long process of incus was necrosed, the incus has already been taken out. The adhesions around TM and stapes head visible (*black arrow*).

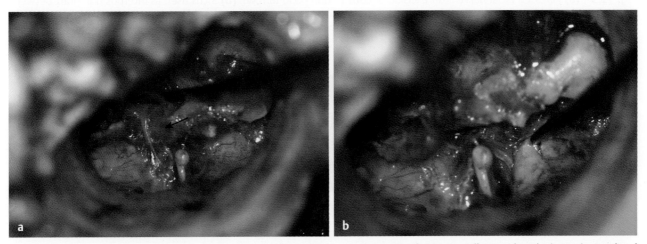

Fig. 11.3 **(a)** Tympanic membrane (TM) elevated from the suprastructure of stapes. Adhesion bands (*arrow*) visualized between TM and promontory. **(b)** Adhesions released. Facial nerve is being decompressed in tympanic segment (TS) after clearing the mucosal bands. Very thin shell of bone covering TS being lifted.

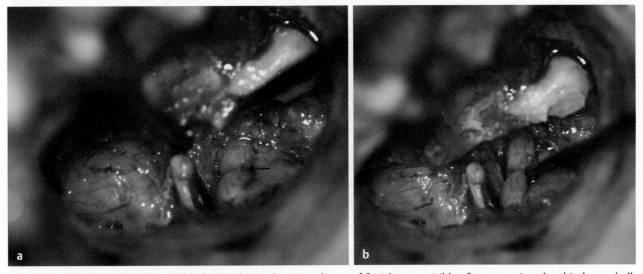

Fig. 11.4 **(a)** Constriction band (*black arrow*) over horizontal part of facial nerve visible after removing the thin bony shell. **(b)** Constriction band around facial nerve being incised with the help of sharp right-angle hook.

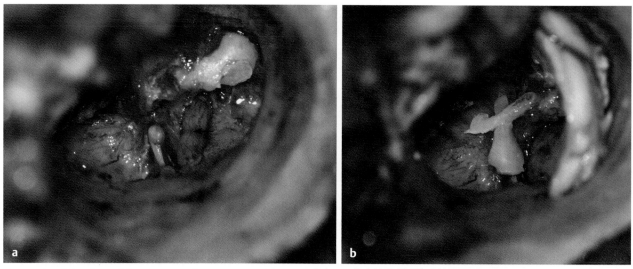

Fig. 11.5   (a) Released facial nerve after excision of constriction band (*arrow*). **(b)** Incus used as interposition graft between head of stapes and handle of malleus for ossiculoplasty reconstruction. The incus should not be touching the exposed facial nerve. The posterior bony canal wall reconstructed with tragal cartilage graft, keeping a space of few millimeters between it and the exposed and decompressed facial nerve.

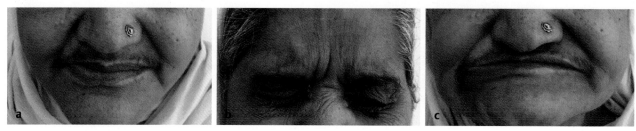

Fig. 11.6   (a–c) Facial nerve improvement to grade I after 9 months of surgery.

Chronic Suppurative Otitis Media with Cholesteatoma

Pathophysiology

Cholesteatoma which is also known as "epidermal inclusion cyst" of middle ear and mastoid is an invagination of keratinizing squamous epithelial layer of external auditory canal (EAC) and TM into middle ear. Cholesteatoma has two layers, the acellular debris known as "keratin" in a cavity lined by "matrix." Matrix is the biologically active layer of cholesteatoma and acts through two layers. The outer epithelial layer produces the keratin and inner subepithelial layer called submatrix, containing mesenchymal cells, res orbs the underlying bone by producing proteolytic enzyme, giving invasive property to cholesteatoma. So cholesteatoma grows by passive growth and active destruction. It gradually expands and starts eroding the surrounding bony structures which includes the fallopian canal as well. The bony erosion can lead to facial nerve palsy as well as other complications. Cholesteatoma can directly erode the facial canal and provoke inflammation or can compress on a dehiscent nerve (macro dehiscence) or through the naturally present canaliculi between middle ear and fallopian canal (micro dehiscence). Bony defects may not be visible in such cases. The dehiscence is most commonly seen in tympanic segment (TS) followed by the first genu area, whereas the erosion of fallopian canal is mostly found in its vertical or the mastoid segment (MS) followed by tympanic segment.

The presentation of facial nerve beneath the cholesteatoma sac (CS) can be in different forms (**Figs. 11.7 and 11.8**):

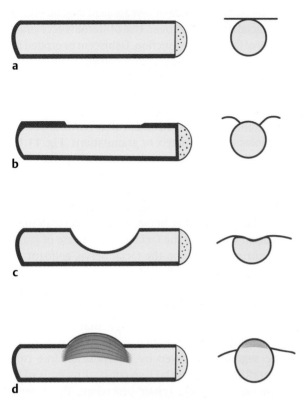

Fig. 11.7 Different presentations of facial nerve underneath the cholesteatoma sac. **(a)** In intact fallopian canal, **(b)** lying dehiscent, **(c)** compressed under infective exudate, and **(d)** protuberant, with fibers inflamed and bulging.

- Lying in intact fallopian canal
- Dehiscent nerve (congenital dehiscence or erosion by the disease)
- Compressed nerve
- Protuberant nerve (reddish inflamed nerve)

Clinical Presentation

The patient presents with complaints of chronic, foul-smelling scanty discharge from ear with slow-onset facial weakness which mostly is less than grade VI. The discharge can be blood stained due to superadded inflamed granulation tissue.

Routine radiological findings (HRCT of temporal bone axial and coronal sections using 1 × 1 mm cuts) unfortunately cannot differentiate between CS and co-presence of granulation tissue, mucosal edema, or effusion. Although cholesteatoma shows a lower attenuation than granulation tissue, the difference is subtle. Magnetic resonance imaging (MRI) has shown potential role to differentiate the two, although it is rarely performed in routine. The exact clinical findings are mostly visualized

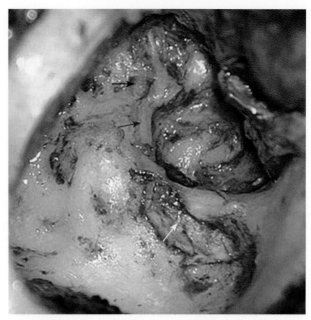

Fig. 11.8 Natural dehiscence of facial nerve in the first genu area (*black arrow*), facial nerve lying in intact fallopian canal in tympanic segment (TS) (*red arrow*) and exposed, protuberant, and inflamed in vertical segment (*white arrow*).

during mastoid exploration only; still routine radiological assessment prior to mastoid surgery is deemed necessary. It can show relevant anatomy, nature and extent of disease, and the exact location of involvement of facial nerve, which is very important for the surgeon to know. It facilitates the surgeons regarding surgical approaches and prepare them for suspected complications.

Culture sensitivity of discharge is another mandatory investigation to be performed in every case of cholesteatoma so as to guide the surgeon for starting accurate antibiotics before and after surgery.

Treatment

Medical treatment in the form of specific antibiotics and steroids are to be started before surgery.

Facial palsy associated with cholesteatoma should be treated as early as possible. Complete recovery can be achieved if corrective procedure is performed within3 months of onset of palsy or paresis. Further delay can lead to incomplete recovery of the nerve.

Surgical intervention in the form of inside-out mastoidectomy is to be performed at the earliest. The surgery includes exposure of the CS in all directions by removing all bony ledges lateral to it. After complete exposure, the debulking of the CS is carried out toward the middle ear by lifting the CS from all directions gently with the help of a curved needle and a small cotton ball soaked in adrenaline. By pushing the cotton ball underneath the edge of the CS, the right plane is created, and the matrix layer is lifted gently without tearing it. Once close to important structures, the adrenaline-soaked gelfoam or cotton ball can be kept for few minutes for decongestion to take place, so as to avoid injuring the underlying dehiscent structure (**Fig. 11.9**). Extreme caution is required while peeling off the sac layer from all important structures in the vicinity like lateral semicircular canal (LSC), fallopian canal, dura (in case of erosion of tegmen or posterior fossa dural plate), sigmoid sinus (in case of erosion of sinus plate), stapes area, round window etc.

Accurate assessment of facial nerve intraoperatively is required. Preoperative CT scan is to be corelated with the operative findings. The CT will clearly show the location and extent of involvement of facial nerve and rest of important structures in the vicinity. In every case of cholesteatoma with facial nerve paresis/palsy, erosion or dehiscence of fallopian canal may not be visualized intraoperatively; these are cases of micro dehiscence in facial nerve. Facial nerve function will recover after clearance of cholesteatoma and control of infection, and most of the times decompression of the facial nerve is not required as clearance of disease load is good enough for the facial nerve to recover. Use of steroids accelerates recovery of facial nerve function. Dehiscent or eroded fallopian canal with compressed or protuberant facial nerve (edematous and congested facial nerve) underneath the CS (**Figs. 11.7–11.9**) will require decompression of the facial nerve intraoperatively. The nerve is decompressed for few millimeters on both sides after removal of overlying cholesteatoma matrix or granulations (**Fig. 11.10**). Whenever granulation tissue is covering the facial nerve, complete clearance of the granulation tissue with decompression of the facial nerve in either direction is required (**Fig. 11.11**). Decompression also helps in finding the plane of cleavage between the cholesteatoma or granulation tissue and the facial nerve. In case of granulations sitting directly on the facial nerve, gelfoam and cotton ball soaked in adrenaline or steroids is placed over it and kept for few minutes for decongestion to happen making the right plane of separation visible.

Very rarely, long-standing disease may lead to fibrosis of the facial nerve, which needs resection of the fibrotic segment, followed by interposition free cable nerve grafting between the two cut healthy ends of the facial nerve. After any repair procedure, the exposed nerve fibers need to be protected by placing boomerang-shaped cartilage so as to avoid fibrosis and adhesions.

Case 1: Cholesteatoma with Facial Nerve Palsy Grade V HBS and Lateral Rectus Palsy (Left Side)

A patient presented with foul smelling, scanty, intermittent ear discharge with hearing loss for 3 years. Facial nerve weakness of the left side started developing from 2 months and diplopia from 4 weeks (**Fig. 11.12**). On examination, posterosuperior canal wall sagging was present along with plastered TM (**Fig. 11.13**). Left-sided facial nerve palsy of grade V with left lateral rectus palsy was noted.

Pus was collected from EAC on left side and sent for culture and sensitivity. HRCT temporal bone was performed, which showed extensive erosion of the mastoid bone, posterior canal wall, lateral part of vertical fallopian canal, sigmoid sinus plate, presigmoid dural plate, and tegmen plate.

Surgery Planned

Under the cover of appropriate antibiotics and steroids, left sidedinside-out mastoidectomy with facial nerve decompression was planned.

Preoperative HRCT of temporal bone depicted erosion of mastoid cortex, posterior canal wall, and lateral wall of vertical fallopian canal (**Fig. 11.14**).

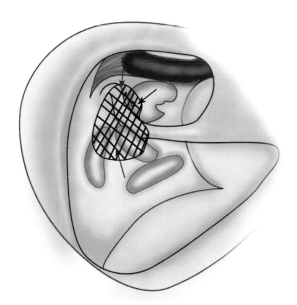

Fig. 11.9 Appearance of cholesteatoma matrix draped on intact or dehiscent facial nerve, stapes footplate, and intact or dehiscent lateral semicircular canal. The matrix can be lifted from the facial nerve by starting from the margin of footplate in inferior to superior direction and creating a plane between the matrix and underlying structures (*black arrow*). If the footplate is not visible, the matrix can be lifted anteriorly from processus cochleariformis (*red arrow*) or posteriorly from the antrum toward the attic and middle ear (*purple arrow*).

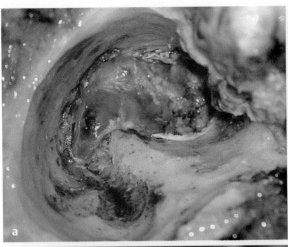
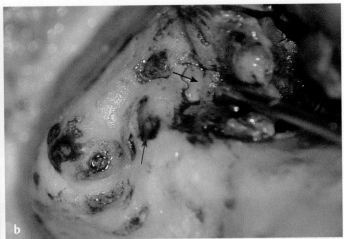
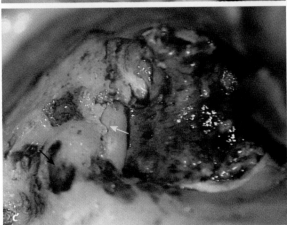

Fig. 11.10 Right sided inside out, canal wall down mastoidectomy for cholesteatoma removal **(a)** cholesteatoma sac (CS) exposed till its extension in the antrum. It is tightly draped over important structures like lateral semicircular canal (LSC), fallopian canal, stapes footplate area, and middle ear. **(b)** CS being lifted from the antrum toward the middle ear, taking care to create the right plane between the CS and underlying structures. The LSC (*red arrow*) is found eroded and facial nerve (*black arrow*) seems dehiscent while lifting the CS. **(c)** By lifting the edge of the CS, the whole sac without tearing is peeled off the underlying tympanic segment (TS), footplate, and semicircular canals. The different structures visible after peeling off the CS are eroded LSC (*black arrow*), dehiscent and slightly inflamed facial nerve in the TS (*yellow arrow*).

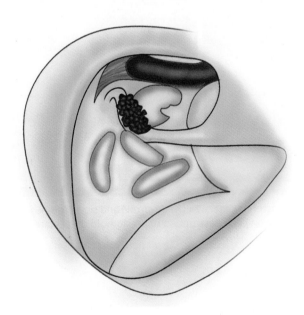

Fig. 11.11 In case of granulations sitting directly on the facial nerve, gelfoam and cotton ball soaked in adrenaline or steroids is placed over it and kept for few minutes for decongestion to happen making the right plane of separation visible.

Surgical Steps

Postaural incision was made, temporalis fascia graft harvested, and posteroinferiorly based musculoperiosteal flap elevated. Posterior canal wall skin was elevated in three-fourths of the circumference and retracted anteriorly. Cholesteatoma matrix was seen eroding the posterior canal wall (**Fig. 11.15**).

Inside-out mastoidectomy with canaloplasty and atticotomy was performed. Drilling was performed along and around the cholesteatoma matrix (**Fig. 11.16a**).

Atticotomy extended to the antrum in inside-out manner. Drilling was carried out lateral to the CS toward sinodural angle and mastoid tip area. Lowering and thinning of facial ridge were performed along with saucerization of the mastoid cavity. After exteriorizing the CS in complete circumference, the CS along with the matrix was debulked from the mastoid cavity up to the antrum(**Fig. 11.16**). Extensive granulation tissue was visualized in the mastoid cavity, over the exposed sigmoid sinus and tegmen dura. Exposed vertical part of the facial nerve was visualized along with residual CS posterior to it and inferior to the labyrinthine block (**Fig. 11.17**).

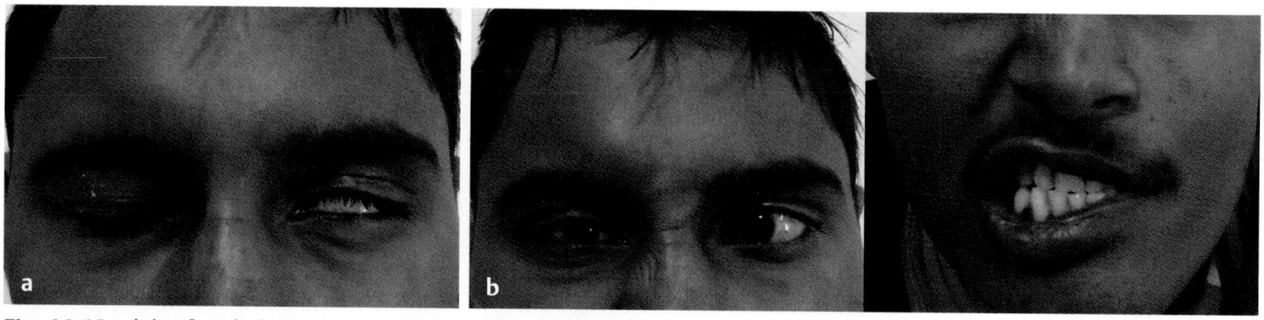

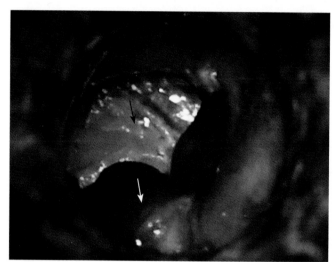

Fig. 11.12 **(a)** Left-sided grade V facial nerve weakness. **(b)** Left lateral rectus palsy.

Fig. 11.13 Sagging of posterior canal wall (*white arrow*) with plastered tympanic membrane (*black arrow*).

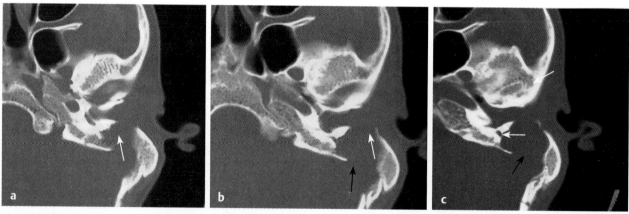

Fig. 11.14 **(a)** Erosion of mastoid cortex (*white arrow*). **(b)** Erosion of posterior canal wall (*white arrow*) and sigmoid sinus plate (*black arrow*). **(c)** Erosion of lateral wall of vertical fallopian canal (*white arrow*) and destruction of presigmoid dural plate (*black arrow*).

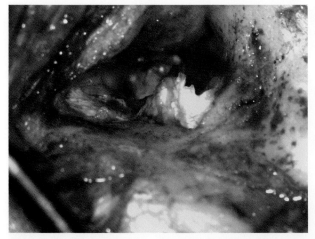

Fig. 11.15 Cholesteatoma eroding the posterior bony canal wall visualized.

Polishing of mastoid cavity was performed, and residual cholesteatoma from infralabyrinthine and retrofacial area was removed. Granulation tissue from exposed sigmoid sinus and tegmen dura was debulked and bipolarized (**Fig. 11.18a**).

The CS was elevated and removed from the antrum toward the aditus. Osteitic bone around the vertical facial nerve was polished along with lowering and thinning of the facial ridge. Thinning of the LSC in the form of blue lining was visualized (**Fig. 11.18b**).

The CS was elevated from the attic and horizontal fallopian canal (**Fig. 11.19a**). Plastered TM was elevated from the stapes head and promontory after incising the adhesion band, malleus denuded off epithelium. Further decompression of vertical facial nerve was performed in both directions (**Fig. 11.19b**).

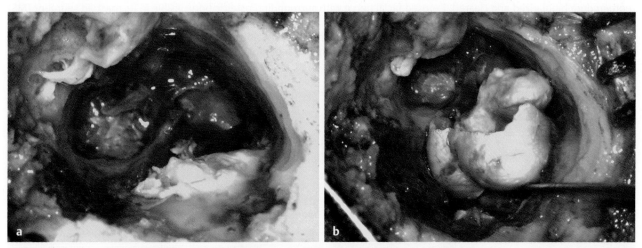

Fig. 11.16 **(a)** Canaloplasty followed by atticotomy and antrostomy cholesteatoma (*black arrows*) visualized further eroding the mastoid cortex. **(b)** Cholesteatoma sac being mobilized and elevated from the mastoid tip and sinodural angle area to be finally debulked.

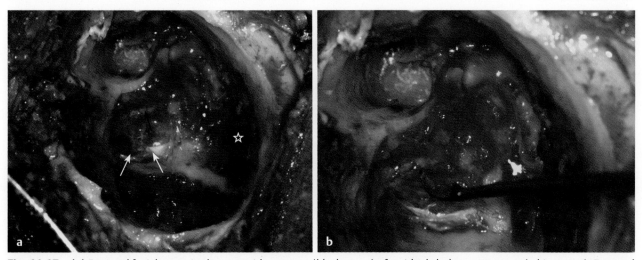

Fig. 11.17 **(a)** Exposed facial nerve in the mastoid segment (*black arrow*) of residual cholesteatoma sac (*white arrow*). Exposed sigmoid sinus lateral wall with granulations (*black asterisk*) and exposed middle fossa dura with granulations (*white asterisk*) are visualized. **(b)** Exposed vertical facial nerve being pointed.

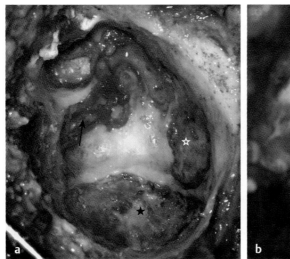
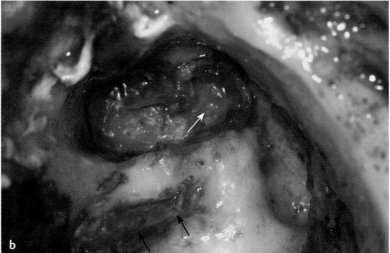

Fig. 11.18 **(a)** Mastoid cavity polished and residual cholesteatoma sac removed. Granulation tissue over sigmoid sinus and tegmen dura bipolarized and cleared. Exposed facial nerve with surrounding osteitic bone visible in its mastoid segment (MS) (*black arrow*). Cleared sigmoid sinus lateral wall (*black asterisk*) and exposed middle fossa dura (*white asterisk*) after removing granulations are visualized. **(b)** Cholesteatoma sac cleared till the attic. Osteitic bone around vertical facial nerve (*black arrow*) polished after lowering and thinning of the facial ridge. The tympanic segment covered with a layer of cholesteatoma sac (*white arrow*).

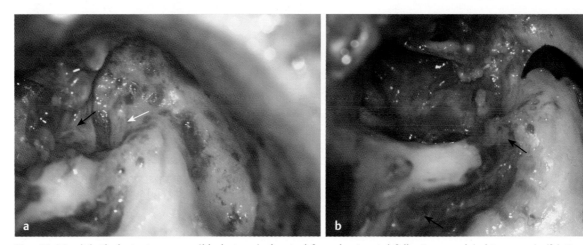

Fig. 11.19 **(a)** Cholesteatoma sac (*black arrow*) elevated from horizontal fallopian canal (*white arrow*). **(b)** Decompression of the vertical segment of facial nerve was performed in both proximal and distal directions till healthy looking nerve was achieved (*black arrows*). Plastered tympanic membrane has been elevated from the stapes head and promontory after incising the adhesion band. Dehiscence in tympanic segment (TS) visualized and pointed out with instrument.

The defect in the tegmen bone was repaired with tragal cartilage graft. For ossiculoplasty, the incus was reshaped and placed as interposition graft between the head of stapes and handle of malleus. The incus should not be touching the exposed facial nerve (**Fig. 11.20**). Also, the sheath of the exposed facial nerve is not incised as it may lead to infection entering the facial nerve fibers

(**Fig. 11. 20**). Pedicle postaural muscle flap was mobilized and used to cover the exposed sigmoid sinus and to obliterate posteroinferior part of the cavity (**Fig. 11.21**).

Postsurgery facial nerve improvement was up to grade II in 3 months (**Fig. 11.22**) and complete recovery to grade I in 1 year (**Fig. 11.23**). The neotympanum was completely healed.

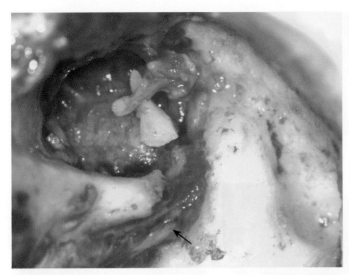

Fig. 11.20 Reshaped incus placed from the head of stapes to handle of malleus. The incus is not touching the exposed facial nerve. The sheath over the exposed mastoid segment (MS) is intact (*black arrow*).

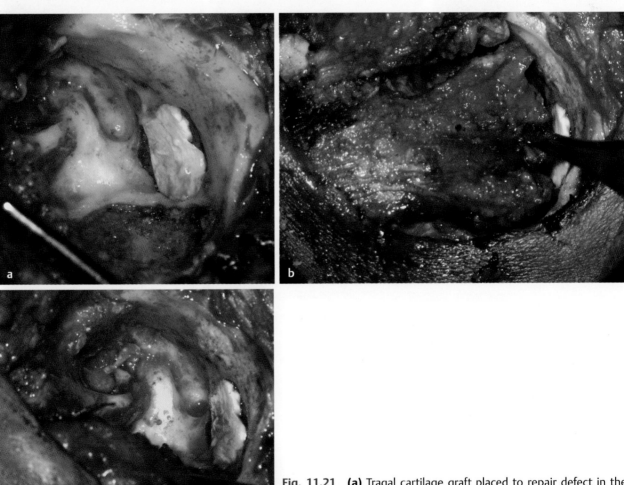

Fig. 11.21 **(a)** Tragal cartilage graft placed to repair defect in the tegmen bone. **(b)** Pedicled postaural muscle flap being mobilized. **(c)** Postaural muscle placed to cover exposed sigmoid sinus and obliterate posteroinferior part of the cavity.

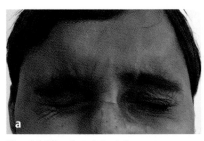
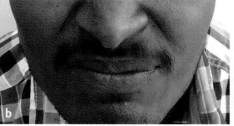
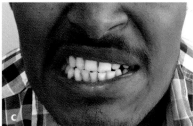

Fig. 11.22   (a–c) Facial nerve recovery up to grade II after 3 months of surgery.

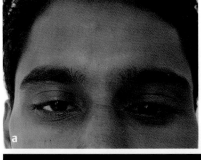
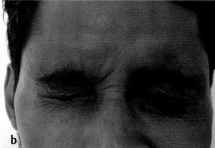
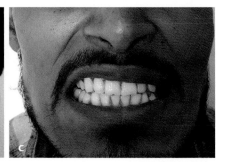

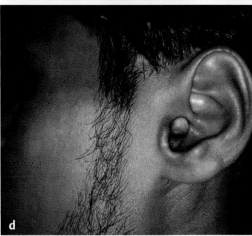

Fig. 11.23   (a–c) Recovery of facial nerve up to grade I after 1 year of surgery. **(d)** Healed neotympanum.

Case 2: Case of Extensive Cholesteatoma Involving Middle Ear, Attic, and Antrum with Facial Nerve Palsy Grade III HBS (Right Side)

A patient presented with chronic ear discharge with profound hearing loss and facial weakness on the right side. The otoendoscopy picture showed big polyp filling the EAC. Pure tone audiometry showed profound sensorineural hearing loss on the right side.

HRCT of temporal bone showed cholesteatoma eroding the LSC, bony wall of TS and second genu, internal carotid artery (ICA), and round window (**Fig. 11.24**).

Surgical Planning

Canal wall down mastoidectomy with repair of fistula and decompression of the facial nerve on the right side was planned.

Surgical Steps

Inside-out canal wall down mastoidectomy performed. The CS was exposed in all directions up to the antrum. All ossicles other than footplate were absent. Gentle lifting of the epithelium of the CS from the underlying LSC and fallopian canal was performed with the help of curved needle and cotton ball, keeping in mind the CT scan finding of LSC fistula and dehiscent tympanic segment of facial nerve underneath the CS. Fistula in the LSC was noticed underneath the sac. Further lifting of epithelium exposed dehiscent facial nerve in the TS. After separating the epithelium from the facial nerve, it was further lifted and separated from underlying footplate and round window without breaking the continuity of the epithelium. Further separation of the epithelium exposed dehiscent carotid canal in the vertical segment (**Figs. 11.25–11.27**).

The facial nerve was decompressed without incising the sheath from the first genu to the second genu. Once all the disease was cleared, the repair was performed. Bone dust was placed to cover the ICA. The fistula, which was deep up to the membranous labyrinth (grade II), was repaired in three layers, namely, free muscle graft, bone dust, and bone wax (**Fig. 11.28**). As the hearing loss is profound, no ossiculoplasty was performed. A big-sized cartilage piece was placed lateral to the exposed facial nerve and covering the whole middle ear. Postoperative results are shown in **Fig. 11.29**.

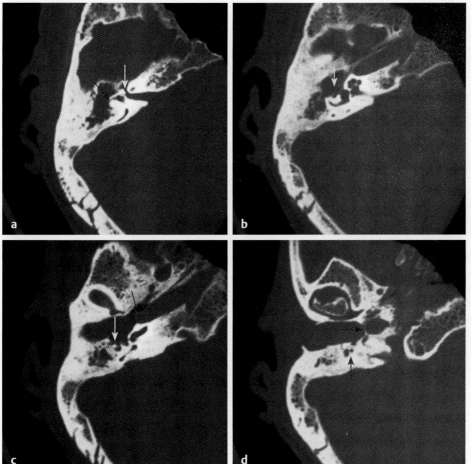

Fig. 11.24 High-resolution computed tomography (HRCT) of temporal bone, right side, axial cut from inferior to superior, showing **(a)** fistula (*red arrow*) in the lateral semicircular canal (LSC) underneath the soft tissue shadow involving the antrum. **(b)** Bony erosion of the fallopian canal in the tympanic segment (TS) (*yellow arrow*). **(c)** Bony dehiscence in the second genu area (*yellow arrow*) along with soft tissue mass filling the external auditory canal (EAC), middle ear, attic, and antrum. Dehiscent internal carotid artery (ICA) canal (*red arrow*) is visible. **(d)** Mastoid segment (MS) of the facial nerve (*yellow arrow*) seen unaffected by the disease. Bony erosion of the vertical portion of carotid canal visualized.

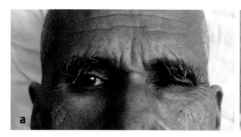
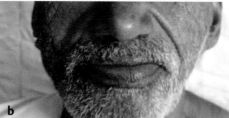

Fig. 11.25 **(a, b)** Preoperative pictures of the patient showing grade III facial palsy of the right side.

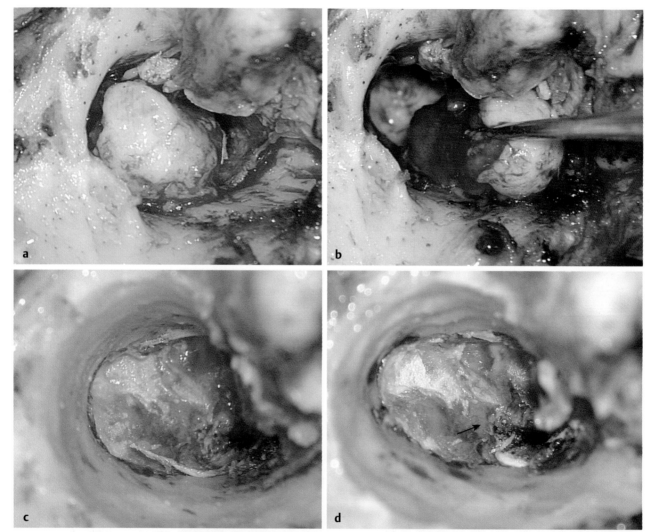

Fig. 11.26 **(a)** A big polyp filling the external auditory canal (EAC) and middle ear. **(b)** The polyp is being excised and delivered from the EAC. **(c)** Inside-out mastoidectomy in progress. The cholesteatoma sac (CS) extending from the middle ear toward the attic and antrum visualized. **(d)** The tympanic membrane and CS seen plastered to the underlying structures including the tympanic segment (TS) of the facial nerve (*black arrow*). *(Continued)*

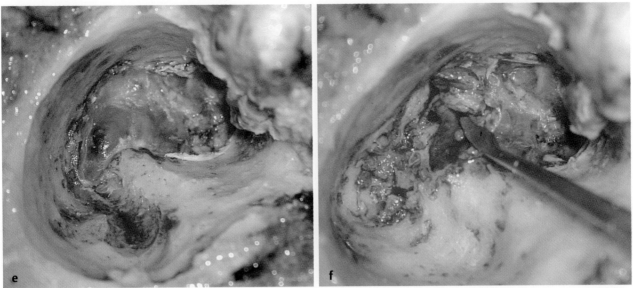

Fig. 11.26 *(Continued)* **(e)** Outermost extent of the CS up to the antrum after exposing the sac in all directions. **(f)** The plastered epithelium is being lifted from underlying dome of the lateral semicircular canal (LSC), fallopian canal, and footplate by creating the right plane between the sac and underlying structures.

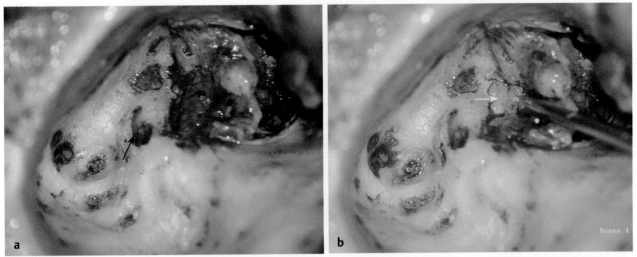

Fig. 11.27   **(a)** Fistula in the dome of lateral semicircular canal (LSC) *(black arrow)*. **(b)** Dehiscent fallopian canal (FC) in the tympanic segment (TS) *(yellow arrow)* underneath the epithelium. *(Continued)*

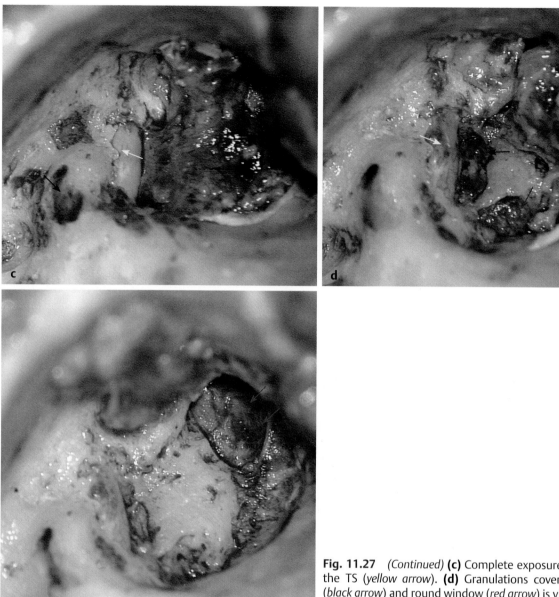

Fig. 11.27 *(Continued)* **(c)** Complete exposure of dehiscent the TS (*yellow arrow*). **(d)** Granulations covering footplate (*black arrow*) and round window (*red arrow*) is visualized after lifting of plastered epithelium. **(e)** Dehiscent internal carotid artery in its vertical segment (*red arrows*).

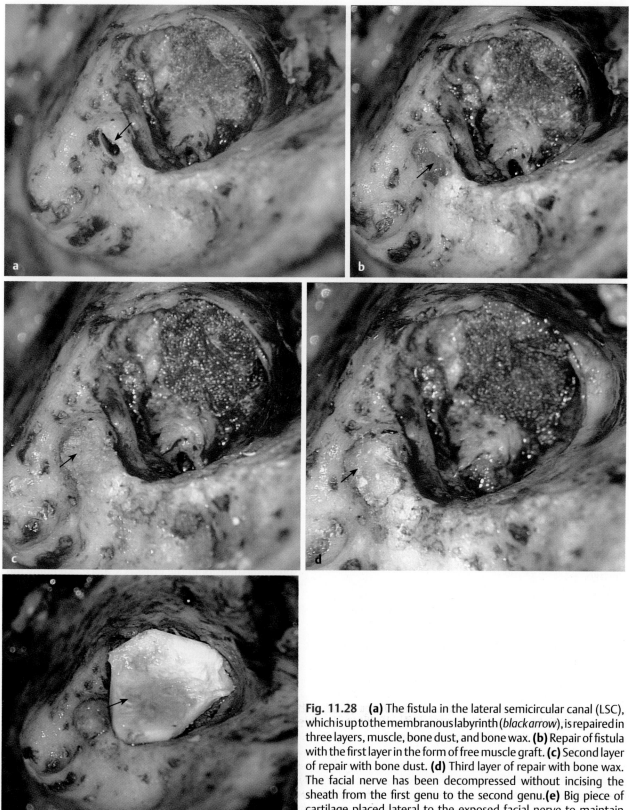

Fig. 11.28 **(a)** The fistula in the lateral semicircular canal (LSC), which is up to the membranous labyrinth (*black arrow*), is repaired in three layers, muscle, bone dust, and bone wax. **(b)** Repair of fistula with the first layer in the form of free muscle graft. **(c)** Second layer of repair with bone dust. **(d)** Third layer of repair with bone wax. The facial nerve has been decompressed without incising the sheath from the first genu to the second genu.**(e)** Big piece of cartilage placed lateral to the exposed facial nerve to maintain the middle ear space.

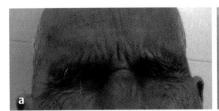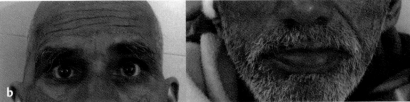

Fig. 11.29 **(a, b)** Complete recovery of the facial nerve to grade I after 21 days of surgery.

Congenital Cholesteatoma

Congenital cholesteatoma (CC) is believed to arise from embryonic epithelial cell rests within the middle ear cleft. They rarely present at an early age. Their late presentation is because the CC with intact TM often remains asymptomatic and undetected for many years until it has grown into a considerable size or has caused complications. So, patient of CC actually may present with one of its complications and that can be facial palsy (Case 3). Hearing loss may not be the first presenting symptom as the CS causes a bridging effect in transmitting and conducting sound in the middle ear despite damage to the ossicular chain. The patient my present with sensorineural hearing loss, indicating inner ear involvement either caused by the toxins secreted or direct invasion.

Regarding the facial nerve involvement, as the epicenter of CC remains in the middle ear, the TS of the facial nerve is mostly at risk. The TS is either congenitally dehiscent, or the enzymatic activity of the cholesteatoma causes osteoclastic activity, leading to bony erosions of the facial canal. As the same osteoclastic activity can lead to pathological dehiscence in the bony labyrinth, apart from facial paralysis, the patient may at times present with occasional giddiness and positional vertigo.

HRCT of temporal bone remains the only important investigation. It delineates the CS as a soft tissue density filling the Prussak's space extending into the middle ear cavity, involving the mesotympanum and epitympanum causing displacement of normal ossicular configuration with an intact but bulging TM. In case of facial nerve involvement, it will show the involved segment of the facial nerve which most of the times is dehiscent TS or eroded MS.

Case 3: Congenital Cholesteatoma of Middle Ear and Mastoid with Facial Palsy Grade IV HBS (Left Side)

A patient presented with complaint of headache, vomiting, fever, and signs of meningitis along with severe hearing loss and grade IV facial palsy of the left side (**Fig. 11.30**). He was admitted in neurology department and started on intravenous antibiotics depending on culture and sensitivity report of cerebrospinal fluid (CSF). CT scan was suggestive of pathology in the middle ear, attic, aditus, and mastoid on the left side. In spite of the conservative management in the form of intravenous antibiotics for 15 days, the patient persisted with facial palsy and hearing loss, although there was improvement in signs and symptoms of meningitis. The patient was referred to ENT department for exploration of mastoid. The patient did not have any history of ear discharge.

Otoscopic examination revealed a whitish mass medial to an intact left TM (**Fig. 11.31**). His pure tone audiogram assessment demonstrated severe conductive hearing loss on the left side.

A provisional diagnosis of left CC was made at this point. HRCT of the temporal bone delineated extensive soft tissue density in the Prussak's space extending into the left middle ear cavity, involving the mesotympanum and epitympanum causing displacement of normal ossicular chain with intact but bulging TM (**Fig. 11.32**).

Surgery Planned

Modified radical mastoidectomy with removal of disease with canal wall reconstruction left side was planned.

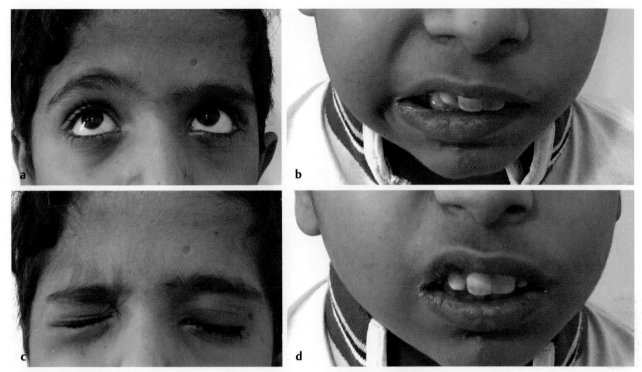

Fig. 11.30   (a–d) Preoperative images of the patient showing left-sided facial palsy of grade IV HBS.

Surgical Steps

Postaural and musculoperiosteal incision was made. Temporalis fascia graft was harvested. Posteroinferiorly based musculoperiosteal flap was elevated. EAC skin was elevated in three-fourths of the circumference and separated at the level of annulus. Intact TM with subepithelial cholesteatoma was visualized after canaloplasty. Cortical mastoidectomy was performed. Upon opening of the mastoid antrum, the CS was visualized (**Fig. 11.33**).

The TM was elevated and cholesteatoma visualized under it (**Fig. 11.34**). As the cholesteatoma was seen extending under the ossicles and posterior canal wall, bony posterior canal wall was removed after making superior and inferior osteotomies in posterior canal wall (**Fig. 11.35**).

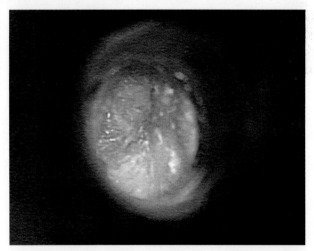

Fig. 11.31   Intact tympanic membrane (TM) with subepithelial cholesteatoma.

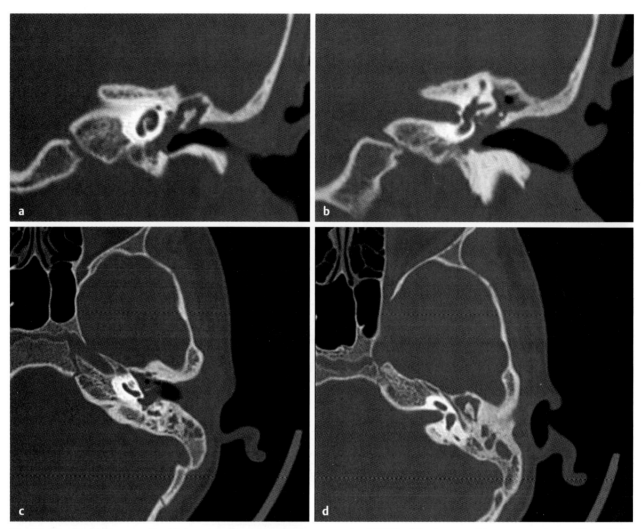

Fig. 11.32 **(a, b)** Preoperative high-resolution computed tomography (HRCT) of the temporal bone coronal cuts: The middle ear and attic found filled with soft tissue, surrounding and pushing head of malleus and body of incus with intact tympanic membrane (TM). **(c)** The axial cuts depict soft tissue in the middle ear with intact, bulging TM. **(d)** Axial cuts depicting soft tissue in the attic around the head of malleus and body of incus lateral to intact horizontal fallopian canal.

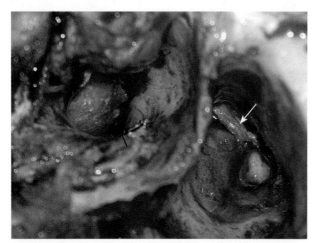

Fig. 11.33 Intact tympanic membrane (*black arrow*) with subepithelial cholesteatoma. Cortical mastoidectomy and cholesteatoma sac in the antrum (*white arrow*).

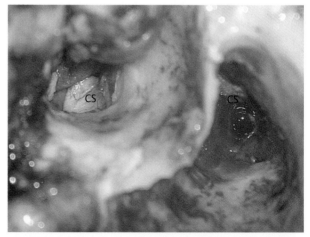

Fig. 11.34 Tympanic membrane elevated; cholesteatoma sac (CS) seen in the middle ear. Continuity of the congenital cholesteatoma visualized in the antrum also. The sac extending under ossicles and posterior canal wall.

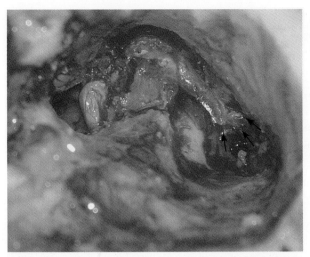

Fig. 11.35 Partial lowering and thinning of the facial ridge performed; cholesteatoma sac (CS) extending from the attic toward the middle ear visualized better. *Black arrows* showing posterior extent of the CS.

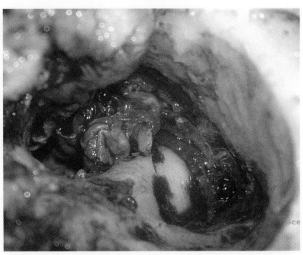

Fig. 11.36 Cholesteatoma sac being lifted toward the attic and middle ear (*black arrows*). Short process of incus (Is) visible.

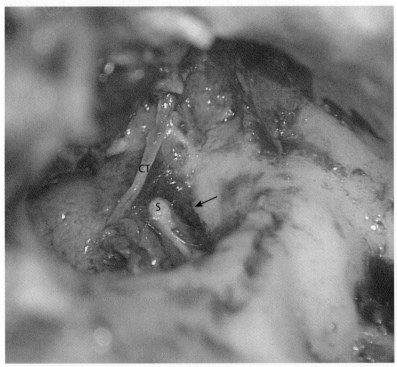

Fig. 11.37 Whole of the cholesteatoma sac removed from the antrum, attic, and middle ear. Dehiscence in the inferior part of the tympanic segment of the facial nerve (*black arrow*) visualized. Head of stapes (S) and chorda tympani (CT) are shown.

After removal of the posterior canal wall, extension and continuity in the CS were seen from the middle ear to the attic, aditus, and antrum (**Fig. 11.35**). The whole CS was exteriorized.

The CS in aditus and attic was excised. As the CS was seen extending under and anterior to the malleus, so the incus was removed and the head of malleus was amputated (**Figs. 11.36** and **11.37**). The CS in the anterior attic was excised, and clearance of anterior ventilation pathway was performed. Intact stapes was present with preserved chorda tympani. Residual CS was removed from the antrum, attic, and middle ear. Horizontal fallopian canal was found dehiscent along the length of the inferior part of TS of the facial nerve, which was the cause of facial paresis (grade IV) (**Fig. 11.37**).

Post-surgery, facial nerve recovery up to grade I could be achieved in 5 months (**Fig. 11.38**).

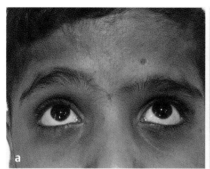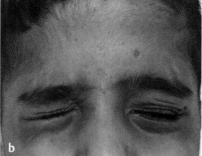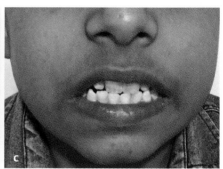

Fig. 11.38 **(a–c)** Facial nerve recovery up to grade I after 5 months of surgery.

Malignant Otitis Externa/Malignant External Otitis (MEO) with Facial Paresis/Palsy

MOE remains a serious and life-threatening infection of the temporal bone and surrounding soft tissue structures. Most of the times, it is seen in immunocompromised patients, classically elderly patients with diabetes mellitus, and the infecting organism remains *Pseudomonas aeruginosa*. The disease process starts in EAC, and spread of the disease outside the EAC occurs through the fissures of Santorini and the osseocartilaginous junction. From posteroinferior quadrant of the EAC the infection reaches the mastoid part of fallopian canal mostly around the stylomastoid foramen (SMF). Facial paralysis usually results from presence of necrotizing granulation tissue eroding the fallopian canal and affecting the MS of the facial nerve at and around the SMF.

Clinical Features

The patient gives a history of local trauma in the form of ear cleaning with some unusual applicators. The bacterial invasion starts at the trauma site and progresses through suture lines in the EAC to reach the mastoid part of the fallopian canal. The presentation remains a deep-seated pain in the affected side ear, out of proportion to the clinical picture along with facial weakness in case the facial nerve is involved.

On Examination

The EAC is found inflamed and bulging, and granulation tissue is found filling the EAC mostly in its posteroinferior quadrant. Progressively increasing facial nerve paresis in different stages is noted and it may be associated with other lower cranial nerves paresis/palsy as

the infection traverses inferiorly into the skull base. The TM, middle ear, and mastoid are usually found free of the disease.

Investigations

Differentiating facial nerve palsy due to cholesteatoma from MEO is quite difficult when inflamed EAC hides the intact TM. HRCT temporal bone remains the best modality to differentiate and diagnose case of MEO with facial nerve palsy. It demonstrates erosion of the bony EAC with adjacent soft tissue and sparing of the middle ear and mastoid other than slight fluid opacification.

However, HRCT temporal bone may not be able to differentiate carcinoma of EAC from MEO. In case of doubt, preoperative or intraoperative biopsy from granulation tissue in the EAC is sent for histopathology examination to rule out malignancy.

Treatment

Medical management in the form of therapeutic dose of systemic antibiotics remains the preferred treatment. The choice of antibiotics remains fluoroquinolones (primarily ciprofloxacin and ofloxacin) and antipseudomonal parenteral antibiotics which are given for a long time along with management of diabetes, and the patient should expect good to excellent recovery of facial nerve. Fluoroquinolones are DNA-gyrase inhibitors that are effective against *P. aeruginosa* and well tolerated by patients. They are used in high dose (ciprofloxacin is given 750 mg twice daily) due to poor vascularization of the target area. Due to emergence of ciprofloxacin-resistant pseudomonal strains, culture sensitivity becomes the most important investigation before topical or systemic antimicrobial therapy is initiated. The conservative treatment should be continued for at least

4 weeks, but the duration of therapy should be customized according to the signs and symptoms and severity of the disease.

Surgery has an important role but is treatment of choice for few limited situations.

Surgical Management

Surgical debridement is performed in few situations where the progression of the disease continues in spite of continuous medical therapy, evidenced by any one of the following:

- Persistence of severe excruciating pain and granulation tissue in the EAC
- Deterioration of facial nerve functioning and development of lower cranial nerve paresis/palsy during treatment
- Other signs or symptoms of active infection for more than 2 weeks after institution of therapy

Any one of these criteria is considered an indication for radical surgical intervention.

Surgical procedure ranges from intact canal wall mastoidectomy with facial nerve decompression in the affected part to subtotal temporal bone resection in cases of extensive osteomyelitis. The aim of extensive exposure is to gain access to the primary focus of infection and provide adequate drainage.

In usual cases, there is osteomyelitis of bone around the MS, and after clearing the osteitic bone the facial nerve is found intact. Clearing the diseased tissue and decompressing the facial nerve are good enough for facial nerve recovery up to grade I. In very few cases, if the surgery is delayed, or the infection is aggressive, it may lead to congestion, necrosis, and finally fibrosis of affected segment of the facial nerve. In such cases the involved segment of the facial nerve is excised, and the repair of the nerve is taken up in the second stage, after complete control of the infection. The second-stage repair can be planned after few months and it can be interposition cable nerve grafting with end-to-end anastomosis, once the proximal stump is found viable. In case the viability of the proximal stump is doubtful, the repair is in the form of motor nerve transfer which can be either facio-hypoglossal anastomosis or facio-masseteric anastomosis in case the MEO has traversed to lower cranial nerves. The two-stage surgery has been described in detail in Chapter 7 titled "Facial Nerve Palsy of Short Duration with Proximal Stump Unavailable").

Case 4: Malignant Otitis Externa with Grade VI Facial Palsy (Right Side)

A diabetic patient presented with ear discharge, hearing loss, and headache with excruciating pain around the pinna on the right side. At the time of presentation, the patient had minimal weakness of right-sided facial nerve. The patient was given intravenous antibiotics after culture and sensitivity testing, and antibiotics continued for 6 weeks. Discharge reduced but pain persisted with deterioration of facial nerve function to grade V HBS (**Fig. 11.39**). Along with repeat culture and sensitivity of persisting ear discharge, granulation tissue from external canal was sent for histopathology examination to rule out malignancy and the patient was taken up for surgery.

Surgery Planned

Debridement for the skull base osteomyelitis with facial nerve decompression through transmastoid approach was planned.

Surgical Steps

Postaural and musculoperiosteal incision was made and flap mobilized. Canal skin was elevated in three-fourths of the circumference. The TM was mobilized anteriorly. Granulation tissue from floor of the canal was excised. This granulation tissue was extending posteriorly along the vertical course of the fallopian canal. Simple mastoidectomy was performed and granulation tissue visualized in the retrofacial area. It was found extending along the facial nerve in complete circumference in the lower half of the MS. The granulation tissue and all of the osteitic bone were excised. Osteitic bone over jugular bulb was polished till healthy bone was visualized. Facial nerve was decompressed further toward the second genu till healthy noninflammed facial nerve was visualized. The bony defect in the floor of the external canal and middle ear was reconstructed with a piece of tragal cartilage. Facial nerve was protected with a piece of floor cartilage which also covered the socket in retrofacial area. Temporalis fascia graft was placed to reconstruct the TM. The residual TM was reposited (**Figs. 11.40–11.46**).

Postoperatively, antibiotics were given for prolonged period according to culture and sensitivity report of the sample collected from the pus and granulation tissue in the SMF area intraoperatively. Postoperative results are depicted in **Figs. 11.47** and **11.48**.

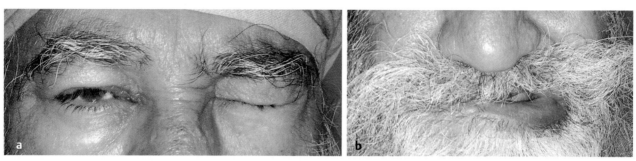

Fig. 11.39   (a, b) Preoperative pictures demonstrating right facial palsy grade V.

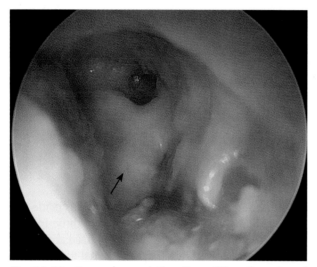

Fig. 11.40   Pus and granulation tissue filling the external auditory canal (EAC), more toward the posteroinferior side.

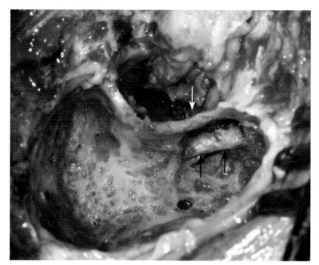

Fig. 11.41 Cortical mastoidectomy with lifting of tympanomeatal flap already performed. The granulation tissue is visible in the floor of the canal (*white arrow*); granulation tissue seen around the facial nerve (*black arrows*).

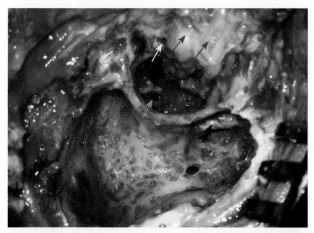

Fig. 11.42 Granulation tissue cleared from the floor of the canal; elevated tympanomeatal flap (*red arrows*) and denuded malleus (*white arrow*) with intact incudostapedial complex (*green arrow*) seen. Exposed facial nerve in its mastoid segment (MS) toward the stylomastoid foramen (SMF) is visualized (*black arrow*).

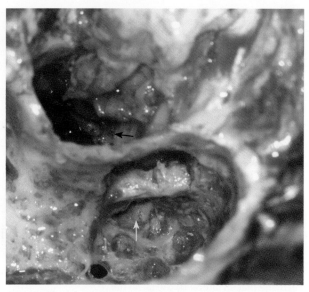

Fig. 11.43 Floor of the canal polished (*black arrow*); jugular bulb is seen (*yellow arrow*).

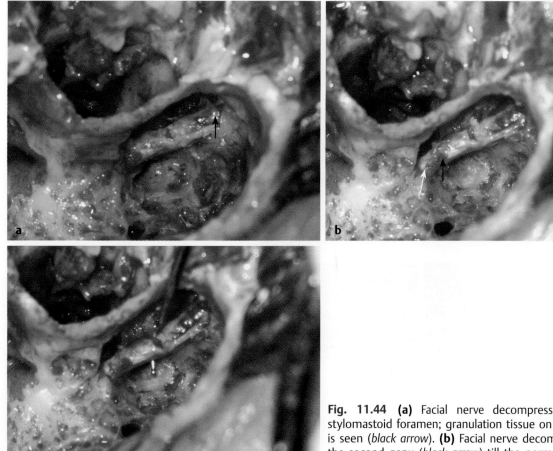

Fig. 11.44 **(a)** Facial nerve decompressed toward the stylomastoid foramen; granulation tissue on the facial nerve is seen (*black arrow*). **(b)** Facial nerve decompressed toward the second genu (*black arrow*) till the normal healthy nerve appeared (*white arrow*). **(c)** Granulation tissue from the under surface of facial nerve cleared.

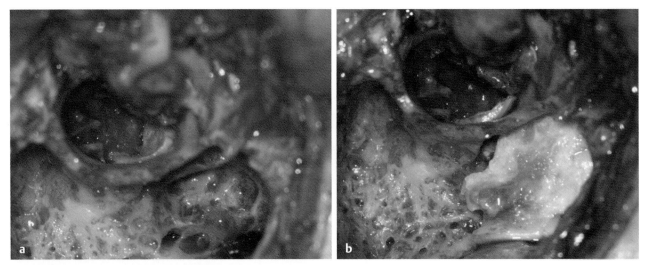

Fig. 11.45   (a) Piece of tragal cartilage placed to cover the defect in the floor; intact ossicular chain visible. **(b)** L-shaped cartilage placed lateral to the facial nerve.

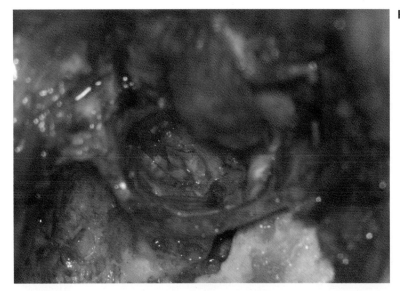

Fig. 11.46   Temporalis fascia graft in place.

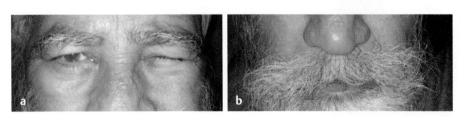

Fig. 11.47   (a, b) Postoperatively, after 3 months minimal improvement is seen.

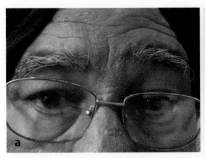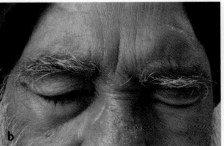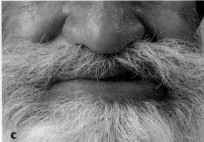

Fig. 11.48   After 6 months of surgery, facial nerve recovery was up to grade I, forehead wrinkling and nasolabial fold improved, eyes closure was complete, and angle of the mouth improved.

Case 5: A Similar Case of MEO of Right Side, Where the Disease Was Found Located in Floor of EAC and Along the Whole Length of Vertical Part of Fallopian Canal Leading to Grade VI HBS Facial Palsy on Right Side

In this case, the surgical treatment was performed in the form of transmastoid decompression of facial nerve in its MS up to the SMF where pus pockets were found. The different finding from the previous case is that the extent of facial nerve involvement was more. The facial nerve in the MS showed areas of necrosis in between areas of congestion, but it was not fibrosed. The granulations around the exposed facial nerve cleared in its complete circumference and the disease was removed in toto. The facial nerve was decompressed in both directions till normal healthy nerve could be reached on both sides. The nerve sheath was kept intact all along, and the patient was put on long-term parenteral antibiotics based on culture report. The recovery of the facial nerve could be achieved up to grade II. So, the important message is that unless until the facial nerve is completely fibrosed in full thickness, the resection of segment is to be avoided, as the clearance of infected tissue with specific antibiotics will help facial nerve to recover and regain function almost up to grade I which cannot be achieved by performing interposition free cable grafting once the infected segment of the facial nerve is resected (**Figs. 11.49–11.53**)

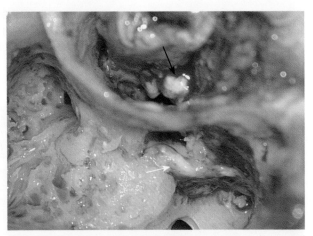

Fig. 11.49   After lifting of tympanomeatal flap and performing cortical mastoidectomy, the granulations and the necrotizing tissue involving posteroinferior quadrant of the external auditory canal (EAC) (*black arrow*) are visualized.

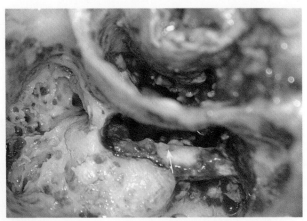

Fig. 11.50   Facial nerve decompression in its mastoid segment (MS) (*white arrow*) is in progress. The middle ear and mastoid seen free of disease.

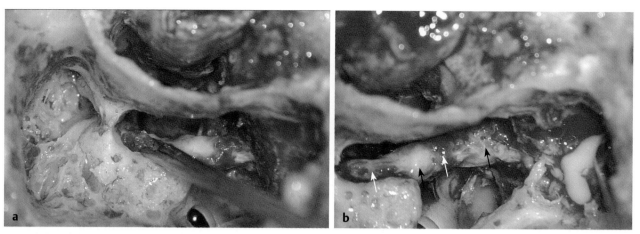

Fig. 11.51 **(a)** Clearance of granulation tissue from around the facial nerve close to the second genu. **(b)** The exposed facial nerve from the second genu till its exit at the stylomastoid foramen (SMF) showing patches of congestion (*white arrow*) and necrosis (*black arrow*) as well. Pus visualized at the SMF.

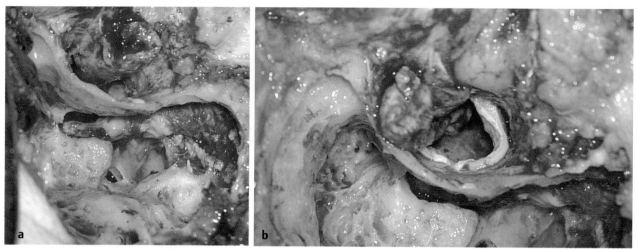

Fig. 11.52 **(a)** All pus cleared and decompression of facial nerve achieved from the second genu till the stylomastoid foramen (SMF) without incising the facial nerve sheath. **(b)** A piece of tragal cartilage placed to cover the defect in the floor and posterior wall of the external auditory canal (EAC).

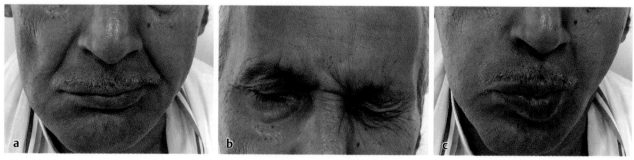

Fig. 11.53 Recovery of facial nerve up to grade II after 1 year of surgery.

Case 6: A Different Case of Skull Base Osteomyelitis/Malignant Otitis Externa with Complete Facial Nerve Palsy Grade VI (HBS) (Left Side)

Another case of a 57-year-old patient presenting with excruciating pain and grade VI facial palsy of left ear which progressed over 2 months and chronic ear discharge on the same side for 3 months. She was a known diabetic and on antidiabetic treatment since long. She had already been treated with antibiotics based on culture sensitivity report of ear discharge. As the condition did not improve after medical treatment and facial nerve palsy (grade VI HBS) persisted, surgical intervention was planned.

HRCT of temporal bone depicted the extent of osteomyelitic lesion in the left temporal bone (**Fig. 11.54**).

Preoperative clinical assessment showed grade VI facial nerve palsy on the left side (**Fig. 11.55**).

Surgical Planning

Middle ear exploration with cortical mastoidectomy with facial nerve exploration in the first stage followed by facio-hypoglossal anastomosis in the second stage.

Surgical Steps

Middle ear exploration with cortical mastoidectomy was performed. Excessive granulation tissue with polypi was found filling the mastoid cavity and the middle ear along with complete blockage of ventilation between the mastoid air cell system and the middle ear (**Fig. 11.56**). All polypi, granulation tissue, and hypertrophic mucosa from the mastoid cavity and middle

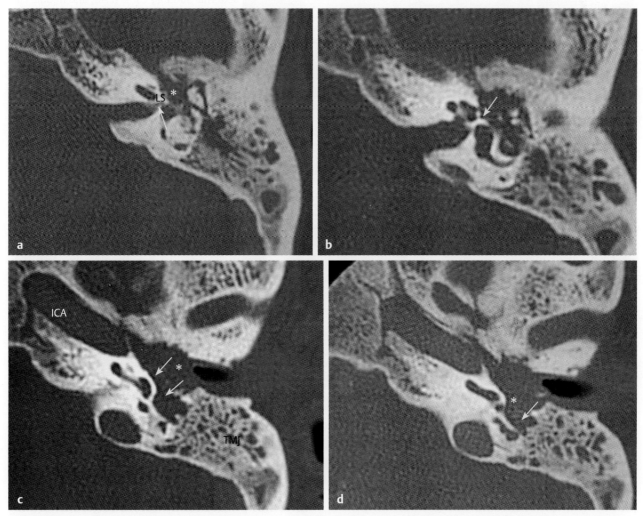

Fig. 11.54 (a–d) High-resolution computed tomography (HRCT) of temporal bone axial cuts of left side showing soft tissue shadow filling medial part of the external auditory canal (EAC), middle ear, attic, and antrum (*asterisk*). Anteriorly, the soft tissue shadow is seen involving the labyrinthine segment (LS) of the facial nerve and reaching up to the internal carotid artery (ICA). The fallopian canal is eroded from **(a)** the LS to **(b)** the first genu, **(c)** tympanic segment (TS), and **(d)** second genu and the whole length of the mastoid segment (MS) (whole of intratemporal course shown by *yellow arrows*).

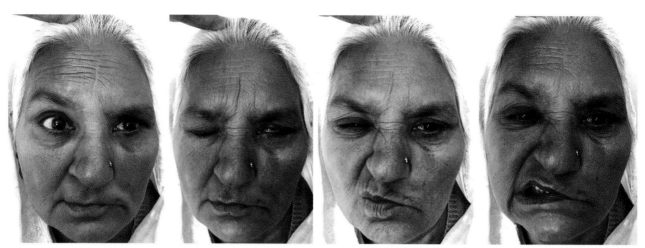

Fig. 11.55 Preoperative pictures of the patient showing grade VI facial nerve palsy (House-Brackmann's scale) on the left side.

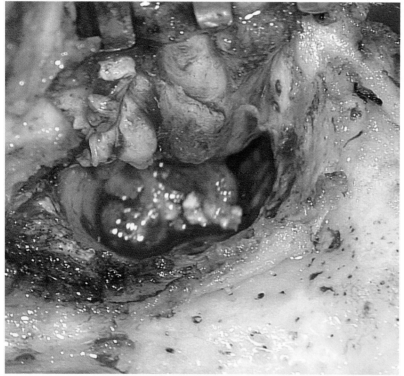

Fig. 11.56 Picture showing polyp filling the external auditory canal (EAC) and middle ear.

ear were excised (**Fig. 11.57**). While decompressing the facial nerve, it was found that there was ischemic necrosis of complete intratemporal segment of the facial nerve from the LS up to the MS till the SMF (**Fig. 11.58**). As the facial nerve functioning is not expected to return once ischemic necrosis is involving the maximum length of intra temporal segment with doubtful viability of proximal stump, facial nerve management was postponed to second stage surgery after a sufficient period of wait and watch and confirmation of the clearance of complete disease tissue from the attic, antrum, and mastoid cavity (including the disease reaching up to ICA and TMJ), reconstruction of the ossicular chain was performed by placing tragal cartilage graft between the stapes and bony annulus, and the tympanic membrane was repaired with temporalis fascia. Repair of the facial nerve was planned for the second stage, after settling down of infection and inflammation.

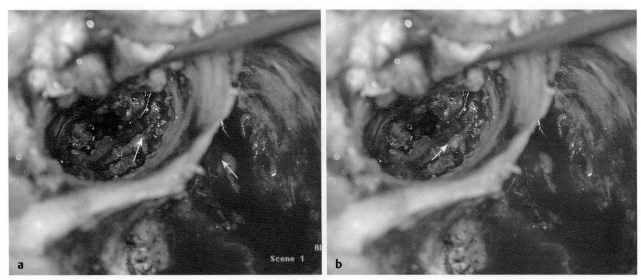

Fig. 11.57   (a, b) Cortical mastoidectomy performed to clear all granulations (*yellow arrow*) filling the antrum and mastoid cavity and achieve patency between the middle ear and mastoid. Multiple polypi with hypertrophic mucosa filling the middle ear (*white arrow*) visualized.

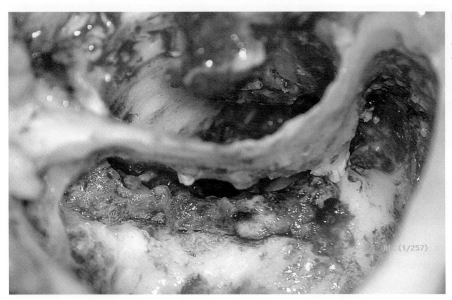

Fig. 11.58 After clearing all the hypertrophic tissue and granulations from the middle ear and mastoid, facial nerve decompression was performed from the labyrinthine segment (LS) till the mastoid segment (MS). The facial nerve decompression in progress. The whole intratemporal segment of the facial nerve found ischemic and necrosed.

Postsurgery Results

After 6 months of surgery, the osteomyelitis got cured, the graft was taken up well, but complete facial nerve palsy grade VI persisted (**Fig. 11.59**).

Second-Stage Surgery: Classical End-to-End Facio-hypoglossal Anastomosis (Left Side)

Surgical Planning

As the osteomyelitis had caused complete avascular necrosis of the facial nerve up to the labyrinthine part,

the proximal stump was nonviable up to the LS. As the sensorineural hearing was well preserved on the ipsilateral side, translabyrinthine approach to reach the proximal healthy stump of the facial nerve could not be performed. So the procedure of choice for facial reanimation here was motor nerve transfer in the form of facio-hypoglossal anastomosis (**Figs. 11.60** and **11.61**).

Surgical Steps

Details of the steps of faciao-hypoglossal anastomosis are described in Chapter 8 titled "Short Duration Flaccid Facial Palsy with Proximal Stump Unavailable."

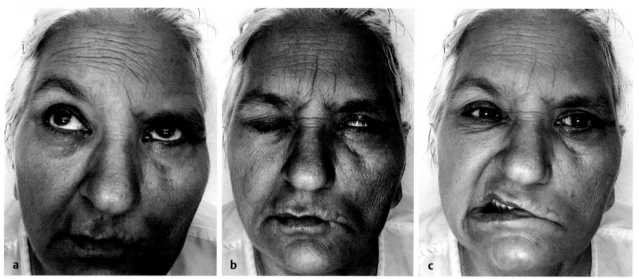

Fig. 11.59   (a–c) Complete grade VI (House-Brackmann's classification [HBC]) facial nerve palsy persisting after 6 months of surgery.

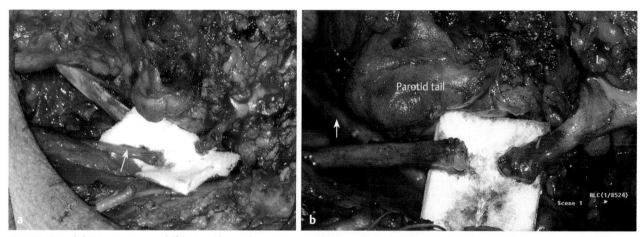

Fig. 11.60   (a) Direct view and **(b)** view through microscope: Transection of the hypoglossal nerve (as distal as possible) and the facial nerve (as proximal as possible) has been performed. Both cut ends brought together and placed on a piece of gelfoam. Posterior belly of digastric is visible (*white arrow*). Tail of parotid visible.

Postsurgery Results

After 1 year of surgery, the recovery of facial nerve function is up to grade I (HBC) (**Fig. 11.62**), but there is atrophy of left-sided tongue (**Fig. 11.62**). The patient felt difficulty in swallowing for the first few months which improved over 6 months. The tongue paresis also improved over time.

The important point conveyed through this case is, once ischemic necrosis of the facial nerve sets in, the nerve becomes nonviable and nonfunctioning. Simple decompression will not help and free cable nerve grafting, if proximal stump is available, and motor nerve transfer, if proximal stump is not available, become the procedure of choice.

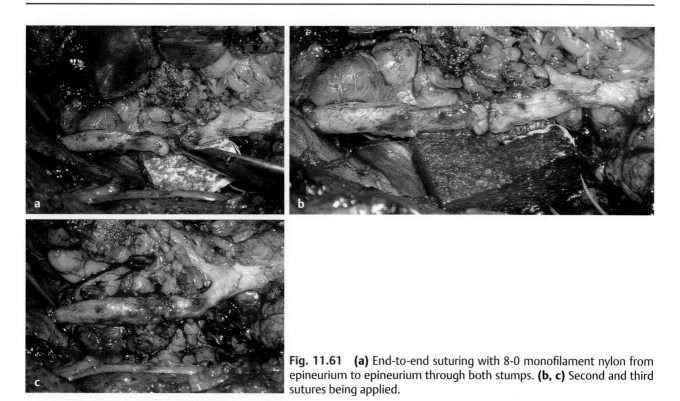

Fig. 11.61 **(a)** End-to-end suturing with 8-0 monofilament nylon from epineurium to epineurium through both stumps. **(b, c)** Second and third sutures being applied.

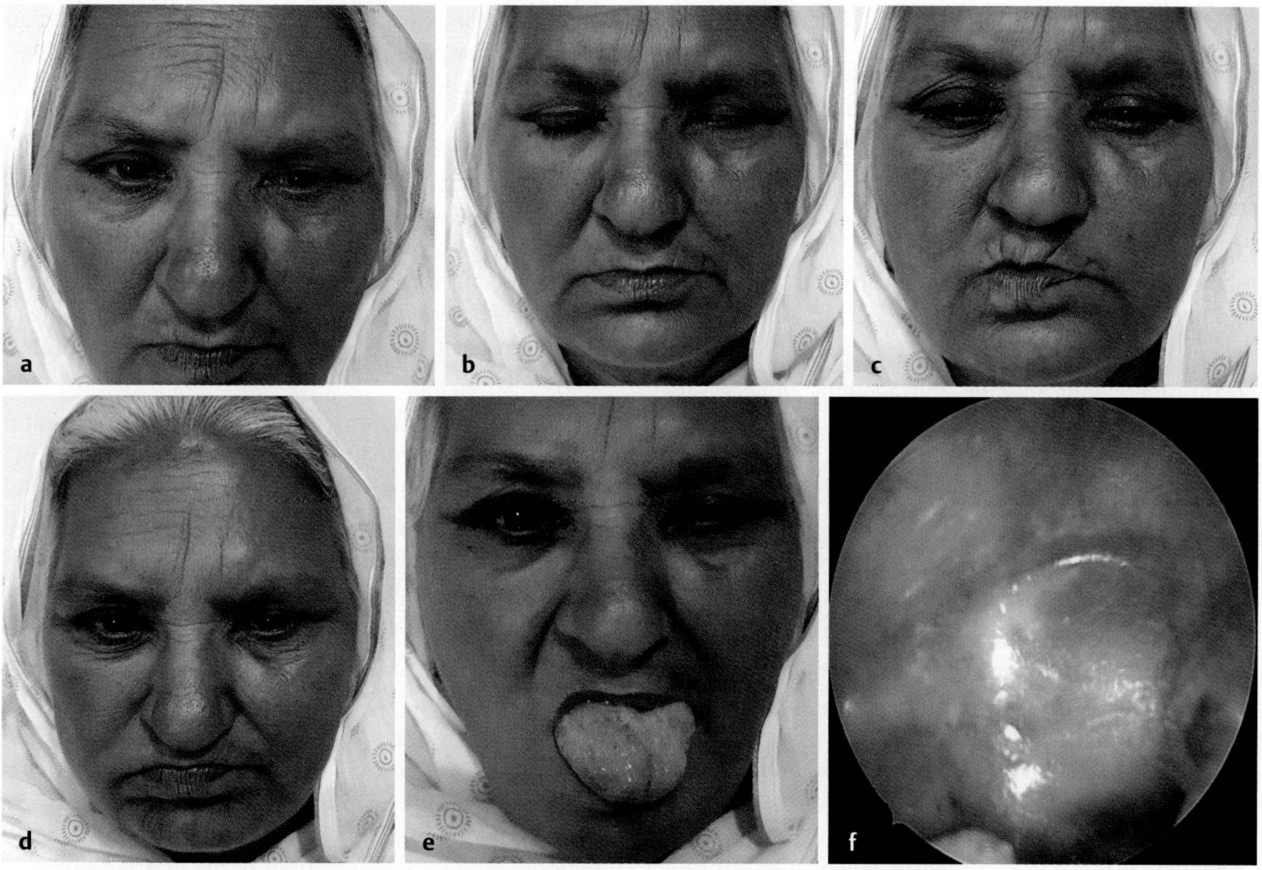

Fig. 11.62 **(a–d)** After 1 year of surgery, facial nerve recovery to grade I. **(e)** Left-sided tongue atrophy and mild paresis, although the patient has learned to swallow with the help of self-training and physiotherapy. **(f)** Healthy intact neotympanum.

Tubercular Otitis Media

Tuberculosis (TB) is a very common contagious infectious disease potentially affecting various organs and tissues. Tuberculous otitis media (TOM) is an uncommon, slow growing, and frequently a missed diagnosis. TOM is usually secondary to direct transmission from adjacent organs (i.e., the nose, larynx, pharynx, and lungs) and the primary form has rarely been seen. Most of the cases don't even give any history of current tubercular infection or in the past, which causes delay in diagnosis leading to delay in starting antitubercular treatment.

Clinical Presentation

Early diagnosis of TOM is dependent on a high index of suspicion. The patient classically presents with a triad of intractable, antibiotic-resistant, scanty, profuse, or blood stained, painless discharge from the ear, single or multiple perforations in the TM with rapidly progressing facial nerve palsy. Middle ear mucosa is found pale, and the cavity is filled with pale, soft granulation tissue. The clinical manifestation may not always be in a classical pattern. That makes TOM difficult to be definitively diagnosed on the basis of clinical manifestations only. The final diagnosis is made on the basis of histological and microbiological tests (gene amplification techniques such as real-time polymerase chain reaction [PCR]). Histological report of biopsy from granulation tissue showing granulomas, Langhans giant cells, and caseation necrosis, in association with positive (TB PCR), confirms the diagnosis of TOM.

These are methods for rapid diagnosis and detecting tuberculous bacilli, which usually present in very low numbers or at times are not even detected.

Early diagnosis is essential for the prompt initiation of antituberculous therapy and avoiding unnecessary treatments and sequelae.

Treatment

Treatment of TOM includes anti-TB treatment for at least 6 months. Surgical intervention is considered for the treatment of complications, such as extensive involvement of important structures like facial nerve (sequestrum of complete lateral wall of fallopian canal), inner ear (big fistula or multiple fistulae in semicircular canals and cochlea), subperiosteal abscesses, and cholesteatoma coexisting with TOM, where the picture can be even more confusing. The surgery is usually planned after initiating antitubercular treatment and giving it for at least 1 months followed by surgical removal of disease. Surgery is controversial in case of noncomplicated TOM.

The erosion of fallopian canal, inflammation, or edema of facial nerve may not show the extent of damage to fibers. Time duration of recovery of facial nerve function following surgery may not be proportionate to the clearance of the disease. The antitubercular medication should be started at least 1 month before surgery to have good recovery of facial nerve functioning. Any delay in starting the medication can lead to complete necrosis of facial nerve with irreversible changes.

Case 7: Revision Case of Tubercular Mastoiditis with Iatrogenic Grade VI Facial Palsy of the Right Side

A 27-year-old female patient presented with big postaural fistula, CSOM, and grade VI facial palsy on the right side. She had been operated for CSOM 6 months back.

The diagnosis of TOM was not made during the first surgery. The details of first surgery were not available, though the clinical presentation of patient showed incomplete tympanomastoid surgery with persistence of the disease, presence of grade VI facial palsy, and the occurrence of a large postauricular fistula in the region of the incision. The mastoid bone was partly uncovered and partly lined by granulation tissue and osteitic bone with sequestrum that filled mastoid cavity, involved the whole length of the fallopian canal, and extended in the middle ear region with no TM. Rest of the ENT examination was found normal. Hearing test showed severe sensorineural hearing loss on the right side. Blood tests as well as sputum examination were negative. The chest X-ray was normal while HRCT scan of the chest showed some old changes of tuberculosis (Kock's) in lungs bilaterally.

CT scan of temporal bones showed big postaural fistula with inflammatory tissue filling the right EAC, middle ear, and mastoid. The facial nerve was found involved and not separately visible in maximum length of the fallopian canal (from the first genu till the MS up to the SMF) (**Fig. 11.63**).

The histological examination of the granulation tissue showed caseous necrosis, epithelioid cells, and Langhans type giant cells.

The TB PCR test of the secretions and granulation tissue showed detection of *Mycobacterium tuberculosis*. On the basis of the laboratory findings, anti-TB treatment including rifampicin and isoniazid was started together with local medications of the mastoid cavity.

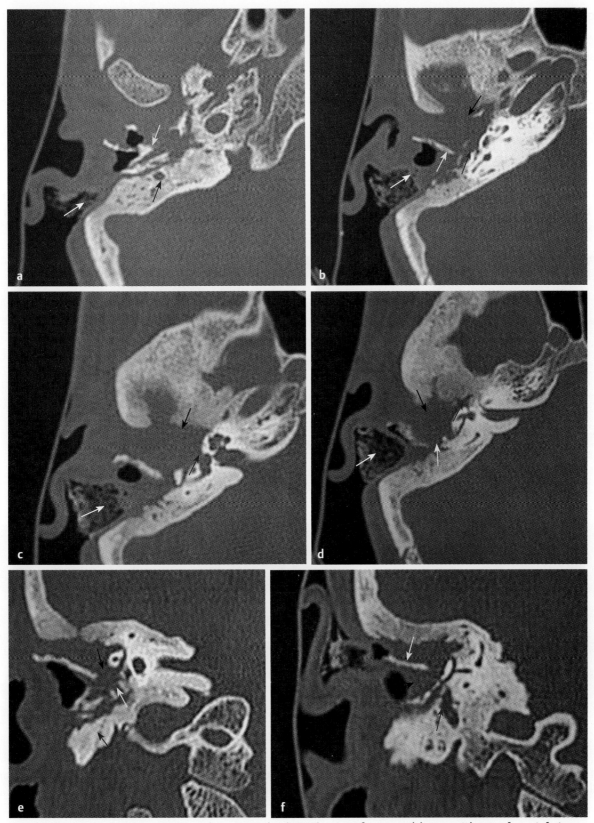

Fig. 11.63 High-resolution computed tomography (HRCT) scan of temporal bone axial cuts, from inferior to superior **(a–d)**, and coronal cuts **(e, f)** from anterior to posterior showing the postaural fistula (*white arrow*), sclerotic mastoid with osteitic bone and sequestrum (*yellow arrow*), and granulation tissue in the middle ear area (*black arrow*). The facial nerve involvement in the mastoid segment, second genu, and tympanic segment is seen (*red arrow*).

Surgical Planning

Radical mastoidectomy with clearance of granulation and sequestrum along with the facial nerve grafting was planned.

Surgical Steps

After 1 month of antitubercular therapy (ATT), the surgery was performed in the form of completion mastoidectomy, clearance of osteitic bone, sequestrum, granulations, and exposure of facial nerve from the first genu till the SMF by drilling away the infected fallopian canal and surrounding bone. The nerve was found fibrosed from the TS up to MS. The fibrotic segment of the facial nerve was resected and interposition free cable grafting performed with great auricular nerve graft. End-to-end anastomosis between cut ends of the facial nerve and free cable graft was achieved by applying sutures and fibrin glue. Reconstruction of the middle ear and mastoid cavity was performed in the same stage and ATT continued for a total of 6 months. On follow-up, the facial nerve started showing recovery in 6 months and after 2 years the facial nerve recovery could be achieved up to grade III. After the second month of therapy, the condition of the mastoid cavity progressively improved, and the postauricular fistula finally healed, and the granulation tissue disappeared (**Figs. 11.64–11.74**)

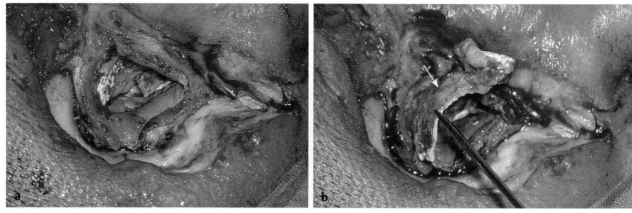

Fig. 11.64 **(a)** Right ear showing a large postauricular fistula in the region of the incision. **(b)** The big mastoid cavity found lined by skin and granulation tissue and osteitic bone with sequestrum (*white arrow*) that is extending into the middle ear.

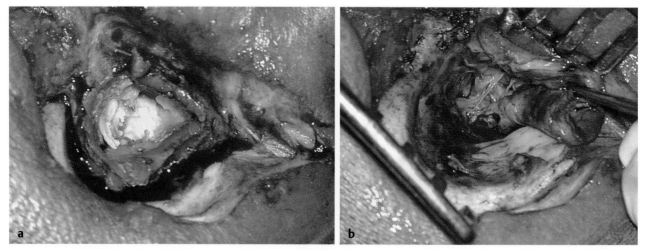

Fig. 11.65 **(a)** Skin lining the fistula and mastoid cavity, bony sequestrum, and whitish necrotic tissue filling the mastoid and middle ear with no tympanic membrane. **(b)** The skin has been lifted and retracted anteriorly.

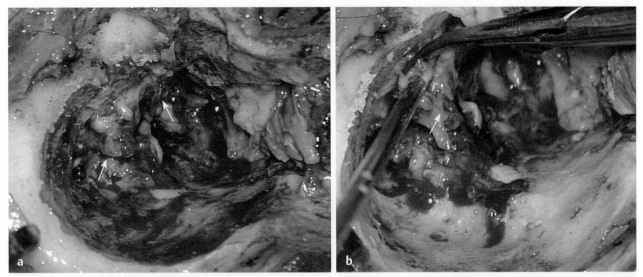

Fig. 11.66 **(a)** Completion canal wall down mastoidectomy in progress. A lot of granulation tissue and bony sequestrum found filling the middle ear and mastoid cavity (*white arrow*). **(b)** Granulation tissue sample collected for histological testing. Region of the facial nerve demarcated with *black arrows*.

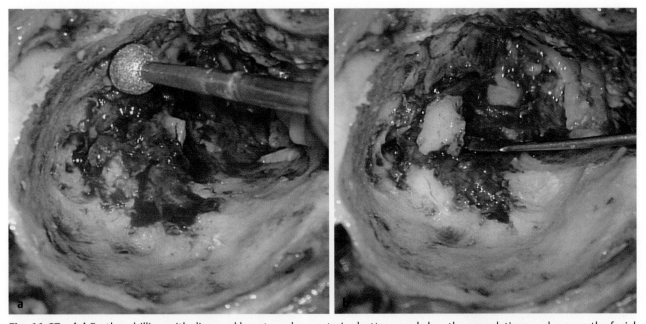

Fig. 11.67 **(a)** Further drilling with diamond burr to reduce anterior buttress and clear the granulations and expose the facial nerve. **(b)** Sequestrum of bone being lifted and removed from the antrum (second genu area of the facial nerve).

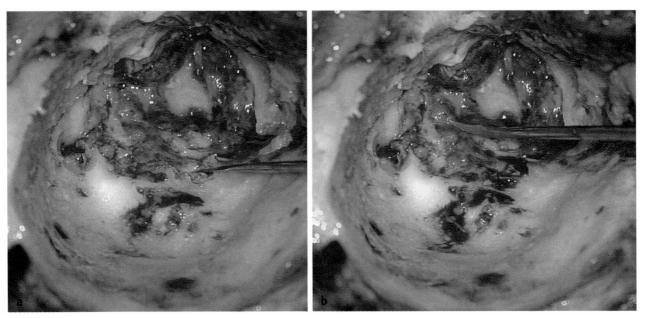

Fig. 11.68 **(a)** Instrument pointing toward lower part of mastoid segment of the facial nerve. **(b)** Instrument pointing toward tympanic segment of the facial nerve.

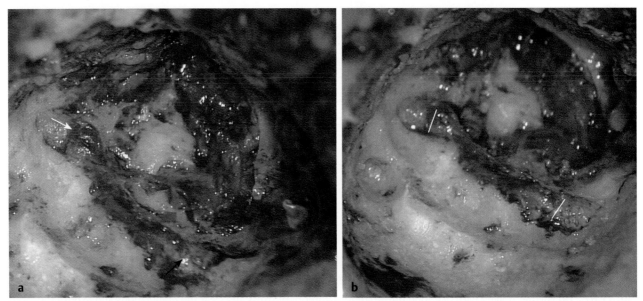

Fig. 11.69 **(a)** Complete canal wall down mastoidectomy performed and facial nerve exposed from the mastoid segment (MS) near stylomastoid foramen (*black arrow*) till the first genu (*white arrow*). **(b)** The demarcation between affected facial nerve and the healthy facial nerve is marked by *white line*.

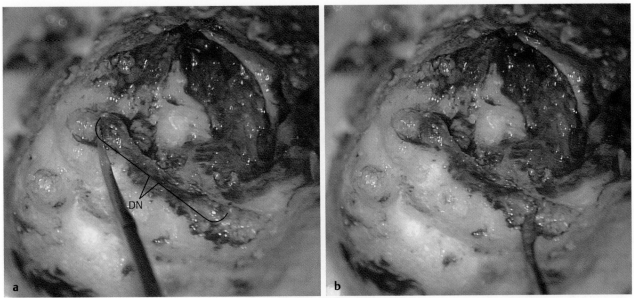

Fig. 11.70 **(a)** Dumbbell neuroma (DN) formation visualized. The instrument pointing toward the proximal level up to which the affected nerve is to be resected. **(b)** The distal level till which the nerve is to be resected is being pointed.

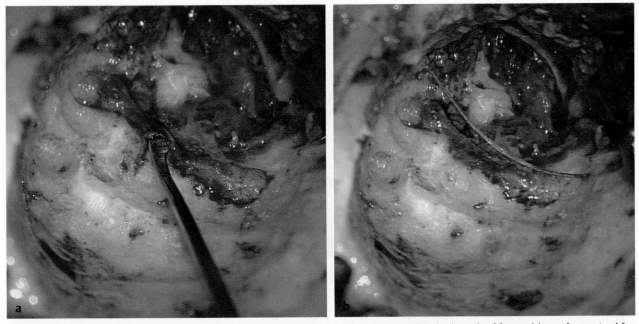

Fig. 11.71 **(a)** The instrument showing the fibrotic segment of the facial nerve. **(b)** The length of free cable graft required for interposition grafting between cut ends of the facial nerve after excising the affected segment.

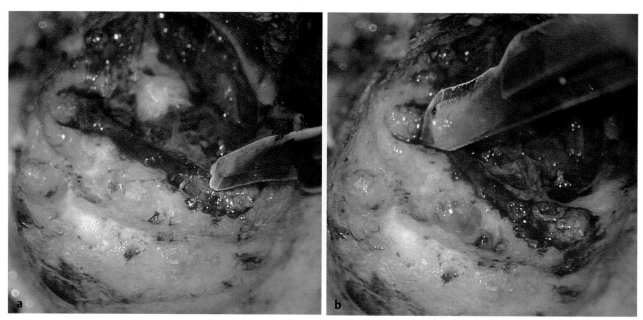

Fig. 11.72 **(a)** Resection of nerve at the distal level with a sharp blade in progress. **(b)** Resection of nerve at the proximal level in progress.

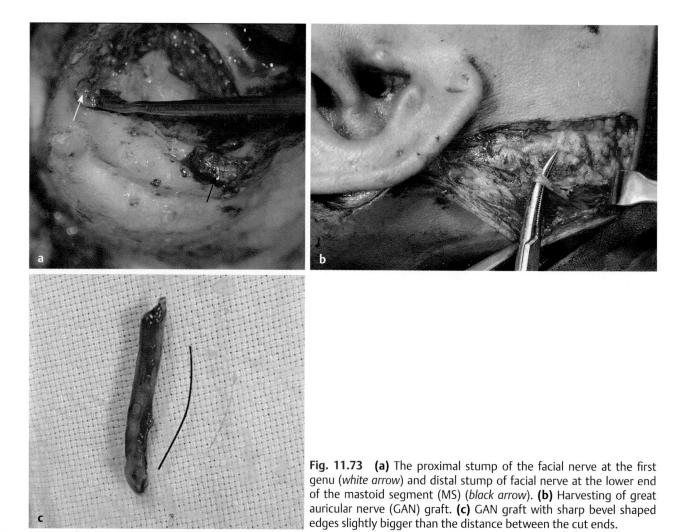

Fig. 11.73 **(a)** The proximal stump of the facial nerve at the first genu (*white arrow*) and distal stump of facial nerve at the lower end of the mastoid segment (MS) (*black arrow*). **(b)** Harvesting of great auricular nerve (GAN) graft. **(c)** GAN graft with sharp bevel shaped edges slightly bigger than the distance between the cut ends.

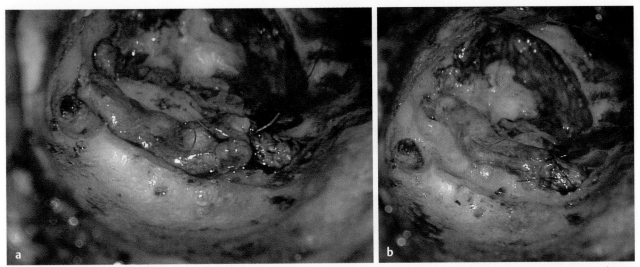

Fig. 11.74 **(a)** Great auricular nerve (GAN) graft placed between the cut ends of the nerve. End-to-end anastomosis with two cut ends of the facial nerve performed by applying sutures on the distal side. **(b)** Three sutures placed. On proximal end, the fibrin glue is applied around approximated cut ends of the facial nerve and graft in place of sutures.

■ Conclusion

The knowledge of the pathogenesis of otitic facial nerve paralysis due to infections is important for accurate and timely management of the actual disease with recovery of the facial nerve functioning. Pathology involves osteitis, bone erosion, external compression, edema, and inflammation of the nerve which if not treated can lead to fibrosis of the facial nerve causing irreversible damage to it.

CSOM causing facial paralysis is most frequently seen in CSOM with cholesteatoma followed by TOM, MOE, and tympanosclerosis and least found in CSOM without cholesteatoma. The facial palsy in cholesteatoma disease is rarely complete, which explains that the disease does not infect the nerve directly. Cholesteatoma can either erode the facial canal and provoke inflammation or can compress on a dehiscent nerve (macro dehiscence) or through the naturally present canaliculi between the middle ear and fallopian canal (micro dehiscence). Early surgical intervention is necessary to attain complete recovery of the facial nerve functioning. In most of the cases, canal wall up or down mastoidectomy with complete eradication of cholesteatoama, its careful lifting from exposed facial nerveis good enough. Most of the times decompression of the facial nerve is not required as clearance of disease load is good enough for the facial nerve to recover. To prevent recurrent cholesteatoma, leading to local destruction of the facial nerve, complete clearance of the disease must be attained in the first attempt only. The surgical procedure on facial nerve is usually facial nerve decompression as the facial nerve palsy is usually due to compression on dehiscent facial nerve or through erosion of bone. and is rarely a complete grade VI palsy.The outcome of surgical intervention is closely related to the gap between the onset of facial palsy and the time of surgery. Long durations of facial palsy can cause more severe deterioration of the facial nerve functioning and poor surgical outcomes. That proves that every case of cholesteatoma with facial weakness (paresis/palsy) should be operated on as early as possible, regardless of the severity of facial function, the extent of cholesteatoma, type of onset, age, and any previous otologic surgical history.

Facial nerve palsy in MEO is an uncommon complication that can be prevented with timely and proper management. This includes early recognition of the disease, appropriate treatments, and optimizing the comorbidities. Medical management is in the form of therapeutic dose of systemic antibiotics in the form of fluoroquinolones and antipseudomonal parenteral antibiotics which are given for a long time along with management of diabetes for achieving good to excellent recovery of the facial nerve. Surgical debridement is performed only in situations where the progression of the disease continues in spite of continuous medical therapy, evidenced by presence of severe excruciating pain and granulation tissue in the EAC, deterioration of facial nerve functioning and development of lower cranial nerve paresis/palsy during treatment, and persistence of rest of the signs and symptoms even after giving medical therapy for 4 weeks.

TB of the ear is a rare entity and, in most cases, the clinical features resemble that of chronic otitis media. The diagnosis is often delayed due to varied clinical presentations and this can lead to irreversible complications. Early diagnosis is essential for prompt administration of ATT and to prevent complications.

Although usual presentation of patient with TOM is in the form of painless otorrhea, multiple tympanic perforations, early severe hearing loss, abundant granulations, bony necrosisetc. but at times facial nerve palsy can also be the presenting symptom. The final diagnosis is made on the basis of histological and microbiological tests. Histological report of biopsy from granulation tissue showing granulomas, Langhans giant cells, and caseation necrosis, in association with positive TB PCR, confirms the diagnosis of TOM.

Treatment of TOM with facial nerve palsy has to include ATT for at least 6 months for early recovery of facial nerve functioning. The surgical intervention is advised in cases of TOM only when it is associated with complications such as extensive involvement of important structures like facial nerve (sequestrum of complete lateral wall of fallopian canal) and inner ear (big fistula or multiple fistulae in semicircular canals and cochlea),

subperiosteal abscesses, and cholesteatoma coexisting with TOM, and the surgery is always preceded by ATT for at least 1 month.

Bibliography

1. Carvalho C, Velankar H, Pusalkar AG. Tuberculous otitis media with facial paralysis—case report and review of literature. Otolaryngol Open Access J 2018;3(2)
2. Quaranta N, Petrone P, Michailidou A, et al. Tuberculous otitis media with facial paralysis: a clinical and microbiological diagnosis—a case report. Case Reports in Infectious Diseases 2011;2011 |Article ID 932608 | https://doi.org/10.1155/2011/932608
3. Othman IA, Abdullah A, Hashim ND. A case report of congenital cholesteatoma in adult patient mimicking as Bell palsy and proposed follow-up schedule for Bell palsy. Egypt J Otolaryngol 2021;37:86
4. Singh J, Bhardwaj B. The role of surgical debridement in cases of refractory malignant otitis externa. Indian J Otolaryngol Head Neck Surg 2018;70(4):549–554
5. Raines JM, Schindler RA. The surgical management of recalcitrant malignant external otitis. Laryngoscope 1980;90(3):369–378
6. Handzel O, Halperin D. Necrotizing (malignant) external otitis. Am Fam Physician 2003;68(2):309–312

12 Management of Post-traumatic Facial Palsy

Introduction

Facial nerve is the commonest cranial nerve involved in cases of trauma sustained on head and face due to different causes, and trauma is the second most common cause for facial palsy (FP) after Bell's palsy. The external trauma includes road traffic accidents (the commonest cause of FP), gunshot wound, blunt injury, burns, and lacerations. The cause may be any but it definitely results in devastating consequences. The cosmetic defects resulting from the trauma renders it one of the most unsettling and hard to accept lesions.

Types of Fractures

Post-traumatic FP is usually associated with temporal bone fractures. Temporal bone fractures are generally classified into longitudinal, transverse, and mixed fractures with respect to the long axis of the petrous bone. Longitudinal fractures run parallel, whereas the transverse fractures cross the long axis of the petrous bone. In mixed fractures, both fracture lines exist together. A different classification given by Jackler in year 1997 is based on temporal bone fractures involving or sparing otic capsule.

In author's experience almost 80 to 85% of post-traumatic temporal bone fractures are longitudinal in nature and mostly follow the path of least resistance toward the petrous apex of the temporal bone. The fracture line passes through the external auditory canal (EAC) and rarely involves the otic capsule or transect the fallopian canal (**Figs. 12.1** and **12.2**). FP occurs in around 20% of these cases and trauma is in mild form like impingement by bony spicules, contusion, extraneural or intraneural hematoma, inflammation of dehiscent segment of facial nerve, etc. Facial nerve palsy may vary from grade II to grade VI depending on the extent of trauma. These fractures tend to result in tympanic membrane (TM) perforation, ossicular disruption, or hemotympanum thus leading to conductive hearing loss.

Transverse fractures on the other hand are less common and account for only 10 to 15% of temporal bone fractures. These fractures usually occur in the occipital and frontal region (front–back trauma) and fracture lines run perpendicular to the long axis of the

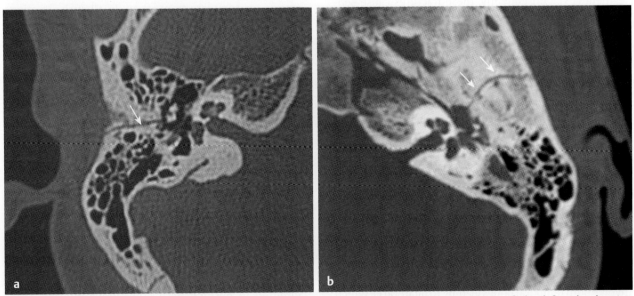

Fig. 12.1 High-resolution computed tomography (HRCT) of the temporal bone coronal cuts of the left side showing longitudinal fracture line (*white arrows*) running parallel to the long axis of the petrous bone. **(a)** Fracture line remaining lateral to ossicles and fallopian canal. **(b)** Fracture line reaching up to but keeping lateral to the fallopian canal at the first genu (*red arrow*).

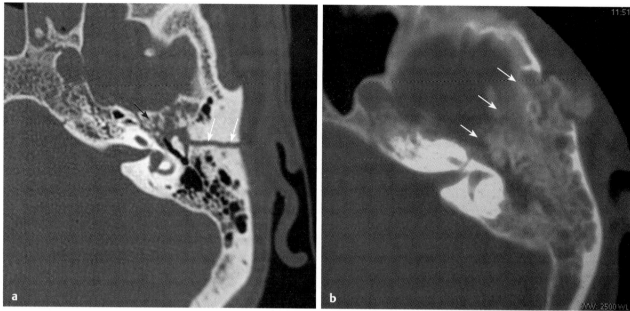

Fig. 12.2 **(a)** High-resolution computed tomography (HRCT) of the temporal bone axial cuts of the left side showing longitudinal fracture line running parallel to long axis of petrous bone extending up to the first genu area (*white arrows*). The fragmentation of bone around the first genu area is visualized (*red arrow*). **(b)** Longitudinal fracture line (*white arrows*) reaching up to the labyrinthine segment (LS) and the first genu area.

petrous bone. They usually originate around the jugular foramen or foramen magnum and extend into the middle cranial fossa. They pass through the labyrinthine capsule leading to transection of the cochlear nerve, damage to the labyrinthine structures, and injury to the footplate of stapes. These fractures mostly lead to transection of facial nerve and the commonest segment to get involved is the first genu and/or the labyrinthine segment (LS). Consequently, these fractures cause sensorineural hearing loss, perilymphatic fistula, and facial nerve palsy which is found in around 70 to 80% of cases.[3] The paralysis is likely to be immediate in onset and grade VI (complete) in severity. The important thing to keep in mind is that in cases of transverse fractures, most of the times facial nerve gets transected and trauma involves mostly the first genu or the labyrinthine segment (LS) (**Fig. 12.3**). So, we have to devise an approach which takes the surgeon directly to the labyrinthine portion without intervening with any important structure. The approach devised by the author and her colleague Prof. K.P. Morwani is "Transzygomatic Anterior Attic Approach," which will be discussed in detail in the chapter.

Mixed type of fractures are very rare, they account for 5% of all temporal bone fractures. Rarely trauma can involve both temporal bones leading to bilateral FP which is discussed in detail in Chapter 16, titled "Management of Bilateral Facial Palsy." All in all, the severity of head trauma decides both the severity of temporal bone fracture and the grade of facial nerve palsy.

Type of Injury to Facial Nerve

Injury to nerve in temporal bone fractures can be mild in the form of impingement by bony spicules, contusion, intraneural hematoma, or inflammation of dehiscent facial nerve, or severe in the form of crush injury, laceration, or complete transection. In all such situations, other than complete transection or severely crushed or lacerated facial nerve, usually decompression suffices along with incision of epineural sheath to relieve edema of the nerve. In cases of intraneural hematoma incision of the perineural sheath is also performed to release the hematoma. In situations where the nerve is transected or badly crushed, multiple procedures are available depending upon the type and extent of injury beyond the site of transection like primary nerve repair, end-to-end neurorrhaphy, interposition grafting, motor nerve transfer, or dynamic or static procedures.

Time of Onset of Facial Palsy

The onset of FP in post-traumatic cases can be immediate or delayed. The immediate onset FP (within few hours of trauma) may go unnoticed if the patient is admitted in hospital with other grave injuries. These patients should be treated as immediate-onset FP to avoid delay in appropriate treatment. The facial nerve

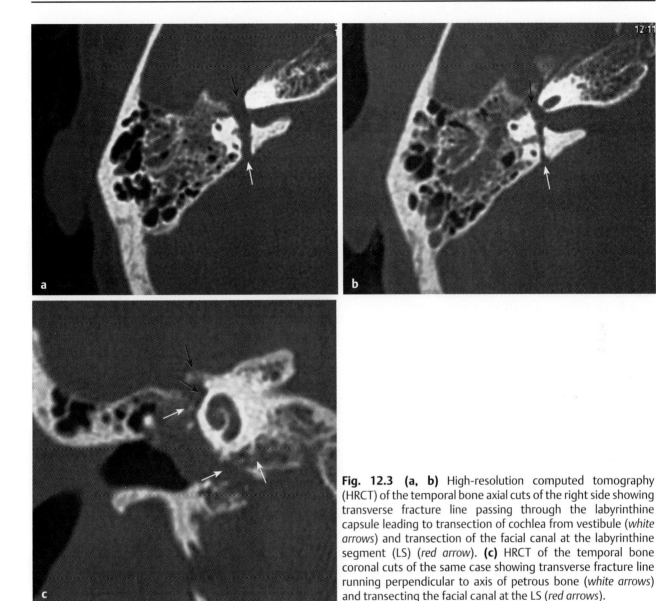

Fig. 12.3 (a, b) High-resolution computed tomography (HRCT) of the temporal bone axial cuts of the right side showing transverse fracture line passing through the labyrinthine capsule leading to transection of cochlea from vestibule (*white arrows*) and transection of the facial canal at the labyrinthine segment (LS) (*red arrow*). **(c)** HRCT of the temporal bone coronal cuts of the same case showing transverse fracture line running perpendicular to axis of petrous bone (*white arrows*) and transecting the facial canal at the LS (*red arrows*).

in these cases is either completely transected, lacerated, or contused at the fracture site leading to grade VI FP. A FP 1 to 10 days after injury is considered to be delayed-onset FP. The pathophysiology of post-traumatic delayed FP is different. As facial canal is occupied by facial nerve and the surrounding vessels with connective tissue loosely arranged around the nerve, delayed FP can be due to either bleeding through these vessels in the facial canal leading to hematoma formation thus compressing the facial nerve and the injury sustained can range from neuropraxia to axonotmesis or neurotmesis or it can be because of the inflammatory reaction in and around the nerve, or a swelling of the nerve in the canal which could lead to ischemic damage to facial nerve.

Evaluation

Clinical Assessment

Given the complexities of post-traumatic FP and its association with head and face injuries, consultation with an otologist at the earliest along with neuroconsultation is required. A thorough history and examination are vital to differentiate complete from incomplete and immediate from delayed FP in time as 75% of all cases of facial nerve injuries are mild and tend to recover spontaneously. Still, we need to know those 25% which require surgical treatment. So, ENT assessment should be started as early as possible (the details are already explained in Chapter 4 titled "Facial Palsy: Evaluation and Diagnosis").

Clinical examination should include a full neurological assessment along with ENT and facial nerve assessment, which includes evidence of skull base fracture like raccoon eyes and battle signs (which develop within a day or two of injury) (**Fig. 12.4**).

Along with FP, the ear examination may reveal trauma to the TM, hemotympanum, or bloody otorrhea/cerebrospinal fluid (CSF) leak. In case of suspected CSF otorrhea, material suspicious for CSF is to be sent for evaluation for beta-2 transferrin.

The time of onset and grade of palsy of the facial nerve are recorded as early as possible so as to decide for appropriate management technique and prepare the prognostic data. The functional assessment of facial nerve is done according to the House-Brackmann Scale (HBS).

Bedside tuning fork testing, if the patient is immobile, or pure-tone audiometry (PTA), if the patient is mobile, is performed for every case of post-traumatic FP to assess the nature of any hearing loss recorded. PTA is an important diagnostic tool in such cases. Sudden-onset sensorineural hearing loss along with transverse fracture and grade VI facial nerve palsy clearly indicates fracture line crossing inner ear and transecting the facial nerve, whereas a conductive loss points toward sparing of the inner ear.

Radiological Assessment

High-resolution computed tomography (HRCT) of the temporal bone (1-mm cut overlapping at 0.5-mm bone window) is the most important investigation which can provide the surgeon with specific details of any temporal bone fracture. Along with location of fractures, it also guides us on whether the fracture line has transected the fallopian canal or not, or if any bony fragment is impinging the facial nerve. It can also show the presence of associated ossicular disruption, extent of injury to inner ear, and suspected injury to tegmen leading to CSF leaks with or without meningoencephalocoele. Magnetic resonance imaging (MRI) is only performed in cases where there is associated intracranial or spinal injury, suspected defect in tegmen with or without meningoencephlocoele, and cases where the fracture line is not visible in grade VI FP.

Electrophysiological Testing

In acute phase of injury, electroneuronography (ENoG) and electromyography (EMG) are performed from 4 and 14 days after injury because Wallerian degeneration of axons takes place in this period only and ENoG is helpful in predicting recovery within this time window of 3 to 21 days. Early signs of denervation on ENoG are a poor prognostic sign because they predict a more severe nerve injury. Surgical intervention is needed when ENoG degenerates by 90% in comparison to the normal side and no volitional EMG is recorded. EMG is most valuable within the time frame of 2 to 3 weeks to 3 months after the onset of a facial nerve injury.

The limitation of these tests is that they do not differentiate the extent of nerve injury beyond neurotmesis and so do not help in classifying the nerve injury according to the Sunderland classification. So, these tests may not help in deciding for accurate right surgical management.

Both Seddon's and Sunderland's classifications are:

- Type 1: Conduction block (neuropraxia).
- Type 2: Axonal injury (axonotmesis).
- Type 3: Type 2 + endoneurium injury (neurotmesis).

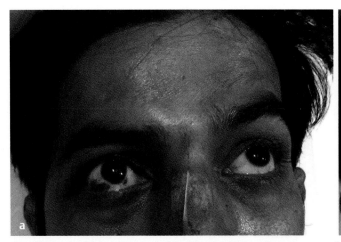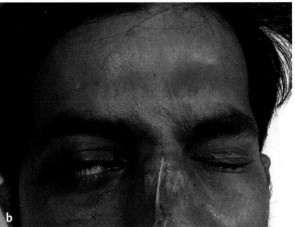

Fig. 12.4 **(a, b)** Appearance of facial palsy (FP) and racoon eye of the right side within hours of head injury.

- Type 4: Type 3 + perineurium injury (neurotmesis).
- Type 5: Type 4 + epineurium injury (neurotmesis).

The electrophysiological tests are only useful in distinguishing injuries that do not cause Wallerian degeneration (type 1) from those that do (types 2–5). The benefit of ENoG is that it can diagnose probable Sunderland type 5 injury with poor prognosis if there is up to or greater than 95% degeneration within 14 days. At the same time it is of no benefit in cases of facial paresis as the nerve is always intact in such cases.

ENoG and EMG tests are not performed in every case of post traumatic cases by the author. They are only performed together in cases of immediate complete (grade VI HBC) FP in the absence of a visible fracture line on HRCT, EMG alone is performed in cases of long standing post traumatic facial plasy to rule out complete atrophy of facial mimic muscles. They are not performed routinely by the author, but only in cases of complete grade VI palsy where the patient has reached very late to the clinician. The utility of EMG is more in long-standing facial nerve palsy cases, where the facial muscles atrophy is suspected. In such situations, based on non-availability of viable facial muscles (a silent graph on EMG indicates atrophy of facial muscles) the primary repair techniques are either performed along with some static and dynamic procedures or only dynamic and static procedures are performed.

Topographic Tests

These tests used to be performed in past to assess the anatomical level of a peripheral lesion and these are *Schirmer's test*, stapedius reflex through impedance audiometry, and electrogustometry or comparison of taste perception. These tests have lost their relevance over time due to their false positive or negative results.

■ Management

Although management of post-traumatic FP is both medical and surgical, there has always been debate and controversy regarding the selection of patients for surgical intervention. According to the author, the factors that play important role in deciding the management are:

- Time of onset—immediate/delayed.
- Degree of FP—complete (grade VI)/incomplete (grade V or less) palsy.
- Type of fracture—longitudinal/transverse/mixed.
- Time of the first visit to the otologist.
- Associated hearing loss, vertigo, CSF leak/ meningoencephlocoele (MEC).

Considering factors 1, 2, and 3 together, for cases with immediate, complete (grade VI HBS) post-traumatic FP with HRCT (temporal bone) showing a transverse fracture line transecting the fallopian canal, surgical repair is the only treatment and it should be performed as early as possible (within 2–3 weeks), depending on the patient's neurologic status.

In other cases, where there is immediate, but incomplete (grade V or less) facial nerve palsy with longitudinal fracture line through temporal bone, the patient is put on medical management in the form of steroids and followed up for at least 3 months or till the time there is improvement up to grade I, in case the recovery has already started. Although all these cases improve over a few months and surgery is not required, associated TM perforation or ossicular disruption may require surgical exploration and repair along with inspection of facial nerve injury as well.

In cases of immediate complete (grade VI HBS) FP in the absence of a visible fracture line on HRCT, a medical treatment with steroids is given. MRI may be required in such cases to confirm the diagnosis and rule out any intracranial cause. The patient is followed up with electrophysiological tests over a period of 3 months starting from day 4 of injury.

In certain cases, where the nerve may not have been transected, but sustained crushing or stretching injuries leading to grade VI FP, surgery may be performed if there is no recovery in terms of both electrophysiological tests and clinical tests latest for up to 4 months after trauma.

In cases of delayed-onset, complete FP (grade VI FP, a few days after trauma), even if a visible fracture line is present on HRCT, the patient is followed up with medical management. The patient is put on steroids (1 mg/kg/d in tapering dosage) to reduce inflammation and edema in the nerve. In case grade VI facial nerve palsy persists even after 3 months, it requires reassessment and surgical correction.

The time gap between onset of FP and patient's first visit to the clinician, in case the patient is not admitted in hospital, is very important. If it is less than 3 months, then the same protocol follows as described above. In case the patient's first visit to the clinician post FP is delayed by more than 4 months, the management may differ. Complete FP persisting even after 4 months needs immediate surgical intervention whatever may be the nature of temporal bone fracture or the time of onset. In case FP has improved to grade V or lesser grade, the patient can be observed for 9 months to 1 year further for the facial nerve to improve.

If there is a delayed diagnosis of paralysis with neural degeneration of 90% or more on ENoG, then also surgical decompression is indicated. Literature suggests the use of a combination of electrodiagnostic testing and computed tomography (CT), especially if the timing of the palsy is not known.

Associated symptoms like sensorineural hearing loss, vertigo, CSF leak/meningoencephalocoele point toward involvement of inner ear or intracranial extension of injury. In these situations surgical intervention becomes necessary even if the FP is grade V or less, and the facial nerve exploration can be performed along with other procedures.

Although a rare situation, some specific head injuries can cause trauma to temporal bones on both sides leading to bilateral FP. Prompt surgical correction of at least on one side is mandatory according to the author as bilateral FP is a severely debilitating condition for the patient. The details of this situation are discussed in Chapter 16 titled "Management of Bilateral Facial Palsy."

The time of surgery remains controversial in post-traumatic FP. The important thing to remember is that, if surgery is performed at the earliest (within 7 days), the functional and aesthetic results are more likely to be better than if the surgery is delayed. If the nerve is transected, the repair of it should be completed within 72 hours from the onset of the trauma. Some studies suggest that, if the nerve does not undergo repair within 3 days, then decompression should be performed after 20 days of trauma as axoplasmic flow and regeneration are the greatest 3 weeks after injury.

To sum up, the indications for surgical management are:

- Immediate, complete (grade VI) facial nerve palsy with fracture line transecting FC.
- Immediate/delayed/doubtful time of onset, grade VI FP not recovering in 4 months.
- Facial nerve paresis with additional sign and symptoms requiring surgery, namely, severe vertigo, profound conductive/mixed hearing loss, and persistent CSF otorrhea.
- Bilateral facial nerve palsy.

The management of the traumatized facial nerve includes general and specific treatments. General management includes treating associated conditions like head injury, injury to other organs, and any other comorbidities. Specific management includes both medical and surgical treatments.

Medical Management

High dose corticosteroids to be started as early as possible in cases of delayed-onset complete paralysis or incomplete paresis. These patients generally demonstrate good prognosis. The rationale is reducing neural edema, which is the cause of facial nerve palsy in such cases.

In cases of CSF leak where chances of infection are there, add prophylactic antibiotics.

In cases of vertigo due to inner ear damage, antivertigo and antiemetic drugs are started.

Eyecare is always involved in every case of facial nerve paralysis. As it takes a long time for an FP to recover, there can be continuous corneal exposure which can lead to corneal ulceration and further complications in the eye. Eyecare in the form of artificial tears, adequate lubricant, and taping the eyes closed at night are to be performed in every case. Ophthalmology referral is essential.

Surgical Management

As with all surgical interventions, the treatment plan must be tailored to the individual patient's requirement. The plan must take into account their age, comorbidities, and etiology, as well as the severity of the paralysis.

There is a systematic stepwise approach for surgical management of facial nerve palsy, which includes primary neurorrhaphy, interposition nerve graft (in case its short-term FP with both ends of facial nerve available for anastomotic repair), motor nerve transfer or cross-facial nerve graft (CFNG), in case proximal end of the nerve is not available, and dynamic procedures in the form of regional muscle transfer or free micro neurovascular muscle transfer (FMMT) along with static procedures in cases of long-term FP. The different procedures can be summed up as follows:

- In cases of contusion, stretch trauma, and intra-neural hematoma, where the nerve continuity is maintained, decompression of nerve 4 to 5 mm on both sides of the site of injury is performed.
- Removal of bony fragment along with decompression of nerve in case bony fragment is impinging on the facial nerve. The epineurial sheath is incised to release hematoma or edema if there is any.
- In case of transected facial nerve, primary nerve repair in the form of end-to-end anastomosis/neurorrhaphy is performed, where the cut ends of nerve lie close to each other (gap <5 mm) and are well approximated. Wherever possible, the clinician should always attempt the primary nerve repair. In case the gap is more but can be covered up through rerouting or mobilization of proximal and/or distal stump is possible, end-to-end anastomosis should always be performed and preferred over interposition graft.

- Interposition cable grafting is performed in case of transection of the facial nerve with significant loss of nerve tissue in between the two cut ends, and even rerouting the nerve does not fill up the gap. A sensory nerve is used as free interposition cable graft, which can be either great auricular or the sural nerve.
- When primary neurorrhaphy or interposition cable grafting is not possible, due to absence of proximal stump and duration of FP is less than 2 years, which means facial mimetic muscles are still viable, motor nerve transfer in the form of faciomasseteric or faciohypoglossal anastomosis is performed. CFNG is another technique which is usually practiced by plastic surgeons. It involves utilizing the peripheral branches of the contralateral intact facial nerve to innervate the paralyzed hemiface.
- Dynamic procedures like regional muscle transfer/elongation (temporalis muscle) are performed with static procedures like upper eyelid gold implant in long-term facial nerve palsy (duration >3 years with negative EMG) where the facial muscles have already atrophied or become nonviable. The other procedure can be FMMT where free gracilis muscle with neurovascular bundle is used as a free graft.
- Static procedures (gold implant, slings) can be used as additional procedures with primary nerve repair where late recovery of nerve is expected.
- Adjunctive procedures (botulinum toxin) are used in cases of complete muscle atrophy, where dynamic reanimation is not possible or they can be used in combination with primary procedures.

All these procedures have been explained in detail in Chapter 5 titled "Facial Palsy: Management Strategy, Surgical Rehabilitation Techniques, and Outcome Tracking," Chapter 7 titled "Management of Flaccid Facial Palsy of Short and Intermediate Duration with Proximal Stump Available," Chapter 8 titled"Management of Flaccid Facial Palsy of Short and Intermediate Duration with Proximal Stump Unavailable," and Chapter 9 titled "Management of Long Duration Flaccid Facial Palsy."

The result depends on the time of surgical intervention and extent of damage to facial nerve. The best results are achieved when surgical intervention takes place within 30 days, still excellent result can be achieved if done within 3 months, fairly good results till 6 months, after which the recovery is incomplete or defective due to collagenization of endoneurial sheath at the cut ends or the injury site. In collagenization, progressive shrinkage in axon diameter occurs over 3 months followed by gradual thickening of the collagen in the endoneurial layer surrounding the nerve fibers. Early repair promotes axons to grow into the collapsing tubules in time, thus expanding them and avoiding collagenization.

Selection of Technique

International criteria for surgical management of post–head injury FP are as follows:

- **Middle cranial fossa approach:** This approach is specifically for grade VI FP cases where injury is proximal to the geniculate ganglion at 1st genu, (LS, or meatal segment) with no sensorineural hearing loss. It is also preferred in patients with contralateral profound hearing loss. This approach requires the creation of a temporal bone flap parallel to the middle cranial fossa with retraction of temporal lobe to reach skull base. Careful dissection is required to prevent bleeding from the middle meningeal artery, which can be embedded in the inner table. Also, there are chances of injuring the superior semicircular canal and basal turn of the cochlea.
  - ➤ **Pitfalls:**
    1. As there is retraction of temporal lobe, it can lead to trauma to the brain due to pressure caused by retractors.
    2. There are chances of injuring middle meningeal artery, superior semicircular canal (SSC) or basal turn of cochlea.
    3. Special surgical expertise is required, as only a skull base surgeon can perform this surgery.
    4. Special instruments are required as it is a lateral skull base procedure.

- **Transmastoid approach:** This is performed for decompression or repair of the tympanic segment (TS) and mastoid segment (MS) up to the stylomastoid foramen (SMF).
  - ➤ **Pitfalls:**
    1. It is an insufficient approach to reach the LS in sclerosed mastoid.
    2. Mild hearing loss (conductive hearing loss) is expected as in this approach, other than decompressing the MS, decompression of all other segments requires removal of incus to reach the fracture site.

- **Combined approach:** In few situations, where decompression or repair of facial nerve is needed in the LS and segments distal to it, both middle cranial fossa and transmastoid techniques are performed together.

- **Translabyrinthine approach:** This approach is performed in cases of injury involving meatal part of facial nerve with profound hearing loss on the same side.

Selection of techniques according to the author is as follows:

Middle cranial fossa approach with all its limitations is not the procedure of choice for the intratemporal portion of facial nerve. The author prefers to do it only in cases of facial nerve palsy associated with meningoencephalocoele and CSF otorrhea secondary to tegmen defect or when the patient is having contralateral profound hearing loss.

The preferred approaches are depicted in **Fig. 12.5**.

- **Transmastoid approach (Fig. 12.5** and **Figs. 12.9–12.13):** This approach is used preferably for the second genu and MS up to the SMF. Perioperatively,

the surgeon just follows the fracture line involving the mastoid or squamous portion, till its medial extent, through posterior tympanotomy approach, until the point of facial nerve injury. If the fracture line is not present, the facial nerve is exposed through posterior tympanotomy approach lateral to the the MS and traced along until the injury site or damage is detected. The advantages of this technique are that no special equipment or surgical training is required. The only training required is the handling of the facial nerve. This remains the best approach to address facial nerve injuries at the second genu and MS.

- **Transmastoid supralabyrinthine approach (Figs. 12.15–12.16):** This approach is for decompressing the LS, first genu, and TS through the trans mastoid approach but only in cases with cellular mastoid and wide supralabyrinthine

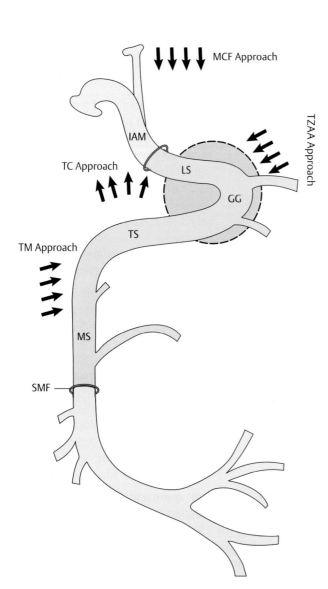

Fig. 12.5 Right sided facial nerve. All four possible approaches, middle cranial fossa (MCF) approach, transmastoid (TM) approach, transcanal (TC) approach, and transzygomatic anterior attic (TZAA) approach. The illustration shows that TZAA approach is the most direct convenient approach to reach the labyrinthine segment (LS) and farthest from important structures like stapes. IAM, Internal auditory meatus; LS, Labyrinthine segment; GG, Geniculate Ganglion; TS, Tympanic segment; MS, Mastoid segment; SMF, Stylomastoid Foramen.

corridor. However, it requires dislocation of the incus to reach these segments. Ossicular reconstruction needs to be performed in these cases. Therefore, this approach is usually preferred in otic capsule sparing fractures with ossicular discontinuity already existing. Also, it is preferred in cases where HRCT of the temporal bone is showing longitudinal fracture line reaching up to but not transecting the fallopian canal in the LS, first genu, TS, or MS, as repairing with nerve graft through this approach is a little tricky and better approaches are available for it. Perioperatively, the surgeon just follows the fracture line through mastoidectomy and epitympanotomy. To reach the TS, first genu, or LS, the incus and head of malleus need to be removed. After reaching the injury site, decompression of nerve is performed for few millimeters beyond the site in both proximal and distal directions, till normal nerve is reached. The epineurial sheath is incised in case of intraneural edema. Ossiculoplasty is performed in every case. The limitation with this technique is it is impossible to perform this technique in sclerotic mastoid. And if there is intact ossicular chain then the patient may suffer conductive hearing loss of up to 10 dB, as incus is first dislocated and used again for ossiculoplasty after facial nerve procedure is done.

- **Transcanal approach (Figs. 12.17–12.19):** This is a very convenient technique for managing injury in the TS, first genu, and LS. This technique can be used to reach up to the LS though chances of injuring ampulla of LSC and SSC and suprastructure of stapes are there.
- **Transzygomatic approach (Figs. 12.23–12.31):** It is specifically designed for the LS but can also be extended distally to decompress the TS and MS till the SMF. This technique is discussed in detail along with the relevant case below.
- **Translabyrinthine approach:** This approach is for the cases where meatal segment of facial nerve is involved in injury, usually in transverse fracture which also lead to the otic capsule disruption resulting in profound sensorineural hearing loss (dead ear). This approach has the advantage of excellent exposure to almost the complete course of the intratemporal facial nerve and the meatal segment as well. The closure in these cases is with abdominal fat grafts and pedicled muscoloperiosteal flaps to obliterate mastoid cavity and thick periosteum with cartilage pieces to obliterate eustachian tube to to minimize CSF leakage.

■ Surgical Cases

Transmastoid Approach

Case 1

A 32-year-old patient presented with sudden immediate onset facial palsy on left side for 6 months post road traffic accident. On examination, there was complete grade VI FP involving the left side with Bell's phenomenon noted (**Fig. 12.6**). Examination showed normal nose, ears, oral cavity, and nervous system. HRCT of the temporal bone (**Figs. 12.7 and 12.8**) showed temporal fracture line running across squamous temporal bone, mastoid bone, and EAC. It is reaching up to mid of the MS of fallopian canal but not cutting across it. The nerve was found to be bifid in its course from the MS up to the posterior half of TS.

The patient had already received conservative treatment in the form of oral prednisolone 1 mg/kg body weight in tapering dosage in the starting 1 month of palsy.

As 6 months had already passed, and grade VI FP persisted, surgical decompression of facial nerve was planned.

Surgical Steps (Figs. 12.9–12.13)

Postaural skin incision was made. Fascia graft was harvested. Anteriorly based musculoperiosteal flap was raised. Meatotomy incision was made at the junction of cartilaginous and bony canal wall in the posterior quadrant and cartilaginous EAC was lifted anteriorly and retracted in mastoid retractor. The TM was found to be intact (**Fig. 12.9**). Fracture line was visualized running across the squamous temporal and the posterior bony wall of the EAC (**Fig. 12.9**). Cortical mastoidectomy was performed and fracture line followed up to its medial-most extent which reached up to vertical part of fallopian canal (**Fig. 12.10**). Posterior tympanotomy was performed and fallopian canal in the MS skeletonized. Decompression of facial nerve at the site of trauma was performed (**Fig. 12.11**). The decompression extended in both directions few millimeters distal and proximal to the site of injury (**Fig. 12.12**). While decompressing, facial nerve was found to be bifid which corelated well with the preoperative CT images (**Fig. 12.13**). The anomaly was visualized starting from the inferior part of the MS reaching up to the TS. **Fig. 12.14** provides the postoperative results with recovery of grade I.

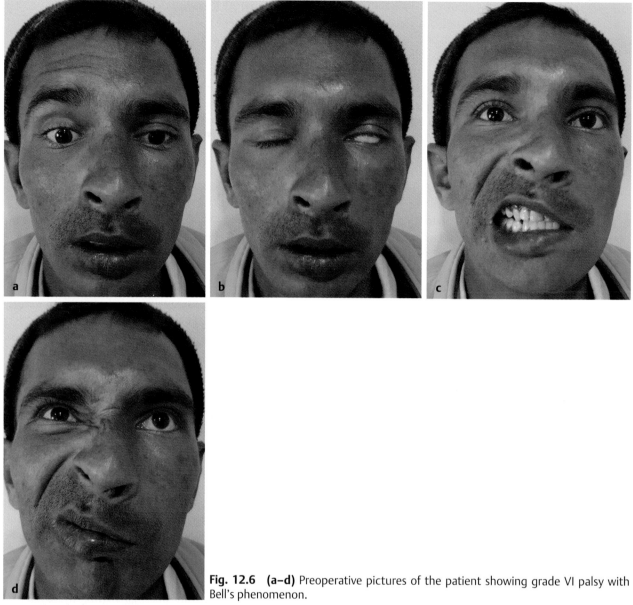

Fig. 12.6 (a–d) Preoperative pictures of the patient showing grade VI palsy with Bell's phenomenon.

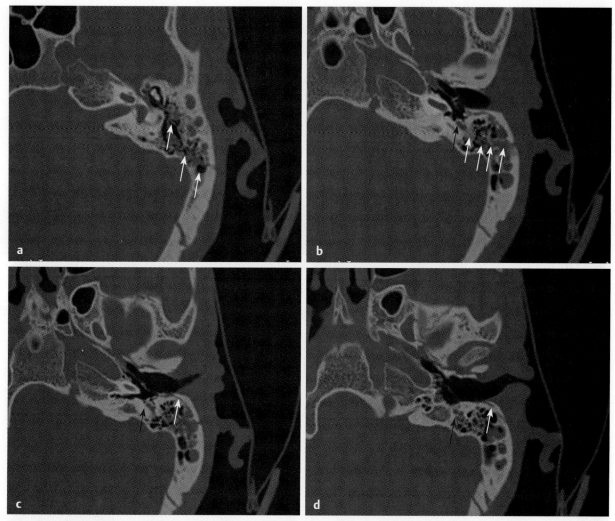

Fig. 12.7 **(a, b)** High-resolution computed tomography (HRCT) of the temporal bone axial cuts of the left side showing fracture line (*white arrows*) along mastoid bone and posterior canal wall reaching up to fallopian canal in the mastoid segment. The bifid facial nerve in the mastoid segment (MS) is also visualized (*red arrow*). **(c, d)** HRCT of the temporal bone axial cuts of the same case showing longitudinal fracture line (*white arrow*) and bifid facial nerve in the MS (*red arrow*).

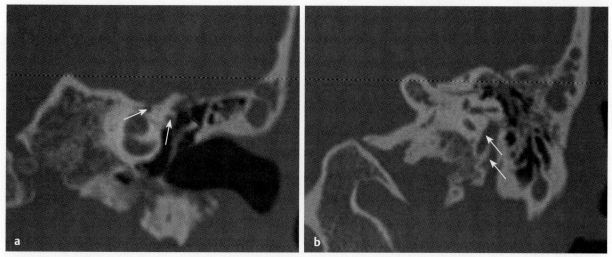

Fig. 12.8 **(a)**HRCT of the temporal bone coronal cuts of the same case showing fracture line (*red arrow*) reaching up to the cut section of LS and TS are shown by *white arrows*. **(b)** Coronal cut showing bifid facial nerve in the MS (*white arrows*).

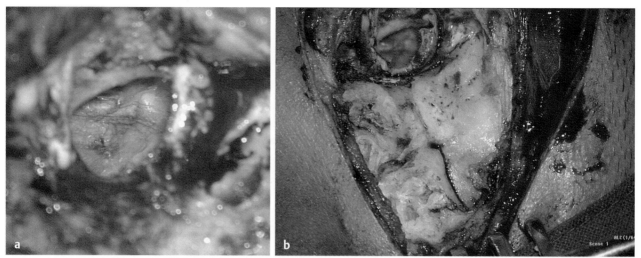

Fig. 12.9 Left side: **(a)** Meatotomy already performed with intact tympanic membrane. **(b)** Fracture line running across the mastoid bone reaching up to the posterior bony external auditory canal (EAC).

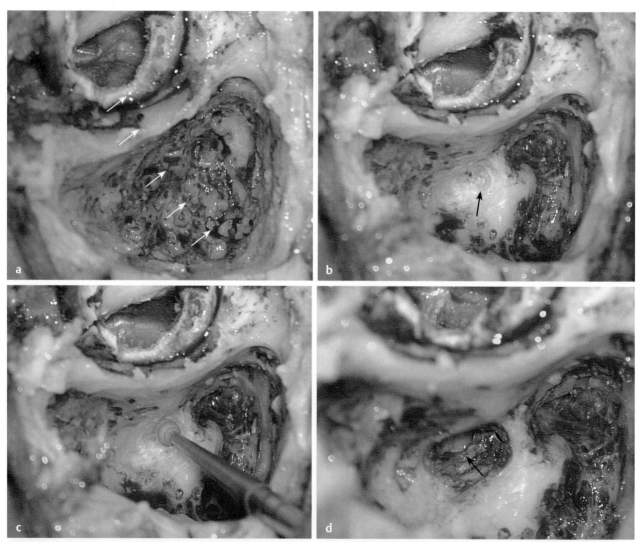

Fig. 12.10 **(a)** Cortical mastoidectomy performed and fracture line followed up to its medial-most extent which reached up to the mastoid segment of fallopian canal (*white arrows*). **(b)** Posterior tympanotomy in progress (*black arrow*). **(c)** Fallopian canal to be skeletonized and facial nerve to be exposed in the mastoid segment (MS). **(d)** The facial nerve seems bifid in the MS (*black arrow*).

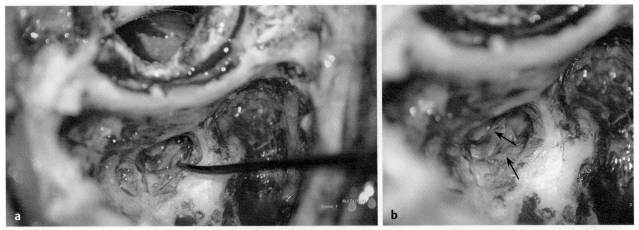

Fig. 12.11 **(a)** The bony chip between two parallel running facial nerve segments is being lifted. **(b)** Appearance of bifid facial nerve (*black arrows*).

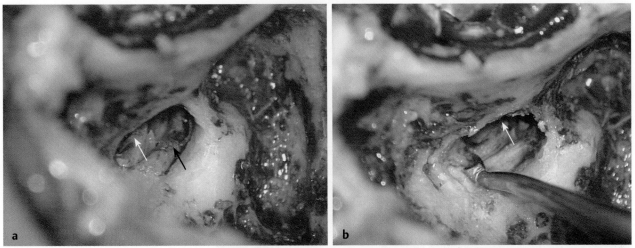

Fig. 12.12 **(a)** The double facial nerve is visible in the mastoid segment (MS). The true facial nerve segment is decompressed up to the second genu distally (*black arrow*), the second part of mastoid segment is shown with *white arrow*. **(b)** Bone over the distal part of the MS being curetted out to decompress the facial nerve a few millimeters distal to the site of injury.

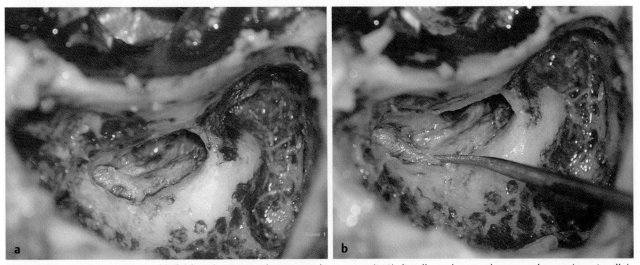

Fig. 12.13 **(a)** Decompressed bifid facial nerve in the mastoid segment (MS) distally and up to the second genu (proximally). **(b)** Duplication of facial nerve in the MS visualized.

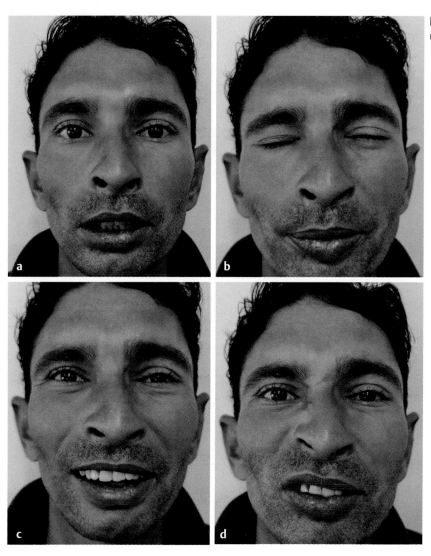

Fig. 12.14 (a–d) Facial nerve recovery up to grade I after 1 year of surgery.

Transmastoid/Supralabyrinthine Approach

Case 2

A 40-year-old patient presented with sudden immediate onset of facial palsy on right side post road traffic accident 3 months back. On examination, there was complete grade VI FP involving the right side. Examination showed normal nose, ears, oral cavity, and nervous system. HRCT of the temporal bone on right side showed temporal fracture line running through mastoid bone, and EAC. reaching up to anterior part of TS. a bony fragment was seen impinging on anterior part of TS.

Surgical Steps (Fig. 12.15)

After lifting the skin and mucoperichondrial flap and performing meatotomy, tympanomeatal flap was raised and TM separated from handle of malleus. Mastoid cortex also exposed. Longitudinal fracture line could be seen running across mastoid bone and posterior wall of the EAC. Cortical mastoidectomy with epitympanotomy was performed and fracture line followed. Body and short process of incus were exposed and the incus was removed. Head of malleus was also nipped off to expose the area of tympanic segment, geniculate ganglion, and labyrinthine segment.

Facial nerve decompression was performed after drilling away the supralabyrinthine and suprafacial cells. This step was possible because of wide supralabyrinthine corridor in this case. The injury was found to be involving anterior part of TS, caused by the impingement of a small bony fragment. So, after removing the bony fragment, decompression performed at the injury site and 4-5mm beyond it which means, decompression up to first genu proximally and second genu distally. For ossiculoplasty, incus was reshaped and placed as interposition graft between stapes head and handle of malleus. Finally, tympanomeatal flap replaced back. As the TM was intact, repair was not required.

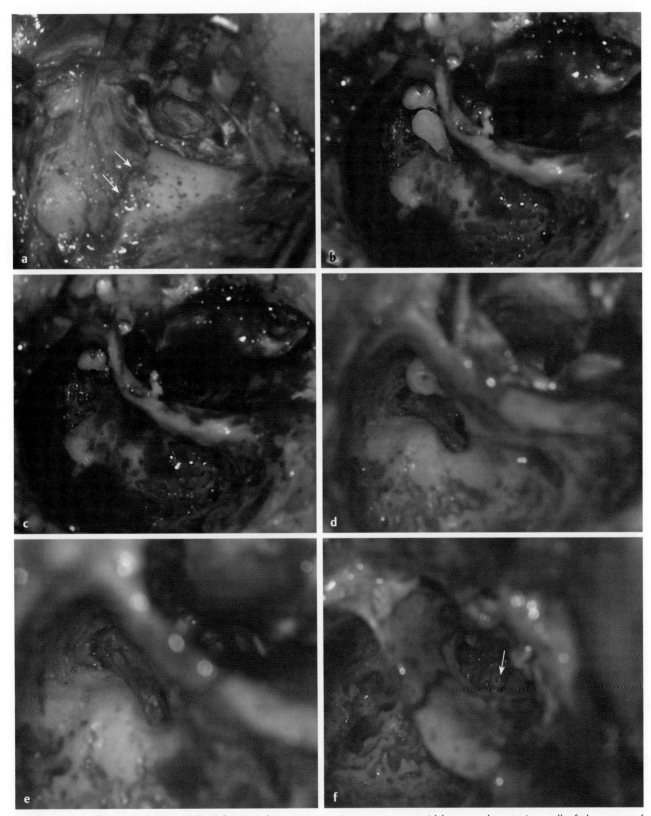

Fig. 12.15 Right ear: **(a)** Longitudinal fracture line seen running across mastoid bone and posterior wall of the external auditory canal (EAC) (*white arrows*). **(b)** Cortical mastoidectomy with epitympanotomy performed and fracture line followed medially. Body and short process of incus with head of malleus exposed. **(c)** Incus removed. **(d)** Facial nerve decompressed distal to the site of injury till the second genu and tympanic segment (TS). Head of malleus visible. **(e)** After removal of head of malleus, decompression was achieved proximal to the site of injury up to the first genu. **(f)** Head of stapes visualized (*white arrow*).(*Continued*)

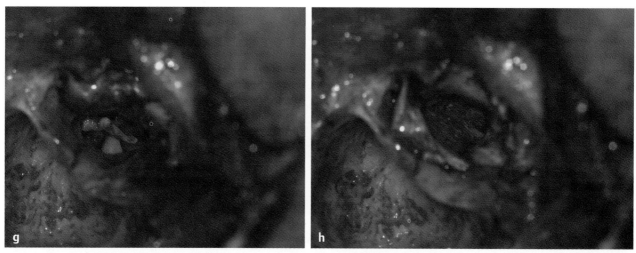

Fig. 12.15 (*Continued*) **(g)** For ossiculoplasty, incus was reshaped and used as interposition graft between head of stapes and handle of malleus. **(h)** Intact tympanic membrane replaced back.

Case 3

Surgical steps (Fig. 12.16)

This is a case of decompression of right-sided facial nerve from the LS to MS including both genus (**Fig. 12.16**). As it was a large cellular mastoid with wide supralabyrinthine corridor, the LS could be reached easily through transmastoid supralabyrinthine approach.

Transcanal Inside-Out Technique

This approach has been explained in detail in case 1, Chapter 7 titled "Management of Flaccid Facial Palsy of Short and Intermediate Duration with Proximal Stump Available." This technique is used for inside out mastoidectomy procedure commonly by the otologists, So no special training or equipments are required. However, the surgeon should have training in the handling of facial nerve.

Case 4

The patient presented with post head injury immediate complete facial palsy which had not improved in 4 months. Grade VI FP was persisting when the patient visited the surgeon. The CT Scan temporal bone right side showed longitudinal fracture line reaching up to anterior part of TS and a bony spicule impinging on TS.

Surgical Steps (Figs. 12.17–12.19)

Postaural incision with posteroinferiorly based musculoperiosteal flap was raised. Skin of the EAC was lifted in three-fourths of the circumference and retracted anteriorly in the self-retaining mastoid retractor. Canaloplasty was performed to expose tympanic annulus in its whole circumference. The fracture line was followed from

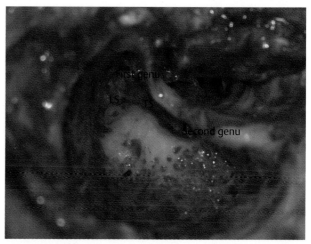

Fig. 12.16 Decompression of right-sided facial nerve from the labyrinthine segment (LS) to the mastoid segment (MS) including the first genu and second genu through transmastoid supralabyrinthine technique is visualized.

lateral-most part of the canal wall to its medial-most extent where it reached up to the ossicles. Lateral wall of the scutum drilled away to expose the incus up to the long process and neck of malleus. The incus was then disarticulated and removed. The injury was found involving the TS which lies medial to body of incus. Head of malleus was also nipped off and removed, so as to expose complete length of the TS and first genu area.. Further atticotomy was performed and lateral attic wall was drilled from anterior to posterior direction to expose the nerve beyond the site of injury. Once the site of injury was located, the decompression of nerve from first genu to second genu performed. Ossiculoplasty, reconstruction of lateral attic wall with cartilage graft, and reinforcement of the TM with temporalis fascia followed the facial nerve decompression.

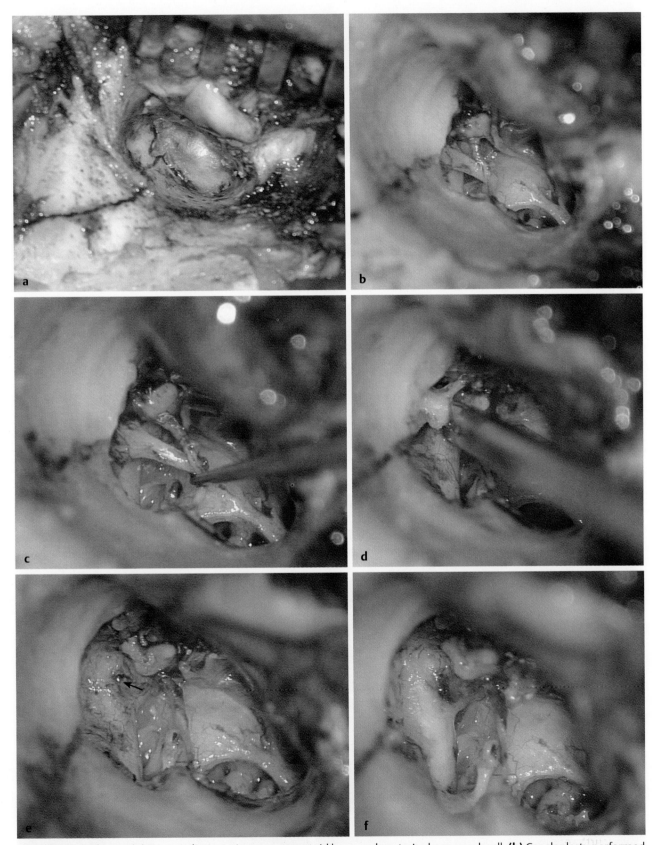

Fig. 12.17 Right ear: **(a)** Fracture line running across mastoid bone and posterior bony canal wall. **(b)** Canaloplasty performed and scutum wall drilled away to expose the long process of incus and neck of malleus. **(c)** Incus is being removed after disarticulating from incudostapedial and incudo malleal joint. **(d)** Head of malleus nipped off. **(e, f)** Trauma involving anterior part of the tympanic segment (TS) (*black arrow*) can be visualized. (*Continued*)

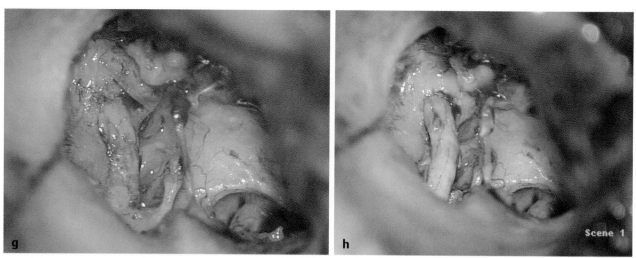

Fig. 12.17 (*Continued*) **(g)** Bony canalcovering the TS is drilled away by using diamond burr. **(h)** Epineurial sheath covering the TS incised.

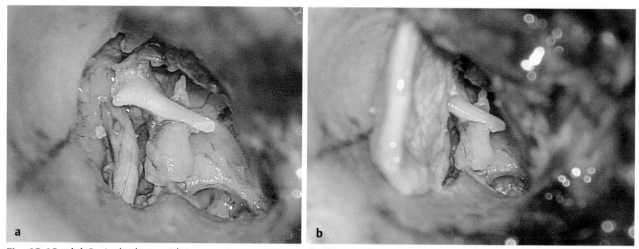

Fig. 12.18 **(a)** Ossiculoplasty with incus as interposition graft. **(b)** Tragal cartilage graft to reconstruct posterosuperior canal.

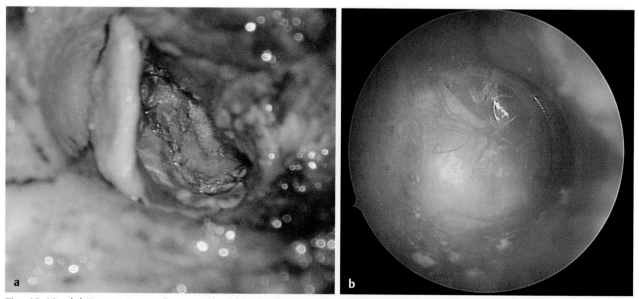

Fig. 12.19 **(a)** Tympanic membrane replaced back. **(b)** Otoendoscopy showing well-healed tympanic membrane (TM) with interposition incus ossiculoplasty showing through the TM 1 year post surgery.

Transzygomatic Anterior Attic Approach for Facial Nerve Decompression

Although this technique has been specifically devised by the author's colleague and improvised by the author, to access the labyrinthine segment of facial nerve, it can be extended up to the SMF distally depending up on the segment which requires addressal.

Common situations where labyrinthine segment needs exposure are:

- Post head injury immediate grade VI facial palsy involving the first genu or LS.
- Bell's palsy not responding to medical line of treatment for adequate period, that is, 3 to 4 months (as already explained in Chapter 6 titled "Evaluation and Management of Acute Facial Palsy").
- Excision of neuroma or hemangioma involving the first genu.

In short, this technique is suitable for any pathology of reasonably small size in and around the first genu and LS of facial nerve.

It is quite a simple technique where rather than approaching the ear from the posterior side, it is approached from the anterior side, keeping in mind that the LS is the anterior-most part of facial nerve in its intratemporal course. No special instruments are required and it can be performed by any experienced ENT surgeon with sufficiently good surgical expertise. The only limitation is that, to reach the TS, the first genu or the LS, incus needs to be dislocated and after managing the facial nerve, it is reused as interposition ossiculoplasty, so the patient suffers mild conductive hearing loss.

The surgeon while tracing facial nerve from the anterior side reaches directly on the first genu and labyrinthine portion of the facial nerve without any important structure intervening. It can be performed in sclerosed mastoid also.

In this approach, position of both the surgeon and patient is unique in a way that the patient lies in lateral position inspite of supine position and the surgeon sits in front of the patient and starts drilling from the posterior root of the zygomatic process of the temporal bone which lies just in front of the anterosuperior wall of the EAC. The drilling is from lateral to medial direction and the cells cleared on the way are: transzygomatic cells, supratubal cells, anterior and posterior attic cells along with cog, supralabyrinthine cells, and suprafacial cells.

In all other approaches, to reach the LS, while drilling the mastoid air cells from posterior to anterior direction, there is always a risk of injuring the ampulla of SSC and to reach the TS, we can injure the ampulla of LSC as can be seen in **Figs. 12.20a** and **b**, due to angle of hand piece and shaft of burr. Whereas when we come from the anterior side, there is no such risk associated as we keep away from these important structures while drilling around the LS, first genu, and TS, as can be visualized in **Fig. 12. 20c**.

The position of the patient is unique in a way that the patient lies in lateral and not supine position (**Fig. 12.21a**) and the surgeon sits in front of the patient (**Fig. 12.21b**). The patient is strapped to the table so head rotation is possible in both directions.

Early surgical steps where surgeon operates from the posterior side are:

- It is mostly performed under general anesthesia.
- The patient lies strapped in lateral position.
- Extended end aural (EER) or extended post aural route (EPR) is followed, extended end aural incision in case of decompression of the LS and first genu and extended post aural incision if we need to decompress facial nerve distal to the first genu.
- Cartilaginous external auditory canal (EAC) skin is retracted anterosuperiorly.
- The TM with handle of malleus (the head of malleus is cut from the handle of malleus) is retracted inferiorly from 3 o'clock to 9 o'clock position.
- Incus is taken out.
- The surgeon shifts in front of the patient.

Surgical steps from the anterior attic side are:

- Drilling starts anterior to the middle ear at the posterior root of the zygomatic process of temporal bone which lies just in front of anterosuperior wall of the EAC.
- Cells to be drilled are zygomatic, supratubal, anterior attic, supralabyrinthine, and suprafacial cells.
- Specific segment of facial nerve is delineated depending on the site of fracture/injury.
- Decompression/anastomosis/nerve grafting is performed.
- Reconstructive procedures in the form of ossiculoplasty, posterosuperior canal wall reconstruction, and repair of the TM are performed.

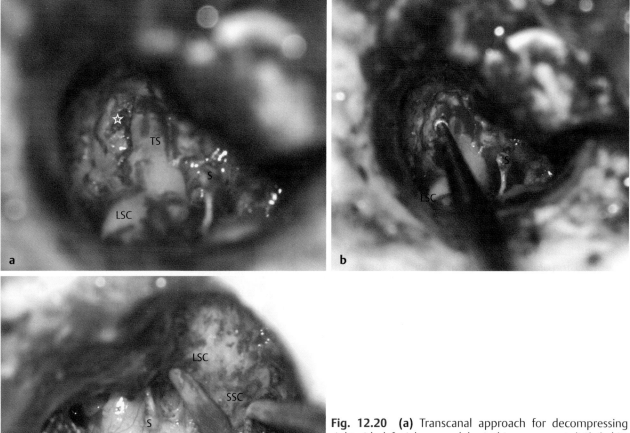

Fig. 12.20 **(a)** Transcanal approach for decompressing right-sided facial nerve, labyrinthine segment (LS) (*white astrisk*). The tympanic segment (TS) Lateral semicircular canal (LSC) and stapes (S) are also visualized. **(b)** Decompressing the first genu and LS through transcanal route carries risk of injuring the LSC and stapes. **(c)** Transzygomatic anterior attic approach for decompressing right-sided LS and TS. As sharp instruments like burr remain anterior and away from these important structures, so there are least chances of injuring them.

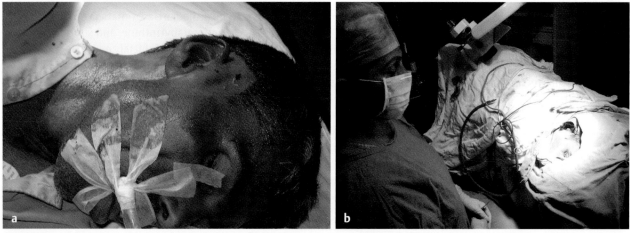

Fig. 12.21 **(a)** Lateral position of the patient, right ear to be operated. **(b)** The surgeon sits in front of the patient.

Case 5

A 25-year-old patient presented with sudden immediate onset right-sided facial palsy for 4.5 months, which developed after she met with an accident on road. On examination, there was complete grade VI FP involving the right side of face (**Fig. 12.22**). Examination showed normal nose, ears, oral cavity, and nervous system. HRCT of the temporal bone (**Fig. 12.23**) showed longitudinal fracture line running across squamous temporal bone, mastoid bone, and EAC on the right side. It reached up to the first genu of fallopian canal. There were bony fragments at the site of injury. The patient had already received conservative treatment in the form of oral prednisolone 1 mg/kg body weight in tapering dosage in the starting 2 months of palsy.

As 4.5 months had already passed, and grade VI FP persisted, surgical decompression of facial nerve was planned.

Surgical Steps (Fig. 12.23–12.31)

Extended post aural incision was made. Fascia graft was harvested. Posteroinferiorly based musculoperiosteal flap was raised. EAC skin was lifted in three-fourths of its circumference up to the annulus, mobilized anterosuperiorly and retracted in self-retaining mastoid retractor. Annulus of the TM was elevated from 3 o'clock to 9 o'clock position. Dislocation of incudostapedial joint was done. Malleus was cut at the level of its neck. The TM along with handle of malleus was retracted inferiorly. Incus and head of malleus were removed and preserved in saline. Posterior root of zygomatic process of

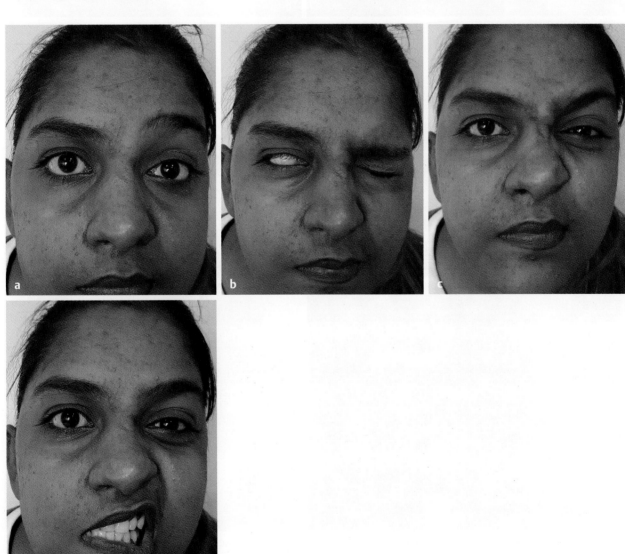

Fig. 12.22 (a–d) Preoperative pictures of the patient showing grade VI facial palsy on the right side.

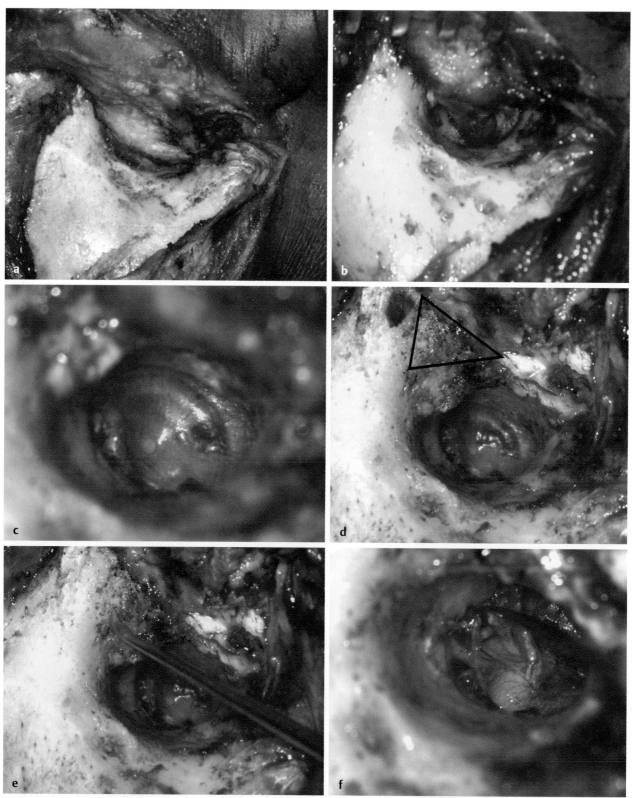

Fig. 12.23 Right side: **(a)** Postaural incision made, posteroinferiorly based musculoperiosteal flap lifted, and mastoid bone exposed. **(b)** External auditory canal (EAC) skin lifted in the three-fourths of its circumference up to the annulus. **(c)** EAC skin retracted anterosuperiorly in self-retaining mastoid retractor. Intact drum visualized. **(d)** Posterior root of zygomatic process of temporal bone (*black outlined triangle*) exposed. It forms the triangle of attack/drilling to reach the labyrinthine segment (LS). **(e)** The area where drilling will be started is pointed out with a sickle. **(f)** TM being elevated from 3'o clock to 9'o clock position to be shifted inferiorly *(Continued)*

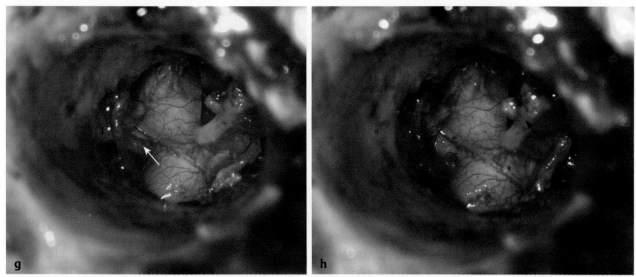

Fig. 12.23 *(Continued)* **(g)** Tympanic membrane (TM) with malleus handle and fibrous annulus elevated from 3 o'clock to 9 o'clock. **(h)** Incus removed after disarticulating I–S joint (*white arrow*). Malleus has already been cut at neck and handle (*black arrow*) lifted with the TM. CT, chorda tympani; I, incus; S, stapes.

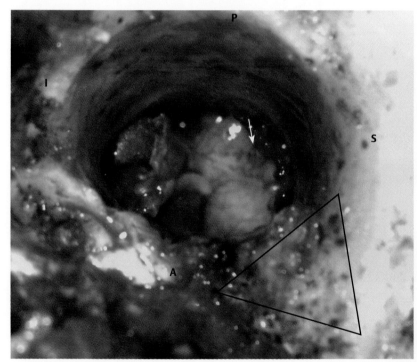

Fig. 12.24 Surgeon has shifted and sitting in front of patient. *Triangular* demarcation for posterior root of zygomatic process of temporal bone which lies just in front of anterosuperior wall of the external auditory canal (EAC) with surgeon sitting in front of the patient. The drilling to be started in the *triangular* area demarcated. The tympanic membrane (TM) with handle of malleus retracted inferiorly. Chorda tympani (*black arrow*) and stapes (*white arrow*) can be visualized. The orientation of surgical field is shown by "S" as superior, "I" as inferior, "A" as anterior, and "P" as posterior.

temporal bone was exposed by further lifting the soft tissue in anterosuperior direction.

At this stage, the surgeon shifts to anterior position and sits in front of the patient. Bone work was started at the posterior root of zygomatic process of temporal bone by drilling away transzygomatic cells (**Figs. 12.24** and **12.25**). Widening of the anterior attic was achieved after drilling away supratubal and anterior attic cells.

Thinning of tegmen tympani was performed in complete attic (**Fig. 12.26**).

Further drilling carried out superior to tensor tympani tunnel to expose greater superficial petrosal nerve (GSPN). Once GSPN was exposed, dissection was carried out further to expose the first genu and LS (till fundus of the internal auditory canal (IAC) if required) (**Figs. 12.27** and **12.28**).

Now the egg shell bone over the facial nerve in the TS and first genu area was removed with the help of a fine pick or blunt hook (**Figs. 12.27** and **12.28**).

After decompression of the nerve, incising the epineurial sheath was performed to release edema around facial nerve in the exposed portion. The sheath was incised till normal healthy looking nerve at least few millimeters beyond the inflamed portion on both sides was exposed (**Fig. 12.29**).

In case there is complete laceration of nerve, grafting of facial nerve can also be performed through this approach. Graft is usually harvested from great auricular nerve or sural nerve.

Reconstruction of superior canal wall was performed with the help of tragal cartilage graft with intact perichondrium on the side facing neotympanum (**Fig. 12.30**). As the TM shrinks by one-third of its size after retraction, an added temporalis fascia graft is required to reinforce the posterior part of the TM. The TM was replaced after placing temporalis fascia graft underneath.

Ossiculoplasty was performed with head of malleus over stapes, (other techniques can be incus as interposition graft between head of stapes and handle of malleus or cartialge strip between head of stapes and groove on bony annulus) (**Fig. 12.31**). Temporalis fascia graft was lifted to check placement of head of malleus over stapes head. EAC skin was replaced (**Fig. 12.31**). Canal was filled with gelfoam. Wound was sutured in two layers.

Postsurgery facial nerve pictures show complete recovery of facial nerve functioning up to grade I (**Fig. 12.32**).

After 1 year of surgery otoendoscopic image showed complete healing of the TM with reconstructed posterosuperior canal wall and ossicular chain (**Fig. 12.33**). 1 year post surgery face showing facial nerve recovery up to grade I (Fig. 12.32) and otoendoscopy showing perfectly healed tympanic membrane with tragal cartilage for superior canal wall reconstruction visible through the neotympanum.

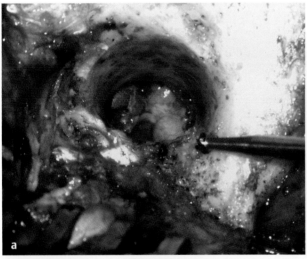
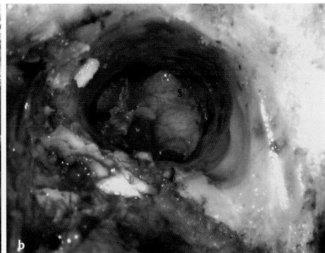
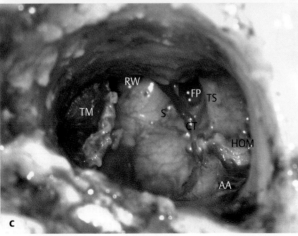

Fig. 12.25 Surgeon sitting in anterior position. **(a)** Drilling through the zygomatic process sitting in the anterior position is started. **(b)** Drilling in progress. The tympanic membrane (TM) from 3 o'clock to 9 o'clock position shifted inferiorly can be visualized. CT, chorda tympani; S, stapes. **(c)** Anterior attic (AA), head of malleus (HOM), chorda tympani (CT), stapes (S) with footplate (FP), tympanic segment (TS), round window (RW), and tympanic membrane (TM) can be visualized.

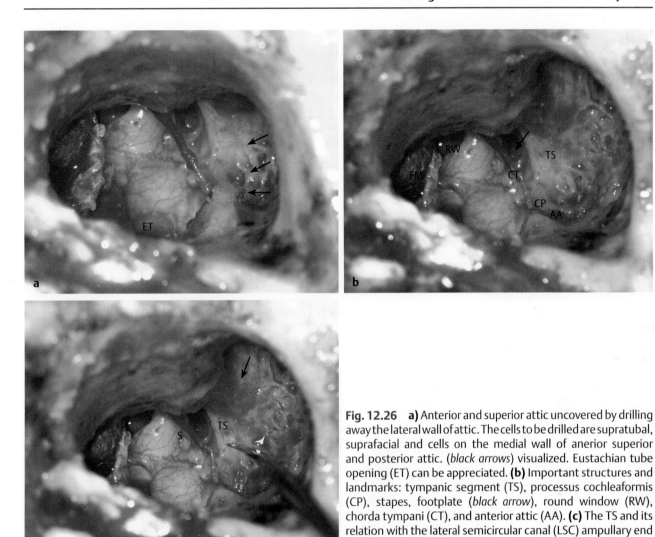

Fig. 12.26 **a)** Anterior and superior attic uncovered by drilling away the lateral wall of attic. The cells to be drilled are supratubal, suprafacial and cells on the medial wall of anerior superior and posterior attic. (*black arrows*) visualized. Eustachian tube opening (ET) can be appreciated. **(b)** Important structures and landmarks: tympanic segment (TS), processus cochleaformis (CP), stapes, footplate (*black arrow*), round window (RW), chorda tympani (CT), and anterior attic (AA). **(c)** The TS and its relation with the lateral semicircular canal (LSC) ampullary end (*black arrow*). In transzygomatic approach, there is minimal risk to the LSC and stapes (S).

Fig. 12.27 **(a)** Drilling superior to tensor tympani tendon (TT) in progress. Tegmen plate (*white arrows*), processus cochleariformis (CP), stapes (S), round window (RW), tympanic segment (TS), and lateral semicircular canal (LSC) (*black arrow*) are the important structures visualized. **(b)** Drilling around the first genu (*black arrow*) and labyrinthine segment (LS) of facial nerve in progress. Removal of suprafacial cells (*white arrow*) close to the dura to expose the LS in progress. *(Continued)*

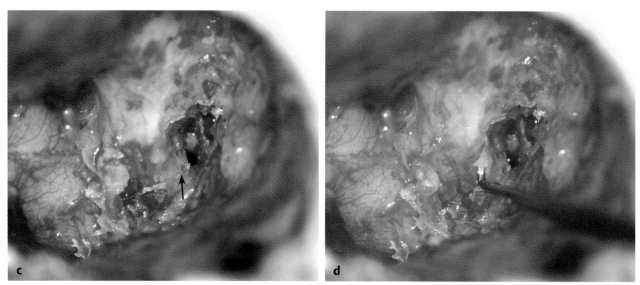

Fig. 12.27 *(Continued)* **(c)** Further clearance and exposure of the first genu (*black arrow*) in process. **(d)** Egg shell bone over the TS and first genu area being removed.

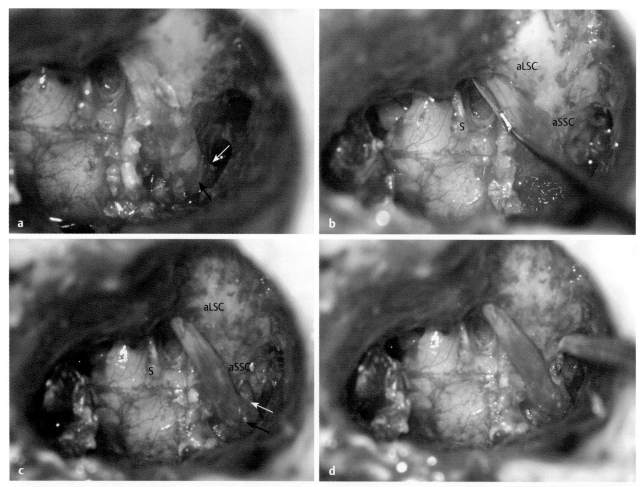

Fig. 12.28 **(a)** Anterior half of the tympanic segment (TS) (*red arrow*) and first genu (*black arrow*) part decompressed. The bent from the labyrinthine segment (LS) to first genu visualized (*white arrow*). **(b)** Thin bony shell over the posterior half of the TS being lifted to be removed. Stapes (S), ampulla of lateral semicircular canal (aLSC) and superior semicircular canal (aSSC) can be visualized. The TS lies anteromedial to aLSC and LS lies just anteromedial to aSSC. **(c)** The first genu (*black arrow*) and LS (*white arrow*) are visualized. **(d)** Exposed and decompressed facial nerve from the LS up to second genu. Instrument pointing toward the LS. *(Continued)*

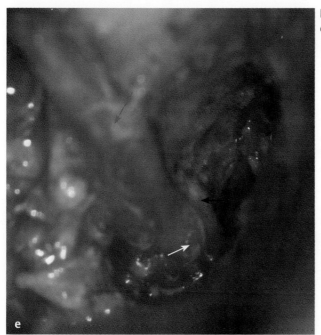

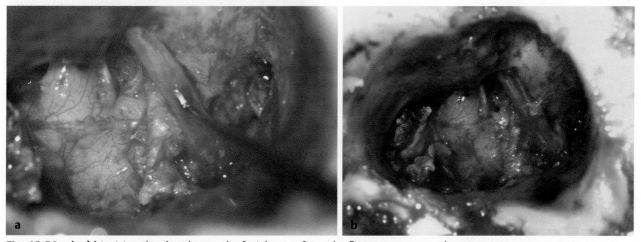

Fig. 12.29   **(a, b)** Incising the sheath over the facial nerve from the first genu to second genu.

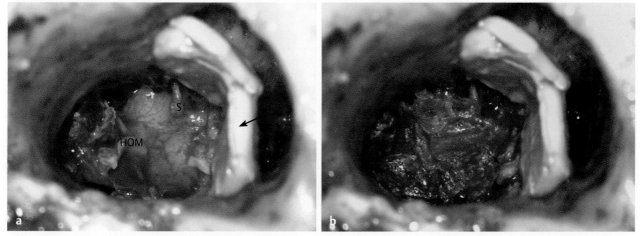

Fig. 12.30   **(a)** Reconstruction of superior wall of the external auditory canal (EAC) with tragal cartilage. Make sure that there is space between medial end of tragal cartilage graft and decompressed facial nerve. Tragal cartilage graft (*black arrow*), stapes (S), and tympanic membrane (TM) with handle of malleus (HOM) visualized. **(b)** Replacing the retracted TM.

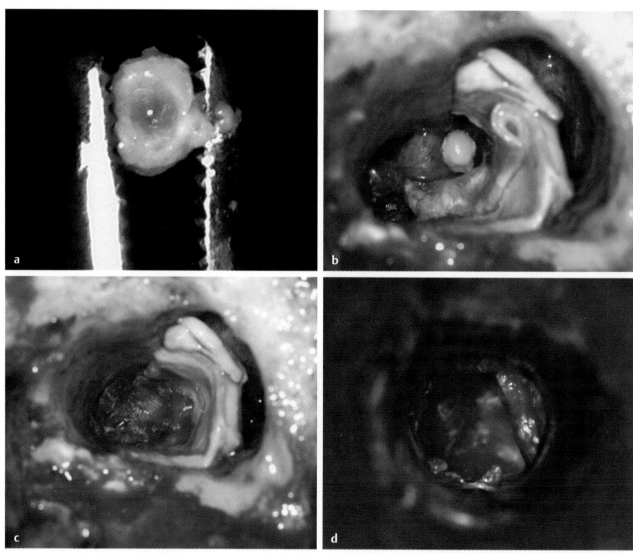

Fig. 12.31 **(a)** Facet drilled on the surface of head of malleus to fit on head of stapes. **(b)** For Ossiculoplasty head of malleus fitted over stapes head, and temporalis fascia placed to reenforce the tympanic membrane in posterior quadrant and to cover the tragal cartilage graft. **(c)** Tympanic membrane (TM) replaced back over ossiculoplasty. **(d)** External auditory canal (EAC) skin replaced.

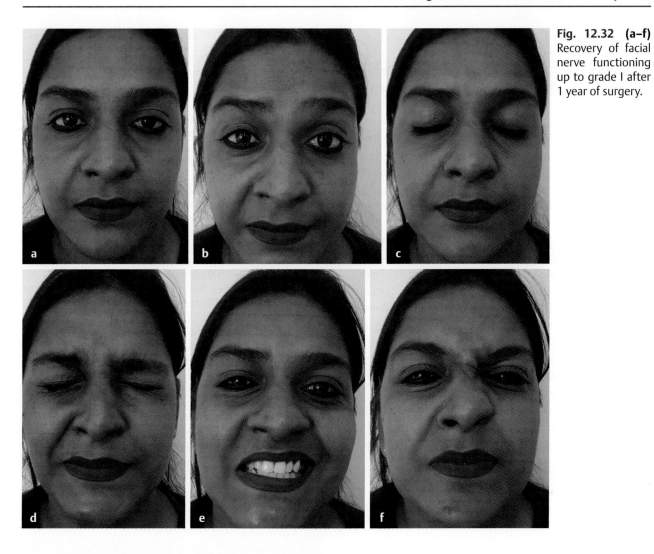

Fig. 12.32 (a–f) Recovery of facial nerve functioning up to grade I after 1 year of surgery.

Fig. 12.33 After 1 year of surgery otoendoscopic image showing complete healing of the tympanic membrane (TM) with reconstructed posterosuperior canal wall and ossicular chain visible through the neotympanum.

■ Conclusion

By handling post-traumatic facial palsy in time and through appropriate technique and approach, maximum benefit of facial nerve recovery can be passed on to the patient, but few important things are to be kept in mind. These are: diagnosing the right etiology, type and site of injury, extent of injury, time factor, and finally the skills and experience of the operating surgeon in handling the facial nerve. Almost 75% of post-traumatic FP improve on their own, requiring only conservative treatment and regular follow-up, whereas the rest 25% require surgical intervention and the technique can be decided depending upon various factors. Prognosis of post-traumatic FP depends on the timely surgical intervention and repairing the nerve at the earliest. Delayed or incomplete post-traumatic FP usually has a good prognosis, whereas immediate, complete FP which usually require surgical correction may show recovery up to different grades. A decompression, end-to-end repair, or motor nerve transfer can give complete facial nerve recovery whereas an interposition cable graft gives maximum recovery of up to grade II (HBS) only. To conclude, transzygomatic anterior attic approach is a novel approach devised by the author and her colleague to reach the LS directly without risk of injuring important structures like the LSC, SSC, and stapes.

Bibliography

1. Gordin E, Lee TS, Ducic Y, Arnaoutakis D. Facial nerve trauma: evaluation and considerations in management. Craniomaxillofac Trauma Reconstr 2015;8(1):1–13
2. Mistry RK, Al-Sayed AA. Facial nerve trauma. Treasure Island (FL): StatPearls Publishing; 2021
3. Dahiya R, Keller JD, Litofsky NS, Bankey PE, Bonassar LJ, Megerian CA. Temporal bone fractures: otic capsule sparing versus otic capsule violating clinical and radiographic considerations. J Trauma 1999;47(6):1079–1083
4. Ishman SL, Friedland DR. Temporal bone fractures: traditional classification and clinical relevance. Laryngoscope 2004;114(10):1734–1741
5. Little SC, Kesser BW. Radiographic classification of temporal bone fractures: clinical predictability using a new system. Arch Otolaryngol Head Neck Surg 2006;132(12):1300–1304
6. Fisch U. Facial paralysis in fractures of the petrous bone. Laryngoscope 1974;84(12):2141–2154
7. Diaz RC, Cervenka B, Brodie HA. Treatment of Temporal Bone Fractures. J Neurol Surg B Skull Base 2016; 77(5):419–429
8. Ghorayeb BY, Yeakley JW. Temporal bone fractures: longitudinal or oblique? The case for oblique temporal bone fractures. Laryngoscope 1992;102(2):129–134

13 Iatrogenic Facial Palsy

Introduction

Facial nerve is the most important neural structure traversing through the temporal bone. Performing surgery on or around the facial nerve is an art, which is to be mastered by learning its anatomy and complete course through temporal bone dissection courses. The right training helps in avoiding inadvertent injury to the nerve. Regular temporal bone dissections also help the surgeon in gaining hand–eye coordination skills to perform microsurgeries of ear and lateral skull base. The facial nerve has quite a predictable though tortuous course within the temporal bone so accidental injuries are rare in trained hands. Challenges arise when there is dehiscence of facial nerve in any of its segments or any variation in its anatomy. So, the surgeon should be well versed with these situations as well, The facial nerve monitor can be of great help in surgeries around and involving the facial nerve, though it is still not accessible in many institutions in developing countries.

The interesting fact remains that, we as otologists don't get the chance to see the complete normal course of the facial nerve in live patients. As the facial nerve is a deep-seated structure, covered by thick bony fallopian canal, it cannot be visualized, other than in cases of extensive disease, where it lies exposed. Its only through regular practice on temporal bones, that the surgeon can learn the facial nerve anatomy, its placement and orientation in the temporal bone along with the important landmarks surrounding it. the facial nerve as its seen in three-dimensional orientation in the temporal bone. Its operating field is to be seen repeatedly to be imprinted in the mind. The surgeon should also know the usage of right instruments and be able to identify the cases at risk of injury to the facial nerve. This chapter will brief about various aspects of iatrogenic facial nerve palsy under the following headings:

- Important aspects of surgical anatomy of the facial nerve.
- Causes of iatrogenic trauma to the facial nerve.
- Type of injury to the facial nerve.
- Injury involving to the facial nerve in different surgeries.
- Management of iatrogenic facial palsy.
- Prevention of iatrogenic facial palsy.

Important Aspects of Surgical Anatomy of the Facial Nerve

Length of Different Segments of the Facial Nerve in: (Fig. 13.1)

- Cerebellopontine angle (CPA): 23 to 25 mm (its exit from the brain stem till the porus of internal auditory meatus [IAM]).
- IAM: 8 to 10 mm (from the porus till the fundus of IAM).

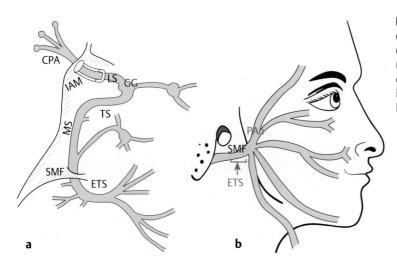

Fig. 13.1 (a, b) Diagrammatic depiction of different segments of the facial nerve. CPA is cerebello pontine angle, IAM is internal auditory meatus, LS is labyrinthine segment, GG is geniculate ganglion, TS is tympanic segment, MS is mastoid segment, SMF is stylomastoid foramen, ETS is extra temporal segment, PAn is pes ansarinus

a   b

- Fallopian canal: 28 to 30 mm:
  - Labyrinthine segment (LS): 3 to 5 mm (from the fundus of IAM till the proximal end of geniculate ganglion [GG]).
  - Tympanic segment (TS): 11 mm (from the GG till the second genu up to pyramid).
  - Mastoid segment (MS): 13 to 15 mm (from the second genu up to the stylomastoid foramen (SMF).
- Extratemporal segment (ETS): 15 mm (from the SMF to the pes anserinus). Pes anserinus (PAn) is the main bifurcation of the facial nerve into the upper (temporofacial) and lower (cervicofacial) branches.

Important Landmarks for the Facial Nerve in the Intratemporal Course

Cochlea, vestibule, semicircular canals, cog, processus cochleariformis, incus, oval window (OW), round window (RW), digastric ridge (DR), tragal pointer, posterior belly of digastric muscle, and root of styloid process are the important landmarks for the facial nerve in the intratemporal course.

Relationship between Different Segments of the Intratemporal Facial Nerve and the Surrounding Landmarks (from Proximal to Distal Segment)

- The LS lies anterior to the ampulla of superior semicircular canal (SSC) and posterior to the cochlea (**Fig. 13.2a**).
- Anterior ends of the TS and GG lie approximately 2 mm above and medial to the processus cochleariformis (PC) (**Fig. 13.2b**).
- The cog is a bony ridge from the tegmen tympani (TT), 1 mm superior and posterior to the PC and directs toward the facial nerve (TS).
- Short process of incus: The second genu of the facial nerve lies approximately 2 mm inferior to it (**Fig. 13.2b**).
- OW: The second genu of the facial nerve lies approximately 1 mm superior to it. The MS lies approximately 4 mm posterior to the OW (**Fig. 13.2b**).
- Ampulla of the lateral semicircular canal (LSC): The MS lies approximately 2 mm antero-inferomedial to the ampulla of LSC.
- Ampulla of posterior semicircular canal (PSC): The MS lies anterolateral to the ampulla of PSC.
- RW: The MS lies approximately 4 mm posterior to the RW (**Fig. 13.2b**).
- DR: The MS at the SMF lies just anteromedial to the DR (**Fig. 13.2c**).

- Tragal pointer: At the SMF the facial nerve lies approximately 1 cm inferior and medial to it.
- Superior border of posterior belly of digastric muscle: The facial nerve after its exit from the SMF lies just superior and parallel to it.
- Root of styloid process: The facial nerve lies lateral to it in the neck.

Important Distances to be Borne in Mind

- Second genu to the ampulla of LSC: 2 ± 0.76 mm.
- Posterior border of the OW to the facial nerve: 4 ± 1.29 mm.
- RW to the facial nerve: 4 ± 1.22 mm.
- Angle at the first genu between the LS and TS is around 90 degrees.
- Angle at the second genu between the TS and MS: 110 degrees (range 95–125).
- Just distal to the second genu, the nerve suddenly takes a turn in a posterolateral direction inferior to the ampulla of LSC. This is the site most prone to injury by accidental slippage of burr.
- Mean depth of the facial nerve at the second genu to outer mastoid cortex: 21.6 ± 2.62 mm.
- Mean depth of the facial nerve at the SMF to the outer mastoid cortex: 12.8 ± 2.42 mm.
- Site of origin of chorda tympani (CT): 4 to 8 mm proximal to the SMF.
- Lower one-third of the MS to DR: 3.8 ± 0.8 mm.

■ Causes of Iatrogenic Trauma to the Facial Nerve

The important causes of iatrogenic facial nerve trauma are as follows:

- Anomalies of the facial nerve like dehiscent facial nerve or bifid or trifid facial nerve (**Fig. 13.3**).
- Anomalous course of the facial nerve with or without congenital anomalies of pinna, external auditory canal (EAC), and middle ear.
- Destruction/distortion of landmarks for identification of the facial nerve in cases with extensive disease or revision surgery.
- Displacement of material used for reconstruction of ossicular chain or bony canal wall with underlying dehiscent facial nerve.
- Faulty equipment and operative techniques which include:
  - Insufficient knowledge of surgical anatomy of the facial nerve and concept about the disease.
  - Quality and magnification of microscope or endoscope not up to the mark.

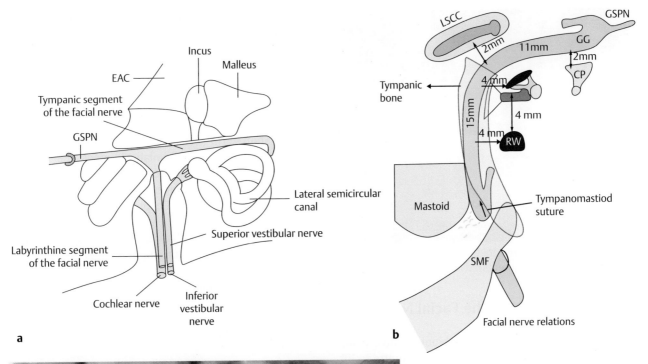

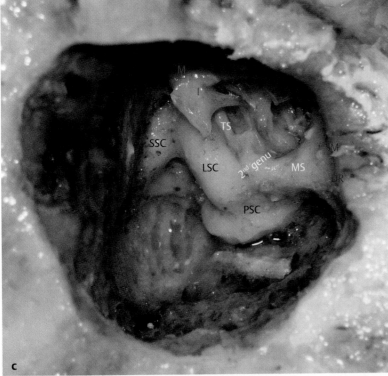

Fig. 13.2 **(a)** After its exit from the internal auditory meatus (IAM), the facial nerve as the labyrinthine segment (LS) lies posterior to the basal turn of the cochlea and anterior to the ampulla of superior semicircular canal (SSC). **(b)** Relationship of the facial nerve with the surrounding structures. **(c)** Course of the facial nerve in the middle ear and mastoid. CP, cerebellopontine; DR, digastric ridge; EAC, external auditory canal; GG, geniculate ganglion; I, incus; LSC, lateral semicircular canal; M, malleus; MS, mastoid segment; PSC, posterior semicircular canal; RW, round window; SSC, superior semicircular canal; SMF, stylomastoid foramen; TS, tympanic segment.

> Quality of drill machine and burrs not up to the mark.
> Use of cutting burr in place of diamond burr.
> Direct mechanical trauma from tip, side, or shaft of moving burr or heat generated from the drilling burr.

> Improper size of burr for that given area.
> Improper size, quality, and use of suction tip; big-sized, sharp-edged, worn-out suction tips can cause trauma to dehiscent facial nerve.
> Surgical acumen of surgeon not up to the mark.

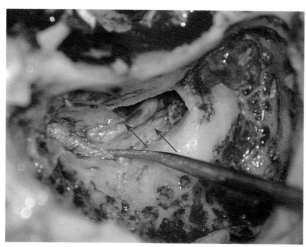

Fig. 13.3 Left cortical mastoidectomy showing bifid facial nerve in the mastoid segment (*red arrows*).

Types of Injury to the Facial Nerve

- Compression, caused due to blunt trauma, while using certain instruments like bone curette to lift thin shell of bone from the facial nerve or tight packing against a dehiscent nerve. Usually, compression leads to facial paresis rather than facial palsy.
- Stretch trauma can be caused while manipulating the facial nerve in lateral skull base surgery for anterior or posterior transposition. In the extratemporal part, the stretch to the facial nerve can happen while clearing parotid tumor from one of its branches. As long as the nerve continuity is maintained, the patient should be reassured about the complete spontaneous recovery of facial function. If in doubt, the electrodiagnostic testing can be performed and if response remains greater than 10% of the normal side beyond 14 days following the surgical injury, spontaneous recovery is anticipated though steps must be taken to avoid synkinesis formation.
- Crush injury can happen while using burr, microforceps to clear granulations or sharp-edged big suction tip over the facial nerve in the middle ear, mastoid, and skull base surgery, or using hemostat to control bleeding during parotidectomy. The decision to resect crushed segment of the facial nerve requires great acumen and clinical judgment during the primary surgery. Small injury can be repaired without resection, but if it involves more than 50% of fibers, it is better to resect that segment and repair with either end-to-end anastomosis or free cable grafting.
- Injury can be inflicted by the use of cautery while controlling bleeding close to the facial nerve.

Injury to the Facial Nerve in Different Surgeries

Iatrogenic facial nerve palsy can be part of any of the following procedures:

- Middle ear and mastoid surgery.
- Lateral skull base surgery (Chapter 7 titled "Short-term Flaccid Facial Nerve Palsy with Proximal Stump Available" under the heading "Intracranial Facial Nerve Reconstruction", chapter 10 tittled ' Management of Nerve Regeneration Complications' and Chapter 15 titled "Facial Nerve Schwannoma").
- Parotid surgery (Chapter 11 titled 'Management of Facial nerve in Extratemporal segment'.)
- Surgery around the ear like preauricular (temporomandibular joint surgery) or infra-auricular region (congenital sinuses especially in pediatric patients). Lateral Skull Base Surgery is discussed in Chapter 11.

Middle Ear and Mastoid Surgery

The risk of iatrogenic injury to the facial nerve in primary tympanomastoid surgeries is substantially high and this risk is doubled in revision surgeries.

Iatrogenic Facial Palsy in Canal Wall up Mastoidectomy with Tympanoplasty

- Injury to the TS during the process of clearing granulations medial to the incus while performing posterior epitympanotomy (**Fig. 13.4a**).
- Injury to the second genu and vertical course while performing cortical mastoidectomy in small, sclerosed mastoid with low-lying TT and anteriorly located sigmoid sinus (SS) (**Fig. 13.4b**).
- Injury to the MS just distal to the second genu (where the nerve takes sudden posterolateral turn), while locating or identifying the antrum (**Fig. 13.4c, d**) or mid of the MS while performing posterior tympanotomy in cochlear implantation (**Fig. 13.4e–g**).
- Injury to dehiscent or decompressed TS while performing ossiculoplasty or placing graft for reconstructing bony canal wall (**Fig. 13.4h, i**).
- Injury to TS or second genu while clearing tympanosclerotic plaques in case of extensive tympanosclerosis (**Fig. 13.4j–p**).
- Injury to the MS at its exit from the SMF, while giving post aural incision, in children less than 4 years of age, due to superficially located facial nerve at the SMF (mastoid tip not developed till then).

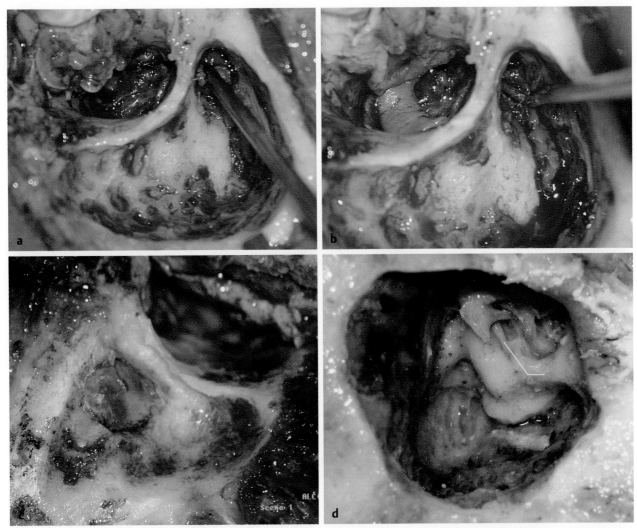

Fig. 13.4 **(a, b)** Epitympanotomy performed on the left ear. Granulations filling antrum and epitympanum. Clearance of granulation tissue medial to the body of incus can cause trauma to the dehiscent tympanic segment (TS). **(c)** Anteriorly located sigmoid sinus (*white arrow*), left ear. The mastoid cavity and antrum are very small and sclerosed, increasing the chances of traumatizing the mastoid segment (MS) while locating the antrum. **(d)** Right ear cortical mastoidectomy showing the relationship of the MS of facial nerve in the middle ear and mastoid. The sudden posterolateral turn of the facial nerve inferior to fossa incudis (FIn) and ampulla of lateral semicircular canal (LSC) (distal to the second genu) can be well appreciated (*yellow line*). Distance between the pyramid and facial nerve is 1 mm. Distance between the stapes head (S) to facial nerve is around 2 mm. Distance between the tip of short process of incus and the dome of LSC is around 2 mm. Distance between the tip of short process of incus to the second genu of the facial nerve is around 2.5 mm. Distance between the dome of LSC and the second genu of facial nerve is around 2.5–3 mm. (*Continued*)

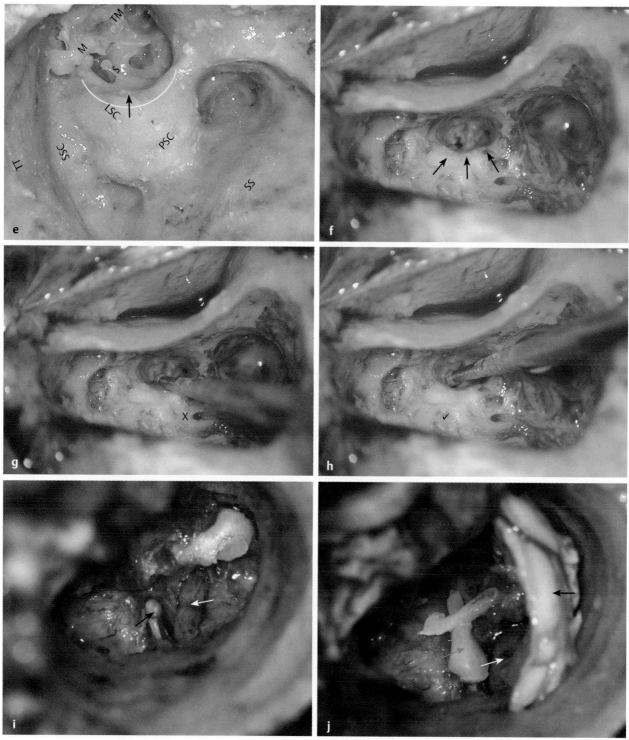

Fig. 13.4 (*Continued*) **(e)** The course of the facial nerve after removal of the incus. Distance between the cochleariform process (CP) to the second genu of the facial nerve is around 2.5 mm. Distance between the dome of LSC and facial nerve is around 1.25 mm. **(f)** Left ear, posterior tympanotomy in progress. The bony fallopian canal covering the MS can be visualized separately due to its thick texture and milky white color (*black arrows*). **(g)** the wrong angle of burr used for drilling the bone medial and anterior to MS for reaching the round window or performing cochleostomy. **(h)** The right way to use the burr in same situation. **(i)** Inside out atticotomy left ear showing decompressed TS (*white arrow*) performed with incising of the nerve sheath. Stapes is shown with *black arrow*. **(j)** Incus (*green arrow*) used as interposition graft for ossiculoplasty should not touch or press upon the decompressed facial nerve in the TS (*white arrow*). Tragal cartilage graft (*black arrow*) used for reconstructing posterosuperior bony canal wall should not be touching the decompressed TS (*white arrow*) and there should be a gap of at least 4 to 5 mm between the two structures. (*Continued*)

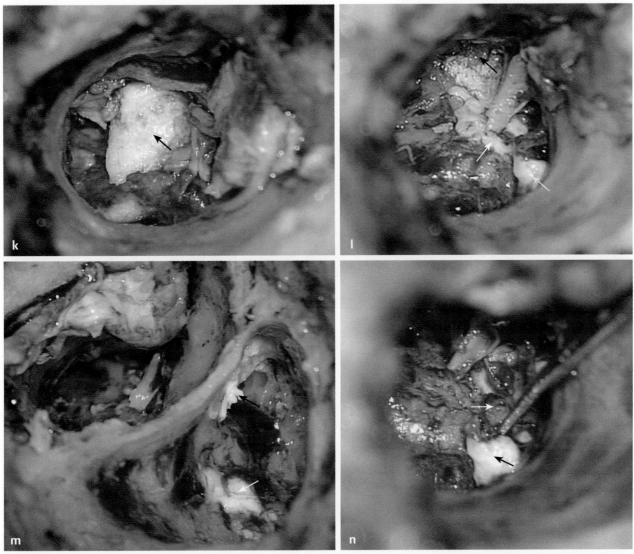

Fig. 13.4 (*Continued*) **(k)** Left ear: canaloplasty in progress showing tympanosclerotic plaques (TSP) involving mesotympanum (*black arrow*). **(l)** TSP involving supratubal area (*black arrow*), stapes area (*yellow arrow*), and promontory (*white arrow*). **(m)** TSP involving fossa incudis (*black arrow*) and mastoid cavity (*white arrow*). **(n)** In mesotympanum, Clearance of TSP (*black arrow*) from around the stapes (*white arrow*) with curved needle. Suprastructure of stapes found fragile with necrosed crura; so it was excised. (*Continued*)

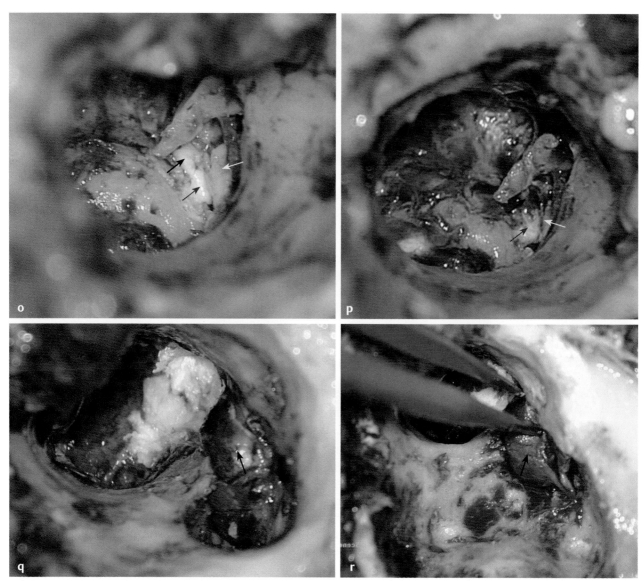

Fig. 13.4 (*Continued*) **(o)** TSP involving the promontory (*black arrow*), footplate (*red arrow*), and TS (*yellow arrow*). **(p)** Clearance of TSP from the promontory and TS. The footplate is obliterated, so a second stage stapedotomy was planned. **(q)** Left ear revision surgery for cholesteatoma disease with iatrogenic facial palsy showing meningoencephalocele (MEC) (*black arrow*) due to iatrogenic trauma to the tegmen tympani in the previous surgery by the slippage of moving bur. **(r)** MEC reduced with bipolar cautery and repaired in layers. (*Continued*)

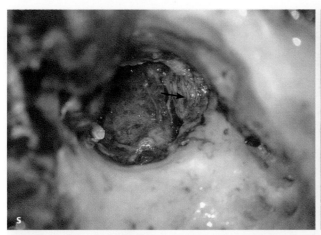 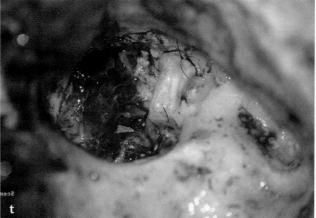

Fig. 13.4 (*Continued*) **(s)** After repair of tegmen defect, iatrogenic trauma to the facial nerve assessed in its TS. More than 90% of fibers in the TS found damaged due to injury by moving burr (*black arrow*). **(t)** After resecting the affected part of the nerve, interposition free cable nerve graft placed between the cut ends of the facial nerve and sutured by placing two sutures on each side, with 8-0 monofilament nylon.

- Slippage of moving burr leading to trauma to the facial nerve at the second genu, and/or TS. Usually in such injury there is associated trauma to tegmen bone leading to CSF otorrrhoea or meningoencephlocoele or injury to semicircular canal (mostly LSC) leading to fistula. In such cases, canal wall up mastoidectomy may need conversion to canal wall down mastoidectomy to completely eradicate the disease and repair the facial nerve along with repairing the defect in tegmen bone and/or labyrinth.

Iatrogenic Facial Palsy in Stapes Surgery

The congenital stapes ankylosis/fixation forms around 20 to 30% of all ossicular malformations. Surgical management in these cases can give good results regarding hearing improvement, but special attention is to be paid to exclude anomalous facial nerve or its aberrant location, and specialized care is needed to avoid injuring it while performing the stapes surgery (**Fig. 13.5**).

Anomalous facial nerve is very common in cases undergoing surgery for congenital stapes fixation. Failure to recognize the malpositioned facial nerve can be devastating to the patient. The common forms of facial anomaly include a dehiscent or displaced facial nerve. The dehiscent facial nerve can be present either at normal anatomical location (**Fig. 13.5a**) or with antero-inferior displacement (**Fig. 13.6a**). The displaced facial nerve can either be covering the OW partially or completely, bifurcating around the OW or crossing over the promontory (**Fig. 13.6b, c**).

Concomitant stapes malformation is found in the form of rudimentary stapes suprastructure with nondevelopment of anterior crus, *atresia*, or stenosis of the OW or absence of both stapes and OW. Along with malformed stapes, the long process of incus is also found short and medially rotated, which is not fit for anchoring the piston as in traditional stapedotomy, so in such cases we use a specialized piston called malleovestibulopexy piston (MVP) which is anchored between fenestra in footplate and handle of malleus bypassing the incus long process.

In such cases the presence of microtia (small malformed pinna) or atresia should warn the surgeon regarding presence of aberration in facial nerve. A preoperative computed tomography (CT) is mandatory to evaluate the anomalies well in advance. Imaging assessment of middle ear structures, particularly the anatomic relationship between facial nerve and stapes/OW, helps in selecting the right surgical procedure for optimal hearing improvement. The whole course of intratemporal facial nerve from the LS till the MS is traced in high-resolution computed tomography (HRCT) of temporal bone (fine cuts). Accordingly, the choice of surgery for hearing improvement in such cases can be preplanned.

Depending upon the anomaly of the facial nerve and OW, different surgical procedures, for the purpose of hearing improvement, are performed. In case the facial nerve is covering the OW partially, stapedotomy + MVP implantation between fenestra in fixed footplate and handle of malleus is performed. If facial nerve covers the footplate completely, don't try to shift or manipulate the facial nerve superiorly, as it will definitely give facial paresis/palsy to the patient and it can last for quite a long time. In such case, after locating the lower edge of the OW, a fenestra is created just inferior to it and MVP implantation is performed (**Figs. 13.5d–j** and **13.7a–h**).

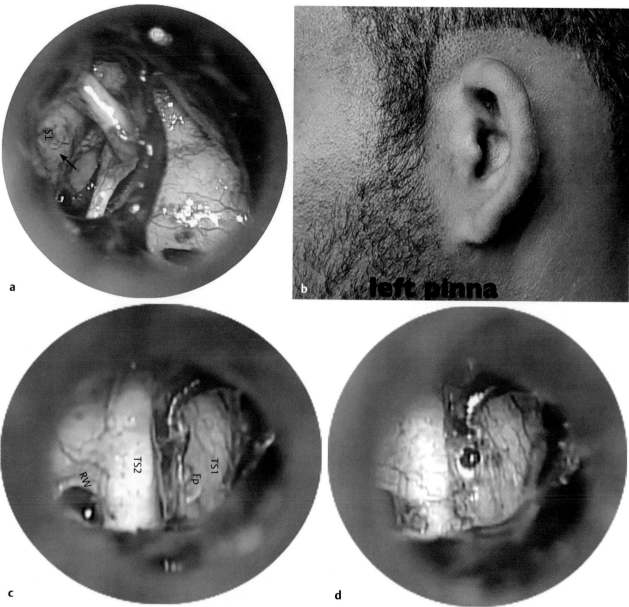

Fig. 13.5 **(a)** A case of stapedotomy of the right ear showing dehiscent facial nerve in the tympanic segment (TS) shown by *black arrow*, a cause for iatrogenic trauma to the TS during creation of fenestra in footplate or while placing the piston. **(b)** A case of congenital stapes showing microtia of left pinna. **(c)** After lifting tympanomeatal flap for stapedotomy, the anomalous course of the TS of facial nerve in the form of bifurcated TS (TS1 and TS2) around oval window, rudimentary suprastructure of stapes (S), and incus (I) visible. The lower division of bifurcated TS can be seen passing between the footplate (FP) and round window (RW). **(d)** Fenestra created in the footplate. (*Continued*)

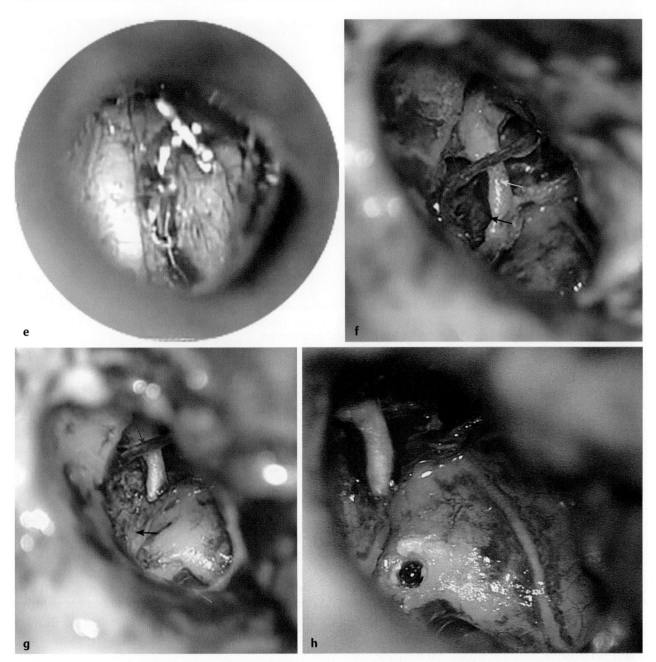

Fig. 13.5 (*Continued*) **(e)** Titanium clip piston between fenestra and long process of incus. **(f)** A case of congenital stapes (right ear) showing rudimentary suprastructure of stapes (only head and posterior crus present) (*orange arrows*) and the anomalous course of the facial nerve in the form of low-lying nerve (*black arrow*) covering the oval window (*blue arrow*) associated with anomaly of incus (short and medially rotated long process of incus) (*yellow arrows*). The TS lying inferior to chorda tympani (*red arrow*) covering the oval window completely. Oval window is absent in this case. Round window is depicted by *green arrow*. **(g)** The same case after removal of rudimentary stapes suprastructure. **(h)** Fenestra created just inferior to inferior margin of anticipated location of the oval window. (*Continued*)

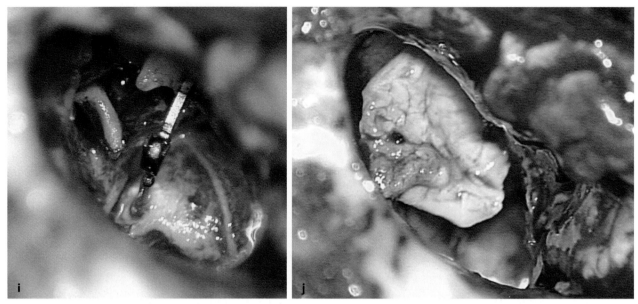

Fig. 13.5 (*Continued*) **(i)** Malleovestibulopexy piston (MVP) in place bypassing the rudimentary long process of incus. **(j)** A split-thickness cartilage graft placed lateral to piston to prevent its extrusion.

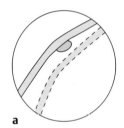
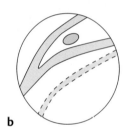
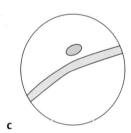

a   b   c

Fig. 13.6 Various locations of congenitally displaced facial nerve in the tympanic segment (TS): **(a)** partially covering the oval window, **(b)** bifurcating around the oval window, and **(c)** crossing over the promontory.

In case of bifurcated TS, once we identify the situation, it is easy to make fenestra in footplate and perform MVP implantation as bifurcated facial nerve crosses OW superiorly and inferiorly but does not cover it (**Fig. 13.5b–e**). Fenestration of the scala vestibule below the facial nerve with either total ossicular replacement prosthesis (TORP) or MVP implantation is performed in case there is complete atresia of stapes and footplate, with facial nerve completely covering that area. Fenestra in *scala tympani* drill-out technique combined with TORP implantation is also tried in case the footplate and OW are absent. The fenestra corresponds to the promontory wall anterior–inferior to the RW membrane. This location is found most optimal for sound vibrations to be conducted through the fenestra to the *perilymph* in the scala tympani.

Despite the anomalous course of facial nerves in such patients, if planned in advance, all procedures mentioned above give good audiometric outcome to the patient, without facial nerve damage. Lately, new hearing implants are being used if the patient is not ready to

take risk of complications associated with opening the inner ear and facial nerve injury. These are active *middle ear implants*, active *bone conduction* implants, and passive bone conduction implants. Never force the patients for surgery, if they are not convinced and not prepared for complications as devastating outcomes can be faced by the patients as well as the surgeon.

Iatrogenic FP in Canal Wall Down Mastoidectomy

- In congenitally anomalous ear presenting with cholesteatoma, there are chances of injuring the facial nerve due to its anomalous presentation (**Fig. 13.8a–f**). HRCT of temporal bone is mandatory in such situations to have a preoperative evaluation of the location of the facial nerve to avoid inadvertent injury to the facial nerve.
- Injury to the TS and MS while performing canaloplasty.
- Injury to the TS and second genu while performing inside-out mastoidectomy in extensive disease with necrosed ossicles.

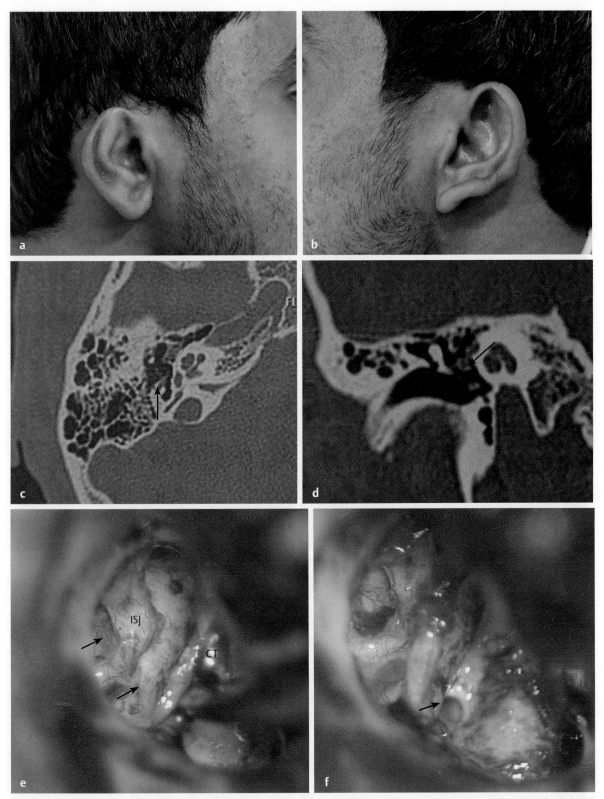

Fig. 13.7 **(a)** Microtia of right pinna and **(b)** normal left pinna. **(c, d)** High-resolution computed tomography (HRCT) of temporal bone right side axial cut showing inferiorly placed bifid facial nerve (*black arrow*) bifurcating around rudimentary suprastructure of stapes (as in **Fig. 13.6b**) and covering footplate completely. **(e)** Right ear per meatal picture after lifting of tympanomeatal flap for stapedotomy showing middle ear with incudostapedial joint (ISJ) and bifid facial nerve surrounding rudimentary stapes (*black arrows*). Chorda tympani (CT). **(f)** Fenestra created along the lower margin of hidden footplate (*black arrow*) inferior to inferior margin of bifid tympanic segment (TS) of facial nerve. (*Continued*)

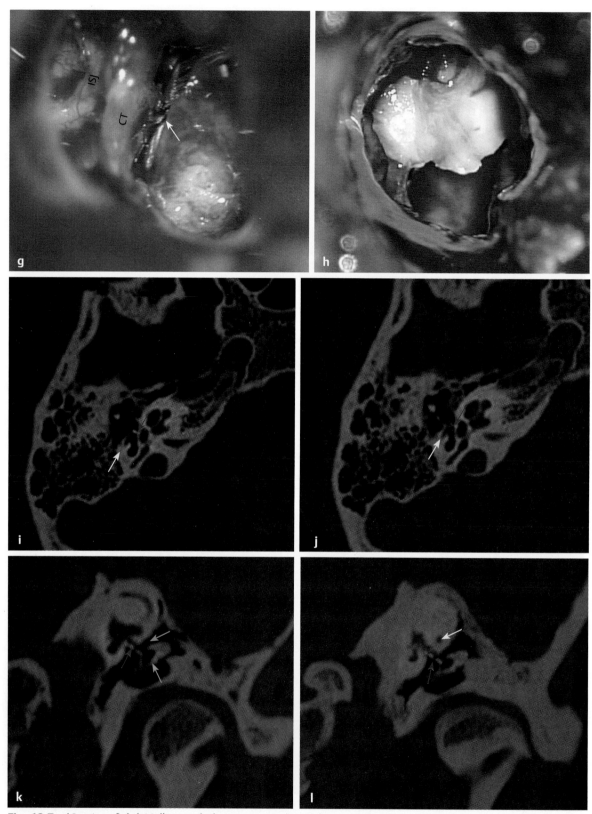

Fig. 13.7 (*Continued*) **(g)** Malleovestibulopexy piston (MVP) between fenestra in footplate and handle of malleus (*white arrow*). **(h)** Split-thickness cartilage placed lateral to the piston to avoid its extrusion. **(i–l)** Post-surgery HRCT of temporal bone scans highlighting the titanium MVP in place and intact facial nerve. **(i, j)** axial cuts showing MVP (*red arrow*) in place, between fenestra in footplate and handle of malleus (*blue arrow*). Bifid facial nerve (*yellow arrow*) also visible. **(k, l)** Sagittal cuts showing MVP set at an angle of 90 degrees fitting around handle of malleus (*blue arrow*). Rudimentary long process of incus is visible (*green arrow*). CT, chorda tympani; ISJ, incudostapedial joint.

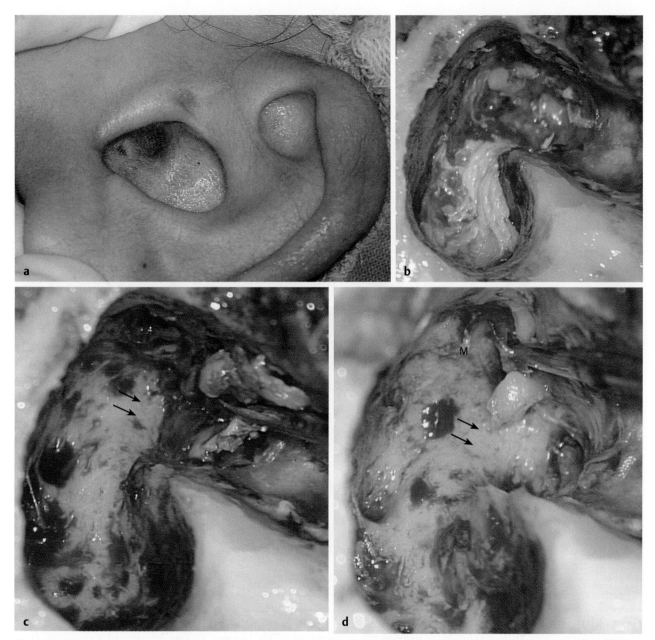

Fig. 13.8 **(a, b)** Congenital anomaly of right pinna with cholesteatoma involving the middle ear and mastoid. **(c, d)** After exposing the cholesteatoma sac (CS) in all directions, CS is being lifted in toto toward the middle ear up to the location where tympanic segment of facial nerve is normally located (*black arrow*) tympanic segment of facial nerve, but not found in this case. Incus is rudimentary and stapes and footplate are absent; only malleus (M) visible. (*Continued*)

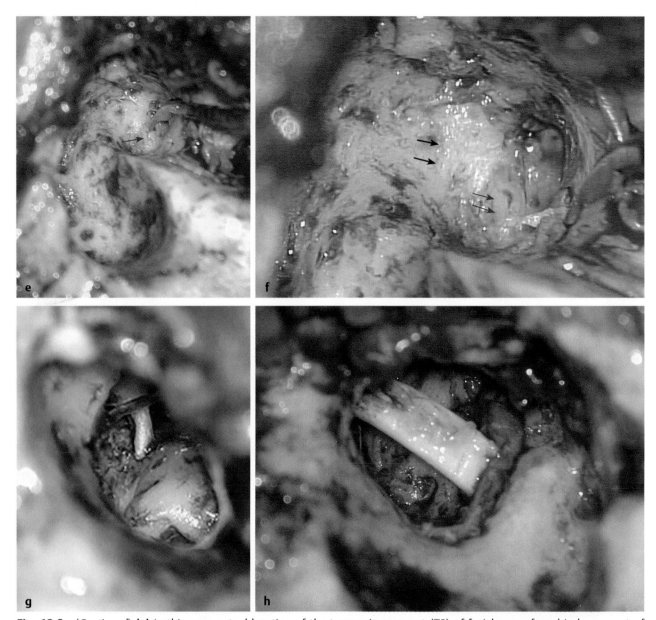

Fig. 13.8 (*Continued*) **(e)** In this case, actual location of the tympanic segment (TS) of facial nerve found in lower part of mesotympanum close to hypotympanum pointed out by instrument. **(f)** Exposed TS (*red arrow*). **(g)** Canal wall down mastoidectomy of left ear showing dehiscent facial nerve in the TS of left ear (*black arrow*). Lifting of cholesteatoma sac can cause accidental trauma to dehiscent nerve in such cases. Any mishandling with suction tip or instrument tip can also cause trauma to the nerve. **(h)** Left ear, canal wall mastoidectomy showing decompressed facial nerve from the first genu till the second genu. Cartilage graft for ossiculoplasty placed between footplate and bony annulus can cause compression trauma to the exposed facial nerve. (*Continued*)

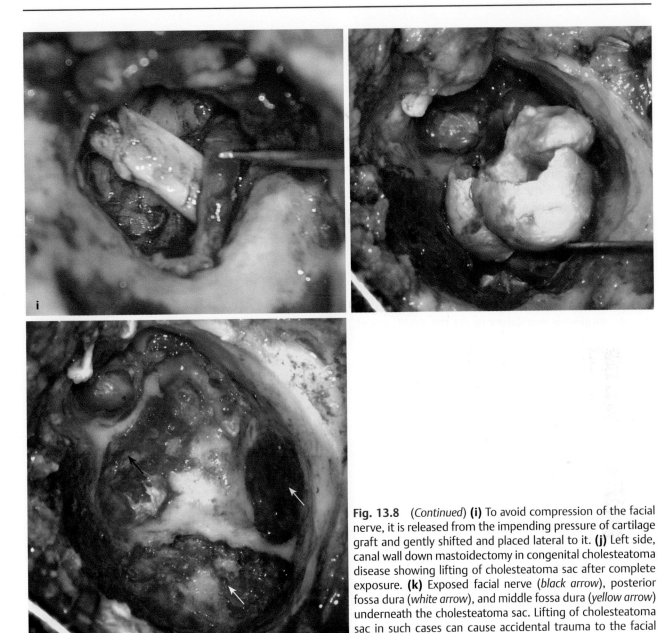

Fig. 13.8 *(Continued)* **(i)** To avoid compression of the facial nerve, it is released from the impending pressure of cartilage graft and gently shifted and placed lateral to it. **(j)** Left side, canal wall down mastoidectomy in congenital cholesteatoma disease showing lifting of cholesteatoma sac after complete exposure. **(k)** Exposed facial nerve (*black arrow*), posterior fossa dura (*white arrow*), and middle fossa dura (*yellow arrow*) underneath the cholesteatoma sac. Lifting of cholesteatoma sac in such cases can cause accidental trauma to the facial nerve, sigmoid sinus, and middle cranial fossa dura.

- Injury to dehiscent TS while lifting the cholesteatoma sac or placing ossicular prosthesis (autologous, homologous, or alloplastic) (**Fig. 13.8g–i**).
- In congenital cholesteatoma due to intact tympanic membrane there is late presentation to the clinician, and mostly the patient presents with FP only. As important landmarks are already damaged, chances of injuring the facial nerve while lifting cholesteatoma sac from underlying exposed facial nerve are quite high (**Fig. 13.8j–k**).

- Injury to any or all the facial nerve segments in extensive disease like tubercular mastoiditis, with excessive destruction of bone surrounding different segments of the facial nerve.
- Injury to the MS while lowering and thinning the facial ridge in cholesteatoma surgery.
- There can be associated trauma to the TT leading to MEC formation and fenestra in the lateral or posterior semicircular canal leading to labyrinthine fistula.

Management of Iatrogenic Facial Palsy

Following are the protocols to be followed in the management of iatrogenic FP:

- Proper detailed consent prior to surgery.
- Supportive management:
  - In case it is the primary surgeon:
    1. Explain the exact situation to the patient and the attendant.
    2. Inform regarding the time and quality of recovery of nerve function expected.
    3. Take immediate positive decision.
    4. Include a senior surgeon with experience and expertise in the team.
  - In case the first surgery was performed by different surgeon. Consultation with the first surgeon is mandatory to get the details about the first surgery and rest is same as above.
- Investigations:
  - Pure tone audiometry (PTA) to see the status of hearing, as the iatrogenic trauma might have involved internal ear leading to irreversible sensorineural hearing loss which the patient needs to be informed about.
  - Imaging: HRCT of temporal bone for evaluating the level and extent of injury to the facial nerve and for diagnosing associated lesions like residual cholesteatoma, cerebrospinal fluid (CSF) otorrhea, MEC, labyrinthine fistula etc. MRI is advised in case of additional signs and symptoms.
  - Electrodiagnostic tests to evaluate the extent of injury to the facial nerve.
  - Ear swab for culture sensitivity is mandatory as it guides us in using the right antibiotics in pre-, intra-, and postoperative periods.
- Management:
  - Supportive treatment.
  - Medical Management: Steroids, antibiotics, and ear drops according to culture sensitivity report and added treatment in case of injury to the TT and/or CSF otorrhea.
  - Eye care: Before the actual surgery, eye care and tarsorrhaphy are to be performed according to the requirement of the case. This has already been described in detail in Chapter 9 titled "Management of Long Duration Facial Palsy."
  - Surgical Management.
  - Combination of all four.

Surgical Management: Selection of Time of Exploration and the Surgical Procedure

Selection of time of exploration and surgical procedure depends on time of onset and extent of injury to the facial nerve along with period between onset of palsy and patient's first visit to the clinician.

Selection of Time of Exploration

For selection of time of exploration, the situation can be categorized into:

- Immediate FP/paresis.
- Delayed FP.
- Post palsy first visit to otologist.

Immediate Facial Palsy or Paresis

- No direct trauma according to surgeon:
  - Local anesthesia effect: Immediate, complete, or incomplete FP can be due to infiltration of local anesthesia in case of dehiscent facial nerve (seen in almost 30% of cases). In all such cases observation is advisable for 4 to 6 hours for effect of local anesthesia to wean off. It is better to assess the grade of facial nerve palsy after removing the mastoid bandage. The surgeon should develop the habit of recording all cases, as it always help in identifying the true cause of FP.
  - Immediate grade V or VI FP can happen, even after minimal handling of facial nerve like elevating plastered epithelium from the facial nerve, removal of granulation tissue from around the facial nerve, accidentally touching the dehiscent facial nerve with needle, suction cannula, or slight damage to the nerve sheath. In these situations, usually facial nerve paresis is expected postoperatively rather than grade VI palsy. Immediate grade V and VI FP in such cases will need surgical intervention unless the first surgeon has video recording of the procedure, and the competent surgeon has not noticed any significant damage to the facial nerve on review of the video. Unfortunately, the grade of the facial nerve palsy is not proportionate to the degree of damage to the facial nerve. If video recording of these cases are available, upon review of the video recording, the extent of facial nerve damage or mishandling can be reconfirmed and assurance can be given to the patients and relatives regarding complete recovery of facial nerve function. Occasionally

the patient is given the choice of facial nerve decompression to hasten the recovery and avoid negligible mismatching of fibers as the author believes that decompression will help in reducing the edema of the nerve fibers and its consequences. In spite of good result expected in all abovementioned situations, if no video recording is available, the author strongly recommends re-exploration of cases with grade VI palsy at the earliest in presence of experienced surgeon or in institute well equipped with experienced team and infrastructure to manage facial nerve injury.

- Actual trauma incurred by the surgeon:
  - ➤ Trauma recognized during surgery: Intraoperative repair in the same stage is always advised. As the trauma is fresh, and the surrounding tissue is healthy, the traumatized ends can be repaired without any loss of nerve tissue or infection. The planes are well-maintained, and minimal handling of surrounding tissue is required. The patient's attendants are informed about the repair of the nerve and the time required for the recovery of functioning which can be from 4 to 5 months (in case of minimal injury and up to 2 years in case of repair of completely transected nerve).
  - ➤ Trauma recognized postoperatively: The facial nerve is always evaluated in the immediate postoperative period to determine the integrity of the facial nerve. This evaluation can begin on the operation table once the patient is out of general anesthesia, then in the recovery room, followed by postoperative ward after 24 hours of surgery. The closure or approximation of eyelids is of little value in evaluating facial function in immediate postoperative period as the closure of eyelids may remain for up to 3 to 5 days post injury due to sympathetic activity, postoperative edema, limitation of mobility, mastoid bandage, or effect of gravity due to lying in supine position. Once it is clear that it is grade VI FP, exploration is mandatory. Although the dictum says that "the sun should not set on an immediate postoperative facial palsy," the author feels that a sufficient waiting period is required to assess the cause, location, and extent of injury. Exploration with facial nerve repair has to be performed in a well-equipped setup by an experienced surgeon. In incomplete FP (less than grade VI), the waiting period can be prolonged as chance of spontaneous recovery in such cases is almost sure. In case no improvement is noted in 3 months, exploration is must.

Delayed Facial Paresis or Palsy (After 24 Hours)

In delayed facial nerve paresis/palsy (which appears after 24 hours of the first surgery) the causes can be:

- Commonest cause is congenital micro or macro dehiscence of horizontal fallopian canal, leading to edema of facial nerve causing temporary FP.
- Bell's palsy or herpes zoster oticus. The cause in such cases is viral reactivation after surgery.

Delayed FP can occur as late as up to 14 days after primary surgery.

All such cases do not require any surgical intervention as these are self-limiting situations and start improving within 3 weeks, so they can be managed with conservative treatment, although care must be taken to avoid development of synkinesis later on.

Post Palsy First Visit to Otologist

Many a times the patient reaches late to the clinician after iatrogenic FP. The time period between the onset of palsy and the surgical management is very important. In case it is late but less than 24 months multiple procedures are available. Once the time period crosses 24 months, the role of electrodiagnostic tests like electromyography (EMG) becomes important. Surgical procedures are different for situations where EMG shows positive graph and where EMG shows negative silent graph. All these procedures have been explained in detail in Chapter 3.

Selection of the Surgical Procedure

The selection of the surgical procedure depends upon the following factors:

- Duration of palsy:
  - ➤ Up to 3 weeks: Primary procedure like nerve decompression or nerve repair.
  - ➤ 3 weeks to 2 years: Primary procedure like decompression, nerve repair or nerve transposition/transfer.
  - ➤ More than 2 years with fibrillations in EMG: Decompression, nerve repair or nerve transposition.
  - ➤ More than 2 years with electric silence in EMG: Specifically in Iatrogenic cases, the primary repair is always performed along with dynamic procedures, static procedures and adjuvant therapy.

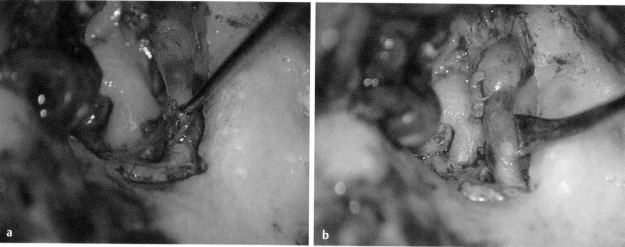

Fig. 13.9 **(a)** Incising the sheath of facial nerve to release edema. **(b)** The released facial nerve.

- Extent of damage to the facial nerve which can be:
  - ➢ Damage to the nerve sheath (epineurium) and/ or minimal nerve fibers (<10%).
  - ➢ Damage to 10 to 50% of the nerve fibers.
  - ➢ Damage to >50% of the nerve fibers.
  - ➢ Complete transection of facial nerve with <5 mm gap between the two cut ends after trimming the lacerated fibers (during intraoperative repair) or fibrosed end (in the second stage repair) margins.
  - ➢ Complete transection of facial nerve with >5 mm gap after trimming the lacerated margins (during intra operative repair) or fibrosed segment of nerve (in the second stage repair).

Surgical procedure depending upon the extent of damage to the facial nerve are classified into:

- Decompression:
  - ➢ Injury to the nerve sheath:
    1. At the site of injury, decompress 3 to 4 mm of facial nerve on either side till healthy normal-looking nerve appears on both sides.
    2. Incise the sheath only in case of gross edema of the facial nerve (**Fig. 13.9a, b**).
    3. Avoid incising sheath in case of infection.
  - ➢ Injury to <10% of fibers:
    1. After decompressing the facial nerve for 3 to 4 mm on either side of the injury site, the nerve sheath is incised and traumatized fibers are approximated if possible.
    2. Exposed nerve fibers need to be protected so as to avoid fibrosis and adhesions. Boomerang-shaped cartilage graft is placed lateral to exposed nerve (**Fig. 13.10**) with space in between in a way that it avoids any contact with dehiscent nerve and, at the

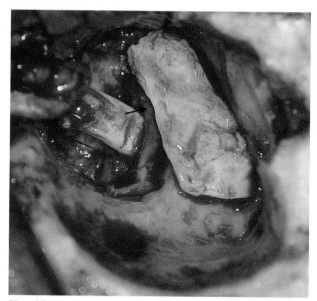

Fig. 13.10 Boomerang-shaped cartilage graft placed to cover the decompressed facial nerve. The *black arrow* shows the space of around 5 mm between the nerve and the graft.

same time, avoids retraction of neotympanum which otherwise can cause fibrosis and adhesions between the nerve and temporalis fascia leading to ischemia of nerve with further delay in recovery or incomplete recovery of the nerve.

3. The author prefers to avoid incision of the sheath if there is infection in mastoid cavity.

- ➢ Injury with neuroma in continuity (NIC): Minimal injury to the nerve can lead to formation of NIC. In case neuroma is involving minimal thickness of the nerve, only decompression of the nerve at and around the neuroma site along with excision of hypertrophic and fibrotic tissue covering the neuroma is performed. Neuroma in such cases is not excised.

- Partial-thickness nerve grafting:
  - ➤ Injury to around 10 to 50% of fibers: Excision of damaged part of nerve fibers with partial-thickness cable grafting with great auricular nerve (GAN) or sural nerve (SN) graft is performed (**Fig. 13.11**). Most often GAN is used as grafting material due to its proximity to surgical site. A minimum of one or two sutures are applied on either side whenever it is technically possible to suture. When it is not possible fibrin tissue glue is used.

- End-to-end anastomosis with/without rerouting: End-to-end anastomosis is only possible when trauma is recognized intraoperatively. In long-term FP, an incomplete transection usually leads to end on neuroma along with fibrosis of the distal segment of the facial nerve. When the neuroma with distal fibrosed segment is excised, there is a big gap between the two ends, so end-to-end anastomosis is not possible.
  - ➤ In cases of damage to more than 50% of nerve fibers: If it is an intraoperative situation, the minimal intact fibers are also transected followed by either end-to-end anastomosis or rerouting with end-to-end anastomosis between the ends of the facial nerve (in case of gap between the ends) is performed.
  - ➤ In case of complete transection of facial nerve at the site of trauma: In case the gap between the cut ends is less than 5 mm, the cut ends can be approximated and anastomosed by suturing or applying fibrin glue. Rerouting with end-to-end anastomosis is performed if approximation of cut ends is not possible. Rerouting with single neurorrhaphy is better than the full-thickness cable grafting with two neurorrhaphies as the recovery expected is to grade I or II, whereas in grafting with two neurorrhaphies, the maximum recovery can be up to grade II only.

- Full-thickness cable grafting:
  - ➤ In case of complete transection with gap after trimming the lacerated (in case of fresh trauma) or fibrosed (in case of old trauma) ends of the nerve is more than 5 mm, full-thickness nerve grafting is performed. Sutures between the cable graft ends and healthy facial nerve stumps are placed. Minimum one to two sutures are placed on either side if technically possible. If not possible, fibrin glue can be used. The disadvantage of full-thickness nerve graft is that there are two neurorrhaphies, reducing the recovery

to up to grade III or maximum up to grade II. Suture line should be protected with pieces of perichondrium or periosteum wrapped around the anastomotic site in 270 degrees.

In long-term iatrogenic FP, if injury has caused incomplete transection (damage to >50% of fibers), it leads to formation of dumbbell-shaped neuroma or end on neuroma with fibrosis of segment distal to it (**Fig. 13.12a**) (explained in detail in Chapter 3 tilled "Facial Nerve Unit, Structure, Lesions, and Repair" under topic "Traumatic Neuromas").

- ➤ The neuroma along with fibrotic segment and distal edematous end of the nerve should be completely excised, even when it means creating a large gap (**Fig. 13.12b**). The healthy nerve ends are to be reached on either side. This is followed by placing interposition free cable graft between the two healthy ends of the facial nerve. The rule says that the healthy ends are more important than the gap between them.
- ➤ Important tips for end-to-end anastomosis/full-thickness cable grafting: Edges of the graft to be cut sharp and bevel-shaped. Length of the graft should be 10% longer than the defect to avoid tension on the suture line. The graft should form a lazy "S" or "C" in final position. Reversing the polarity of the nerve before grafting is optional; this is facilitated by placing the suture at one end.

The ends of the facial nerve are freed up for few millimeters on both sides. The epineurium is stripped back for few millimeters on both ends. Suturing of cut ends can be either epineurium to epineurium (in case it is a fresh trauma where cut ends are fresh and healthy) or perineurium to perineurium (in old injuries where epineurium at cut edges has got thickened preventing the regenerating nerve fibers to grow). Suturing at both anastomotic sites is performed with 8'0 monofilament; minimal two sutures on either side with protection of suture line to avoid fibrosis and adhesions is crucial. In technically difficult situation, use of fibrin glue gives comparable results as described earlier.

In case where fallopian canal is there to support the anastomotic site, suturing or use of glue gives equally good results. In case fallopian canal is not there, pedicled musculoperiosteal flap can be used as bed to support the anastomotic sites. Here sutures work better than fibrin glue, as chances of accidental separation or slippage of cut ends is there. SN, which is a sensory nerve, can be used if greater auricular

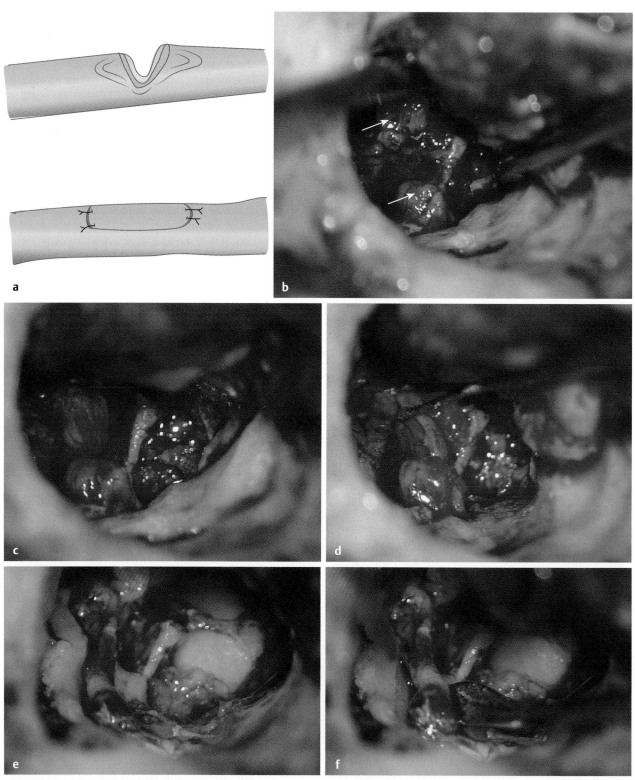

Fig. 13.11 **(a)** Diagrammatic depiction of partial-thickness nerve injury and grafting (G). **(b)** Right side revision mastoid surgery showing damage to almost 50% of fibers in the first surgery. The cut ends are lacerated with edema. **(c)** The cut ends are kept in approximation. **(d)** The level up to which the trimming of cut ends is required is marked by a sickle knife. **(e)** After trimming the unhealthy margins, the gap between the two ends is >5 mm. **(f)** The continuity of the rest of the thickness of the nerve is checked by lifting the nerve. (*Continued*)

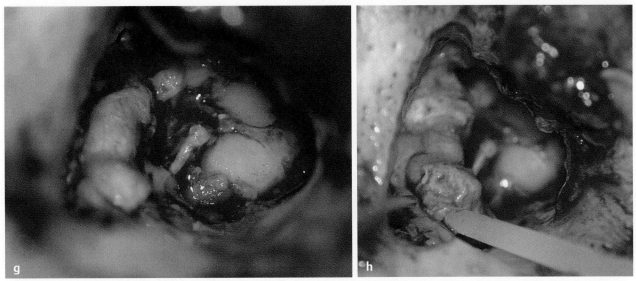

Fig. 13.11 (*Continued*) **(g)** Great auricular nerve (GAN) is used as a cable graft between the cut ends and fibrin glue applied on the approximated edges. **(h)** Placing a piece of perichondrium with glue to cover both the anastomotic sites.

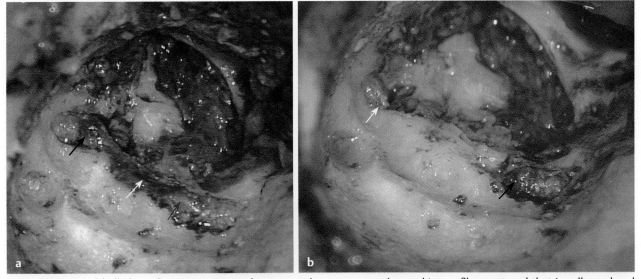

Fig. 13.12 Dumbbell-shaped neuroma. Beyond neuroma the nerve gets changed into a fibrous strand that is collapsed and collagenized at the distal end, leading to complete blockage of nerve impulse. **(a)** End on neuroma (*black arrow*) with fibrosis in distal segment (*white arrow*) with edematous nerve distal to fibrosed segment (*red arrow*) to be excised before free nerve grafting. **(b)** The facial nerve proximal stump (*white arrow*) and distal stump (*black arrow*) after excision.

nerve is not available (revision facial nerve grafting). Cable graft never becomes part of the nerve. It acts as a bridge or tubule through which the regenerating nerve fibers from the proximal stump grow across. So, the size of the cable graft should be optimal. It should neither be too short leading to tension at the suture line nor too long delaying the recovery by making the nerve fibers to grow through extra length.

- **Dynamic reconstruction procedures:** These procedures are performed in delayed presentation by patient where the facial muscles have atrophied and EMG shows silent graph.

  These include the following:

  ➤ Free micro-neurovascular muscle transfer (FMMT) with masseter nerve transfer in single stage or cross-face nerve graft in two-stage surgery.

> Muscle transposition or dynamic transplant.
>   1. Temporalis muscle.
>   2. Masseter muscle.
>   3. Lengthening temporalis myoplasty (Labbe's technique).
>   4. Anterior belly of digastric muscle transplant (Refer Chapter 9).

- Static procedures (upper eyelid implant, slings) with or without adjunctive procedure (botulinum toxin): Static and adjuvant procedures are performed in combination with dynamic reanimation or situations where dynamic procedures are not possible (refer Chapter 9).

Surgeries

- Intraoperative same-stage repair of iatrogenic facial palsy: This is explained clinically in case 1.
- Second-stage surgery for iatrogenic FP: This is explained clinically in cases 2 to 6.

Case 1: Perioperative Iatrogenic Injury to Facial Nerve with Lateral Semicircular Canal Fistula, Left Side

This is a case of extensive tympanosclerosis involving tympanic membrane, attic, and antrum. The surgeon while locating antrum in cortical mastoidectomy mistook the thick layer of tympanosclerotic plaque occupying the antrum to be tegmen and drilled quite inferior to the actual antrum (**Fig. 13.13**). During the process, the surgeon drilled into the LSC and MS of fallopian canal and damaged the nerve sheath and minimal facial nerve fibers (**Fig. 13.13**). After realizing the mistake, the surgeon stopped. The case was immediately taken up by the second, more experienced surgeon.

The situation was analyzed in detail and surgical field was assessed. The actual antrum was located superior to the site of injury and wide cortical mastoidectomy with antrostomy was performed. The exact site of trauma was located. It was found to be involving the inferior part of the LSC and fallopian canal in the MS. Posterior tympanotomy was performed to expose the site of injury at the MS (**Fig. 13.14**). The injury to both the facial nerve and LSC was assessed (**Fig. 13.15**). The facial nerve sheath with a few nerve fibers was found damaged at the site of trauma in the MS and breach in bony labyrinth of LSC was found. The facial nerve was decompressed on either side of site of the trauma till normal nerve was reached on both sides (**Figs. 13.16–13.18**). The fistula in the LSC was only bone deep and the endosteum was found intact, so repair was performed with bone pete and bone wax (**Fig. 13.18**).

Postoperative Results

- The patient suffered from mild giddiness and vertigo in immediate postoperative period with grade IV facial paresis on the left side 24 hours post-surgery (**Fig. 13.19**). Vertigo improved within few days.
- After 3 months of surgery, facial nerve recovery was up to grade II (**Fig. 13.20**).
- After 6 months of surgery the facial nerve recovery reached up to grade I (**Fig. 13.21**).

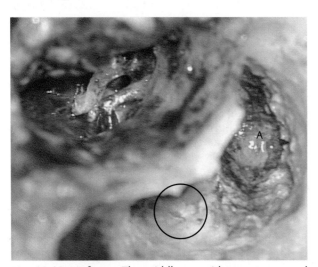

Fig. 13.13 Left ear: The middle ear with tympanomeatal flap lifted; malleus, incus, and stapes are visible. Antrum (A) located and opened and the site of iatrogenic trauma to the facial nerve and lateral semicircular canal (LSC) (*black circle*). The middle ear with tympanomeatal flap lifted; malleus, incus, and stapes are visible.

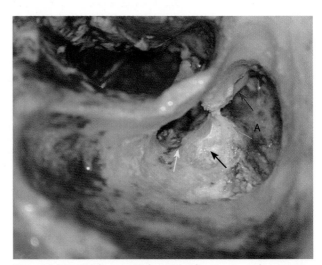

Fig. 13.14 Wide cortical mastoidectomy and posterior tympanotomy performed to clearly identify the site of injury. Body of incus (*red arrow*) and ampulla of lateral semicircular canal (LSC) (*green arrow*) with injury site (*black arrow*) on LSC and site of injury on the fallopian canal (*yellow arrow*).

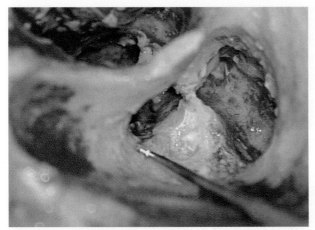

Fig. 13.15   Injury site in fallopian canal pointed by sickle knife. The bony canal covering the facial nerve drilled with diamond burr.

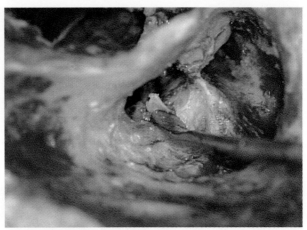

Fig. 13.16   The thin shell of fallopian canal bone lifted.

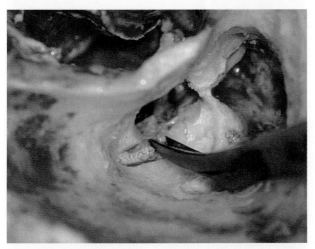

Fig. 13.17   Injured nerve sheath (epineurium) being trimmed with iris scissors.

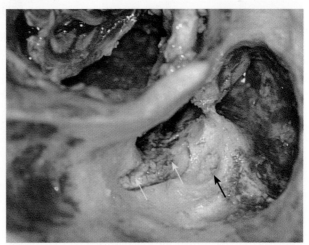

Fig. 13.18   Decompression of facial nerve at and beyond the site of injury on both sides performed (*yellow arrow*). Lateral semicircular canal (LSC) fistula repaired with bone pete (*black arrow*).

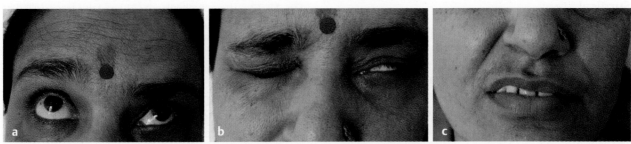

Fig. 13.19   (a–c) Immediate postoperative facial nerve paresis of the left side (grade IV).

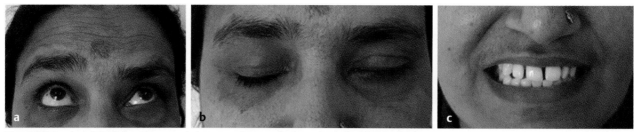

Fig. 13.20 **(a–c)** Facial nerve paresis improved to grade II on the left side 3 months post-surgery.

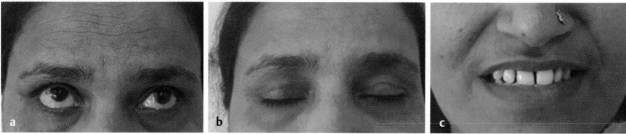

Fig. 13.21 **(a–c)** Facial nerve functioning improved to grade I on left side 6 months post-surgery.

Case 2: Iatrogenic Immediate Grade VI FP, Left Side, Addressed 1 Month Later

This is a case of 1-month-old iatrogenic FP, grade VI, operated for chronic otitis media by another surgeon. Complete FP was noted immediately after surgery. The surgeon felt he had not gone even close to the facial nerve so waited for 1 month for facial nerve to improve. For the first 3 days the left eye could close due to sympathetic activity which gave a false perception to the surgeon who mistook it for grade III facial paresis rather than palsy. The audiometry showed minimal conductive hearing loss on the left side. Otoendoscopy showed central perforation.

Surgical Steps

The surgeon while looking for antrum during cortical mastoidectomy had drilled inferior to the actual antrum and drilled into the MS of the fallopian canal and damaged the whole thickness of the facial nerve in the MS (**Figs. 13.22** and **13.23**). Thinking he had opened the antrum, and cleared the disease, he completed the surgery and placed the temporalis fascia graft.

Presently, the otoendoscopy showed central perforation. In the second surgery, after making post-aural incision, harvesting temporalis fascia, and lifting the musculoperiosteal flap and the tympanomeatal flap, the

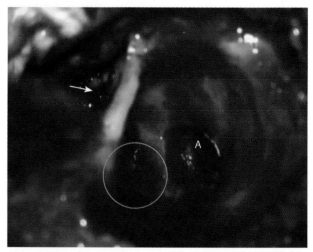

Fig. 13.22 The actual antrum (A) and false tract drilled in the first surgery (*green circle*). The intact incudostapedial joint visible (white arrow) on lifting the tympanomeatal flap

perforation margins freshened up. The ossicular chain was found intact (**Fig. 13.24**). Cortical mastoidectomy was started. The false tract could be located below the actual antrum (**Fig. 13.22**). After opening up the actual antrum and performing wide cortical mastoidectomy, the injury site was assessed. Drilling around the false tract, in both superior and inferior directions, showed the facial nerve totally missing in its MS. The area was found filled with hypertrophic fibrotic tissue and

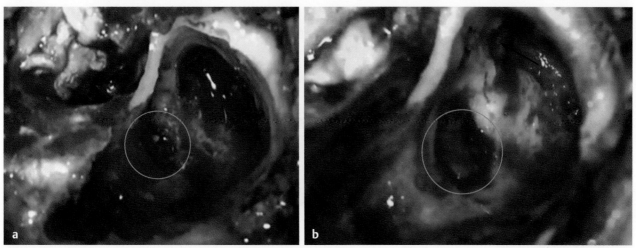

Fig. 13.23 **(a)** Antrum widened and wide cortical mastoidectomy performed. The false tract leading toward the mastoid segment (MS) of the fallopian canal visualized. **(b)** Body of the incus and fossa incudis exposed (*black arrow*). False tract is shown with *green circle*.

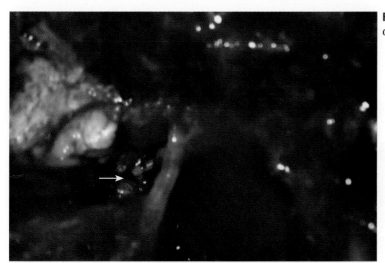

Fig. 13.24 Tympanomeatal flap lifted, intact ossicular chain with incudostapedial joint visualized.

granulations which were cleared carefully. The proximal and distal ends of the facial nerve were located, and the nerve decompressed and freed up to 5 mm on each side for repair (**Figs. 13.25** and **13.26**). The fibrotic and unhealthy tissue at the cut ends was trimmed. The gap was found to be around 2 cm, so free cable graft in the form of GAN was harvested and used to repair the facial nerve as interposition free cable graft between the two cut ends of the facial nerve (**Fig. 13.27**). Before placing the cable graft, a piece of periosteum was placed around both the proximal and distal ends (**Fig. 13.28**).

Fibrin glue applied around the approximated ends on both the anastomotic sites (**Figs. 13.29** and **13.30**) and the piece of periosteum wrapped around the anastomotic sites in 270 degree of circumference (**Fig. 13.31**).

Postoperative Results, Left Side

- After 6 months of surgery facial nerve functioning recovered up to grade IV.
- After 2 years of surgery the facial nerve functioning improvement is up to grade II (**Fig. 13.32**).

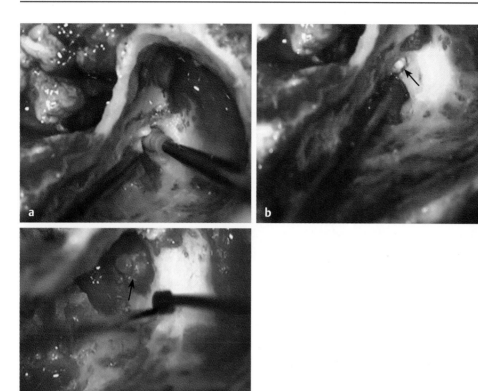

Fig. 13.25 (a) Drilling with diamond burr in proximal direction from the site of injury to reach and expose the facial nerve proximal to the injury site is in progress. **(b)** Proximal stump located at the level of the second genu (*black arrow*). **(c)** The proximal stump is freed up to 5 mm length and epineurium peeled back to expose the perineurium for repair.

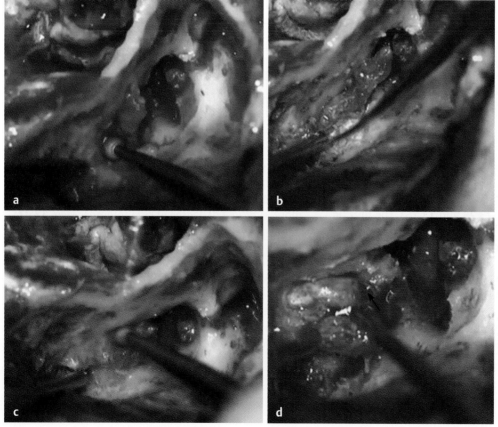

Fig. 13.26 (a) Drilling started with diamond burr in inferior direction from the site of injury for locating the distal stump of the facial nerve. The fibrous tract at the injury site followed inferiorly to reach the distal stump of the facial nerve. **(b)** The fibrous tract followed did not lead to facial nerve stump, as it is leading quite medially, which is not the direction of the facial nerve. **(c)** Drilling started lateral to the fibrotic band with diamond burr to locate the distal stump of the facial nerve. **(d)** The distal stump located lateral to the fibrous tract. The unhealthy cut end of the stump (*black arrow*) to be trimmed.

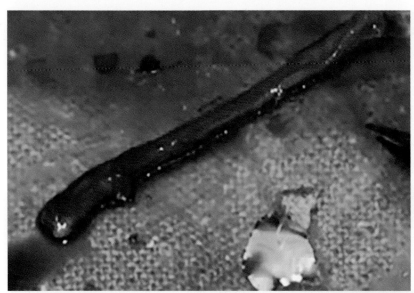

Fig. 13.27 Great auricular nerve (GAN) graft harvested with all branches trimmed.

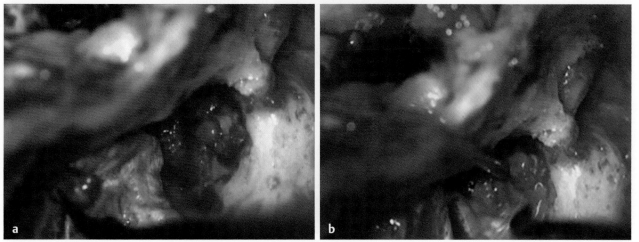

Fig. 13.28 **(a)** A piece of periosteum placed beneath the distal stump. **(b)** A piece of periosteum placed beneath the proximal stump.

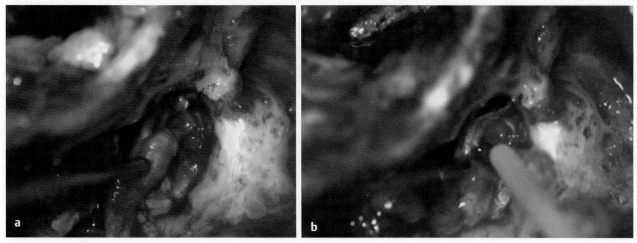

Fig. 13.29 **(a)** Approximation between the cut ends of the great auricular nerve (GAN) graft and proximal stump of the facial nerve in progress. **(b)** Fibrin glue applied at the anastomotic site.

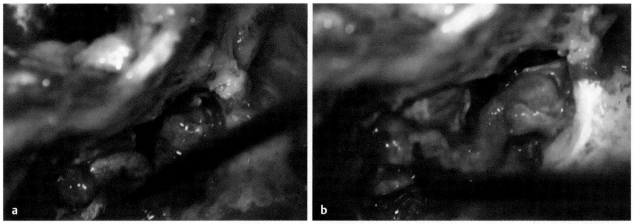

Fig. 13.30 **(a)** Approximation of the great auricular nerve (GAN) graft with the distal stump of the facial nerve. **(b)** Glue applied at the inferior anastomotic site.

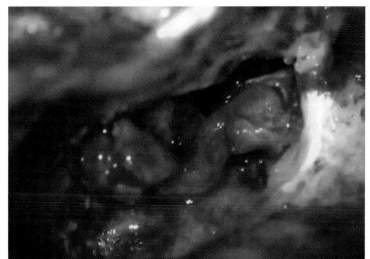

Fig. 13.31 Periosteal flaps wrapped around both the anastomotic sites.

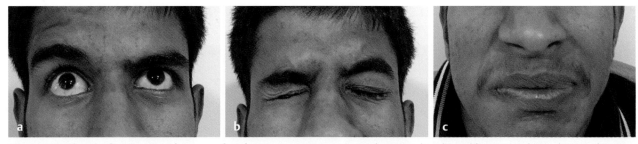

Fig. 13.32 **(a–c)** After 2 years of surgery, facial nerve recovery up to grade II. Forehead wrinkling not achieved. Complete eye closure, lifting of angle of mouth, and appearance of nasolabial fold are achieved.

Case 3: Iatrogenic, Immediate, Grade VI FP with Residual Cholesteatoma, Right Side Addressed After 2 Months

This patient presented with profuse foul-smelling ear discharge on the right side with immediate grade VI facial nerve palsy (House-Brackmann's classification) of 1-month duration which developed after the first surgery. Local and systemic antibiotics were started according to the culture sensitivity report along with steroids and local ear toilet with vinegar and normal saline (1;1) for 1 month, till the ear became dry. As facial nerve function did not improve after 1 month, the patient was taken up for surgery after 2 months of the first surgery.

HRCT of temporal bone (**Fig. 13.33**) showed normal facial nerve in the LS and first genu; dehiscent facial nerve visualized in the TS up to the second genu area. Soft tissue was visualized in the middle ear. The intensity of soft tissue in the middle ear and facial nerve was different. The second genu and the MS had intact bony canal..

Surgical Steps, Right Side

(Corelate with **Figs. 13.34–13.42**).

Postoperative Results

After 6 months of surgery, recovery in facial nerve functioning is up to grade I (**Fig. 13.43**).

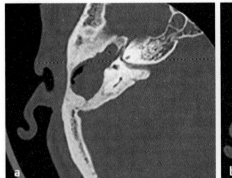 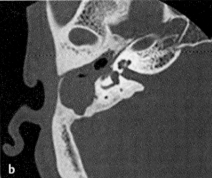 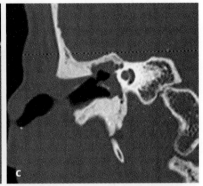

Fig. 13.33 High-resolution computed tomography (HRCT) of temporal bone axial cuts on left side showing normal facial nerve till the first genu. The tympanic segment (TS) is exposed and without bony canal covering in its lateral part. Soft tissue opacity filling the middle ear and mastoid. Ossicles are necrosed and there is incompletely drilled mastoid cavity.

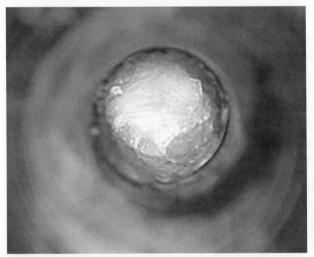

Fig. 13.34 Intact thickened tympanic membrane.

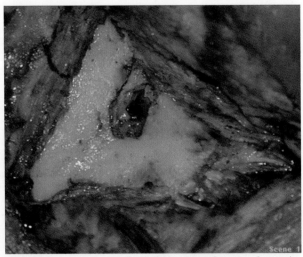

Fig. 13.35 Incompletely drilled mastoid cavity from the previous surgery.

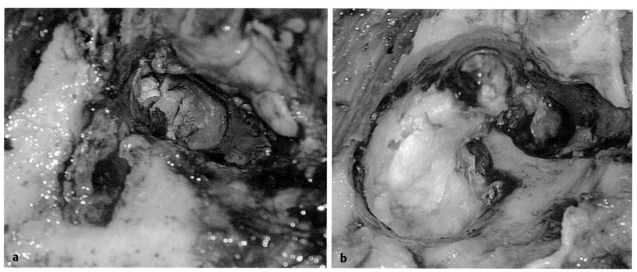

Fig. 13.36 **(a)** Outside in mastoidectomy in progress. **(b)** Cholesteatoma found filling the middle ear, attic, and mastoid.

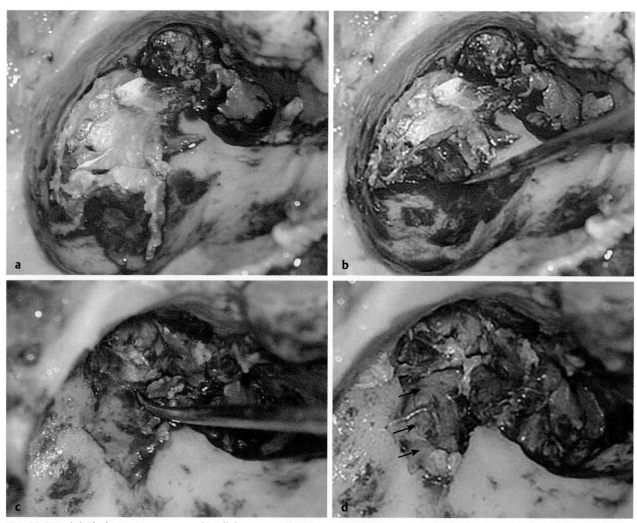

Fig. 13.37 **(a)** Cholesteatoma exposed in all directions. **(b)** The whole cholesteatoma sac is lifted in toto toward the middle ear and excised. **(c)** The cholesteatoma sac lifted up to the tympanic segment (TS) of the facial nerve which seems dehiscent and covered with fibrous tissue due to trauma in previous surgery. **(d)** False epithelium gently lifted from the surface of dehiscent TS (*black arrows*). (*Continued*)

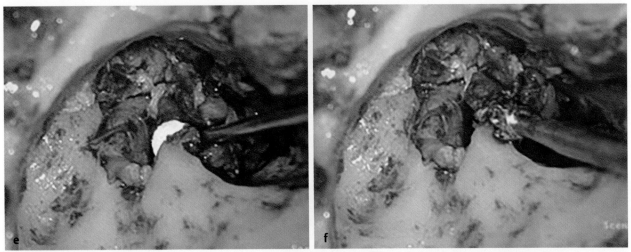

Fig. 13.37   (*Continued*) **(e, f)** To expose facial nerve at second genu and distal to it, the facial ridge bony overhang is assessed and drilled.

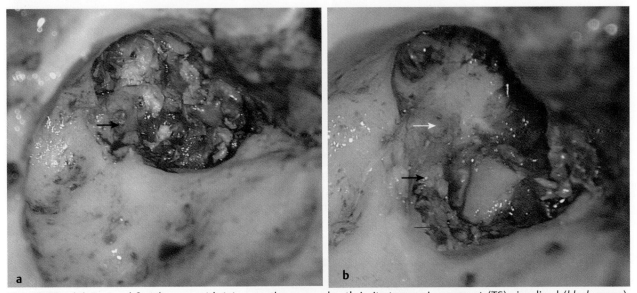

Fig. 13.38   **(a)** Exposed facial nerve with injury to the nerve sheath in its tympanic segment (TS) visualized (*black arrow*). Cholesteatoma sac visualized in anterior attic (*orange arrow*) yet to be cleared. **(b)** All residual cholesteatoma sac cleared, facial nerve exposed from the first genu (*white arrow*) to up to the second genu (*red arrow*).

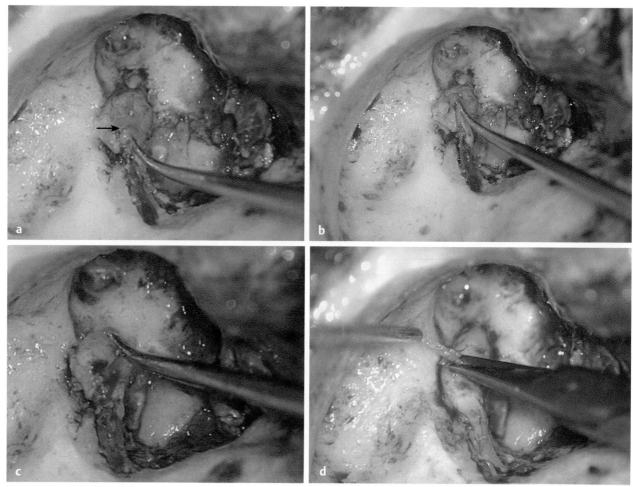

Fig. 13.39 **(a)** After clearing the surrounding hypertrophic fibrous tissue, dehiscent tympanic segment (TS) with neuroma in continuity (NIC) (*black arrow*) visualized and the nerve sheath incised distal to the NIC. **(b)** Over the neuroma **(c)** incising nerve sheath proximal to the NIC up to the first genu. **(d)** All hypertrophic fibrous tissue being cleared from around the nerve.

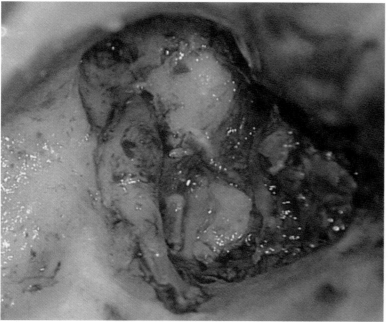

Fig. 13.40 Completely decompressed facial nerve from the first genu up to the second genu.

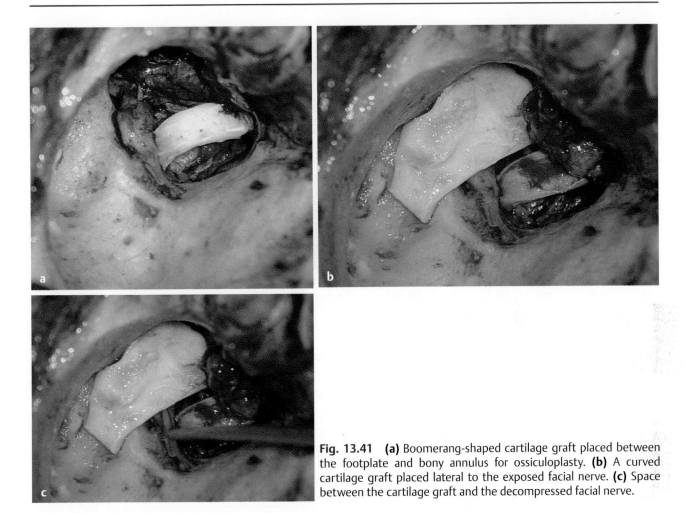

Fig. 13.41 **(a)** Boomerang-shaped cartilage graft placed between the footplate and bony annulus for ossiculoplasty. **(b)** A curved cartilage graft placed lateral to the exposed facial nerve. **(c)** Space between the cartilage graft and the decompressed facial nerve.

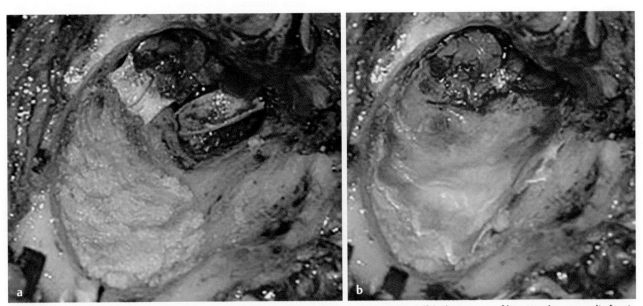

Fig. 13.42 **(a)** Obliteration of mastoid cavity with bone pete and cartilage pieces. **(b)** Placement of big-sized temporalis fascia covering the middle ear and mastoid cavity.

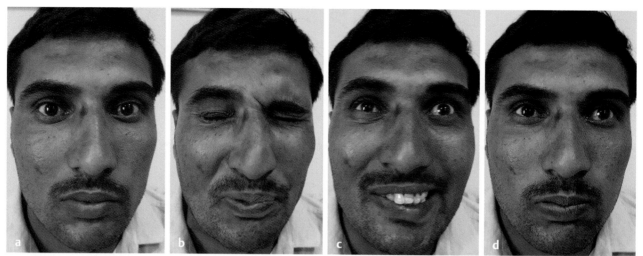

Fig. 13.43 **(a–d)** After 6 months of surgery, recovery of facial nerve, right side up to grade I (normal tone at rest, complete eye closure, lifting of angle of mouth, and wrinkles on forehead achieved).

Case 4: Iatrogenic, Immediate Grade III FP with LSC Fistula, Left Ear Addressed After 6 Months

This patient presented with history of surgery left ear 8 months back. On examination the patient had left ear discharge, facial nerve palsy grade III with slight imbalance on changing posture, and left-sided profound mixed hearing loss on audiometry. Immediately after first surgery the patient had developed complete FP of grade VI, which improved to grade III (House-Brackmann's classification) over few months. The patient also gave a history of severe giddiness and imbalance immediately after the first surgery which improved in 4 to 5 months and presently only complained of imbalance while changing posture. The patient had complete hearing loss on the left side after the first surgery. Pure tone audiometry showed profound sensorineural hearing loss left side. Presently, there is no nystagmus noted. Otoendoscopy of the left ear showed big central perforation with discharge in the EAC and middle ear.

HRCT of temporal bone (**Fig. 13.44**) showed postoperative cavity opacified by soft tissue. Soft tissue was visualized in the antrum extending up to the mastoid cavity. Fallopian canal was seen dehiscent in the MS and

was not separately seen from soft tissue. Labyrinthine fistula was visualized in the LSC.

The patient was put on antibiotics according to the culture sensitivity report along with steroids and local ear toilet, performed with vinegar and normal saline (1;1) till the ear became dry and taken up for surgery.

Surgical Steps, Left Side (Figs. 13. 45-13.50)

Tympanomastoidectomy was performed. Facial nerve NIC found involving the middle part of MS (**Fig. 13.45**). Further exploration showed that the neuroma involved only minimal thickness of the facial nerve, so it was not excised (**Fig. 13.46**). Decompression of the nerve in whole of the MS till the second genu on proximal side and up to the SMF on distal side was performed till normal healthy nerve could be reached on both sides (**Figs. 13.47** and **13.48**). The sheath over the NIC and decompressed nerve were incised (**Fig. 13.49**). The fistula in the LSC was located and repaired with bone pete and bone wax (**Fig. 13.50**).

After 3 months of surgery, the facial nerve recovery is up to grade I (**Fig. 13.51**) and the vertigo completely disappeared.

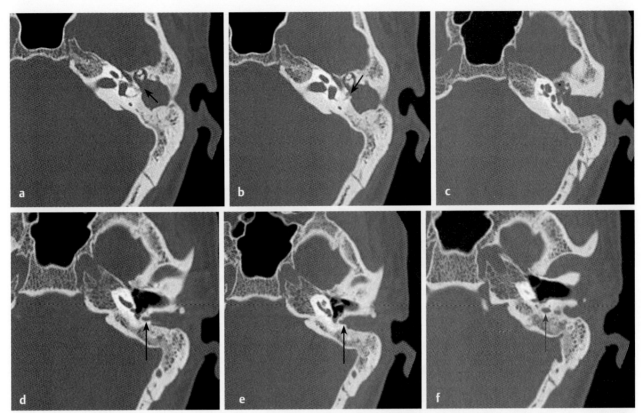

Fig. 13.44 **(a, b)** High-resolution computed tomography (HRCT) of temporal bone axial cuts showing lateral semicircular canal fistula (*black arrow*). The facial nerve found normal till the first genu and tympanic segment (TS). **(c–e)** Intact TS. Mastoid cavity filled with soft tissue connecting to the mastoid segment (MS), which is found dehiscent (*black arrow*). **(f)** Normal distal part of the MS (*red arrow*).

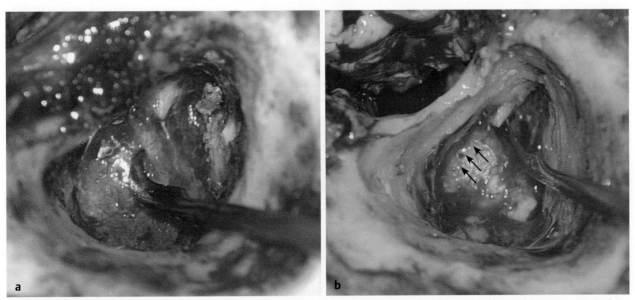

Fig. 13.45 **(a)** Left ear. Cortical mastoidectomy performed. Soft tissue mass in the region of the mastoid segment (MS) of the facial nerve assessed. **(b)** Sickle pointing toward short process of incus. The bony fallopian canal of the MS found breached from previous surgery (*black arrows*).

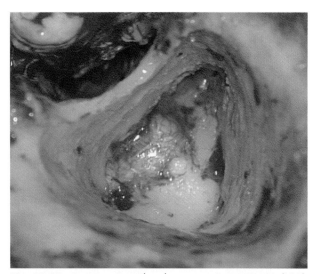

Fig. 13.46 Incus removed and neuroma in continuity (NIC) involving the mastoid segment (MS) visualized.

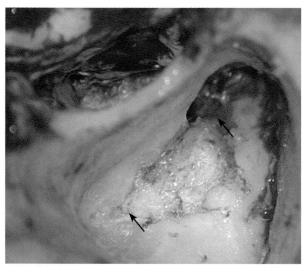

Fig. 13.47 Decompression of the facial nerve beyond neuroma in continuity (NIC) on both sides in progress (*black arrows*).

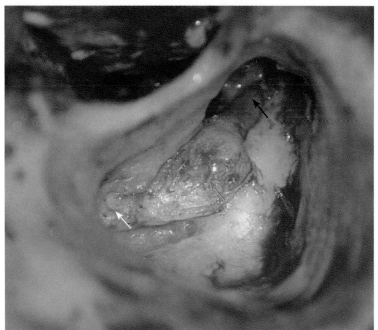

Fig. 13.48 Decompression of the facial nerve up to the tympanic segment (TS) on proximal side and complete length of the mastoid segment (MS) up to stylomastoid foramen (SMF) on the distal side achieved. Normal nerve exposed on both sides till 4 to 5 mm; proximal side shown with *black arrow* and distal side with *white arrow*. Neuroma in continuity (NIC) shown with *green arrow*.

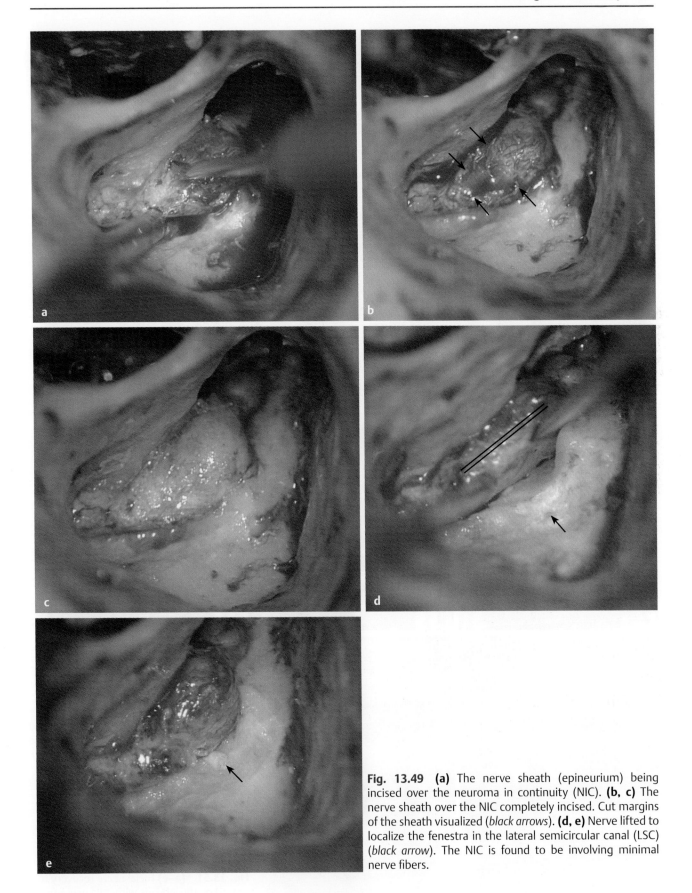

Fig. 13.49 **(a)** The nerve sheath (epineurium) being incised over the neuroma in continuity (NIC). **(b, c)** The nerve sheath over the NIC completely incised. Cut margins of the sheath visualized (*black arrows*). **(d, e)** Nerve lifted to localize the fenestra in the lateral semicircular canal (LSC) (*black arrow*). The NIC is found to be involving minimal nerve fibers.

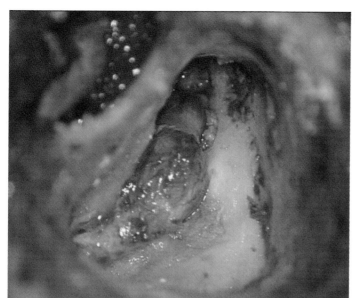

Fig. 13.50   Fistula repaired with bone pete.

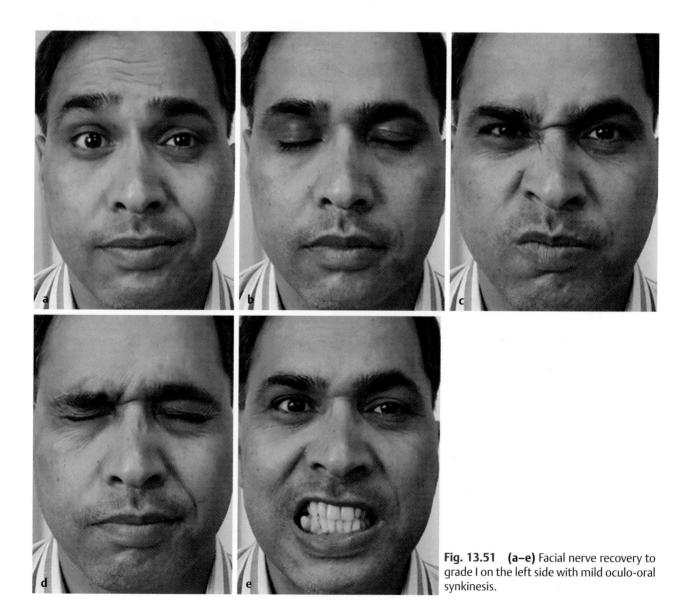

Fig. 13.51   (a–e) Facial nerve recovery to grade I on the left side with mild oculo-oral synkinesis.

Case 5: Iatrogenic, Immediate Grade VI FP with Profound Sensorineural Hearing Loss of Left Side Addressed After 3 Months

The patient presented with grade VI facial nerve palsy of the left side which developed immediately after the first surgery 3 months back. The left ear was still discharging.

Surgical Steps, Left Side (Figs. 13.52–13.60)

After post-aural incision, harvesting of temporalis fascia, and lifting of musculoperiosteal flap, skin of cartilaginous and exteriorized mastoid cavity was lifted and retracted anteriorly in self-retaining mastoid retractor. Tympanic flap was lifted (**Fig. 13.52**). The facial nerve was found exposed in its MS, second genu, and TS (**Figs. 13.53** and **13.54**). The nerve was assessed in its exposed length. Drilling was performed on either side of the site of injury involving the MS to expose normal healthy facial nerve on both sides (**Fig. 13.55**). The exposed part of the nerve was found edematous and there was thick hypertrophic tissue and fibrotic band compressing the inferior half of the MS (**Fig. 13.55**), so it was excised and nerve released. Facial nerve was exposed till the first genu in

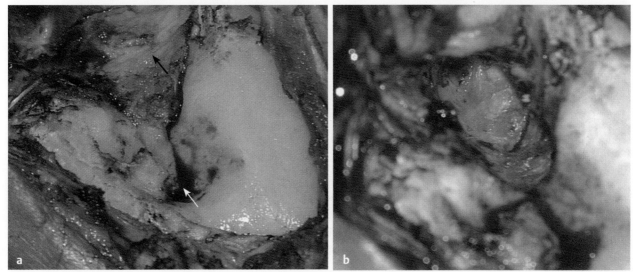

Fig. 13.52   (a) Left ear: Skin of cartilaginous external auditory canal (EAC) along with skin covering exteriorized and mastoid cavity lifted (*black arrow*). The drilled mastoid cavity from previous surgery visualized (*white arrow*). **(b)** Neotympanum covering the middle ear and mastoid cavity visualized.

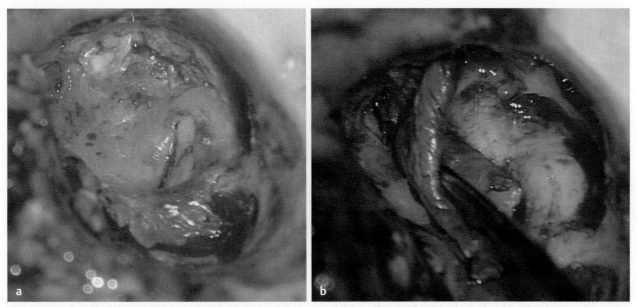

Fig. 13.53   (a) The neotympanum to be lifted along with the meatal flap. **(b)** The flap lifted gently with a flag knife, taking care to avoid injury to underlying exposed facial nerve.

its proximal side and thin bony shell over the TS and first genu removed to expose normal healthy nerve on the proximal side and upto SMF on distal side (**Fig. 13.56**). The facial nerve after clearing the hypertrophic scar tissue from the MS was lifted to assess for any neuroma or fistula in the labyrinth beneath the edematous facial nerve (**Figs. 13.57** and **13.58**). The epineurial layer was incised in whole length of the exposed facial nerve to release the edema (**Fig. 13.59**). As there was profound sensorineural hearing loss, ossiculoplasty was not attempted and strips of cartilage graft was kept over the bony annulus to create middle ear height and temporalis fascia placed lateral to the cartilage strips as neotympanum (**Fig. 13.60**).

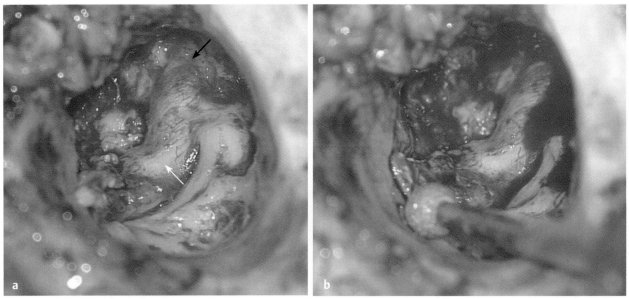

Fig. 13.54   (a, b) The facial nerve lying exposed from the first genu (*black arrow*) to the mastoid segment (MS) (*white arrow*) till the stylomastoid foramen (SMF). Exposed facial nerve seems edematous.

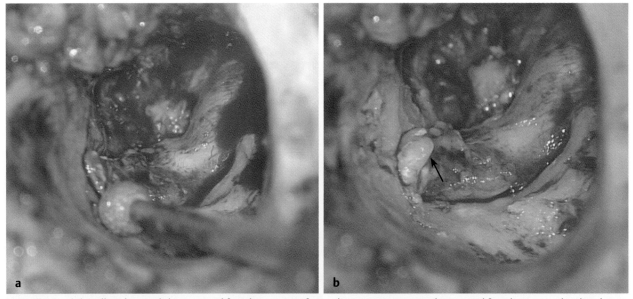

Fig. 13.55   (a) Drilling beyond the exposed facial nerve in inferior direction to expose the normal facial nerve in the distal part. **(b)** Thick fibrotic tissue and band around the distal part of mastoid segment (MS) visualized (*black arrow*).

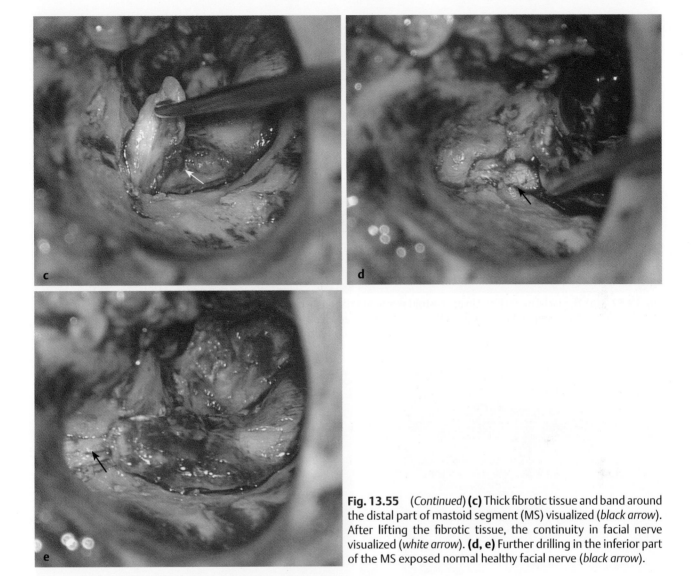

Fig. 13.55 (*Continued*) **(c)** Thick fibrotic tissue and band around the distal part of mastoid segment (MS) visualized (*black arrow*). After lifting the fibrotic tissue, the continuity in facial nerve visualized (*white arrow*). **(d, e)** Further drilling in the inferior part of the MS exposed normal healthy facial nerve (*black arrow*).

Fig. 13.56 Thin bony shell lifted from the first genu of the facial nerve and healthy facial nerve visualized.

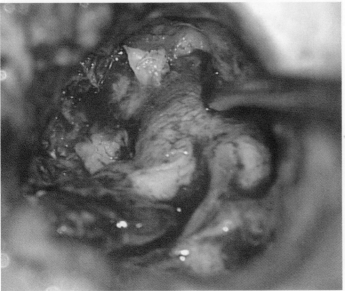

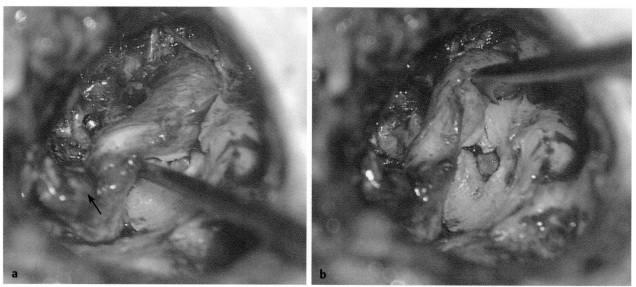

Fig. 13.57 **(a)** The facial nerve lifted in its mastoid segment (MS) and examined for any neuroma. The hypertrophic tissue and fibrotic band surrounding and compressing the facial nerve need to be excised (*black arrow*). **(b)** The nerve lifted to examine for any labyrinthine fistula.

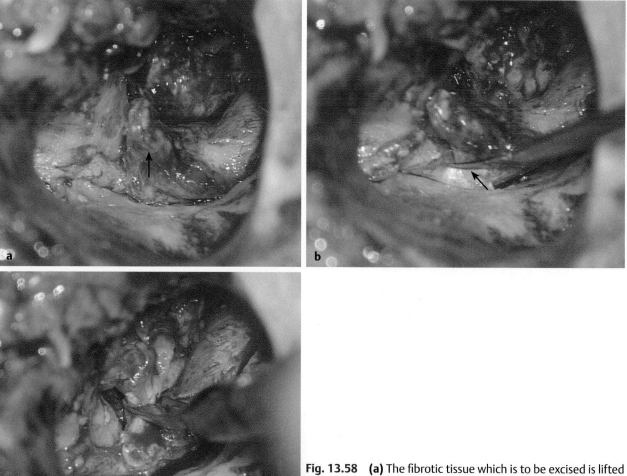

Fig. 13.58 **(a)** The fibrotic tissue which is to be excised is lifted from the underlying facial nerve (*black arrow*). **(b)** The intact nerve under hypertrophic fibrous tissue band is visualized (*black arrow*). **(c)** The hypertrophic tissue which is part of the injured nerve sheath is being excised.

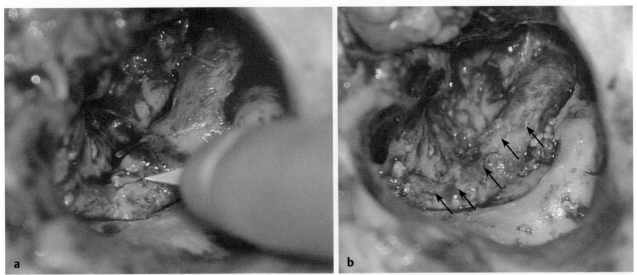

Fig. 13.59 **(a)** The hypertrophic epineurial layer is being incised at the site of injury. **(b)** The nerve sheath (epineural layer) is incised in the whole length of exposed facial nerve (*black arrows*).

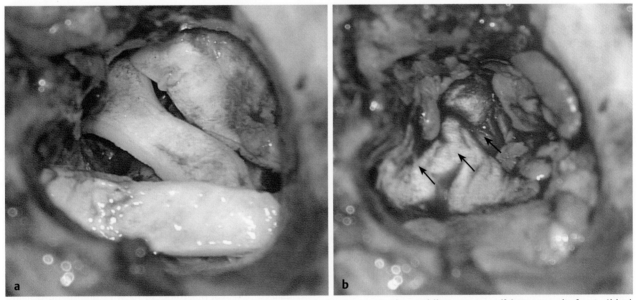

Fig. 13.60 **(a)** Cartilage palisades placed across the bony annulus to create the middle ear space. **(b)** Temporalis fascia (*black arrows*) placed to cover the middle ear. The skin of external auditory canal and exteriorized mastoid cavity replaced over the temporalis fascia and exposed bone of canal and cavity.

Case 6: Iatrogenic, Immediate FP (Grade VI House-Brackmann's Classification), with Residual Cholesteatoma (Right Side)

The patient presented with right-sided iatrogenic grade VI facial nerve palsy following tympanomastoidectomy performed 2 months back with discharging ear and profound hearing loss on the same side. The case was re-explored for completion tympanomastoidectomy and repair of facial nerve.

On clinical examination, grade VI facial nerve palsy noticed and recorded on the right side (House-Brackmann's classification) (**Fig. 13.61**).

Otomicroscopy was suggestive of subepithelial cholesteatoma in the middle ear.

Surgical Steps, Right Side (Figs. 13.62–13.75)

After making postural incision, harvesting of temporalis fascia graft, and lifting posteriorly based

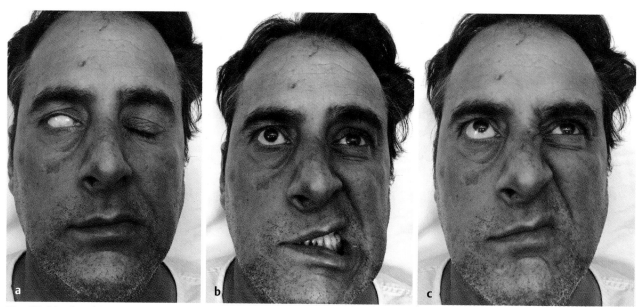

Fig. 13.61 (a–c) Preoperative pictures of the patient depicting grade VI facial palsy (FP) of the right side.

musculoperiosteal flap, the skin of the EAC was lifted and retracted anteriorly in mastoid wound retractor. Evidence of previous cortical mastoidectomy with granulation tissue was noticed (**Fig. 13.62**). Neotympanum with subepithelial cholesteatoma was visualized (**Fig. 13.62**). Tympanic membrane was elevated and cholesteatoma sac under it was mobilized and excised. Cholesteatoma was visualized in the attic and posteriorly under the annulus (sinus tympani) (**Fig. 13.62**).

Inside-out atticotomy was performed (**Fig. 13.63**). As cholesteatoma sac was extending toward the antrum, outer atticoantral wall was drilled (**Fig. 13.63**). Further canal wall down mastoidectomy was performed as cholesteatoma sac was found extending up to the mastoid cavity (**Fig. 13.64**). Residual bony overhang of posterior buttress drilled along with further lowering of facial ridge. Granulation tissue with cholesteatoma sac elevated from the mastoid cavity and antrum toward the aditus (**Fig. 13.65**) and debulked till the TS of the facial nerve (**Fig. 13.66**).

The residual cells of mastoid tip and cells lateral to the SS were polished (**Fig. 13.66**).

Further lowering and thinning of facial ridge was performed (**Fig. 13.67**). Fibrous adhesion band was visualized between the exposed facial nerve and retracted tympanic membrane which is excised with sharp dissection using micro scissors (**Fig. 13.68**). Decompression of facial nerve on both sides of the site of injury was achieved before exposing the nerve at the site of injury (**Fig. 13.69**), so that the right plane between the injured fibers of facial nerve and fibrous tissue is located to avoid damaging the exposed nerve unknowingly. The decompression of the second genu and MS is performed with

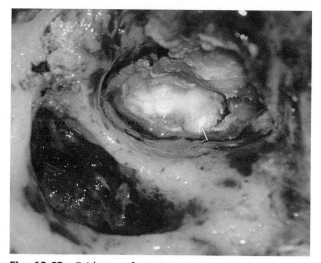

Fig. 13.62 Evidence of previous tympanomastoidectomy visualized. Cortical mastoidectomy with granulations filling mastoid cavity and thickened tympanic membrane with subepithelial cholesteatoma (*yellow arrow*) visualized.

diamond burr and curette (**Fig. 13.70**). Granulation over horizontal facial nerve was excised next (**Fig. 13.71**).

Decompression of facial nerve proximal to the site of injury was also achieved (**Fig. 13.72**). The second genu area and TS were found covered with granulations (**Fig. 13.72**). The facial nerve was decompressed further in its vertical course till normal healthy facial nerve appeared (**Fig. 13.73**). The sheath over the facial nerve was incised in either direction. Finally, decompression of the facial nerve on either side of the site of injury was achieved with incising of the nerve sheath till normal healthy nerve appeared on both sides (LS on proximal side and MS on distal side, **Fig. 13.74**).

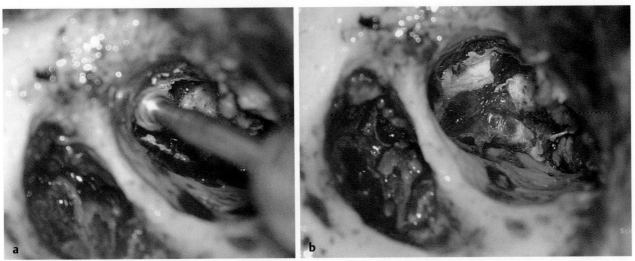

Fig. 13.63 **(a)** Inside out atticotomy in progress. **(b)** Cholesteatoma sac extending from attic toward aditus.

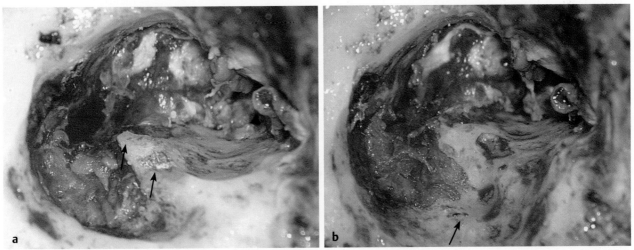

Fig. 13.64 **(a)** Canal wall down mastoidectomy in progress. Residual bony overhang of posterior buttress to be drilled (*black arrows*). **(b)** The bony overhang drilled with further lowering of facial ridge achieved. Polishing of residual cells of mastoid tip and cells lateral to the sigmoid sinus performed (*black arrow*).

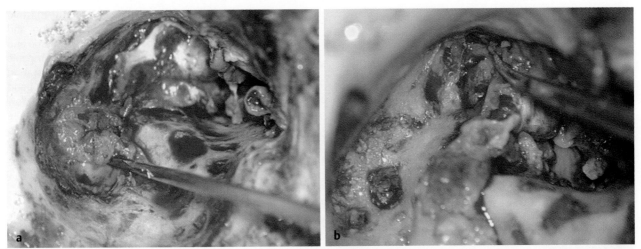

Fig. 13.65 **(a)** Granulation tissue with cholesteatoma sac being elevated from the antrum toward the aditus. **(b)** Cholesteatoma sac being mobilized from the tegmen tympani lifted toward the middle ear.

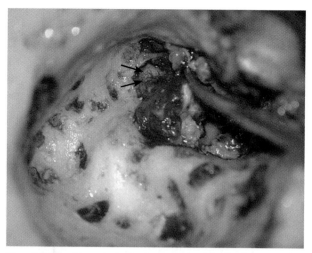

Fig. 13.66 The cholesteatoma sec debulked up to the tympanic segment (TS) of the facial nerve. Anterior part of the TS lying dehiscent is visible (*black arrows*).

Adequate decompression of the facial nerve was achieved on both sides of the site of injury in the TS. Edema of facial nerve regressed.

For reconstruction after complete removal of residual cholesteatoma and decompression of facial nerve, cartilage graft was placed few millimeters lateral to the decompressed facial nerve to prevent adhesion and fibrosis (**Fig. 13.75**). Temporalis fascia graft was placed lateral to cartilage graft to cover the middle ear and bony mastoid cavity (**Fig. 13.75**). Residual tympanic membrane reposited over temporalis fascia (**Fig. 13.75**). Meatoplasty was performed and wound closed in layers.

Postoperative Results

After 6 months of surgery the facial nerve recovered up to grade IV (**Fig. 13.76**). After 1 year of surgery the facial nerve function recovered up to grade II (**Fig. 13.77**).

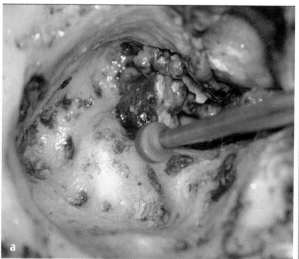
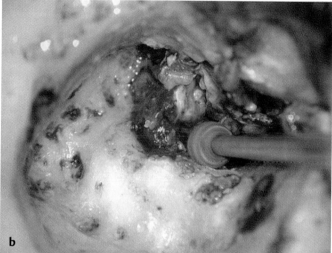

Fig. 13.67 **(a)** Further lowering of facial ridge in progress. **(b)** Further thinning of facial ridge being performed.

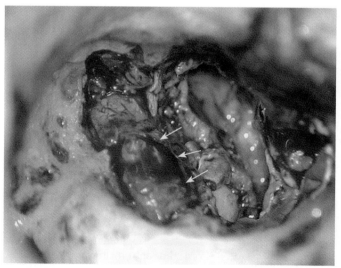

Fig. 13.68 Exposure of the second genu and the mastoid segment (MS) of the facial nerve after lowering and thinning of the facial ridge. There is granulation tissue and fibrosis around the injured second genu and tympanic segment (TS) of the facial nerve. The plane of separation between exposed facial nerve and fibrous adhesion band and tympanic membrane being demonstrated (*yellow arrows*) which are finally incised with microscissors and plane created between facial nerve and plastered tympanic membrane.

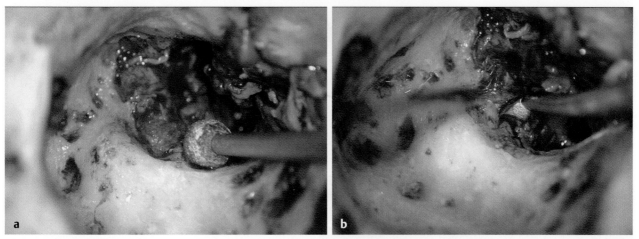

Fig. 13.69　**(a)** Decompression of the mastoid segment (MS) of the facial nerve in progress. **(b)** Thinned out bone lateral to facial nerve being curetted.

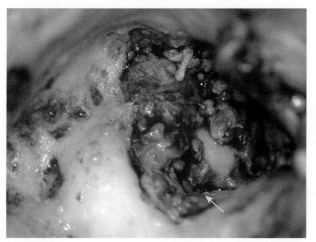

Fig. 13.70　Facial nerve distal to the second genu exposed (*yellow arrow*).

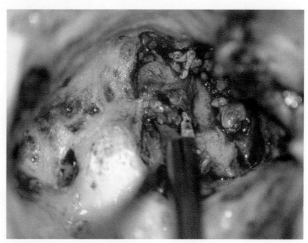

Fig. 13.71　Granulations over exposed facial nerve being excised with microscissors.

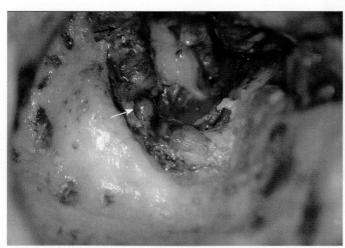

Fig. 13.72　Decompression of facial nerve proximal to the site of injury up to the first genu was achieved (*black arrow*). The affected part of the facial nerve is found edematous in its horizontal course, first and second genu. Damage to the sheath of facial nerve proximal to the second genu is shown by *white arrow*.

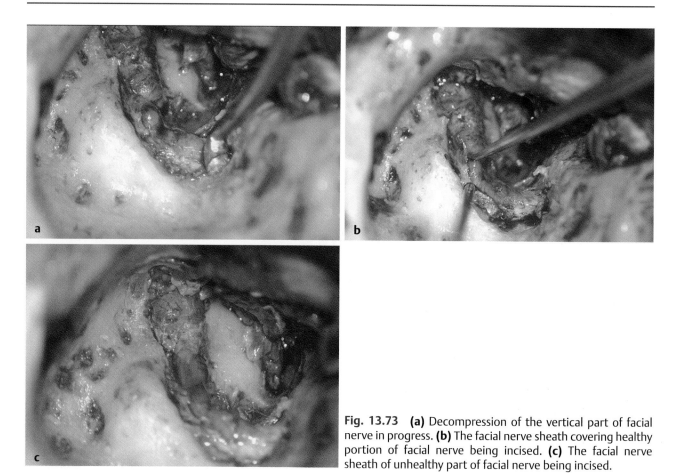

Fig. 13.73 **(a)** Decompression of the vertical part of facial nerve in progress. **(b)** The facial nerve sheath covering healthy portion of facial nerve being incised. **(c)** The facial nerve sheath of unhealthy part of facial nerve being incised.

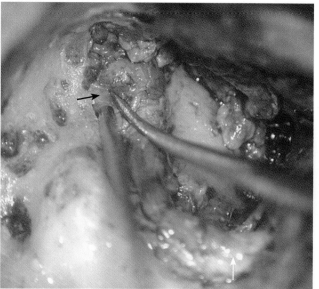

Fig. 13.74 Image showing normal labyrinthine portion (*black arrow*) of facial nerve proximal to the first genu and mastoid segment on distal side (*white arrow*).

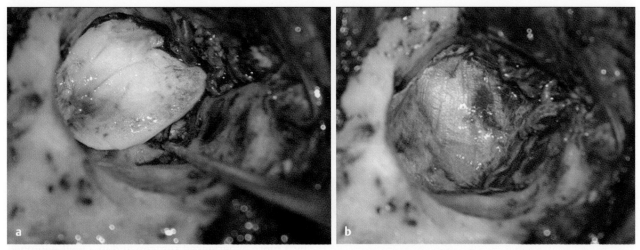

Fig. 13.75 **(a)** Cartilage piece placed few millimeters lateral to exposed facial nerve. Ball probe placed to show space between the facial nerve and cartilage graft. Reconstruction ossiculoplasty is not performed as the patient had profound mixed hearing loss. **(b)** Temporalis fascia graft placed to cover the middle ear and mastoid cavity.

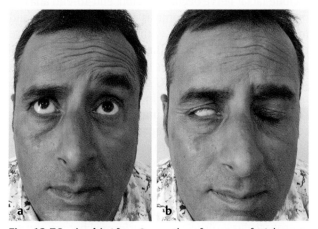

Fig. 13.76 **(a, b)** After 6 months of surgery facial nerve recovery up to grade IV.

▋ Important Tips and Pearls for Prevention of Facial Nerve Injury

- Regular learning through temporal bone dissection courses in lab.
- Knowledge of surgical anatomy and important landmarks for identifying the facial nerve.
- Intraoperative facial nerve monitoring during surgery.
- In the middle ear surgery, the TS is to be always kept in view and be palpated to see whether it is covered with bone or is dehiscent.
- In stapedotomy cases, any congenital anomaly of pinna, middle ear, ossicles, and facial nerve should be diagnosed well in advance and carefully looked for after lifting the tympanomeatal flap. Extra caution is to be taken while making fenestra or

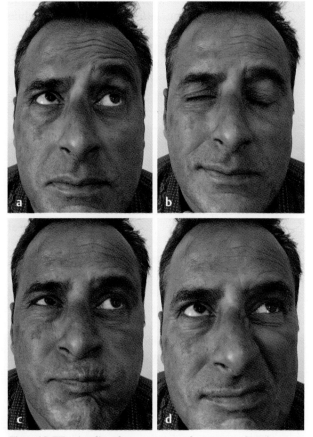

Fig. 13.77 **(a-d)** After 1 year of surgery facial nerve recovery up to grade II.

manipulating the stapes suprastructure in low-lying or dehiscent TS.
- In canal wall up (CWU) mastoidectomy, the antrum location is to be perfected.

- During posterior epitympanotomy procedure, avoid direct drilling close to ossicles. Avoid pulling on tissue medial to the incus.
- In canal wall down (CWD), always outline the landmarks for tracing the facial nerve like the PC, incus, LSC, PSC, and DR.
- Adequate exposure of bony EAC (canaloplasty) and attic in anterior, superior, and posterior parts while performing inside-out atticotomy/mastoidectomy is needed, taking care to keep lateral to the ossicles in the starting steps.
- While lowering and thinning the facial ridge, use diamond burr biggest for that given area. When close to the facial nerve, constant, copious irrigation, small suction, and drilling along the direction of the facial nerve are the enhancing points.
- The risk of mechanical trauma can be reduced by selecting the right size, type, and quality of burr along with speed of rotation. The diameter of burr should be biggest for that given area. This prevents sudden penetration into the facial nerve while drilling on fallopian canal.
- The bleeding close to the facial nerve can be controlled by either placing gelfoam soaked in adrenaline or by just pressing a big-sized static diamond burr over the bleeding point for few seconds. The sentinel bleeding is encountered while approaching the thin bone over the junction of the TS and MS in the area of the second genu, and is due to disruption of the anastomotic site of the petrosal and pharyngeal vessels. This bleeding while drilling in that area is an important warning sign of nerve being in close proximity.
- Always drill parallel to the course of the facial nerve.
- Have a complete control of the burr with clear visualization of the field.
- Copious suction irrigation while drilling is very important to avoid thermal damage. Keep washing the field regularly with saline.
- The facial nerve and all important landmarks are to be kept in clear view all the time.

■ Conclusion

Serious iatrogenic complications can occur in tympanomastoid surgeries and the common ones are injury to the facial nerve (second genu and the TS being the commonest, followed by the of rest of the segments), fenestration of the semicircular canals (commonest being the LSC), and defect in the TT with or without meningoencephalocele. The injury to the facial nerve can occur at any level. Once the injury has occurred, thorough counseling of the patient to address the medical, cosmetic, psychological, and legal consequences of the condition is mandatory.

The management of facial nerve after injury should be prompt and accurate. The time of intervention and the surgical procedure depend upon time of onset and extent of injury to the facial nerve along with the period between onset of palsy and patient's first visit to the clinician.

Once the trauma is recognized by the surgeon, immediate corrective action needs to be taken. Trauma recognized during surgery should be repaired there and then only, but the proper counseling and consent of the patient are mandatory. Also, if possible, it should be performed by a more experienced surgeon and in a well-equipped setup. The TS and pyramid segment are more vulnerable to be injured during mastoid surgery. The injured facial nerve should be explored and repaired. The methods include facial nerve decompression, end-to-end anastomosis, end-to-end anastomosis after nerve transfer, and interposition nerve grafts with the GAN or SN. In case the patient reaches late to the surgeon, the role of electro-diagnostic tests becomes important. FP of more than 2 years duration with EMG test showing silent graph needs a different approach. In such cases proper counseling of the patient is very important regarding limited surgical outcome. Primary repair of nerve is always tried but is always associated with static procedure like upper eyelid implant to protect the eye, as the recovery of the nerve may take very long time. In case there is no return of function of facial muscles, dynamic procedures like muscle elongation, transfer, and free muscle with microneurovascular grafting can be performed but are always associated with upper eyelid implant.

For prevention of disastrous complication like FP, in-depth knowledge of the anatomical features of the facial nerve and the surrounding landmarks in the temporal bone is crucial for all otolaryngologists. Better understanding of this complex structure through regular temporal bone dissection courses will lead to safer ear surgery. Knowledge of the anomalies of the facial nerve is useful in avoiding inadvertent nerve injury. In short, the surgeon must acquire knowledge, develop fine skills to handle the facial nerve, master the meticulous techniques to operate around and on facial nerve, and must know cases at risk.

Bibliography

1. Hao J, Xu L, Li S, Fu X, Zhao S. Classification of facial nerve aberration in congenital malformation of middle ear: implications for surgery of hearing restoration. J Otol 2018;13(4):122–127

2. Kieff DA, Curtin HD, Healy GB, Poe DS. A duplicated tympanic facial nerve and congenital stapes fixation: an intraoperative and radiographic correlation. Am J Otolaryngol 1998;19(4):283–286

3. Yadav SPS, Ranga A, Sirohiwal BL, Chanda R. Surgical anatomy of tympano-mastoid segment of facial nerve. Indian J Otolaryngol Head Neck Surg 2006;58(1):27–30

4. Praveen Kumar BY, Chandrashekhar KT, Veena Pani MK, Sunil KC, Anand Kumar S, Thanzeemunisa, Leivang V. The depth of the facial nerve in the mastoid bone. Int J Otorhinolaryngol Head Neck Surg 2018;4(3): 666–669

5. Fowler EP Jr. Variations in the temporal bone course of the facial nerve. Laryngoscope 1961;71:937–946

6. Gulya AJ. Anatomy of the ear and temporal bone. In: Glasscock ME, Gulya AJ, eds. Surgery of the Ear. 5th ed. Hamilton, Ontario: BC Decker Inc; 2003:35–36

7. Green JD Jr, Shelton C, Brackmann DE. Iatrogenic facial nerve injury during otologic surgery. Laryngoscope 1994;104(8 Pt 1):922–926

8. Shrivastava T, Rajguru R, Baruah D, Kumar S. Surgical anatomy and landmarks of tympanomastoid segment of facial nerve using morphometry as a measurement technique: cadaveric temporal bone dissection study. Int J Anat Res 2020;8(2):7486–7491

9. Yadav SPS, Ranga A, Sirohiwal BL, Chanda R. Surgical anatomy of tympano-mastoid segment of facial nerve. Indian J Otolaryngol Head Neck Surg 2006;58(1):27–30

14 Bilateral Facial Palsy

Introduction

Bilateral facial palsy, which is quite a rare condition, involves facial nerves on both sides, though they might not be having same grade of palsy. The onset of palsy or paresis on both sides may be simultaneous (as in post-traumatic facial palsy) or the second side may get affected within days after the first side (infective or idiopathic). There are multiple causes, and few are similar whereas the rest are different from the ones causing unilateral facial palsy. The situation is more sinister than the unilateral involvement of facial nerve and needs urgent addressal. As mimetic muscles of both sides get paralyzed, it leads to mask-like face with no emotional or volitional activity. The facial paralysis involving upper part of the face causes ocular complications like bilateral lagophthalmos (incomplete closure or total inability to close both eyes) leading to corneal ulceration and further damage to the eyes. There is significant reduction of tear formation on both sides (ageusia). The lower facial paralysis affects the emotional or voluntary smile, speech, and ability to eat. The inability to move the lower part of the face or close the eyes leads to mask-like face and the patients are unable to convey their emotions through facial expression (**Fig. 14.1**). There may be associated drooling of saliva, difficulty in swallowing, and mild slurring of speech.

The situation is quite challenging, so the treatment should be started as early as possible so as to give relief to at least one side. Certain situations are self-limiting, others may require medical treatment, whereas some cases definitely require surgical intervention. These patients warrant admission and prompt laboratory and radiological investigation for evaluation of the underlying cause and deciding for specific management.

Causes of Bilateral Facial Palsy

The causes are many but the commonest one at the author's center has been post-traumatic (road traffic accidents) temporal bone fractures on both sides, followed by Bell's palsy, Ramsay Hunt syndrome, and very rarely Lyme's disease, Moebius syndrome, Guillain-Barre syndrome, sarcoidosis, HIV, and benign bilateral tumors like neurofibromatosis type 2. Moebius syndrome is the commonest congenital cause for bilateral facial palsy.

Evaluation and Assessment

The cause, extent, and time of paralysis decide whether the recovery will be spontaneous with medical treatment or surgical intervention would be required. These same factors influence the course of treatment and prognosis as well.

A thorough history, clinical examination, lab investigations, and imaging are crucial for complete evaluation and assessment of the disease.

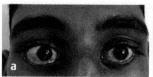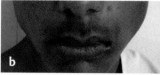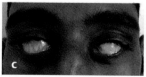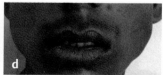

Fig. 14.1 A case of bilateral neurofibromatosis type 2 with bilateral facial palsy. **(a)** The face has become mask-like, and the patient is unable to perform any emotional or volitional activity. **(b)** Inability to put wrinkles on forehead. **(c)** Inability to close both the eyes with Bell's phenomenon visible on both sides. **(d)** Inability to smile and move the angle of mouth on both sides.

History

- Onset of facial palsy:
  - ➢ Recent viral illness, otitis media.
  - ➢ Exposure to tics (Lyme's disease).
  - ➢ History or evidence of any neural tumor.
  - ➢ History of trauma.
  - ➢ Iatrogenic injury following removal of both-sided acoustic neuroma in neurofibromatosis type 2.
  - ➢ Congenital disease.
- Progression and duration of symptoms:
  - ➢ Timing: Sudden onset points toward trauma infective whereas gradual progress points toward tumor.
  - ➢ Duration of symptoms: It can be synchronous or asynchronous palsy which can differentiate between post-traumatic and tumor-inflicted facial nerve palsy. There can be recurrent episodes versus single progressively increasing facial palsy. Recurrent episodes point toward Bell's palsy or facial nerve tumor whereas progressively increasing facial palsy indicates either facial nerve tumor or tumor in vicinity compressing the facial nerve. Any improvement in palsy is a contraindication for surgical intervention.

Examination of Facial Nerve Functioning

As both sides of facial nerves are involved, the examination has to be more thorough and it includes:

- Examination of all distribution of both the facial nerves, evaluating asymmetry between the right and the left sides and examining face at rest and during involuntary and voluntary movements.
- Other than facial nerve, complete ear, nose, throat, and neurological examination is mandatory.
- Topographical evaluation is not of much use in this condition so it is not performed in routine.

Investigations

Laboratory tests are performed to rule out infectious and autoimmune diseases.

Imaging

Computed tomography (CT) scan is performed to evaluate the presence and direction of fracture line in temporal bone and the extent and location of the injury to the facial nerve. Magnetic resonance imaging (MRI) is only considered in cases of bilateral facial palsy associated with tumors involving internal auditory meatus (IAM) or cerebellopontine angle (CPA).

■ Management

Medical Management

In all situations including infective, autoimmune as well as idiopathic pathology, conservative treatment is always given before opting for any surgical intervention, which is usually not required in these cases. The conservative treatment is in the form of steroids, with or without antivirals and antibiotics. Physiotherapy should always form a part of the treatment protocol.

Ocular treatment: Every case, irrespective of the cause and extent of facial palsy, requires eye care and protection. The patient is put on lubricating eye drops and ointments, eyelid taping, glasses for eyes, tarsorrhaphy, and upper eyelid implant (in case the recovery time is long).

Surgical Management

Post-traumatic and neurofibromatosis type 2 lesion leading to bilateral facial palsy and idiopathic facial paralysis not improving in 4 months require surgical intervention. Surgery can be in the form of primary nerve repair, interposition free cable nerve grafting, motor nerve transfer, and certain static and dynamic procedures along with adjuvant therapy. All these procedures have been described in detail in chapters 7, 8, 9, and 10.

Management Protocols for Post-traumatic Bilateral Facial Palsy

A patient with post-traumatic bilateral facial palsy can present with different set of situations and the treatment varies according to that. These can be:

- In case both sides have grade VI facial palsy with longitudinal fracture lines compressing the facial nerve and not transecting it, any one side is to be operated as early as possible so that at least one side of the facial nerve starts improving at the earliest. The other side may improve over the next 3-4 months with conservative management only. Even if there is slow improvement in grades of facial palsy, the wait and watch policy is followed. In case there is no improvement in grade of facial palsy for 4 months, the case is reconsidered for surgical intervention. During recovery time, physiotherapy and nerve reeducation are necessary to avoid synkinesis formation.

- Bilateral facial palsy of grade V or less on both sides is to be treated conservatively and no surgical intervention is required. Self-recovery will take place in few weeks or months.
- When there is transverse fracture line transecting the facial nerve on one side and longitudinal fracture line just compressing the nerve on other side, the side with transected facial nerve should be operated first followed by decompression of the facial nerve on contralateral side, and the gap between the two surgeries should be minimal. The transected nerve is repaired first so as to avoid fibrosis and collagenization around the regenerating fibers at the cut end of facial nerve and have the optimal results. As the repaired or grafted nerve takes a very long time (around 1–2 years) to recover, the other side is to be decompressed at the earliest so that it starts recovering faster. Along with the primary repair or interposition graft, static procedure in the form of upper eyelid implant and facial sling for lifting the angle of mouth should always be performed to protect the eye and symmetry of face at rest.
- In case one side has grade VI palsy and the other side has less than grade VI palsy, then obviously the side with grade VI palsy is to be operated and the other side is expected to recover on its own over a few months. Wherever there is chance of delayed recovery, the upper eyelid implant is always performed along with the primary surgery.
- In case both sides have transected facial nerve (very rare situation), then both sides need to be operated as early as possible, one after the other, along with static procedures like upper eyelid gold implant. Motor nerve transfer is always better than interposition nerve grafting. Because there is one neurorrhaphy or anastomotic site in motor

nerve transfer, it can lead to early recovery of facial nerve and improvement can be up to grade I, whereas in interposition free cable nerve grafting, there are two neurorrhaphies leading to delayed recovery and maximum recovery is up to grade II. Delayed recovery is because the nerve has to grow through the whole length of the cable graft to reach the distal stump.

Case 1

A 4-year-old girl presented with complaint of complete loss of facial expressions for 1 month. The symptoms were insidious in onset and had started with weakness of the right side of the face 45 days ago. The parents noticed deviation of angle of mouth to the left side and incomplete eye closure on the right side (**Fig. 14.2**). Weakness was noticed on the left side as well; a week later when they noticed complete loss of facial expressions and consulted a pediatrician, the patient was finally referred to the otologist. There was no associated history of fever, cough, headache, ear discharge, or reduced hearing. There was no complaint of reduced lacrimation or loss of taste sensation. She had no history of any trauma or surgery in the temporal area. She had no history of skin lesions or contact with any stray animals.

On examination, the child had a dull, expression-less face. She was afebrile with stable vitals. She had bilateral incomplete eye closure even with maximal effort and no wrinkling of forehead on looking up. She was unable to puff her cheeks with air or crinkle her nose. A bilateral grade VI facial palsy (lower motor neuron) was diagnosed (House-Brackmann's scale [HBS]). Other cranial nerves were found normal on clinical examination. Neurological examination was found to be normal. There were no significant findings on ear, nose, and throat examination and hearing was found normal on

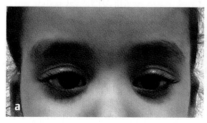
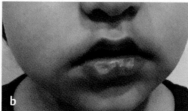

Fig. 14.2 (a, b) Bilateral grade VI (House-Brackmann's classification [HBC]) facial palsy before starting the treatment. Inability to wrinkle the forehead by lifting eyebrow, frowning, closing eyes, lifting nasal ala, showing teeth, lifting the angle of mouth, or pursing the lips on both sides can be visualized.

both sides on pure tone audiogram. She was admitted for evaluation of the cause of facial palsy.

Investigations showed normal hemogram, erythrocyte sedimentation rate (ESR), and blood sugar. Antinuclear antibodies (ANA) and cytoplasmic antineutrophil antibodies (c-ANCA), and IgM EBV (IgM antibodies for Epstein- Barr virus) antibodies to viral capsid antigen (VCA) were negative. Chest X-ray was normal. A high-resolution computed tomography (HRCT) scan of the temporal bone was done which showed normal middle ear space with normal-looking fallopian canal on both sides (**Fig. 14.3**). MRI of the brain showed a normal 7th and 8th nerve complex with no significant findings (**Fig. 14.4**).

With the diagnosis of bilateral Bell's palsy, the child was treated with intravenous antibiotics and steroids along with acyclovir. Eye care for protection of cornea was given. There was no progression of her symptoms during her hospital stay. After a 3 days hospital stay, she was discharged with stable vitals and oral medications for a week.

On subsequent examination after 2 weeks, the child came with a smiling face. Facial weakness had completely recovered on the left side (grade I) with mild weakness (grade II) on the right side persisting (**Fig. 14.5**). When examined 6 weeks later, she had completely recovered (grade I) facial nerve on both the sides and remains asymptomatic till date (**Fig. 14.6**).

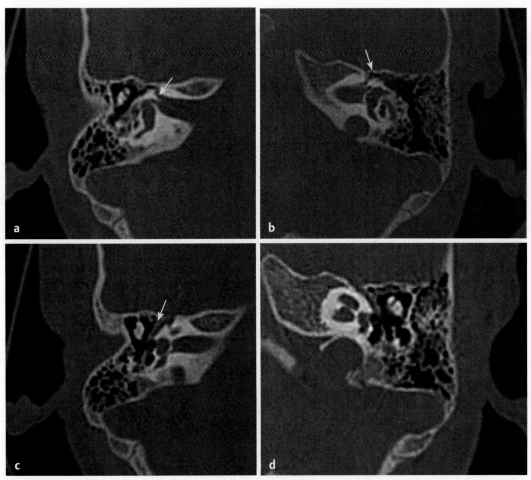

Fig. 14.3 **(a, c)** High-resolution computed tomography (HRCT) of temporal bone. Axial section of the right side showing normal facial nerve (*yellow arrow*). **(b, d)** HRCT of temporal bone. Axial section left side showing normal facial nerve (*yellow arrow*).

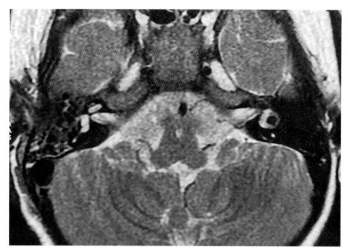

Fig. 14.4 Magnetic resonance imaging (MRI) of the brain. Axial section showing a normal 7th and 8th nerve complex on both the sides.

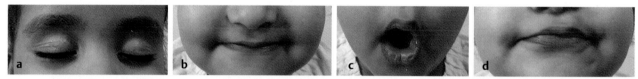

Fig. 14.5 (a–d) Recovery of facial nerve functioning on left side is up to grade I and on right side up to grade II after 2 weeks of treatment.

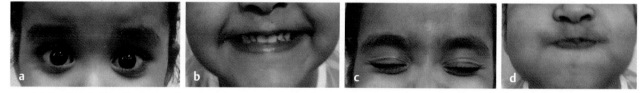

Fig. 14.6 (a–d) After 6 weeks of treatment, the recovery on both sides of face is up to grade I. Wrinkling of forehead, complete closure of eyes on light and tight force, ability to smile and show the teeth, puffing the cheek with air, and complete symmetry of the face on both sides are visible.

Case 2

A 32-year-old patient presented with sudden-onset, immediate, complete bilateral facial paralysis following head injury (post road traffic accident). The patient was under neurological care and treatment for head injury for 10 days. Since day 1, post injury, the patient was unable to have any voluntary or involuntary movement on both sides of the face.

On examination, there was bilateral facial palsy grade VI (HBS) with Bell's phenomenon noted (**Fig. 14.7**). The patient was unable to wrinkle the whole forehead, frown, or close both the eyes. Inability to smile, to show the teeth, or create nasolabial fold was also noticed on both sides of the face.

HRCT temporal bone (**Fig. 14.8**) showed longitudinal fracture line on both the sides. On the right side, the fracture line is seen running across squamous temporal bone, mastoid bone, external auditory canal (EAC), and middle ear and reaching anteriorly up to the first genu. On the left side, it was reaching up to the middle ear but keeping lateral to the tympanic segment (TS).

The patient had already been put on conservative treatment in the form of prednisolone 1 mg/kg body weight.

As 10 days had already passed, and grade VI facial palsy had persisted on both the sides, surgical decompression of facial nerve was planned. The right side was chosen as the fracture line could be seen reaching up to the first genu and a bony fragment seemed to be impinging on the nerve in the first genu area.

Surgical Steps (Right Side)

Facial nerve decompression was performed on the right side through post aural approach and transmastoid supralabyrinthine corridor. The nerve was found to be compressed by bony fragment at the first genu. After removal of bony fragment, decompression was achieved for few millimeters on both sides of the site of injury till healthy normal nerve appeared on both the sides (up to the labyrinthine segment [LS] proximally and the second genu distally) (**Fig. 14.9**). No surgery was performed on the left side.

Postoperative Results

After 3 months of surgery, facial nerve functioning improved to grade I on the right side and grade III on the left side (**Fig. 14.10**).

Left side facial nerve functioning also improved to grade I after one year of surgery on right side (**Fig. 14.11**).

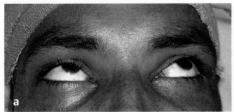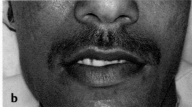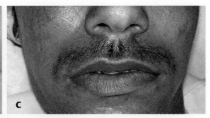

Fig. 14.7 **(a–c)** Bilateral facial palsy grade VI (House-Brackmann's Scale [HBS]) with Bell's phenomenon.

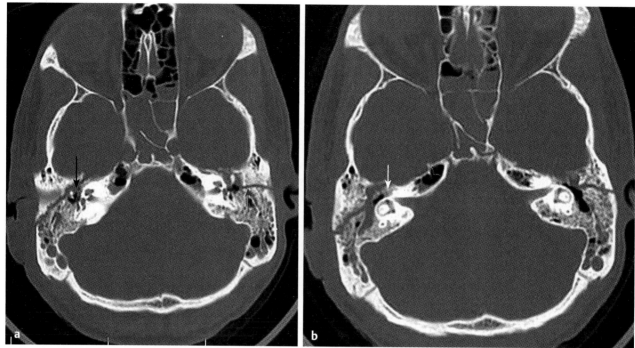

Fig. 14.8   High-resolution computed tomography (HRCT) of temporal bone. Axial section showing temporal bone fracture on both the sides. **(a)** On the right side, longitudinal fracture line (*black arrow*) is running in the direction of petrous apex but reaching up to the first genu in the middle ear. On the left side, fracture line is seen parallel to the axis of petrous bone reaching up to but keeping lateral to tympanic segment (TS) (*red arrow*). **(b)** HRCT of temporal bone. Axial section showing longitudinal temporal bone fracture lines on both the sides. On the right side, a bony fragment (*white arrow*) seems to be pressing on the first genu area, whereas the fracture line on left side is keeping lateral to the facial nerve.

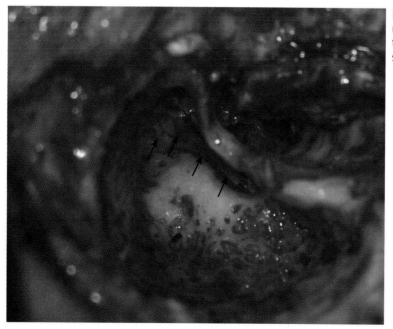

Fig. 14.9   Right side: Decompression of facial nerve from the labyrinthine segment (LS) till the second genu through transmastoid supralabyrinthine approach (*black arrows*).

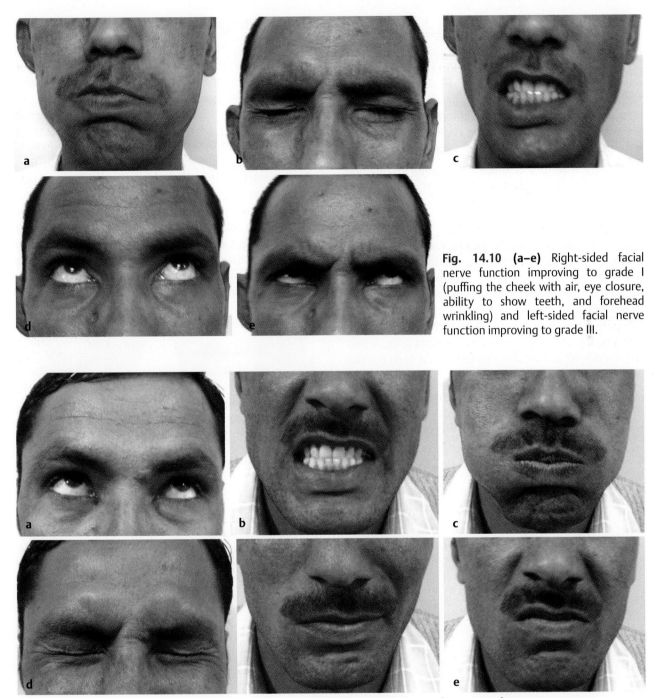

Fig. 14.10 (a–e) Right-sided facial nerve function improving to grade I (puffing the cheek with air, eye closure, ability to show teeth, and forehead wrinkling) and left-sided facial nerve function improving to grade III.

Fig. 14.11   (a–e) Face showing recovery of facial nerve of both sides up to grade I after 1 year of surgery.

Case 3

A 21-year-old patient presented with sudden, immediate, complete bilateral facial palsy post head injury (post road traffic accident). The patient had already got treatment from a neurosurgeon for his head injury. He had a stay of 15 days in intensive care unit (ICU) under neurosurgical care. The patient visited the otologist after 1.5 months of injury.

He gave a history of immediate, complete bilateral facial paralysis since day 1 post injury.

Facial nerve examination showed bilateral facial palsy grade VI (HBS) (**Fig. 14.12**).

HRCT temporal bone (**Fig. 14.13a, c**) on the right side showed a transverse fracture line running through the temporal bone, perpendicular to petrous apex, extending medial to the middle ear and ossicles and seemed to be transecting the nerve just distal to the LS (in the first genu area). On the left side (**Figs. 14.13b, d**), the fracture line is running parallel to the petrous apex, across the middle ear and reaching up to the first genu but not transecting the facial nerve.

The patient had already delayed the surgical treatment by 1.5 month, and had received only conservative treatment, so surgical intervention was planned.

Surgery Planned

As the CT scan showed evidence of transection of facial nerve on the right side, the right side was chosen for the first surgery. As the CT scan showed almost complete transection of facial nerve at the first genu, the surgical route taken in this case was "transzygomatic anterior attic approach" (explained in detail in Chapter 12 titled "Management of Post-traumatic Facial Nerve Palsy"). Facial nerve grafting was performed on the right side. The recovery of the right side was expected to take a minimum of 2 years; hence, the left side was also explored subsequently within days of the first surgery so that there could be early recovery at least on the left side. On the left side also, as the injury was reaching up to the first genu, transzygomatic anterior attic approach was taken, though only decompression was needed to relieve the nerve from compression by bony fragment.

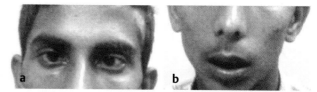

Fig. 14.12 (a, b) Bilateral facial palsy (grade VI). The mask-like face with complete loss of facial expressions on both sides can be noticed.

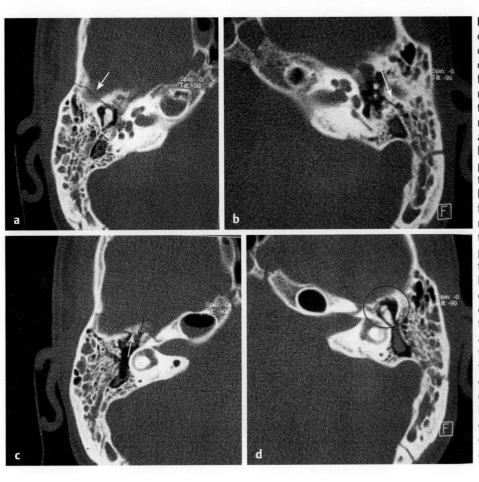

Fig. 14.13 **(a)** High-resolution computed tomography (HRCT) of temporal bone axial section of the right side showing fracture line (*white arrow*) running almost perpendicular to the petrous apex bone, reaching medial to the ossicles and reaching and seeming to be transecting the first genu part of facial nerve. **(b)** HRCT of temporal bone axial cut of the left side showing longitudinal fracture line (*white arrow*) running across the squamous temporal bone, parallel to the petrous apex, reaching up to the middle ear but keeping lateral to the ossicles. **(c)** HRCT of temporal bone axial section of the right side showing fracture line (*yellow arrow*) along with fragments of bone traumatizing the nerve at the first genu (*red arrow*). **(d)** HRCT of temporal bone axial section of the left side showing fracture line extending up to the first genu area. The fragmentation of bone around the first genu area is visualized (*red circle*).

Surgical Steps

Right Side (Figs. 14.14–14.16)

The facial nerve was exposed from the LS up to the second genu through transzygomatic anterior attic approach. The site of injury was identified. The nerve was found transected at the first genu and the TS distal to the site of injury was found completely fibrosed. After trimming the fibrosed TS, up to the second genu, the proximal stump of the facial nerve identified at the LS. The gap between the two cut ends of the facial nerve was more than 1 cm, so interposition free cable grafting (sural nerve) was performed. End-to-end anastomosis between the distal stump of the facial nerve (second genu) and the cable graft on one side and the proximal stump of the facial nerve (LS) and the other end of the cable graft on the other side was

performed. Fibrin glue was applied at the anastomotic sites followed by covering of both the sites with a piece of perichondrium.

Left Side (Fig. 14.17)

On the left side, through transzygomatic anterior attic approach, the facial nerve was exposed at the site of injury which was the first genu. The bony fragment compressing the nerve was removed followed by decompression of facial nerve beyond the site of injury on both sides till healthy facial nerve was reached. In this case facial nerve was decompressed from the LS proximally till the second genu on the distal side.

The patient was lost to follow-up and visited after around 2 years. After 2 years of surgery, the recovery of facial nerve could be achieved up to grade II on the right side and grade I on the left side (**Fig. 14.18**).

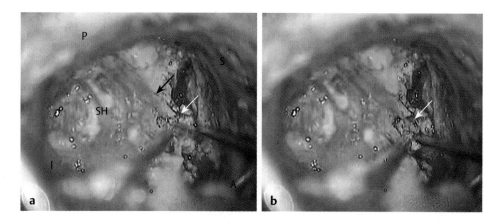

Fig. 14.14 **(a, b)** Right side, transzygomatic anterior attic approach. The surgeon is sitting in front of the patient. The positions have been marked: "S" is superior, "I" is inferior, "P" is posterior, and "A" is anterior. Transection of facial nerve visible at the first genu (*white arrow*). Tympanic segment (TS) is marked by *black arrow*. SH, stapes head.

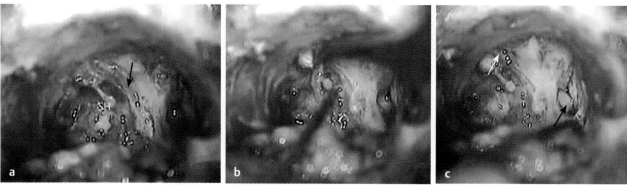

Fig. 14.15 **(a)** Fibrosed tympanic segment (TS) (*black arrow*) up to the second genu. **(b)** Cutting of TS in progress. **(c)** The proximal stump (LS) (*black arrow*) and distal stump of facial nerve (second genu) (*white arrow*) are exposed. SH, stapes head.

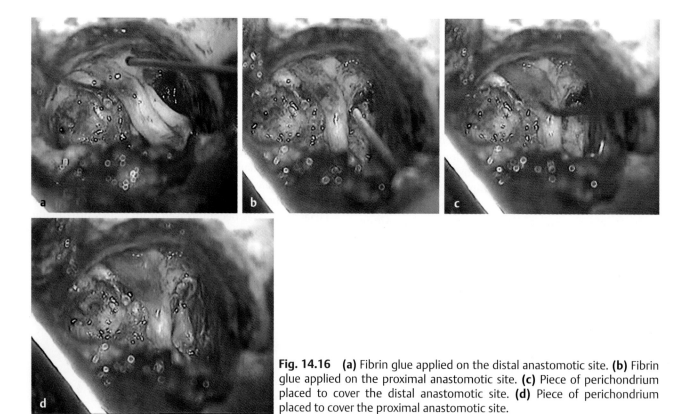

Fig. 14.16 **(a)** Fibrin glue applied on the distal anastomotic site. **(b)** Fibrin glue applied on the proximal anastomotic site. **(c)** Piece of perichondrium placed to cover the distal anastomotic site. **(d)** Piece of perichondrium placed to cover the proximal anastomotic site.

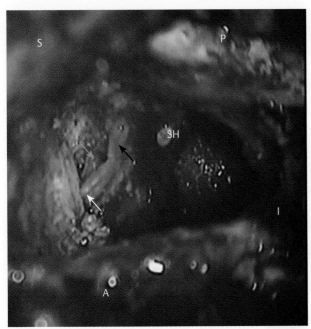

Fig. 14.17 Left side transzygomatic anterior attic approach. The surgeon is sitting in front of the patient. Positions marked: "S" is superior, "I" is inferior, "P" is posterior, and "A" is anterior. Facial nerve exposed and decompressed from the tympanic segment (TS) (*black arrow*) to the first genu (*white arrow*) and the labyrinthine segment (LS) (*blue arrow*). Stapes head (SH) is visible.

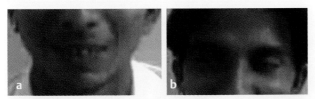

Fig. 14.18 (a, b) Recovery of facial nerve up to grade II on the right side and grade I on the left side.

Case 4

A case of roadside accident with head injury and bilateral facial paralysis presented to us 20 days post injury. On examination, bilateral facial palsy grade VI was noted (**Fig. 14.19**). There was no improvement in facial paralysis on both sides after conservative treatment started by the neurosurgeon.

HRCT of temporal bone (**Fig. 14.20**) showed on right side longitudinal fracture line involving mastoid cortex and posterior canal wall reaching up to facial canal in the tympanic segment. On left side the fracture line could be seen running along the mastoid cortex, middle ear and reaching up to petrous apex and seemed to be involving first genu of facial nerve.

The patient had already been put on conservative treatment in the form of prednisolone 1 mg/kg body weight.

As 20 days had already passed, and grade VI facial palsy had persisted on both sides, surgical intervention was planned.

Surgery Planned

Surgical decompression of facial nerve on the left side through transcanal inside-out approach was planned, as the injury seemed more grave on the left side according to the CT scan.

Surgical Steps (Fig. 14.21)

Transcanal inside-out atticotomy performed following the fracture line up to the middle ear, and decompression of facial nerve was performed at the site of injury which in this case is the first genu where a bony fragment was found to be pressing on the facial nerve. The nerve was decompressed till the LS on the proximal side and the TS on the distal side.

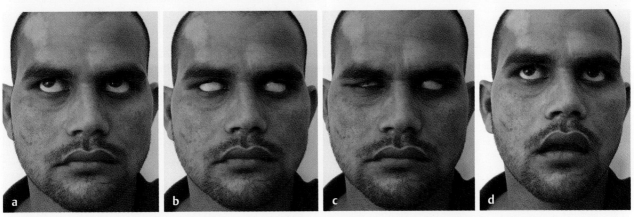

Fig. 14.19 (a–d) Grade VI (House-Brackmann's Scale [HBS]) facial palsy on both sides with Bell's phenomenon.

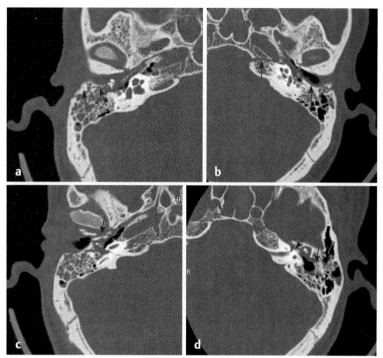

Fig. 14.20 (a, c) High-resolution computed tomography (HRCT) of temporal bone axial cuts of the right side showing longitudinal fracture line involving mastoid cortex and posterior canal wall reaching up to facial canal in the tympanic segment (*red arrow*). **(b, d)** Axial cuts of the left side showing fracture line running along the mastoid cortex, middle ear, and reaching up to petrous apex. The fracture line seems to be involving the first genu area.

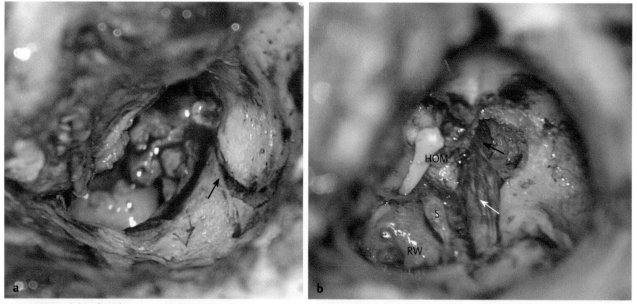

Fig. 14.21 (a) Left side: Fracture line involving posterior canal wall and reaching up to the middle ear anterior to the handle of the malleus (*black arrow*). **(b)** Decompression of facial nerve through transcanal inside-out approach, from the labyrinthine segment (LS) (*black arrow*) up to the tympanic segment (TS) (*white arrow*). HOM, handle of malleus; RW, round window; S, stapes.

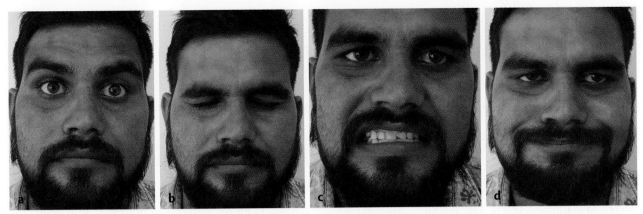

Fig. 14.22 (a–d) Recovery of facial nerve up to grade I on both sides 18 months post surgery.

In 3 months, the recovery on the left side could be achieved up to grade I whereas the recovery on the right side took more than 1 year to reach up to grade I (**Fig. 14.22**).

Conclusion

Bilateral facial palsy is a condition with severe implications especially when seen in children. Due to its functional and aesthetic outcomes, it is a major concern for the patients. Various etiologies have been proposed for the bilateral palsy. A thorough evaluation leading to appropriate differential diagnosis and an early treatment is important as the situation is quite debilitating for the patient. All situations including infective, autoimmune as well as idiopathic pathology being self-limiting, spontaneously remitting, and non-life-threatening, conservative treatment is always given before opting for any surgical intervention, which usually is not required in these cases. Any facial palsy of grade less than VI is always treated conservatively. In post-traumatic, bilateral grade VI facial palsy, at least one side needs immediate surgical intervention so as to hasten the recovery on that side and the other side can be waited upon. If the other side is not improving even after 4 months of injury, the second side also needs surgical intervention. The side with more severe injury shall be taken up first, giving due time to the other side nerve to recover on its own. In case on one side there is transection of facial nerve needing direct repair or repair with interposition graft, the second side should be taken up within few days of first surgery because a repaired nerve will take a minimum 1 year to up to 5 years to show optimal recovery. The recovery on the second side thus hastens the recovery. Situations like bilateral, post-traumatic/iatrogenic facial palsy, neurofibromatosis type 2 lesion leading to bilateral facial palsy, and idiopathic facial paralysis not improving in 4 months require surgical intervention. The situation is more sinister than the unilateral involvement of facial nerve and needs urgent addressal.

15 Facial Nerve Schwannoma

Introduction

This chapter discusses evaluation and diagnosis of facial nerve schwannoma (FNS), the principle involved in managing such tumors, and reanimation of face after resection of FNS.

Skull base tumors in close association with facial nerve are more common than tumors of facial nerve itself. Out of all the facial nerve tumors, schwannoma of facial nerve is the commonest followed by hemangioma, meningioma, and neurofibroma in the benign tumor category. Most of the malignant tumors involving facial nerve are extracranial and usually located and related to parotid gland.

FNSs are rare benign encapsulated tumors that can arise anywhere along the course of the facial nerve, from its origin in the cerebellopontine angle (CPA) to its extracranial division in the parotid gland. The tumor is neuroectodermal in origin, arising from the Schwann cells in myelin sheath which surrounds the axons of facial nerve. FNS has been given different names like facial nerve neuroma, neurinoma, and neurilemmoma. They are typically solitary, unilateral, and sporadic in nature. FNSs may be bilateral as part of neurofibromatosis-2 spectrum.

Histopathology

Macroscopically, schwannomas are pink colored, encapsulated, and have smooth round surface. Cut surface shows yellow colored tissue with occasional areas of hemorrhage. The classic histology shows both Antoni type A and B pictures. The tissue is indistinguishable from vestibular schwannoma, which makes the main differential diagnosis for FNS arising from internal auditory meatus (IAM). Imaging correlation and/or intraoperative confirmation is the best way to differentiate the two tumors.

Microscopically, along with Antoni type 1 and 2 cells, areas of necrosis due to microvascular infarcts, calcification, and chronic inflammatory cell infiltrate may be found. This inflammatory process leads to speedy growth of FNS.

Origin and Growth Pattern

FNS can arise from any segment of facial nerve starting from CPA till its terminal branching in parotid. The commonest site is intratemporal portion out of which geniculate ganglion (GG) is most commonly involved, followed by labyrinthine segment (LS), tympanic segment (TS), mastoid segment (MS), and greater superficial petrosal nerve (GSPN), in that order. Next segment to be involved is meatal segment. CPA and intraparotid neuromas are the rarest of all. At times the tumor may be involving only the branches of facial nerve, namely, the GSPN, chorda tympani, and stapedial nerve. The tumor may not restrict to a single segment but may involve multiple segments like TS, MS, and LS including GG (**Fig. 15.1a**), or it may extend from one segment to other like GG tumor may extend to LS on proximal side and TS on distal side or from MS to TS, GG, etc (**Fig. 15.1b**). Extension of tumor can be from facial nerve to adjacent sites in the form of tumors involving LS usually extending to middle cranial fossa (MCF), tumor from IAM extending to LS and GG taking the shape of a dumbbell (**Fig. 15.1c**), tumor from GG extending to the middle ear, and MCF tumor from CPA can manifest as a lesion of posterior cranial fossa imbibing vestibular schwannoma. The intracranial extension of tumor from the IAM to posterior cranial fossa is another example of extension of tumor. When FNSs track along the GSPN, they may present as a rounded extra-axial mass projecting into the MCF (**Fig. 15.1d**). FNS involving TS preferentially pedunculates into the middle ear cavity (**Fig. 15.1e**), clinically presenting as a middle ear mass behind intact tympanic membrane. When the MS is involved, the tumor margins become irregular and invasive and do not look like classical smooth, lobulated mass on imaging due to tumor invasion in the surrounding mastoid air cells.

The growth pattern of the tumor is as follows:

- The tumor while growing in an eccentric pattern displays and splays the nerve fibers leading to progressive facial paresis/palsy.
- In early stage, the tumor can be separated and resected from the nerve due to well-preserved planes.

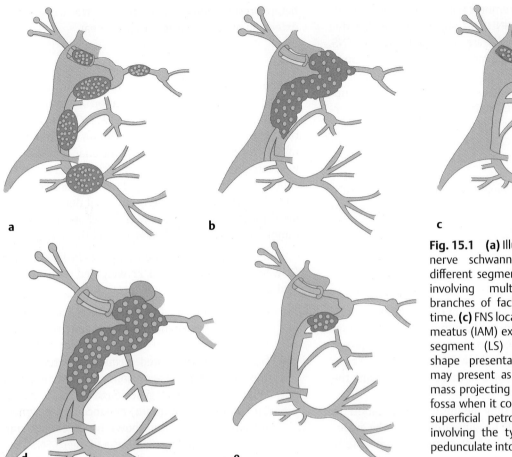

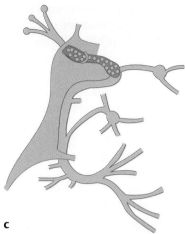

Fig. 15.1 **(a)** Illustration showing facial nerve schwannoma (FNS) involving different segments separately. **(b)** FNS involving multiple segments and branches of facial nerve at the same time. **(c)** FNS located in internal auditory meatus (IAM) extending to labyrinthine segment (LS) leading to dumbbell shape presentation. **(d)** The tumor may present as a rounded extra-axial mass projecting into the middle cranial fossa when it courses along the greater superficial petrosal nerve. **(e)** Tumor involving the tympanic segment (TS) pedunculate into the middle ear (ME).

- In late stages, separation of the tumor from the nerve is not possible due to excessive splaying, ischemia, and pressure necrosis of nerve fiber leading to permanent functional loss of nerve fibers.

Clinical Presentation

- The commonest presentation of FNS is in the form of facial nerve neuropathy which presents either as progressively increasing facial nerve weakness over a span of weeks/months, or the weakness/palsy can be fluctuating and the patient may give a history of recurrent episodes of facial paresis in different stages (House-Brackmann's Scale [HBS]). Or the patient may complaint of a history of transient facial paresis along with other symptoms like facial twitching. The other variety can be development of persistent static facial nerve paresis. There may be associated dysgeusia or dry eye depending upon the presence of tumor proximal to chorda tympani or GSPN respectively. Many a times the facial nerve palsy or paresis may be a late symptom as FNS is a very slow growing tumor and abundant vascularity of the tumor leads to neuronal tolerance of the nerve fibers and in spite of nerve fibers getting stretched, the nerve impulse transmission continues. There can be presence of associated dehiscence of facial canal which also can be the reason for delayed facial paresis or palsy.

- Other presentation could be hemifacial spasm in the form of facial twitching or spasms. It suggests an ongoing degenerative process of facial nerve.

- Hearing loss, which may already be present at the time of patient's first visit, usually presents quite late. It can be either conductive, sensorineural (more common), or mixed depending upon location and spread of the FNS. Profound sensorineural hearing loss (SNHL) happens if the FNS involves IAM or leads to fistula in the basal turn of cochlea due to excessive expansion of the LS involved in FNS. Retrocochlear hearing loss indicates tumor involving intracranial part of the facial nerve. The hearing loss here is different from vestibular schwannoma in a way that the facial palsy/paresis precedes the hearing loss in the FNS. At times even when the tumor is not involving the internal ear (IE) or IAM, SNHL may be found, which is due to intracochlear disease in response to the FNS. Conductive hearing loss occurs in case the tumor involving the LS, GG, or TS starts disrupting the ossicular chain by expansion. Vestibular symptoms may present in the form of dizziness or vertigo, although vestibular involvement is very rare. It is seen specifically in cases of FNS extending or lying completely in the IAM and compressing on the vestibular nerve.

- Middle ear (ME)/external auditory canal (EAC)/parotid mass may be the sole presentation at times.

Investigations

- Full audiological assessment of the patient is to be performed and it includes pure-tone audiogram and speech discrimination score. As explained above, these tests help in differentiating the type of hearing loss, which further helps in making the diagnosis.
- Imaging is the only definitive investigation to diagnose FNS. The imaging protocol for the evaluation of FNS includes both computed tomography (CT) scan and magnetic resonance imaging (MRI) modalities, which are complementary tests and are performed together to know the size, site, and extent of the tumor.

CT Scan

High-resolution CT (HRCT) scan of temporal bone is for diagnosing intratemporal schwannoma and contrast-enhanced CT (CECT) scan of the temporal bone is for extracranial and CPA tumors. In HRCT of temporal bone, the intratemporal FNS is seen as benign-appearing bony scalloping, remodeling, and widening of the facial canal and the surrounding bony boundaries. FNSs do not show true "erosion" of the bony boundaries, but they do demonstrate a more benign osseous expansion of the surrounding bone. The FNS is seen as homogeneous enhancement but it shows heterogeneous enhancement when the size of the tumor becomes large, whereas the FNS involving extracranial or cisternal segment is characteristically seen as homogeneously or heterogeneously enhancing soft tissue attenuation that is isoattenuated to gray matter on CECT and may contain cystic foci.

CT scan clearly displays the site of the tumor and can also pick up tumor in early stage due to extension of the tumor from the LS, GG, or TS into the middle ear even before presentation of facial palsy. It can also display the extension of the tumor into the inner ear.

MRI

Although MRI is complementary to CT scan in diagnosing the FNS, it is more useful for evaluation of extratemporal extensions of the tumor, namely, CPA, MCF, and intraparotid extensions. The classic description of intratemporal FNS on enhanced T1 magnetic resonance is that of a well-circumscribed fusiform enhancing mass along the course of the intratemporal facial nerve. CT scan displays only the dilated part of the facial canal due to involvement by the FNS, whereas MRI can show that part of tumor which has not caused erosion of the bony canal.

MRI sequences used for detecting FNS include T1- and T2-weighted sequences and T1-weighted with contrast (gadolinium) sequences:

- On axial T1-weighted sequences, the tumor appears either isointense or hypointense relative to gray matter.
- On axial T2-weighted sequences, the tumor appears hyperintense or isointense. It may appear heterogeneous for large lesions.
- On contrast (gadolinium) enhanced T1-weighted sequences, the tumor shows homogeneous uniform enhancement whereas larger FNS can undergo a cystic degeneration seen as focal intramural low signal intensity on contrast-enhanced T1 images.

Few Unusual Distinct Imaging Appearances/Situations

- An FNS arising from CPA or IAM cannot be distinguished from vestibular schwannoma (VS) as the symptoms for both remain the same. The only difference is that in FNS, facial palsy precedes the vertigo or hearing loss whereas it is reverse in vestibular schwannoma. Radiologically differentiation can be made in case FNS involving meatal segment extends to and involves the LS demonstrating a dumbbell appearance which is not seen in VS. Another differentiating factor is multisegmental involvement of the FNS in comparison to the VS, which remains restricted to the IAM or extends proximally to the CPA.
- FNSs arising from the GG usually present as the classic tubular description of the lesion, but can also be seen as round mass leading to widening of the fossa itself.
- When an FNS extends along the GSPN, it can present additionally as a rounded extra-axial mass extending into the MCF (**Fig. 15.2a** and **b**).

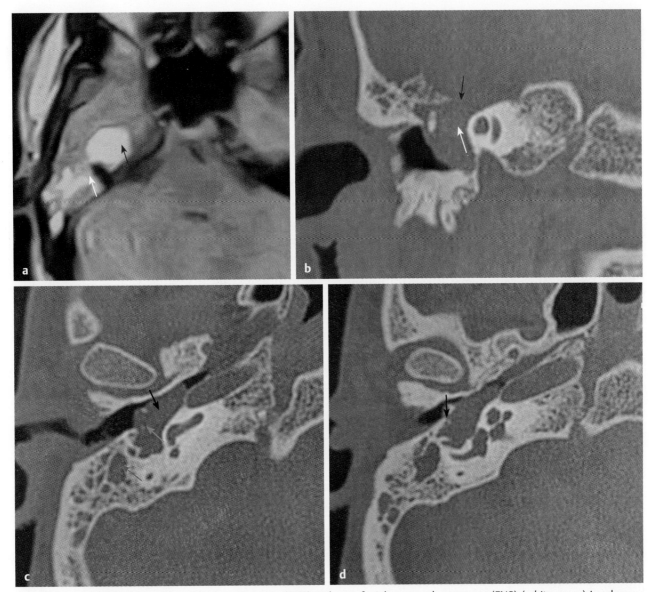

Fig. 15.2 **(a, b)** Axial magnetic resonance imaging (MRI). When a facial nerve schwannoma (FNS) (*white arrow*) involves or extends to the greater superficial petrosal nerve (GSPN), it can present additionally as a rounded extra-axial mass (*red arrow*) extending into the middle cranial fossa. **(c, d)** High-resolution computed tomography (HRCT) of the temporal bone, axial cuts. A tympanic segment FNS which pedunculates into the middle ear cavity loses its tubular configuration and presents as rounded mass filling the middle ear behind the intact tympanic membrane (*black arrow*)). Multisegmental involvement of the FNS (mastoid segment [MS] [*orange arrow*], tympanic segment [TS] [*green arrow*], and geniculate ganglion [GG] [*orange arrow*]).

- A TS FNS which pedunculates into the middle ear cavity loses its tubular configuration and presents as rounded mass filling the middle ear behind the intact tympanic membrane (**Fig. 15.2c** and **d**).
- The MS of the facial nerve is surrounded by fragile, thin-walled septations separating it from the mastoid air cells. An MS FNS could invade the adjacent mastoid air cells, thereby appearing as an irregular and aggressive tumor, especially on MRI. CT explains these margins by showing the FNS breaking into surrounding mastoid air cells.

◼ Differential Diagnosis

- **In IAM:**
  - ➢ Vestibular schwannoma (VS): FNSs involving the CPA–IAM facial nerve segments can be indistinguishable from VSs if no extension into the LS of the facial nerve is present. Extensive CPA–IAM FNS can present with an unusual but distinctive imaging appearance, a "dumbbell" shape due to extension from the IA fundus

through the LS and into the geniculate fossa. This presentation along with T1 magnetic resonance enhancement and sharply scalloped, or fusiform, enlargement of the facial nerve canal is diagnostic of an FNS. Another differentiating factor is multisegmental involvement of FNS in comparison to VS which remains restricted to the IAM or extends to the CPA.

- **Intratemporal segment:**
  ➤ Facial nerve hemangioma: The type of bony destruction or erosion can differentiate the FNS from facial nerve hemangioma which causes a honey comb pattern of bony destruction with irregular bony margins, whereas the FNS causes a smooth expansion leading to smooth remodeling of bony surroundings.
  ➤ Congenital cholesteatoma: It spreads beyond the facial nerve course. It does not enhance on postcontrast, T1-weighted MRI.
  ➤ Glomus tympanicum/mastoidalis: It shows salt pepper appearance on MRI.
  ➤ Bell's palsy: The early stage FNSs with only minor facial nerve symptoms can be frequently misdiagnosed at the clinical level as an idiopathic Bell's palsy. However, CT does not show enlargement of the intratemporal facial nerve canal in Bell's palsy as it shows in FNS. Also, T1-enhanced MRI commonly shows intratemporal facial nerve enhancement of all or part of the facial nerve along with a "tuft" of enhancement in the fundus of the IAM in patients with Bell's palsy.

- **Extratemporal:**
  ➤ Pleomorphic adenoma: There is no extension of tumor (pleomorphic adenoma) up to the stylomastoid foramen (SMF) and further proximal.
  ➤ Parotid malignancy with perineural spread can be seen extending in cephalad direction from an intraparotid invasive mass from distal to proximal along an enlarged facial nerve canal.

Management

Management of FNS is always surgical, although the decision is many a times controversial. Planning and deciding for surgery is a critical and elaborate process as complete resection of the tumor needs to be balanced with the poor outcome of surgery regarding the facial nerve function because grade III is the best that can be achieved through repair after complete removal of the tumor. The decision is especially difficult when the patient's facial nerve functioning is still better or up to grade III. Several factors which are important for

decision-making are: patient's consent, age and general condition, tumor size and location, preoperative facial function, and duration of symptoms prior to presentation. Large-sized tumor or tumor located in the CPA requires immediate addressal as it may prove life threatening due to its complications. At the same time a small-sized tumor in an old patient with facial function better or up to grade III needs to be put on "wait and watch" regime or even gamma knife may become the treatment of choice. On the basis of these observations, the principles of management can be drafted as follows:

- Complete enucleation of the tumor with preservation of the facial nerve in case the tumor is limited to the epineurial sheath and has yet not splayed or stretched the facial nerve fibers. It usually happens when the diagnosis is made at an early stage. In such a situation, surgical intervention gives best results as the tumor can be easily peeled off without compromising on the integrity of the nerve fibers.
- In case the nerve has got affected, complete excision of the tumor along with the affected part of the facial nerve followed by facial nerve grafting or facial reanimation becomes the treatment of choice. The choice between "complete resection with facial nerve repair" versus "wait and watch" can be made as follows:
  ➤ Surgical resection to be performed without delay for:
    1. Progressive facial palsy of grade III or more.
    2. Large CPA tumors compressing brainstem or causing hydrocephalus.
    3. Tumors invading the internal ear leading to sensorineural hearing loss or vertigo.
  ➤ Wait and watch with or without facial nerve decompression is worthwhile in patients who present very early, with facial nerve grade better than grade III. When considering observation as a management choice, the tumor growth/facial weakness is to be kept under observation. If the grade of facial palsy deteriorates in the waiting period or it gets past 1 year after facial palsy started, surgical intervention is immediately undertaken. The average growth of FNS is reported to be around 2 mm per year and large-sized tumor grows more than small-sized tumor (<1 cm). Although the facial nerve functioning can be retained for the maximum time through wait and watch policy, long duration of observation may at times increase the risk of loss of cell bodies in the facial motor nucleus and motor end plates of the facial musculature.
  ➤ The difficulty arises in patients with facial nerve functioning better than grade III facial nerve

palsy, but duration of symptoms has already exceeded 1 year. In such situations, the decision for surgery is taken after counseling the patient in detail about the deterioration of facial nerve functioning expected after tumor resection.

➢ At times the decision may need to be taken intraoperatively when we open up a case anticipating clear removal or excision of the tumor without disturbing the integrity of the nerve fibers and find just the opposite. Whenever the tumor removal needs interruption of the nerve fibers, the surgery needs to be stopped and only continued in the same or second stage after discussing the outcomes with the patient and the attendants.

◼ Surgical Strategy and Approaches for Resection of FNS

The surgical management of facial schwannoma depends not only on the size and anatomical location of the tumor, but also on the patient's hearing status. A tumor proximal to the GG with serviceable hearing should be approached through the MCF provided the tumor does not extend far into the CPA. If the tumor is proximal to the mid IAM with ≤1 cm of a CPA component, an extended MCF approach is best, whereas a retrosigmoid approach gives the best chance of hearing conservation in lesions with a CPA component >1 cm. With nonserviceable hearing, a translabyrinthine approach is the most direct route to the tumor and is the procedure of choice. Involvement of the TS can be reached by a transmastoid approach with facial recess opening. MS tumor alone can be excised through transmastoid approach, whereas additional transparotid approach is the surgical choice for tumor involving both intratemporal and extratemporal segments. These exposures may be used in combination for tumors involving multiple nerve segments.

Depending upon the three important factors, namely, size, location of the FNS, and the hearing status of the patient, the surgical approaches can be classified into:

- In cases of preserved preoperative hearing, the different approaches are:
  ➢ Canal wall up/down mastoidectomy: It is performed in tumors arising from the GG, TS and extending up to the MS with/without conductive hearing loss.
  ➢ Transmastoid + MCF approach: This approach is preferred in FNS involving the IAM/CPA segment with extension up to intratemporal segment with preserved serviceable hearing.

➢ MCF approach: This approach is only performed in tumors limited to the IAM.
➢ Extended MCF approach: This is for FNS involving meatal segment with < or upto 1 cm of CPA component
➢ Retrosigmoid approach: for IAM FNS with >1cm of CPA component.
➢ Transmastoid + transparotid approach: This is performed in tumor based in the parotid gland and extending up to or proximal to the SMF.
➢ Transparotid approach: It is performed in tumors limited to the parotid segment or neck.

- In cases of preoperative profound sensorineural hearing loss, the different approaches can be:
  ➢ Transmastoid + translabyrinthine approach: It is for tumors arising from the IAM/CPA and reaching up to the intratemporal *segment with profound SNHL.*
  ➢ A modified transcochlear approach is added to the translabyrinthine approach: This is performed in case the tumor is extending into the cochlea.

◼ Surgical Techniques for Repair of Facial Nerve and Facial Reanimation

Once the tumor is resected, the next important step is the repair of the facial nerve in case both proximal and distal stumps are available and facial reanimation surgery in case any of the stump is not available.

Primary nerve repair is the treatment of choice once the tumor is excised and it should always be performed in the same stage as the primary surgery. As there is always a gap after the resection of the FNS along with the affected part of the nerve, repair is performed through free cable graft, which is harvested either from the great auricular nerve (GAN) in case the gap is small and a short graft is required or sural nerve (SN). where a longer graft is required (between intracranial to intratemporal or extratemporal segment), (already explained in detail in Chapter 7 titled Management of Flaccid Facial palsy of Short and Intermediate Duration with Proximal Stump Available).

In case the proximal stump of the facial nerve is not available after the resection of the FNS (situation where the FNS involves the cisternal segment), the facial nerve repair is performed through faciomasseteric or faciohypoglossal anastomosis (already explained in detail in Chapter 8 under the heading "Motor Nerve Transfers").

In case the facial nerve palsy associated with the FNS is of more than 2 years duration and electromyography (EMG) shows facial muscles atrophy, the primary repair of the facial nerve may not serve the purpose. In such cases, nerve repair can be performed but it should always be accompanied by certain dynamic and static facial reanimation procedures. The dynamic repair can be in the form of free micro neurovascular muscle transfer (FMMT) or temporalis muscle transfer depending upon the situation. The static procedures performed are upper eyelid implant, lower eyelid surgery, and facial slings (already explained in detail in Chapter 9).

Dynamic reconstruction and static procedures for facial reanimation can be performed separately or as combination of multiple procedures or used along with primary nerve repair.

Case 1

A 28-year-old patient presented with slowly progressing facial paralysis and hearing loss on the right side for 1 year. The patient also complained of heaviness and feeling of mass in the right ear for 7 months.

Otoscopy of the right side revealed intact but bulging tympanic membrane. A reddish mass could be seen behind the intact tympanic membrane. Neurological examination revealed complete grade VI facial palsy (HBS) on the right side (**Fig. 15.3**). Pure-tone audiometry

indicated moderate conductive hearing loss in the right ear with air–bone conduction gap of up to 40 dB. CT showed a lobulated, soft-tissue mass within the right temporal bone corresponding to the location of the GG, LS, TS, and MS of the facial nerve up to the SMF, with bifid facial nerve in inferior portion of the MS. The epitympanum and antrum were found filled with the same soft-tissue mass (**Fig. 15.4**). The mastoid cavity was found free of soft tissue. T2-weighted MRI revealed a mass lesion with high-signal intensity in the same location. The mass had extended to the MCF as extension from the GG/GSPN mass by eroding the tegmen tympani and tegmen antri (**Figs. 15.1d** and **15.5**).

Surgery planned: As the patient's preoperative hearing was preserved, complete excision of the FNS to be performed through transmastoid canal wall down mastoidectomy and facial nerve repair to be performed through faciomasseteric anastomosis in the same stage. As it takes around more than 1 year for to attain optimal facial nerve recovery, both upper eyelid implant and facial sling surgery to be performed in the same or second stage. After 1.5 years, the gold implant could be removed, once the normal voluntary eye closure was achieved.

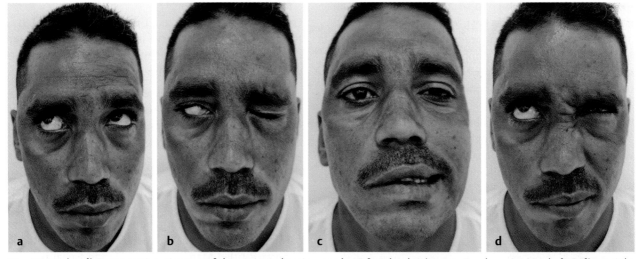

Fig. 15.3 **(a–d)** Preoperative pictures of the patient showing grade VI facial palsy (House-Brackmann's Scale [HBS]) on right side.

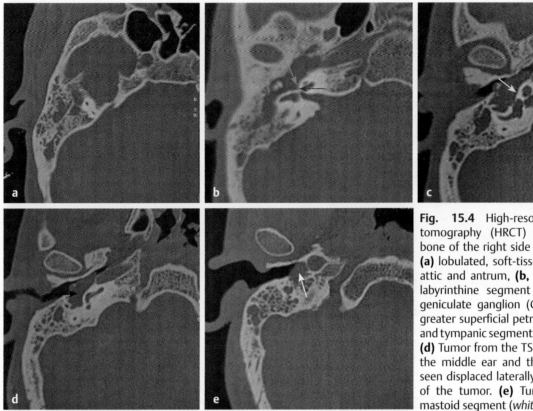

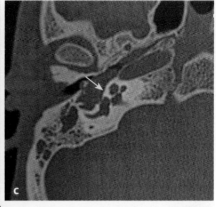

Fig. 15.4 High-resolution computed tomography (HRCT) of the temporal bone of the right side axial cuts showing **(a)** lobulated, soft-tissue mass filling the attic and antrum, **(b, c)** involving up to labyrinthine segment (LS) (*red arrow*), geniculate ganglion (GG) (*green arrow*), greater superficial petrosal nerve (GSPN), and tympanic segment (TS) (*yellow arrow*). **(d)** Tumor from the TS can be seen filling the middle ear and the ossicles can be seen displaced laterally due to expansion of the tumor. **(e)** Tumor involving the mastoid segment (*white arrow*) as well.

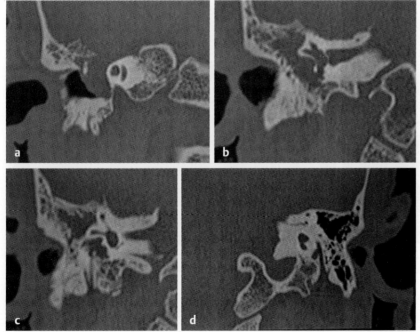

Fig. 15.5 **(a)** High-resolution computed tomography (HRCT) of the temporal bone of the right side coronal cuts showing soft-tissue mass involving the geniculate ganglion and extending into the middle cranial fossa by eroding through the tegmen bone. **(b)** Normal facial nerve in the meatal segment. **(c)** Bifid facial nerve in its mastoid segment on the right side. **(d)** In comparision to the bifid mastoid segment on left side, the opposite normal side is being shown. HRCT of the temporal bone coronal cuts showing normal mastoid segment on the left side in the same patient. *(Continued)*

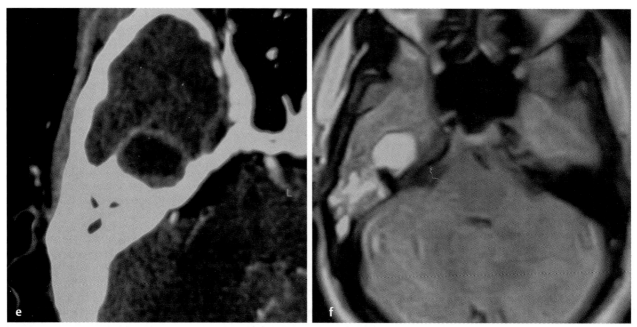

Fig. 15.5   *(Continued)* **(e)** HRCT temporal bone right side axial cuts showing Extension of the mass through the tegmen bone into the middle cranial fossa *(red arrow)* seen on **(e)** HRCT of the temporal and **(f)** MRI, axial cut showing the same extension of mass into the middle crainal fossa on right side .

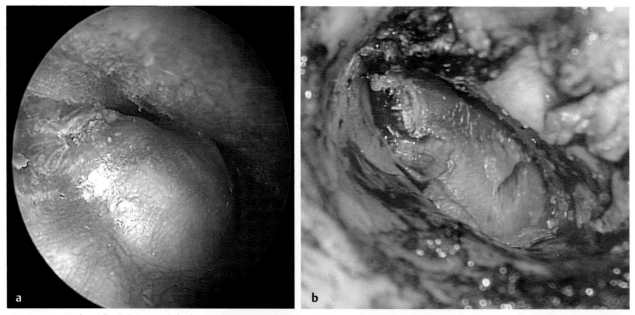

Fig. 15.6   Right side: **(a)** Smooth bulge in intact tympanic membrane due to facial nerve schwannoma (FNS) filling the middle ear. **(b)** Skin of external auditory canal lifted and canaloplasty already performed.

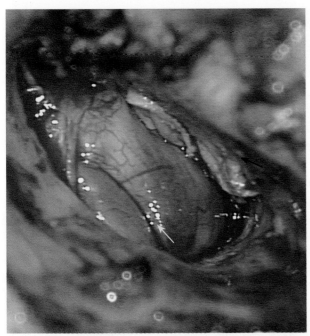

Fig. 15.7 After lifting the tympanic membrane (*black arrow*), the lobulated tumor mass (*yellow arrow*) is visible.

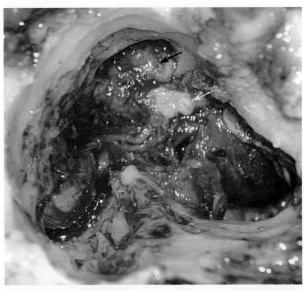

Fig. 15.8 Canal wall down mastoidectomy in progress. The facial nerve schwannoma (FNS) can be seen filling the antrum and epitympanum, and extending beyond the tegmen tympani into the middle cranial fossa (MCF) (*black arrow*). Head of malleus can be visualized (*yellow arrow*).

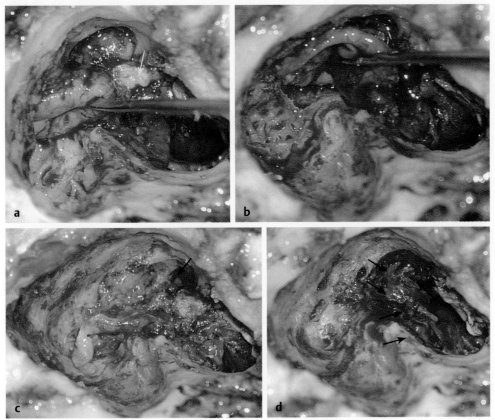

Fig. 15.9 (a, b) The tumor being lifted from the antrum and attic and followed anteriorly. **(c)** Laterally displaced, partially eroded incus has been removed. Head of malleus is visible (*yellow arrow*). Anterior extent of the tumor involving the greater superficial petrosal nerve (GSPN) is visualized (*black arrow*). **(d)** Tumor involving the geniculate ganglion (GG), labyrinthine segment (LS), and tympanic segment (TS) is exposed (*black arrows*).

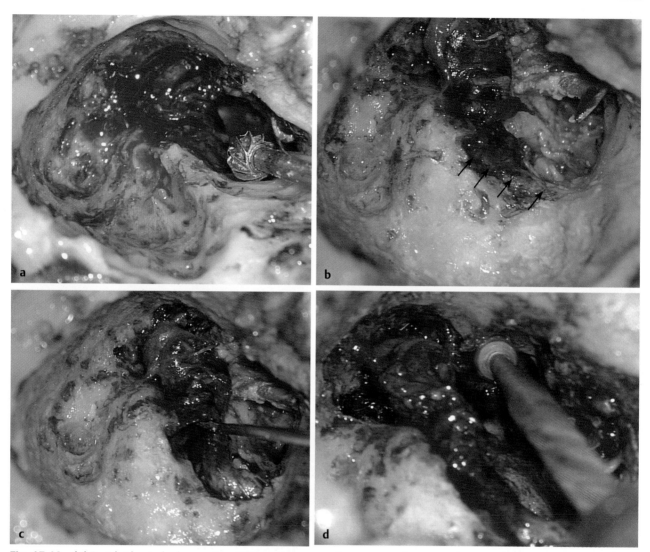

Fig. 15.10 **(a)** Facial ridge to be lowered and thinned to expose the tumor in the mastoid segment. **(b)** Lowering of the facial ridge is achieved and the tumor involving the mastoid segment (MS) is exposed (*black arrows*). **(c)** Extent of the facial nerve schwannoma (FNS) is being assessed. **(d)** Drilling of the anterior buttress to expose the tumor involving the greater superficial petrosal nerve (GSPN) and geniculate ganglion (GG) in progress.

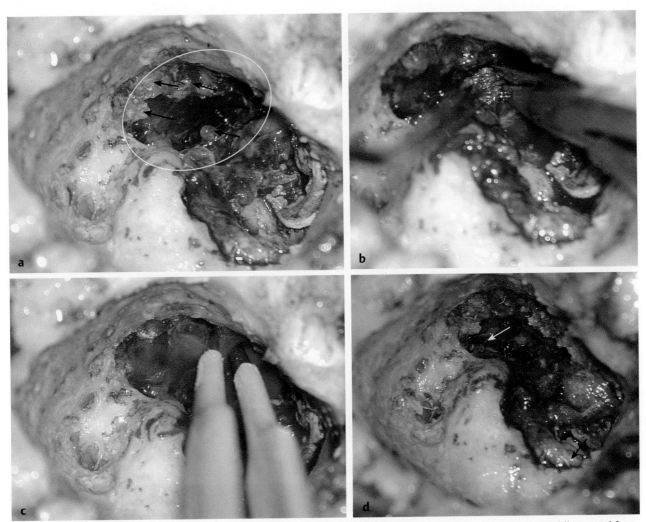

Fig. 15.11 **(a)** The defect in the tegmen bone is visible (*yellow circle*) along with residual tumor lying in middle cranial fossa beneath intact dura (*black arrow*). **(b)** The residual tumor is being excised. **(c)** Final clearance of the residual tumor with bipolar cautery in progress. **(d)** The exposure of the complete tumor from the labyrinthine segment (LS) (*yellow arrow*) to mastoid segment (MS) (*black arrow*).

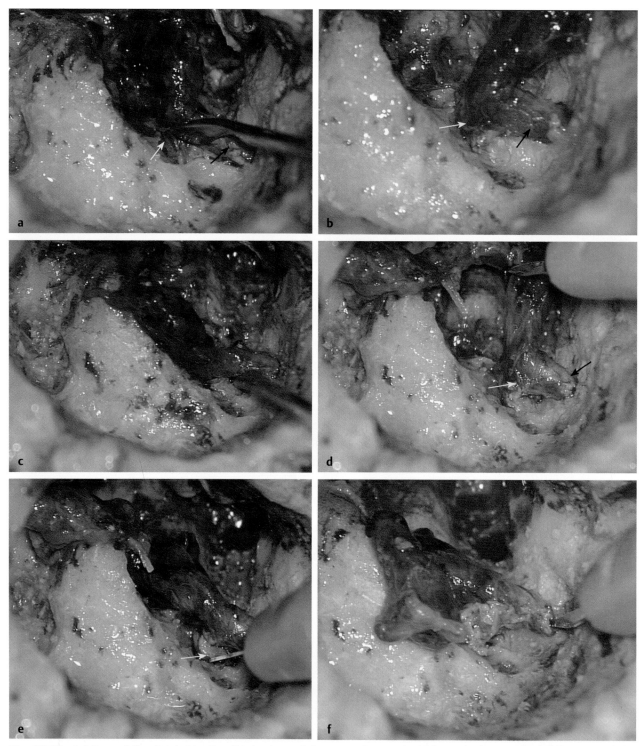

Fig. 15.12 **(a)** Toward the distal side, the distal extent of the tumor is traced which reached up to the bifid portion of the mastoid segment (MS) (*yellow and black arrows*), which is pointed out with a tympanic membrane elevator. **(b)** Tumor involving both the segments of mastoid portion of the facial nerve (primary segment shown with *black arrow*, secondary segment shown with *yellow arrow*). **(c)** The primary segment of the mastoid portion is lifted with a ball probe. **(d)** Both the segments are exposed distally beyond the extent of the tumor (secondary segment shown with *yellow arrow* and primary segment shown with *black arrow*). **(e)** The secondary segment of the mastoid portion facial nerve is being excised. **(f)** The primary segment of the mastoid portion is being excised.

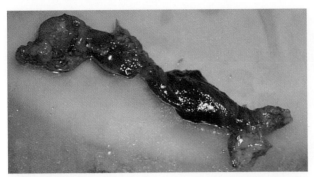

Fig. 15.13 Picture showing excised tumor with healthy cut ends of bifid facial nerve.

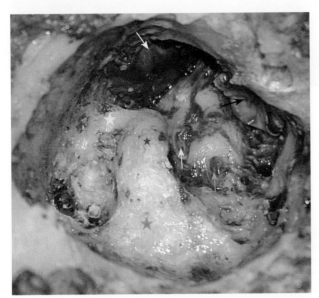

Fig. 15.14 Complete excision of the tumor has been achieved and the involved segments of the facial nerve have been resected. Exposed dura in the middle cranial fossa (MCF) (*white arrow*) through defect in the tegmen antri and tympani, oval window with footplate (*yellow arrow*), round window (*blue arrow*), dome of lateral semicircular canal (*blue asterisk*), dome of posterior semicircular canal (*green asterisk*), and ampulla of superior semicircular canal (*yellow asterisk*) are visualized. Lifted tympanic membrane is also visible (*black arrow*).

Surgical Steps (Figs. 15.6–15.19)

Transmastoid canal wall down mastoidectomy was performed. Complete excision of the tumor along with the affected segments of facial nerve, the mass extending into the middle cranial fossa and few millimeters of normal cuff of facial nerve on both proximal and distal side was performed (**Figs. 15.6-15.15**). The facial nerve was found bifid in its mastoid segment which co-related with the pre operative CT findings. As preoperative

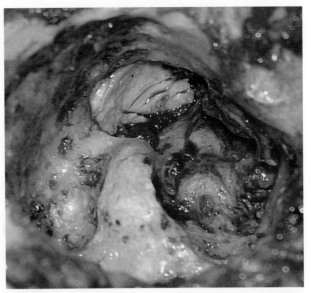

Fig. 15.15 Repair of the tegmen defect: Temporalis fascia as the first layer of repair with tragal cartilage graft as the second layer tucked inside the defect in all directions.

hearing was preserved in this patient, the proximal stump of the facial nerve was not traced further after excision of the LS.

The defect in the tegmen antri, which was around 2 × 1.5 cm in dimension, was repaired in two layers (**Fig. 15.16**). Temporalis fascia was used as the first layer and a big piece of cartilage harvested from the tragal cartilage used as the second layer of repair. Ossiculoplasty was performed by placing boomerang-shaped cartilage strip between footplate and bony annulus (**Fig. 15.16**). Mastoid cavity obliteration was performed with cartilage pieces, bone pete, and pedicled musculoperiosteal flaps created out of the temporalis muscle to obliterate the superior part of the cavity and sternocleidomastoid muscle to obliterate inferior part of the cavity (**Figs. 15.17** and **15.18**). A big-sized temporalis fascia graft was placed to cover the middle ear and mastoid cavity and a wide enough meatoplasty was performed (**Fig. 15.19**). The facial nerve repair was performed through faciomasseteric anastomosis along with upper eyelid gold implant and facial sling in the same stage (the details of nerve repair and secondary procedures have been explained in Chapter 9). Postoperative histopathological examination confirmed the diagnosis of FNS.

The patient's facial palsy recovery could be achieved up to grade II after 2 years (**Figs. 15.20** and **15.21**). Magnetic resonance images found free of disease in the second postoperative year.

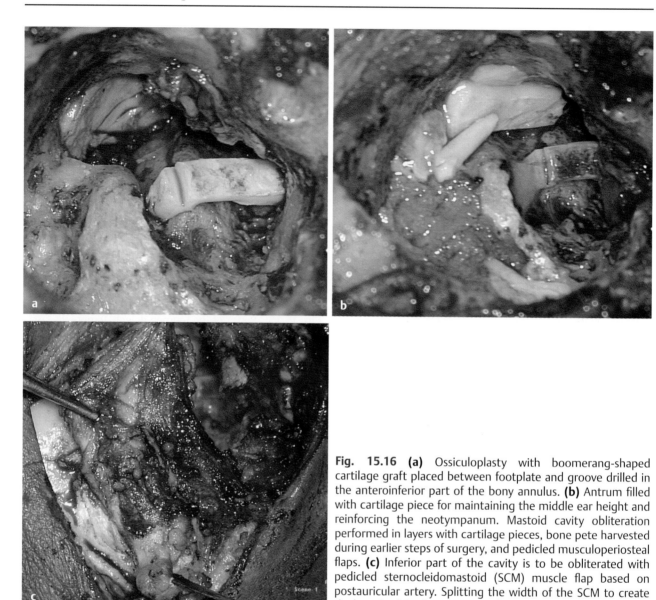

Fig. 15.16 (a) Ossiculoplasty with boomerang-shaped cartilage graft placed between footplate and groove drilled in the anteroinferior part of the bony annulus. **(b)** Antrum filled with cartilage piece for maintaining the middle ear height and reinforcing the neotympanum. Mastoid cavity obliteration performed in layers with cartilage pieces, bone pete harvested during earlier steps of surgery, and pedicled musculoperiosteal flaps. **(c)** Inferior part of the cavity is to be obliterated with pedicled sternocleidomastoid (SCM) muscle flap based on postauricular artery. Splitting the width of the SCM to create the length of the flap. *(Continued)*

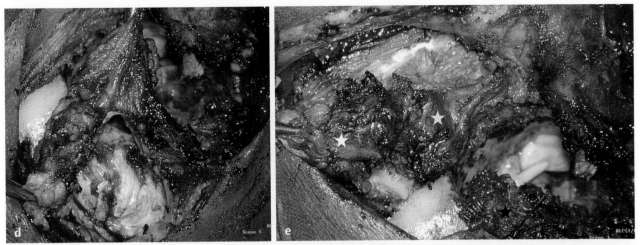

Fig. 15.16 *(Continued)* **(d, e)** The width of the muscle has been split to create the length and is placed in the cavity and sutured to the bony margin (*black asterisk*). The temporalis muscle flap is being created by creating a flap and splitting it in width to create the length to obliterate the inferior part of the mastoid cavity (*yellow* and *white asterix* showing the split parts of the pedicled flap).

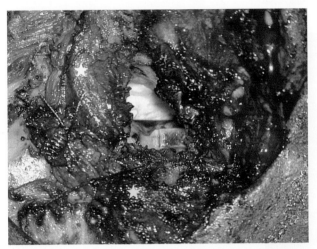

Fig. 15.17 Both pedicled flaps in place temporalis muscle flap, white asterix and sternocliedomastoid muscle flap is *yellow asterix*.

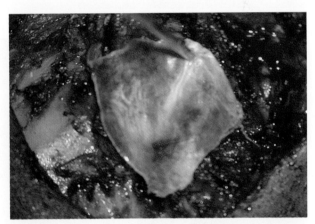

Fig. 15.18 Temporalis fascia placed lateral to ossiculoplasty and the muscle flaps to cover the middle ear and mastoid cavity.

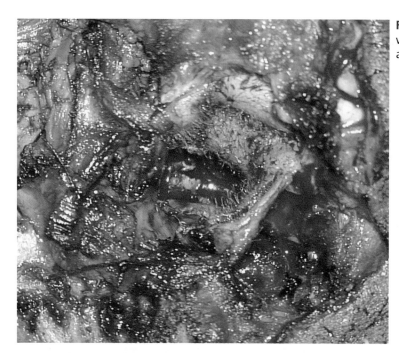

Fig. 15.19 Meatoplasty performed and a widened canal in place of big mastoid cavity is achieved.

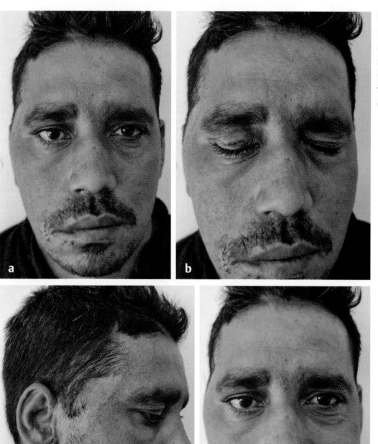

Fig. 15.20 (a, b) After 3 months of surgical procedures which includes facio-masseteric anastomosis, upper eyelid gold implant and fascial sling normal resting tone could be achieved. **(c)** The suture lines for facial sling surgery are visible. **(d)** The voluntary lifting of angle of mouth on right side has not yet been achieved.

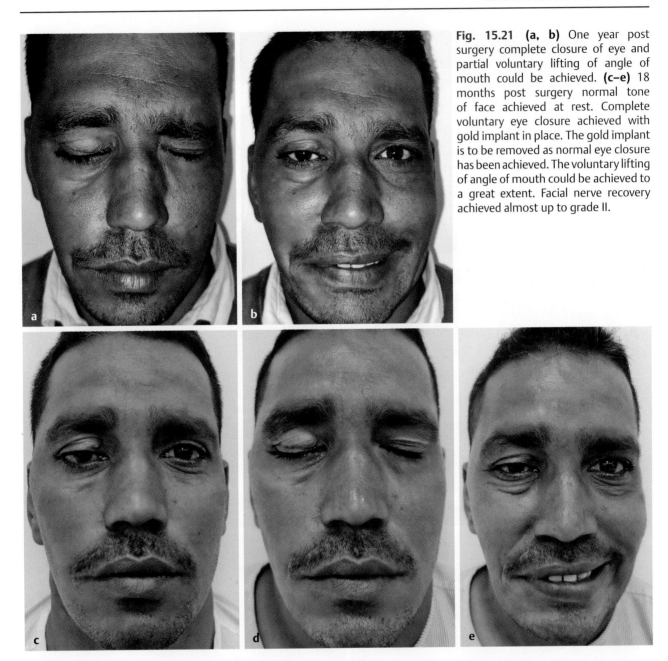

Fig. 15.21 (a, b) One year post surgery complete closure of eye and partial voluntary lifting of angle of mouth could be achieved. **(c–e)** 18 months post surgery normal tone of face achieved at rest. Complete voluntary eye closure achieved with gold implant in place. The gold implant is to be removed as normal eye closure has been achieved. The voluntary lifting of angle of mouth could be achieved to a great extent. Facial nerve recovery achieved almost up to grade II.

Case 2

A 32-year-old patient presented with slowly progressing facial paralysis of the right side for last 3 years. The patient also complained of slowly deteriorating hearing of the right side for last 1 year. Otoscopy showed intact but bulging tympanic membrane. A reddish mass could be seen behind the intact tympanic membrane. Facial nerve examination showed grade VI facial palsy (HBS) on the right side. Pure-tone audiometry indicated moderate conductive hearing loss in the right ear with air-bone gap of up to 45 dB.

CT showed a lobulated, soft-tissue mass within the right temporal bone corresponding to the location of the

GG, LS, TS, and MS of the facial nerve up to the SMF and filling the attic, antrum, and mastoid cavity (**Fig. 15.22**). MRI revealed a mass lesion with high-signal intensity in the same location.

Surgical Steps (Figs. 15.23–15.30)

Transmastoid canal wall down mastoidectomy was performed for complete resection of the tumor with excision of the affected part of the facial nerve (with cuff of normal healthy nerve on both sides). The excised nerve was from mid of the LS to MS up to the SMF. For repair of the facial nerve. Facial nerve grafting was performed in the same stage.

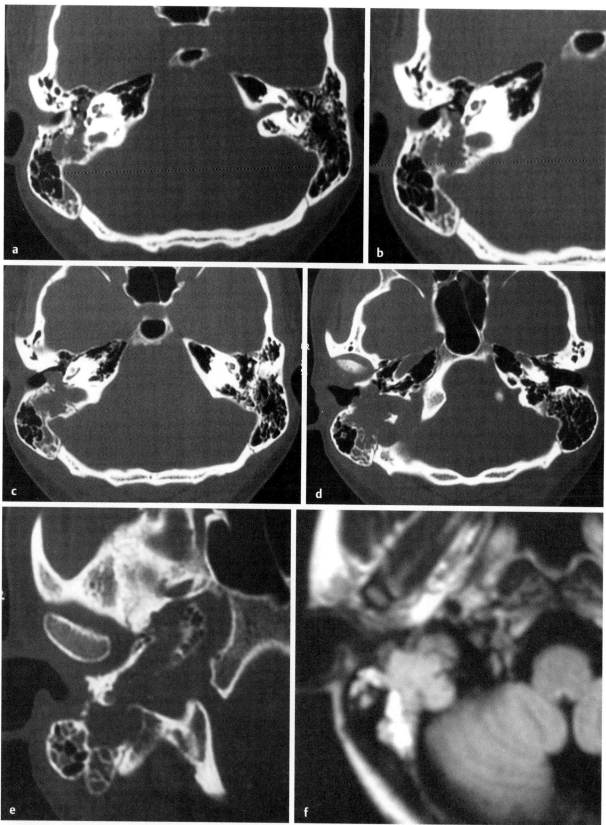

Fig. 15.22 **(a–e)** High-resolution computed tomography (HRCT) of the temporal bone of the right side axial cuts showing lobulated mass involving the geniculate ganglion (GG) and tympanic segment (TS) minimal pushing of the ossicles laterally, and involving the mastoid segment (MS) and mastoid cavity as well. **(f)** Axial magnetic resonance imaging (MRI) demonstrating hyperintense mass in the same locations.

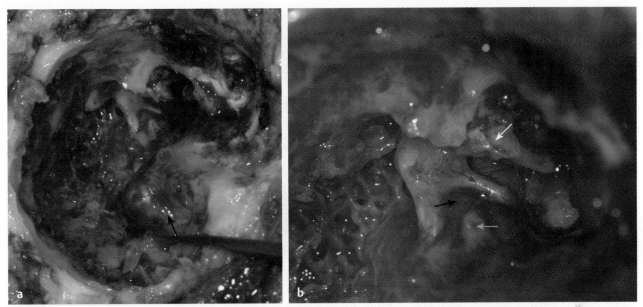

Fig. 15.23 **(a)** Right ear: Canal wall down mastoidectomy already performed. Extent of tumor assessed. Distal extent exposed till the mastoid segment (MS) (*black arrow*). **(b)** Tumor involving the tympanic segment (TS). Swollen TS (*black arrow*) can be visualized medial to the incus (*red arrow*) which has got displaced laterally due to expansion of the tumor in the TS. Head of stapes (*blue arrow*) and malleus (*white arrow*) visualized.

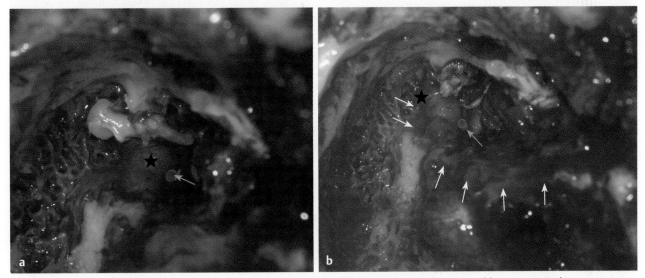

Fig. 15.24 Right side: **(a)** Tumor (*black asterisk*) involving the tympanic segment (TS) exposed by removing the incus, stapes head shown with blue arrow. **(b)** Tumor involving the geniculate ganglion (GG) exposed after removing the malleus (*black asterix*). Stapes head (*blue arrow*) is visible. Tumor (marked with *white arrows*) exposed in its proximal extent (up to the GG) and distal extent (mastoid segment [MS] up to the stylomastoid foramen [SMF]).

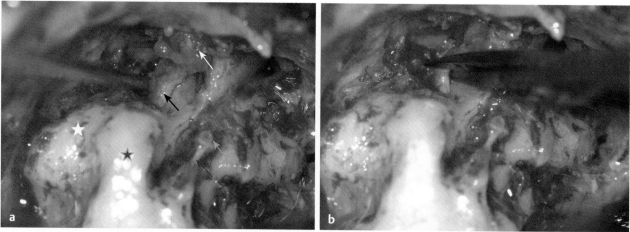

Fig. 15.25 **(a)** The normal healthy facial nerve in the medial half of the labyrinthine segment (*black arrow*) is visualized. The tumor involving the geniculate ganglion (GG) (*white arrow*) can be seen. Dome of the lateral semicircular canal (LSC) (*blue asterisk*), superior semicircular canal (SSC) (*white asterisk*), stapes (*blue arrow*), and stapedial tendon (*red arrow*) are also visualized. **(b)** Facial nerve is transected at mid of labyrinthine segment (LS), few millimeters proximal to the proximal extent of tumor, excising few millimeters of healthy nerve along with the tumor.

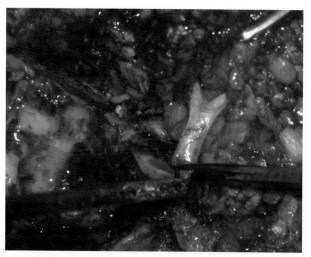

Fig. 15.26 The healthy distal stump of facial nerve after removal of the tumor in distal part, just after its exit from the stylomastoid foramen (SMF). The bifurcation of the facial nerve is visible.

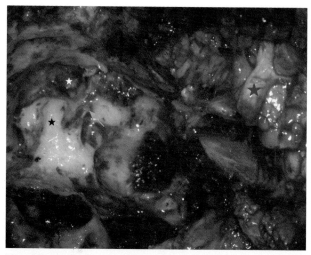

Fig. 15.27 Both proximal (*white asterisk*) and distal (*red asterisk*) facial nerve stumps after excision of the facial nerve schwannoma (FNS). The stapes are shown by *blue arrow* and lateral semicircular canal (LSC) by *black asterisk*.

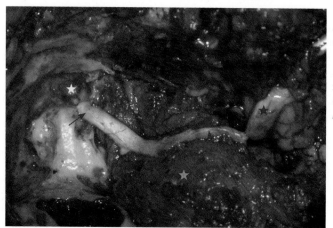

Fig. 15.28 Interposition free cable grafting by placement of great auricular nerve (*red arrows*) as free cable graft between the two stumps of the facial nerve with a bed of pedicled sternocleidomastoid muscle flap (*green asterisk*) underneath the graft and both anastomotic sites to provide stability and vascularity to the graft. The proximal stump is labeled with *yellow asterix* and distal stump is labeled with *red asterix*.

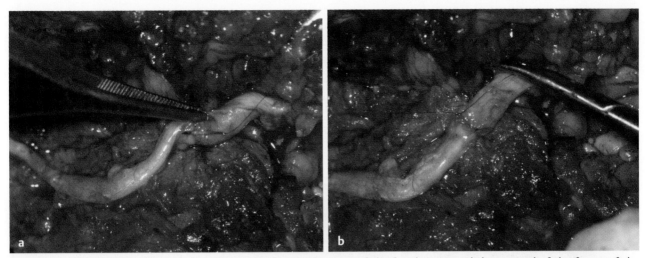

Fig. 15.29 **(a)** End-to-end anastomosis between the distal stump of the facial nerve and the cut end of the free graft by placing sutures with 8-0 monofilament nylon. **(b)** Second suture in progress. At least two to three sutures are to be placed.

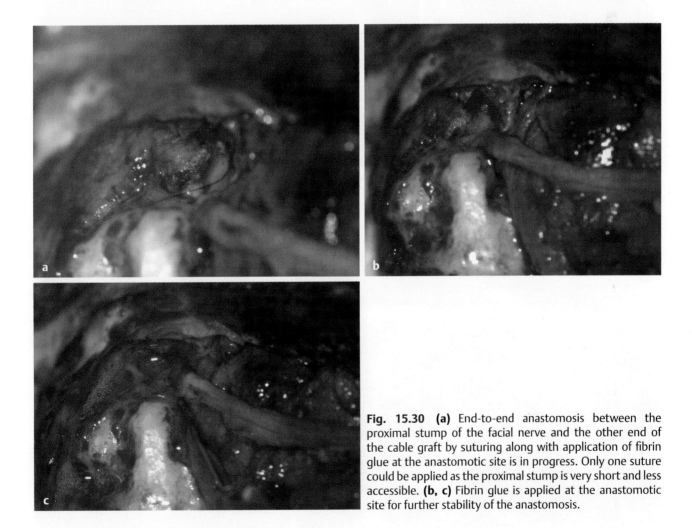

Fig. 15.30 **(a)** End-to-end anastomosis between the proximal stump of the facial nerve and the other end of the cable graft by suturing along with application of fibrin glue at the anastomotic site is in progress. Only one suture could be applied as the proximal stump is very short and less accessible. **(b, c)** Fibrin glue is applied at the anastomotic site for further stability of the anastomosis.

Case 3

It was a case of post gamma knife treated facial nerve schwannoma with complete grade VI facial palsy of the right side.

The patient was 13 years old when he had had received gamma knife treatment for facial nerve schwannoma 2 years back. Presently at 15 years of age, he presented with grade VI facial palsy (HBC) 1.5 years post gamma knife treatment. He visited the present surgeon for the first time with complete grade VI facial palsy and profound mixed hearing loss on right side.

Surgical Steps (Figs. 15.31–15.33)

Surgical management in the form of complete clearance of all diseased tissue was performed through infratemporal fossa type A approach. The surgical exploration showed ischemic and fibrotic changes in the facial nerve

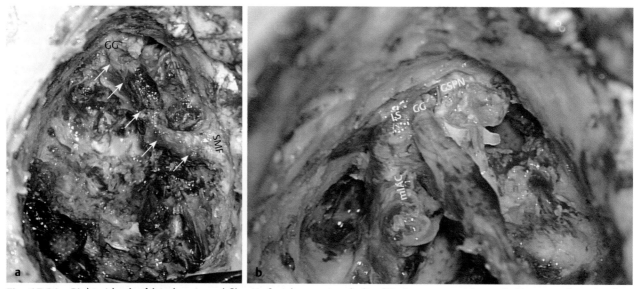

Fig. 15.31 Right side: **(a, b)** Ischemic and fibrotic facial nerve in whole of its intratemporal part (*white arrows*). Geniculate ganglion (GG) and stylomastoid foramen (SMF) visualized. The affected part of the facial nerve exposed from the porus of internal auditory meatus (IAM) till its exit at the SMF. Greater superficial petrosal nerve (GSPN), GG, labyrinthine segment (LS), and meatal segment (mIAM) are visualized.

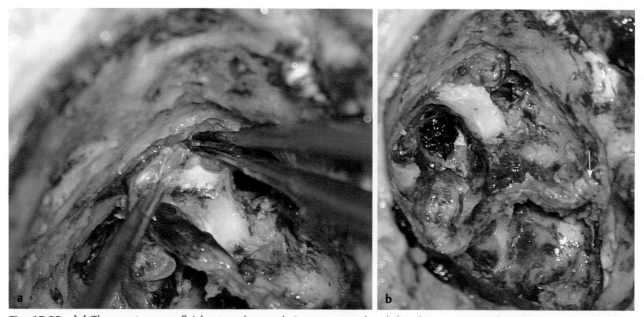

Fig. 15.32 **(a)** The greater superficial petrosal nerve being transected with bipolar cautery so that the nerve can be lifted at the geniculate ganglion (GG). **(b)** Now the nerve involved by the facial nerve schwannoma (FNS) has been lifted from the stylomastoid foramen (SMF) (*White arrows*) till the porus of internal auditory meatus (*red arrow*) for excision.

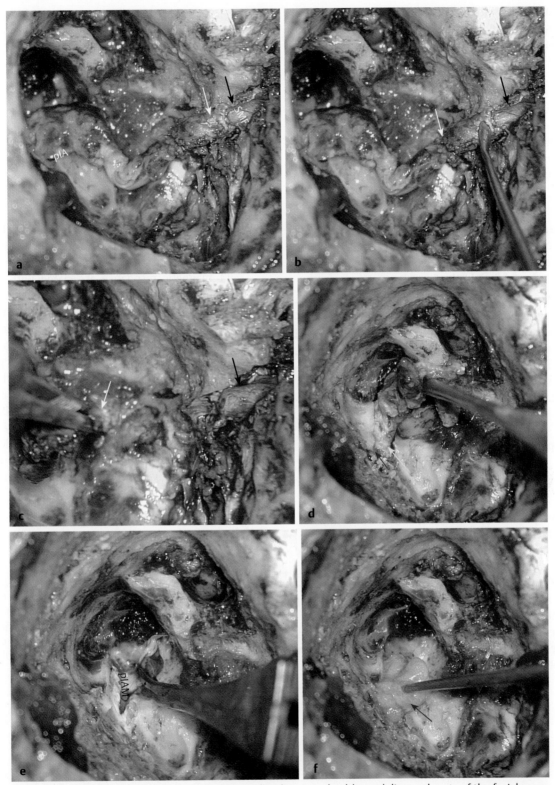

Fig. 15.33 **(a, b)** Pictures showing demarcation line between healthy and diseased parts of the facial nerve at the stylomastoid foramen (SMF). Ischemic nerve is being shown with *white arrow* while healthy nerve is shown with *black arrow*. **(c)** Ischemic facial nerve is excised after cutting distally few millimeters beyond unhealthy mastoid segment (MS) and proximally up tomedial end of IAM (*red arrow*). Unhealthy nerve is shown by *white arrow* and healthy nerve is shown by *black arrow*. **(d)** The proximal nonviable stump of facial nerve (*yellow arrow*) at the porus of internal auditory canal (*red arrow*). **(e)** The proximal unhealthy part of the facial nerve being excised at the porus of internal auditory meatus (pIAM). **(f)** The porus of IAM sealed with fat and fibrin glue (*red arrow*).

in whole of its intratemporal part including meatal segment up to the porus of IAM. As the viability of the proximal stump of the facial nerve after excising the affected part was doubtful, second-stage surgery in the form of motor nerve transfer (faciomasseteric anastomosis) and upper eyelid gold implant (both in the same stage) was performed after 2 months of primary surgery as the patient refused for two major surgeries in one stage. Faciomasseteric anastomosis procedure has been described in detail in Chapter 8 and upper eyelid gold implant surgery has been explained in detail in Chapter 9.

Pre- and postoperative pictures of the face have been depicted in Chapter 8 titled "Flaccid Facial Palsy of Short and Intermediate Duration with Proximal Stump Unavailable" and Chapter 9 titled "Management of Long Duration Flaccid Facial Palsy."

The cavity was obliterated with fat and muscle, eustachian tube obliterated with piece of bone and perichondrium, and external auditory canal was obliterated with blind sac cul de sac closure after removing all skin, tympanic membrane, malleus, incus and supra structure of stapes, and residual mastoid air cells with their mucosa.

Conclusion

Some of the important conclusive remarks of the author are listed below:

- Every sudden-onset facial palsy is not Bell's palsy. A facial nerve tumor should always be ruled out.
- No topographical or electrophysical testing helps in accurate diagnosis of FNS.
- CT and MRI remain the most relevant investigations for diagnosis as well as for visualization of the site and extent of the tumor.
- In early stage of the disease, the schwannoma can be separated and resected from the facial nerve; in late stage, it becomes impossible.

- FNS arising from the IAM cannot be distinguished from VS until it extends to the LS or there is multi-segment involvement.
- Decision for surgical resection should be weighed against "wait and watch" policy as best results with "resection and repair" are not better than grade III or II.
- Surgery is to be delayed till the facial nerve functioning reduced to grade III or more, but proper counseling of the patient is mandatory.
- Always resect around 5 to 6 mm of normal-looking nerve beyond the tumor on both sides to avoid residual tumor.
- The imaging appearance of the facial nerve schwannoma is more varied than originally described. The classic tubular enhancing mass on T1 magnetic resonance associated with smooth enlargement of the facial nerve canal on CT is actually only seen in FNS localized to the CPA–IAM or LS. More extensive FNSs that extend from the CPA–IAM to the geniculate fossa conform to a "dumbbell" shape. GG and GSPN FNSs can present as an extra-axial MCF mass which may get misdiagnosed, so a thorough examination and imaging are required for right diagnosis. Once TS FNSs grow in size, they can present as reddish retrotympanic mass with conductive hearing loss. Finally, MS FNSs can appear on MRI as locally aggressive masses when they invade into the surrounding mastoid air cells.

Bibliography

1. Mundada P, Purohit BS, Kumar TS, Tan TY. Imaging of facial nerve schwannomas: diagnostic pearls and potential pitfalls. Diagn Interv Radiol 2016;22(1): 40–46
2. Wiggins RH, Harnsberger HR, Salzman KL, Shelton C, Kertesz TR, Glastonbury CM. The many faces of facial nerve schwannoma. AJNR Am J Neuroradiol 2006; 27(3):694–699

Introduction

The extratemporal segment of facial nerve starts from the nerve's exit at stylomastoid foramen (SMF) till its terminal branches supplying the facial mimic muscles. The anatomy of this segment and functioning of facial mimic muscles have been described in detail in Chapter 2 titled "Anatomy of Facial Nerve."

Facial paresis/paralysis due to involvement of extratemporal segment can result from blunt, penetrating, or crush injury to the neck and face, or due to accidental iatrogenic trauma while performing surgery or due to involvement by tumor itself. The important conditions where facial nerve may be involved are given below.

Post-traumatic Facial Nerve Injury

Different situations causing trauma to the extratemporal segment of facial nerve have been categorized as follows:

- Blunt trauma.
- Birth (forceps delivery) trauma.
- Penetrating trauma.
- Crush injury.
- Iatrogenic injury.
- Lightening.

Blunt trauma to extratemporal segment in the form of pressure, compression, or stretch injury usually causes neuropraxia and recovery is possible in few days or weeks, so it is managed by conservative treatment and close observation. In case there is no recovery for up to 6 months, surgical correction is required.

Traumatic birth injuries to the facial nerve in the extratemporal segment happen usually after emergency forceps delivery. As the facial nerve lies quite superficial after its exit from the stylomastoid segment (SMF) due to nondevelopment of mastoid tip, the main trunk of the facial nerve is at risk of external trauma. These injuries most of the times heal on their own, so no active surgical treatment is required in such cases.

Penetrating injury on face usually causes more severe trauma such as interruption of nerve segment, leading to immediate, complete facial nerve palsy. In such cases, early surgical exploration and repair are indicated. If the repair is undertaken within 3 days, the nerve ends are identifiable in fresh wound, and the distal cut segment or branches can be identified with nerve stimulator. In case of delay in surgical intervention, a lot of fibrosis takes place, making it really difficult to identify the distal as well as proximal cut ends, more so when injury is away from the main trunk and close to the branches. The technique of repair depends on the extent of injury. In case of transection with both distal and proximal stumps well approximated without anterior segmental loss, end-to-end anastomosis can be performed after identifying the nerve endings, at the earliest. The anastomosis can be achieved through epineurium-to-epineurium or perineurium-to-perineurium suturing or suture-less fibrin glue coaptation. Both give equivalent results. In case there is gap between the two ends after trimming the lacerated ends, which is less than 2 cm, the nerve can be mobilized on either or both sides and end-to-end anastomosis can still be achieved. Excessive mobilization can compromise on vascularity of nerve so only few millimeters on both sides should be mobilized.

In case of crush injury, either a portion of nerve gets crushed or the segment goes missing. In such cases, usually the gap is more than 2 cm, and rerouting or mobilizing the nerve does not suffice. An interposition graft in the form of great auricular nerve (GAN) or sural nerve (SN) cable graft is used as a conduit to bridge the gap between the two cut ends of the facial nerve. If the injury is at the stump level or only one branch is involved, the GAN can be used as free cable graft between the two cut ends. In case the injury is more severe leading to injury to more than one branch, either GAN is harvested with its anterior and posterior branches or SN becomes the nerve of choice, as more length of the graft can be harvested (up to 30 cm) and branches associated with SN can also be used (This situation has been described in details through case 8 showing post surgery iatrogenic transection of facial nerve at pes ansarinus in chapter 7 titled " Management of Flaccid Facial Palsy of short and intermediate duration with proximal stump available").

In case the trauma is so bad that it crushes most of the terminal branches, there is no way a repair can be performed as distal stumps are not available. In such situations, various dynamic procedures with static procedures are performed in different combinations. The same principle applies in case the patient reaches very late to the surgeon (more than 2 years with electromyography

[EMG] testing negative). The silent graph on EMG shows the atrophy of facial mimic muscles, so the only options available for reanimation of face are dynamic and static procedures.

The procedures have already been described in detail in Chapter 9 "Management of Long Duration Flaccid Facial Palsy."

The Iatrogenic injuries can happen while performing surgery on parotid gland (discussed in details in chapter 7 titled " Management of short and intermediate duration flaccid facial palsy with proximal stump available", Case 8.), first branchial cyst/sinus/fistula (case 6, Fig. 16.34–16.42) or any other lesion on face. In case of iatrogenic injury with immediate complete facial nerve palsy, the first surgeon should be asked about the detail of the case. In case the surgeon is sure of not damaging the nerve, and the nerve was always under vision during the surgery, wait and watch policy for local anesthesia effect to wean off is adopted. If the surgeon is not sure regarding the integrity of the facial nerve, or had not visualized it during the surgery, the chances of injuring the nerve are there, so the surgeon should consult a more experienced colleague or go ahead with exploration after detailed counseling with the patient or the attendants.

In case of iatrogenic injury with gradual onset or incomplete facial palsy, the patient is closely monitored for the progression of paralysis. Electrophysiologic tests can be considered once the palsy becomes complete. In case the trauma is due to stretching or traction on the nerve, conservative treatment without surgical intervention is sufficient, whereas direct trauma to nerve requires immediate surgical intervention. If the trauma is recognized intraoperatively, the repair is to be performed at the same stage.

Branchial Cleft Remnant

Facial nerve is anatomically related to the first branchial cleft anomalies.

The risk of facial nerve getting traumatized is great in cases of revision surgery for the first branchial cleft anomaly due to repeated infections and development of fibrosis. These anomalies which develop due to incomplete closure of the ventral portion of the first branchial cleft are closely related to the parotid gland and facial nerve. The anomaly which presents as either cyst or sinus is usually found superficial to the facial nerve whereas lesions with external fistula in neck lie deep to the facial nerve (**Fig. 16.32**). The position of nerve can change due to this abnormal presence of fistulous tract increasing the risk of injury. This grave injury can be best avoided by identifying the type of lesion preoperatively through high-resolution computed tomography (HRCT). Intra

operative, a wide exposure with dissection of the facial nerve after its exit from the SMF is performed in every case to achieve complete excision. Superficial parotidectomy may even need to be performed to accomplish a safe resection.

Benign Lesions of Parotid

Benign lesions of parotid include pleomorphic adenoma, Warthin's tumor, benign myoepithelioma, and benign lymphoepithelioma, and they usually spare the facial nerve. The facial nerve should be well preserved while excising such tumors. Tumors involving the facial nerve, such as facial nerve schwannoma (FNS) or hemangioma, have already been discussed in detail in Chapter 15 titled "Facial Nerve Schwannoma."

FNS has to be clearly demarcated from benign tumors of the parotid preoperatively, as the surgeon may need to sacrifice the facial nerve in such cases due to its involvement by the tumor and a preoperative informed consent is mandatory in all such cases, whereas in benign tumors of parotid, there are least chances of injuring the facial nerve.

Malignant Lesions of Parotid

Poorly differentiated mucoepidermoid carcinomas, malignant pleomorphic adenomas, undifferentiated carcinomas, malignant melanomas, and squamous carcinomas are malignant tumors involving the parotid gland. The patient may present to the surgeon with facial nerve paresis/palsy along with the tumor.

It is mandatory to diagnose the malignant tumor preoperatively and equally important to perform preoperative counseling of the patient and the attendants regarding the facial palsy that may follow the surgery, if it has not already happened. Adenocystic carcinoma needs a special mention here. Adenocystic carcinoma accounts for 2 to 6% of parotid gland tumors. It usually presents as an infiltrating mass with perineural infiltration. Perineural disease can also present with "skip" lesions distally in a nerve that seems to be normal. Facial palsy in such cases may not present in different grades; rather certain areas of face may get paralyzed and certain areas may show weakness or normal functioning.

■ Evaluation of Parotid Tumors

Detailed history, clinical examination along with fine-needle aspiration cytology (FNAC) from the tumor may help in making the diagnosis, and the differentiation between benign and malignant varieties, but it is the imaging modality which plays an important role in clearly differentiating benign from malignant and superficial from deep lobe tumors and help in surgical planning, keeping facial nerve in orientation, once the diagnosis has been made.

The parotid gland is generally subdivided into deep and superficial lobes by the facial nerve and its branches for the purpose of surgical approach; however, there is no anatomical division between lobes. The facial nerve cannot usually be visualized by imaging, so there have to be other criteria to differentiate between superficial or deep lobe tumors. The use of the retromandibular vein (RMV) as a marker for the facial nerve is a sensitive method for identifying the location of parotid gland lesions.

Both benign and malignant salivary gland masses show considerable overlap with regard to imaging appearance such as tumor margins, homogeneity, and signal intensity. Malignancy is suggested if the tumor is found infiltrating into the parapharyngeal space, muscles or bone, and perineural spaces as these findings are not part of benign lesions.

Evaluation through Imaging

To determine the specific location and extent of the lesions affecting the parotid gland, imaging becomes an essential aspect of diagnosis, and it guides the surgeon in deciding the technique of surgery and avoiding damage to the facial nerve during surgery.

Both computed tomography (CT) and magnetic resonance imaging (MRI) can be used for evaluation, though MRI gives more specific information.

For CT imaging, both pre- and postcontrast studies must be performed in order to detect calcifications (precontrast) and enhancement pattern (postcontrast). Coronal and sagittal reconstructions can be helpful in the evaluation of perineural spread.

However, MRI (**Fig. 16.1**) is the investigation of choice for patients with palpable masses with a strong suspicion for malignancy. MRI gives information on the exact location and extent and nature of the lesion and involvement of surrounding structures in the form of perineural spread, bone invasion, and meningeal infiltration.

Imaging findings usually depend on tumor size. Small tumors are more homogeneous and well defined with strong enhancement after contrast-enhanced CT and MRI, whereas larger tumors are heterogeneous due to both necrotic and hemorrhagic areas and tend to have lobulated image which seems like an outgrowth from the main lesion.

Axial T1- and T2-weighted MRI sequences help in assessing the nature and exact extent of the tumor, tumor margins, and its growth patterns, whereas contrast (gadolinium)-enhanced T1-weighted sequences and fat suppression images are used to locate any perineural spread along the facial nerve toward the SMF, the mandibular division of trigeminal nerve through foramen ovale, or the maxillary division of trigeminal nerve through foramen rotundum.

Low-grade, small, benign, mixed tumors are usually homogenous with well-circumscribed margins and are hypointense in T1- and hyperintense in T2-weighted sequences, whereas high-grade large tumors are usually heterogenous and have poor margins with infiltration into surrounding tissues. As already explained, malignancy is suspected once the tumor is infiltrating into the parapharyngeal space, muscles or bone, and perineural spaces. Low signal intensity on T2-weighted images may be observed in carcinoma ex pleomorphic adenomas.

■ Surgical Planning for Parotid Tumors

The parotid tumor can be involving either superficial or deep lobe or both. Differentiation between superficial and deep lobe parotid tumors is important for appropriate surgical planning and avoiding injury to the facial nerve. The parotid duct and RMV (which runs posterolaterally to the mandibular ramus at the level of the parotid gland) are the two vital structures, which can be used to differentiate the two. Mostly it is the RMV which demarcates between the two lobes. The parotid duct is only used in cases where the tumor and the duct are visualized in the same image. Although parotid duct is more accurate than the RMV, it cannot be applied in every case due to its nonvisibility most of the times. So, for diagnosis, the parotid duct criterion is applied first, and for cases in which it cannot be applied, the RMV criterion is used which improves the diagnostic accuracy of parotid tumor location.

Another method proposed for differentiating superficial lobe from deep lobe is drawing certain lines that can do the demarcation very clearly (**Fig. 16.2**). They are:

- Facial nerve (FN) line: A line which connects the lateral surface of the posterior belly of the digastric muscle to the lateral surface of the cortex of the ascending mandibular ramus
- Utrecht (U) line: A line which connects the dorsalmost point seen on the ipsilateral half of a vertebra and the most dorsal point of the RMV

Of the abovementioned lines, good results have been seen with the U line and the FN line, with the FN line being the more reliable and reproducible method of prediction for tumor location on MRI.

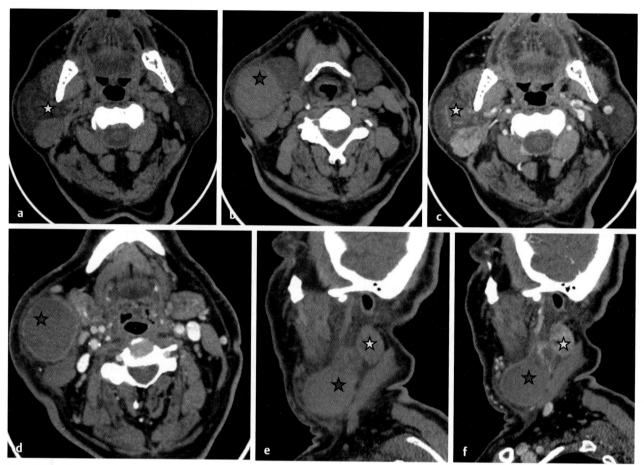

Fig. 16.1 Computed tomography (CT) of neck, plain, right side, showing bilobed parotid tumor. **(a)** Parotid tumor (*yellow asterisk*) involving upper part of superficial lobe. **(b)** Second lesion (*red asterisk*) involving lower part (tail) of parotid. **(c, d)** The same images are shown in CT neck sequences post contrast. **(e)** CT of neck, plain, sagittal view right side, showing the two lesions simultaneously. **(f)** CT of neck with contrast sagittal view showing the two lesions simultaneously.

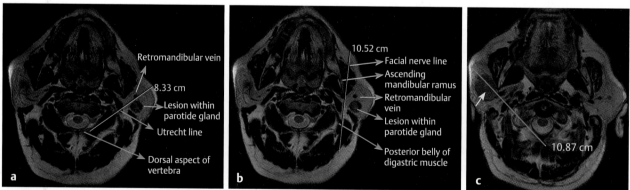

Fig. 16.2 **(a)** Utrecht (U) line (*yellow line*) connecting the dorsal-most point seen on the ipsilateral half of a vertebra and the most dorsal point of the retromandibular vein (RMV) on left side. **(b)** Facial nerve (FN) line (*yellow line*) connecting the lateral surface of the posterior belly of the digastric muscle to the lateral surface of the cortex of the ascending mandibular ramus on left side. The tumor (*yellow asterix*) can be seen lying lateral to both U and FN lines, which means that the tumor is involving superficial lobe of parotid only. **(c)** U line (*green line*) connecting the dorsal-most point seen on the ipsilateral half of a vertebra and the most dorsal point of the RMV on right side. The tumor (*yellow arrow*) can be seen lying lateral and medial to U line, which means that the in this case, tumor is involving superficial as well as deep lobe of parotid.

Surgical Management of Parotid Tumor with Protection of Facial Nerve

The parotid surgery which used to be previously classified into superficial and total parotidectomy has been consistently redefined over time. Different authors have proposed classification systems for parotid surgery depending upon the extent and location of lesion and have defined basically six types of resection: radical parotidectomy (which includes total parotidectomy with resection of the facial nerve), total parotidectomy (facial nerve is saved), complete superficial parotidectomy (whole superficial lobe is resected), partial superficial parotidectomy (with different subdivisions), selective parotidectomy of the deep lobe, and extracapsular dissection (dissection of the normal parotid tissue away from the tumor without searching for the facial nerve followed by mobilization and removal of the tumor).

Complete superficial parotidectomy, partial superficial parotidectomy (with different subdivisions), selective parotidectomy of the deep lobe, and extracapsular dissection are the surgical procedures of choice for benign lesions of parotid, whereas in malignant tumors the patient has to undergo either total parotidectomy which is a more difficult procedure with the surgical risk of facial nerve palsy or radical parotidectomy, where facial nerve has to be sacrificed (depending upon the extent of the tumor).

For benign tumors, the surgical steps are as described in Case 1.

Case 1: Pleomorphic Adenoma Involving Right Parotid Gland. The Tumor is Involving the Upper Part of Superficial Lobe of Parotid

Surgery Performed: Superficial Parotidectomy with Excision of Tumor

Surgical Steps (Figs. 16.3–16.8)

- A lazy, S-shaped preauricular modified Blair's skin incision is made that starts in front of the ear, turns inferiorly, keeping on the medial surface of tragus to hide the incision, passes along the root of the ear lobule from anterior to posterior, and then down along the cervical crease anteriorly in a horizontal direction, keeping approximately 3 cms below the ramus of the mandible. Extreme care is taken while elevating skin over the tragal cartilage to avoid its injury as it can give disfigurement to the face.
- An anterior subplatysmal and subsuperficial musculoaponeurotic system flap is elevated to expose the parotid gland with its capsule. A subplatysmal flap reduces the incidence of developing Frey's syndrome.
- A posterior flap is elevated to expose the cartilaginous part of external auditory canal (EAC), the tip of mastoid process, and the anterior border of sternocleidomastoid (SCM) muscle.
- Fascia over anterior border of SCM is incised and dissection starts in a plane deeper to the parotid tail, which is retracted anteriorly.
- After elevating flaps, GAN is identified as it crosses over SCM. The landmarks for identifying GAN have been described in detail in Chapter 3 "Facial Nerve Unit, Structure, Lesions, and Repair."
- Only the anterior branch of GAN is cut at this stage, preserving the posterior branch, and keeping the sensations of external ear intact. The proximal stump of GAN is kept intact till there is requirement for interposition graft for repairing facial nerve, and is buried underneath the SCM to prevent the development of painful traumatic neuroma postoperatively. The maximum length achieved from GAN as a cable graft is around 9 cm.
- After achieving adequate exposure, dissection is now performed using a cold instrument or bipolar cautery vertically along the anterior surface of the tragal cartilage, separating it from superficial lobe of parotid and exposing the tragal pointer which is a very important landmark for identifying the facial nerve. The dissection is extended inferiorly until the bony anterior wall of the EAC. From here the use of cautery is restricted and dissection is performed with blunt instruments. Dissection is continued vertically downwards along the anterior surface of the bony EAC till the next bony structure, base of styloid, which lies immediately deep to the bony EAC. This is an important landmark for identifying the facial nerve at its exit from the SMF.
- Now the posterior belly of the digastric muscle is identified deep to the SCM after retracting the tail of parotid anteriorly and following to its origin from the groove on mastoid process (digastric ridge). The superior border of the origin of the posterior belly of the digastric forms another landmark for identifying the facial nerve at its exit from the SMF. The landmarks for identifying the facial nerve after its exit from the SMF have been described in detail in Chapter 8 titled " Management of Short and Intermediate duration Flaccid facial palsy with proximal stump unavailable".
- The point where the anterior margin of mastoid process, superior border of posterior belly of the digastric, and cartilaginous EAC meet is the point for exposing the main trunk of the facial nerve emerging from the SMF.

- After exposing the facial nerve after its exit from the SMF, dissection is continued in a plane superficial to the nerve toward the periphery of the gland, keeping the nerve under vision at all times.
- The bifurcation of nerve (pes anserinus) into upper and lower divisions of facial nerve in the parotid tissue is exposed.
- Absolute hemostasis should be maintained.
- Dissection continues along the peripheral branches of the nerve. If tumor is located along the lower branches of the nerve, dissection of parotid tissue along the upper division is done first. It is not necessary to expose all branches of the facial nerve unless required. The gland tissue adjacent to the EAC and zygoma can be divided safely as the nerve lies in a plane deeper to the dissection and is under constant vision.
- The superficial temporal vessels may very rarely be encountered and may need to be ligated.
- To separate the tumor from the facial nerve, a hemostat is inserted superficial to and in the direction of the nerve and its branches, lifted, and spread through the parotid tissue, which is then cut with bipolar cautery or sharp scissors. This step exposes the further segment of the nerve. This is continued throughout the dissection of the nerve and each of its branches, till the tumor is separated from the underlying facial nerve.
- The cut upper half of the gland is retracted anteriorly and held with hemostats.
- Extra attention is required around the buccal branch (**Fig. 16.3**) as it is close to the Stensen's duct (parotid duct). Once the buccal branch is isolated, Stensen's duct is divided, and its stump is ligated.
- The dissection along lower division of the nerve is carried out in a similar fashion, leading to complete removal of the tumor with superficial lobe.
- RMV lies directly beneath the lower division of the nerve entering the deep lobe in 80% of the cases. In rest of the cases, it lies either lateral to the lower division of facial nerve (**Fig. 16.2**), or it can form a loop through which the facial nerve traverses.
- Absolute hemostasis is obtained. Drain is inserted and brought out through the incision behind the ear lobule.
- Incision is closed in two layers. Light is dressing applied.

After 24 hours of the surgery the facial nerve functioning is up to grade I on the right side (**Fig. 16.9**).

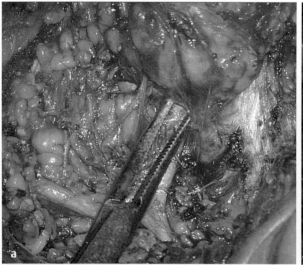
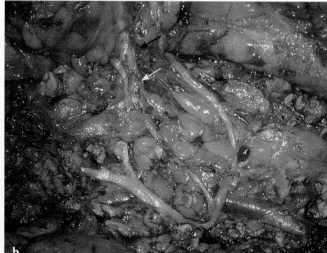
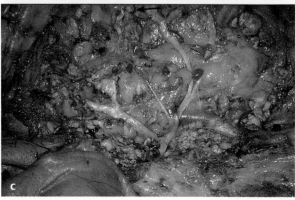

Fig. 16.3 (a) Right side parotidectomy surgery showing Hemostat inserted superficial to and in the direction of the nerve and its branches, and lifted and spread through the parotid tissue which is then cut with bipolar cautery or sharp scissors. **(b)** Parotid duct (*black arrow*) running parallel to buccal branch of the facial nerve (*yellow arrow*) is visualized in right-sided parotid retro mandibular vein (*blue arrow*) can be seen passing beneath the lower division of facial nerve gland. **(c)** The parotid duct is ligated and cut (*black arrow*).

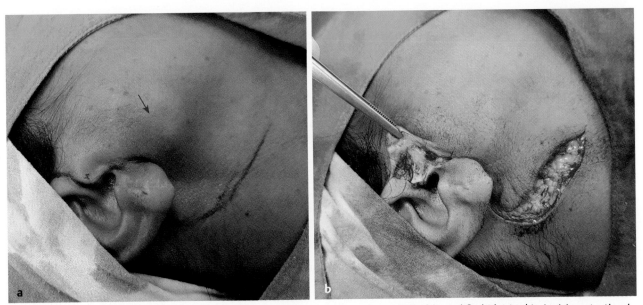

Fig. 16.4   Right side of face with right parotid tumor mass visible (*red arrow*) **(a, b)** Modified Blair's skin incision starting in front of the ear, turning inferiorly, keeping on the medial surface of tragus, passing along the root of the ear lobule from anterior to posterior, and then down along the cervical crease anteriorly in a horizontal direction, keeping approximately 3 cms below the ramus of the mandible.

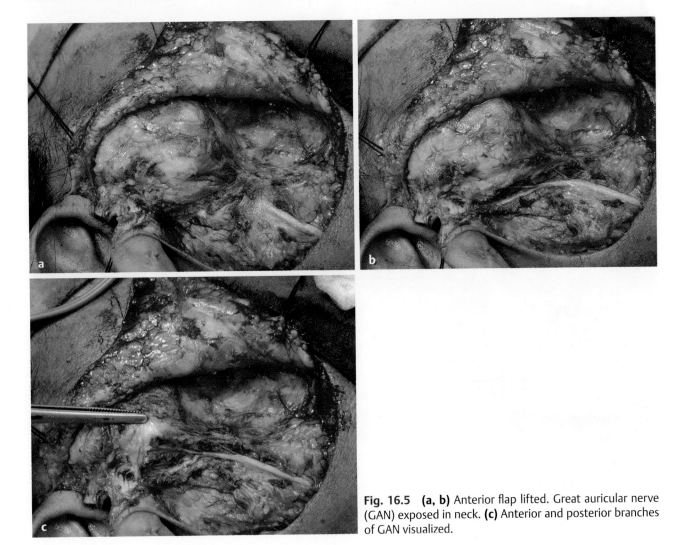

Fig. 16.5   **(a, b)** Anterior flap lifted. Great auricular nerve (GAN) exposed in neck. **(c)** Anterior and posterior branches of GAN visualized.

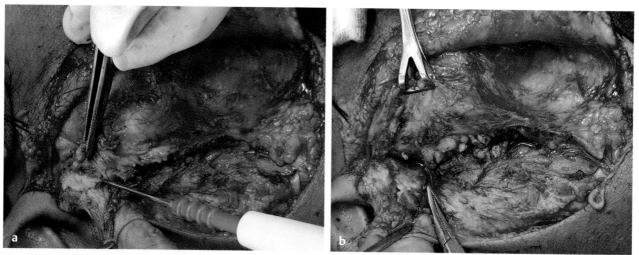

Fig. 16.6 **(a)** Separation of superficial lobe of parotid from cartilaginous part of external auditory canal (EAC). **(b)** Tragal pointer exposed and pointed with an instrument.

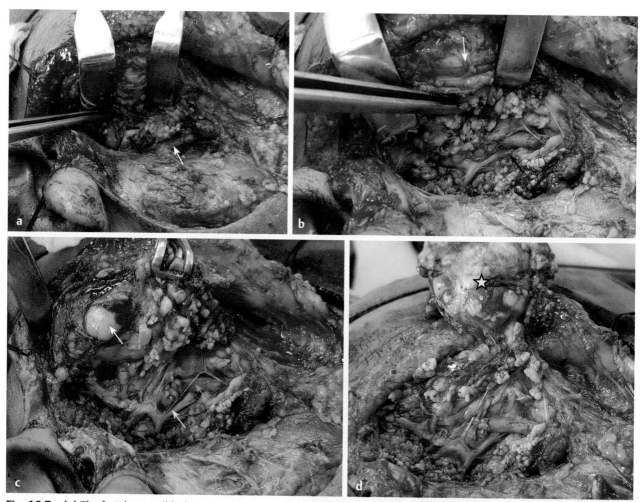

Fig. 16.7 **(a)** The facial nerve (*black arrow*) at its exit from the stylomastoid segment (SMF) exposed, just superior to superior border of posterior belly of the digastric (PBD, *white arrow*). **(b, c)** As the tumor is involving upper part of the superficial lobe, lateral to the upper division of the facial nerve, the cervicofacial branch of the facial nerve is first exposed by lifting the tumor (*white arrow*) along with normal parotid tissue from it. Retromandibular vein (RMV) (*blue arrow*) is visible directly lateral to the cervicofacial division (*yellow arrow*). The tumor is now being lifted from temporofacial division (*red arrows*). **(d)** The tumor with superficial lobe of parotid (*yellow asterisk*) separated from underlying facial nerve and deep lobe, is being excised.

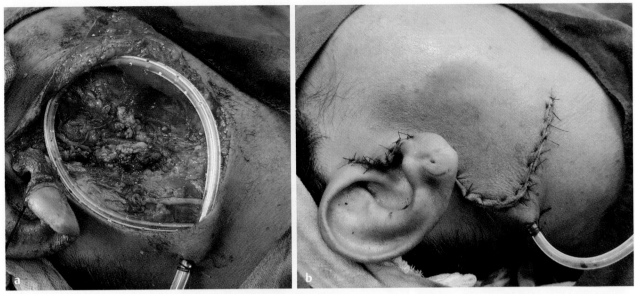

Fig. 16.8   (a) The suction drain in place. **(b)** Final suturing in place.

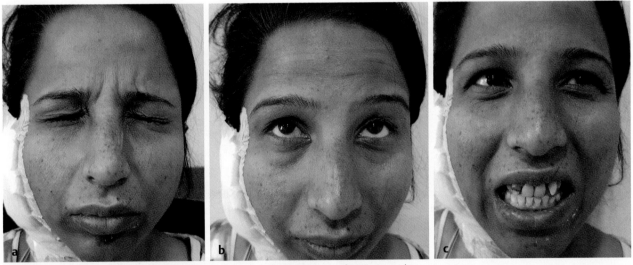

Fig. 16.9   (a–c) Immediate postsurgery facial nerve functioning indicating grade I.

Case 2: Warthin's Tumor Involving Right Parotid Gland Superficial Lobe Lower Part (Tail of Parotid)

Surgery Performed: Superficial Parotidectomy with Excision of Tumor

MRI images showing the tumor involving superficial lobe and is lateral to both the U line and FN line (**Fig. 16.10**).

Surgical Steps

Surgical steps undertaken are shown in **Figs. 16.11–16.13**.

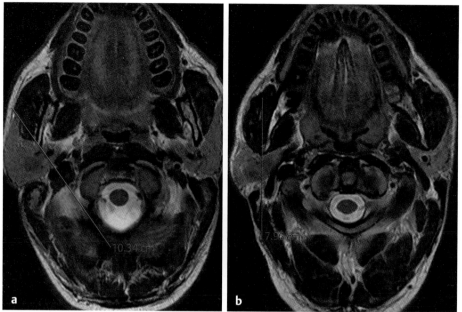

Fig. 16.10 Magnetic resonance imaging (MRI) showing benign parotid tumor of the right side involving superficial lobe in its inferior part. **(a)** Tumor lying lateral to Utrecht's line (*red line*). **(b)** Tumor lying lateral to facial nerve line (*red line*).

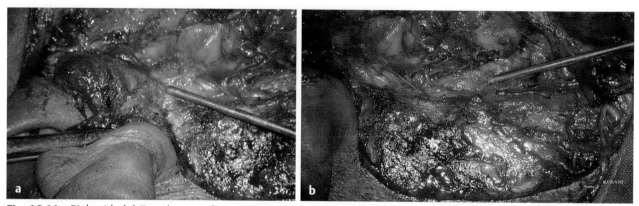

Fig. 16.11   Right side **(a)** Tragal pointer being pointed by instrument. **(b)** Posterior belly of the digastric (PBD) being pointed with an instrument.

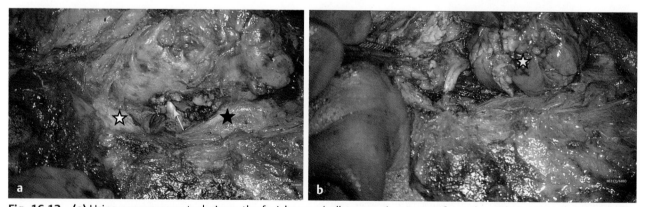

Fig. 16.12   **(a)** Using convergence technique, the facial nerve (*yellow arrow*) at its exit from the stylomastoid segment (SMF) is exposed. Tragal pointer is shown with *white asterisk* and posterior belly of the digastric (PBD) with *black asterisk*. **(b)** As the tumor is involving the lower part of the superficial lobe of parotid, the upper branch of the facial nerve is exposed and the tumor (*yellow asterisk*) is being separated gently from the underlying facial nerve.

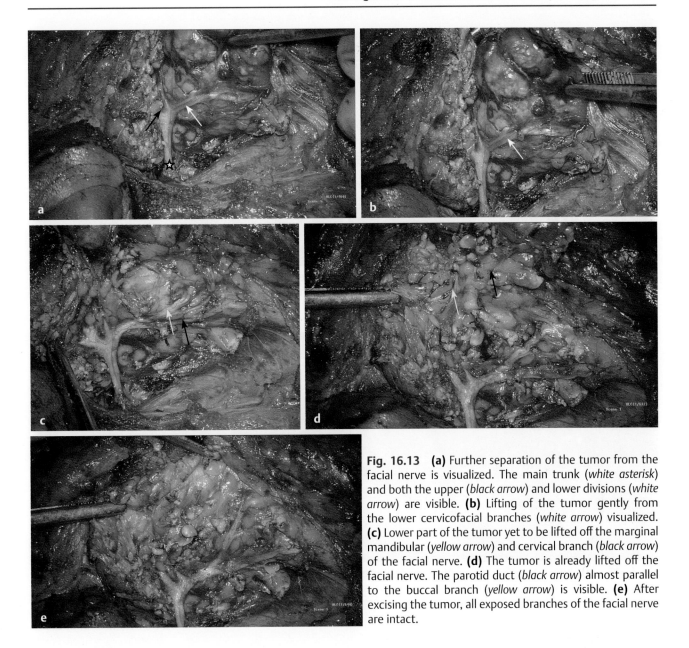

Fig. 16.13 **(a)** Further separation of the tumor from the facial nerve is visualized. The main trunk (*white asterisk*) and both the upper (*black arrow*) and lower divisions (*white arrow*) are visible. **(b)** Lifting of the tumor gently from the lower cervicofacial branches (*white arrow*) visualized. **(c)** Lower part of the tumor yet to be lifted off the marginal mandibular (*yellow arrow*) and cervical branch (*black arrow*) of the facial nerve. **(d)** The tumor is already lifted off the facial nerve. The parotid duct (*black arrow*) almost parallel to the buccal branch (*yellow arrow*) is visible. **(e)** After excising the tumor, all exposed branches of the facial nerve are intact.

Case 3: Warthin's Tumor Involving the Deep Lobe of Left Parotid

Surgery Performed: Selective Parotidectomy of Deep Lobe

Surgical Steps

Surgical steps are depicted in **Figs. 16.14** and **16.15**.

After 24 hours of surgery, the facial nerve functioning is up to grade I on the right side (**Fig. 16.16**).

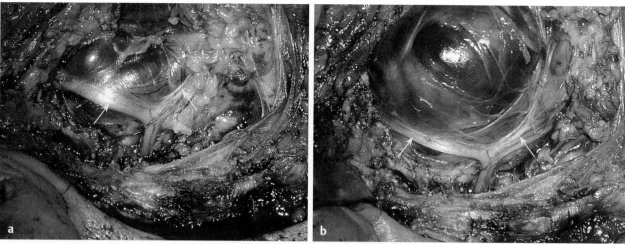

Fig. 16.14 **(a)** Tumor arising from the deep lobe of parotid, lying medial and deep to the temporofacial and cervico facial branches (yellow arrows) of facial nerve. **(b)** Gentle separation of the tumor from the overlying upper and lower divisions of the facial nerve (*yellow arrows*).

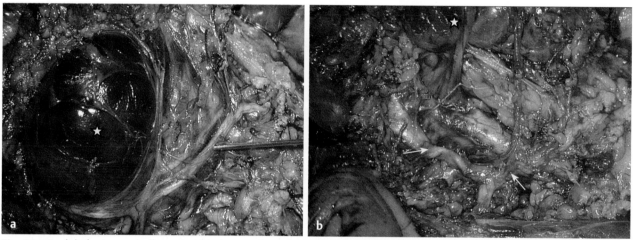

Fig. 16.15 **(a)** The tumor (*yellow asterix*) being gently peeled off the facial nerve branches. **(b)** The final separation and removal of the tumor (*yellow asterisk*) from the deep lobe is in process. Retromandibular vein (RMV) is shown with *blue arrow*, and upper and lower divisions of facial nerve are shown with *yellow arrows*.

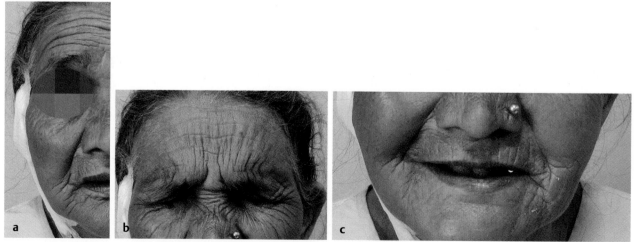

Fig. 16.16 **(a–c)** Immediate postsurgery facial nerve functioning up to grade I.

Case 4: Myoepithelioma Tumor Involving Deep Lobe of Left Parotid Gland

Surgery Performed: Selective Parotidectomy of Deep Lobe Left Side

Surgical Steps

Surgical steps undertaken on the left side are depicted in **Figs. 16.17** and **16.18**.

After 1 year of surgery, pictures of face show facial nerve functioning up to grade I. The patient was kept on follow-up for 5 years and there has been no recurrence of tumor (**Fig. 16.19**).

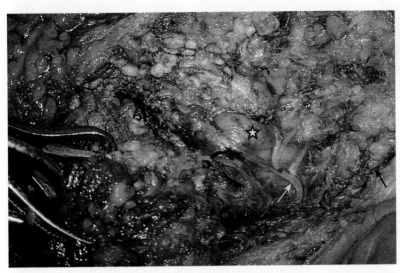

Fig. 16.17 Left side: Tumor (*yellow asterisk*) involving deep lobe of left parotid. The facial nerve with bifurcation (*yellow arrow*) lying stretched over the tumor is visible. Tragal pointer is shown with *black arrow*. Superficial lobe held with Babcock tissue holding forceps.

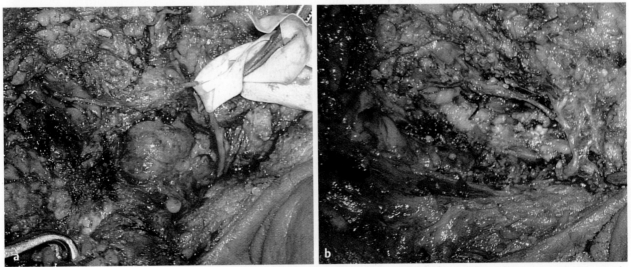

Fig. 16.18 **(a)** Both the divisions of the facial nerve lifted and held gently in cut sleeve of gloves. The tumor is being gently peeled off from the facial nerve. **(b)** Complete removal of the tumor. Both the divisions intact and visible.

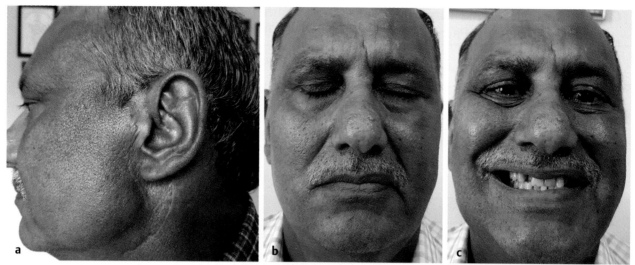

Fig. 16.19 After 1 year of surgery. **(a)** Healed suture line. **(b, c)** Facial nerve functioning up to grade I.

Case 5: Adenoid Cystic Carcinoma Involving Superficial Lobe Left Parotid with Perineural Infiltration of Upper Division of Facial Nerve

The patient presented with tumor left parotid with incomplete closure of upper eyelid of the left side along with inability to lift the angle of mouth on the same side. Plain and contrast-enhanced scans with axial and coronal sections revealed a heterogeneous enhancing soft tissue mass, measuring approximately 4 × 3 × 3 cm in size, seen in the parotid region on the left side of the face. The overall features were suggestive of a neoplastic lesion.

On operation table, facial nerve monitor recording showed presence of nerve impulse only in marginal mandibular branch of the facial nerve on the left side, confirming perineural infiltration of tumor along the facial nerve but in "skip lesion" pattern (**Fig. 16.20**). The extension of lesion is along the upper temporofacial division sparing the cervicofacial division.

The treatment consisted of surgery followed by a course of radiotherapy.

Surgery Performed on the Left Side

Total parotidectomy with sparing of the facial nerve. Interposition grafting was performed between buccal and marginal mandibular nerve as marginal mandibular nerve was found free of tumor invasion and showed nerve impulse on the nerve monitor. Upper eyelid gold implant and facial sling were performed as static procedures in the second stage after the complete course of radiotherapy.

Surgical Steps (Figs. 16.21–16.27)

Facial nerve recovery at different stages is shown in **Figs. 16.28–16.31**.

The patient is free of disease since 5 years post surgery and radiotherapy.

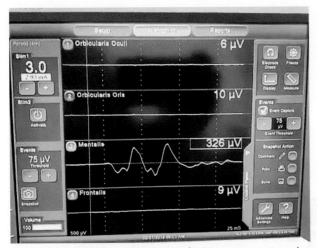

Fig. 16.20 Nerve monitor is showing nerve impulse present only in the marginal mandibular branch.

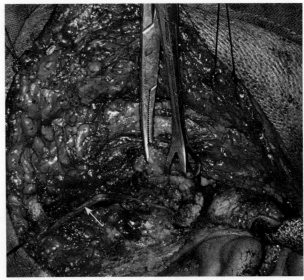

Fig. 16.21 Superficial lobe has been lifted and retracted anteriorly. Great auricular nerve (GAN) visible (*yellow arrow*).

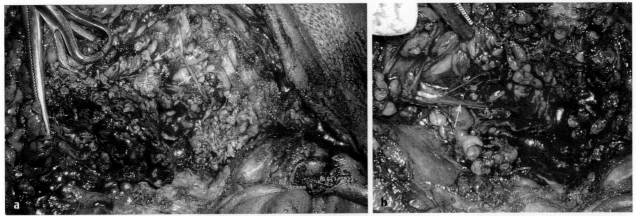

Fig. 16.22 **(a)** The parotid tissue is retracted inferiorly exposing buccal branch of the facial nerve. **(b)** The parotid tissue is retracted superiorly, exposing inferior cervicofacial division (*yellow arrow*).

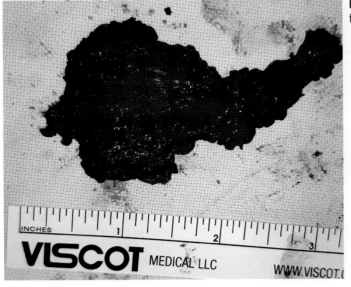

Fig. 16.23 Total parotidectomy performed keeping the facial nerve intact. Excised parotid gland with the tumor.

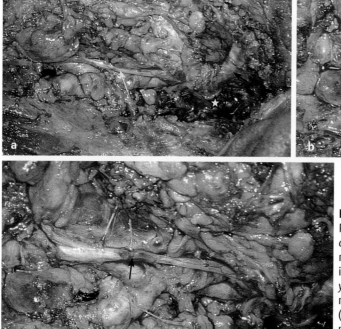

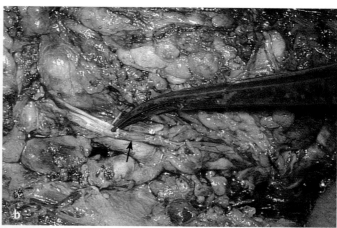

Fig. 16.24 **(a)** Facial nerve with all its branches saved. Perineural spread along temporofacial division (*black arrow*) is there as confirmed on the nerve monitor. Marginal mandibular branch (*yellow arrow*) is spared. Buccal branch is shown with *blue arrow* and main facial nerve trunk with *yellow asterisk*. **(b, c)** For interposition graft between marginal mandibular and buccal branch, Partial thickness (30%) cut is made in the thickness of marginal mandibular nerve (*black arrow*) for end-to-side anastomosis with one end of the great auricular nerve (GAN) graft.

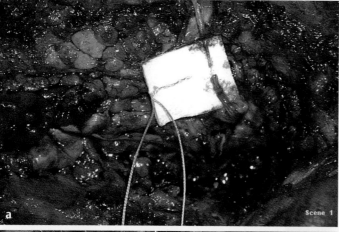

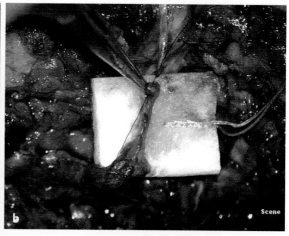

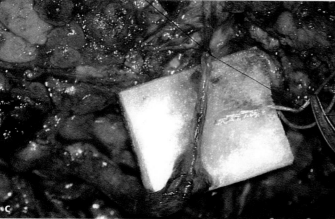

Fig. 16.25 **(a)** Buccal branch transected from the main trunk to be sutured to the other end of the great auricular nerve (GAN) graft as end-to-end anastomosis. **(b, c)** Suturing with 8-0 monofilament suture in progress for end-to-end anastomosis between the cut end of buccal nerve and GAN graft.

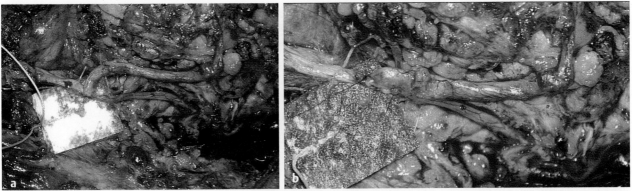

Fig. 16.26 **(a, b)** End-to-side anastomosis between the other end of the great auricular nerve (GAN) and partial cut surface of the marginal mandibular nerve with 8-0 monofilament suture.

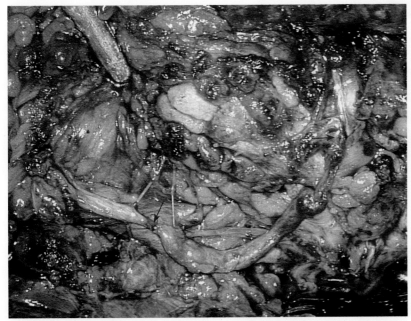

Fig. 16.27 Final interposition grafting with both anastomotic side is visualized (*red arrows*).

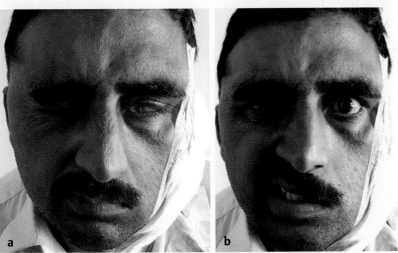

Fig. 16.28 **(a, b)** Immediate (24 hours), postsurgery facial nerve functioning till grade VI.

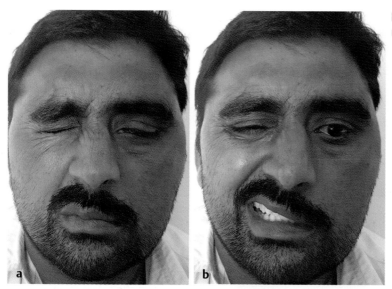

Fig. 16.29 (a, b) Postradiotherapy facial nerve functioning up to grade V persisting.

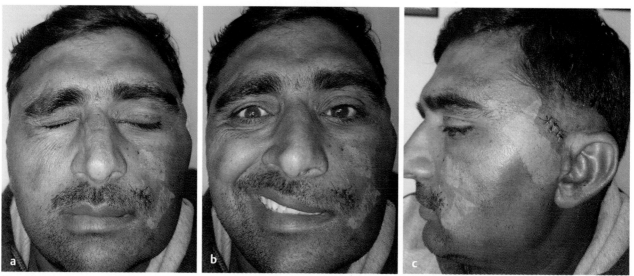

Fig. 16.30 Post second stage surgery which included static procedures like upper eyelid gold implant and fascial sling surgery. **(a)** Complete eye closure has been achieved. Angle of mouth maintained at rest. **(b)** Voluntary lifting of angle of mouth absent. **(c)** Suture line for fascial slings is visible.

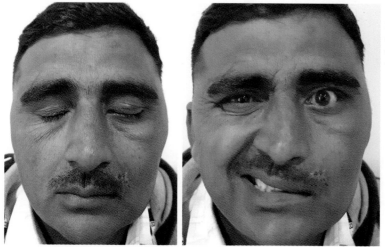

Fig. 16.31 (a, b) After 2 years of the first surgery (3 months post static procedures), eye closure maintained and slight improvement in voluntary lifting of the angle of mouth achieved.

Case 6: Revision Surgery for Branchial Sinus Tract Excision in Neck (After Incomplete Excision of Fistulous Tract in the First Surgery) with Iatrogenic Grade VI Facial Palsy Left Side

A 2-year-old child was operated first for assumed first branchial cleft sinus/fistula in infra-auricular region on left side (operative notes not available) (**Fig. 16.32**). After the first surgery, the sinus persisted along with a lot of fibrosis at the surgical site. The revision surgery was performed after 5 months of the first surgery. CT scan of temporal region performed before the surgery did not add any further information. While excising the residual sinus, surgical dissection of the facial nerve in neck was not performed.

HRCT temporal bone scan before the revision surgery showed intact mastoid segment (MS) of the facial nerve with soft tissue shadow around the facial nerve after its exit from the SMF and this shadow seemed inseparable from the nerve (**Fig. 16.33**).

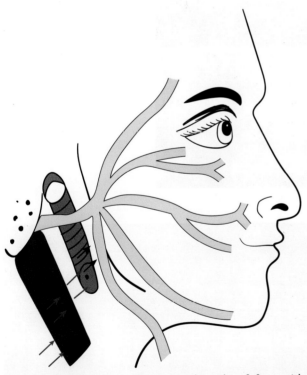

Fig. 16.32 Illustration showing right side of face with exposed facial nerve after its exit from the SMF along with fistulous tract (*black arrows*) extending from the right external auditory canal down along the anterior border of sternocleidomastoid muscle (*red arrows*). The fistulous tract is running deep to the facial nerve and displacing the nerve laterally.

Post revision surgery, immediate complete facial palsy up to grade VI developed as the facial nerve was not exposed before excising the residual fistulous tract. The surgeon was not sure of injury inflicted to the nerve during surgery, so a trial with medical treatment in the form of high dose steroids and antibiotics was given to the patient and finally surgical exploration of the facial nerve in the neck was performed after 15 days when no improvement was noticed.

Pictures after revision surgery show grade VI facial palsy on the left side (**Fig. 16.34**).

Surgical Steps, Left Side (Figs. 16.35–16.40)

Modified Blair's incision made in the neck (left side) and skin with subplatysmal flap lifted. Exploration of the facial nerve after its exit from stylomastoid foramen started, and a proximal stump of the facial nerve could be identified after great effort (**Fig. 16.35**). Fibrotic changes noticed at the cut end of the proximal stump of the facial nerve. It showed that the facial nerve got transected accidentally in the previous surgery. The literature says that mostly the first branchial cleft sinuses lie superficial to the facial nerve, while fistulous tracts usually pass deep to the facial nerve. As the nerve courses over the fistula tract, it can lie more inferior than usual, rendering it at risk for trauma during surgery. In dealing with the first branchial cleft anomalies, it is mandatory to perform the surgical exploration and identification of the facial nerve in neck before excising the sinus or fistulous tract, so as to avoid such iatrogenic trauma to the facial nerve.

After further exploration in neck, the distal end of the facial nerve could also be traced just before its bifurcation in the parotid tissue (**Fig. 16.36**). Both the proximal and distal stumps after separating from the surrounding tissue were brought close together and approximated to each other. There were fibrotic changes with start of collagenization process noticed around the cut ends of the facial nerve (**Fig. 16.37**).

After approximating the cut ends, the unhealthy portions from cut ends of both stumps were excised till healthy nerve was exposed at the cut surface (**Fig. 16.38**). End-to-end anastomosis was performed between the two cut ends by placing sutures with 8-0 monofilament nylon. Maximum five sutures were passed to strengthen and stabilize the anastomosis site (**Fig. 16.39**). The parotid tissue was sutured back to SCM muscle in the neck to provide protection as well as vascularity to the anastomotic site (**Fig. 16.40**).

After 6 months and 9 months of surgery resulting recovery of facial nerve is shown in **Figs. 16.41** and **16.42**.

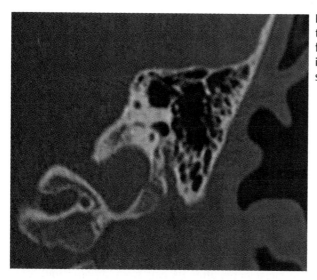

Fig. 16.33 High-resolution computed tomography (HRCT) temporal bone coronal cut left side is showing intact MS of the facial nerve with soft tissue shadow around the facial nerve after its exit from the stylomastoid segment (SMF) and this shadow seems inseparable from the nerve.

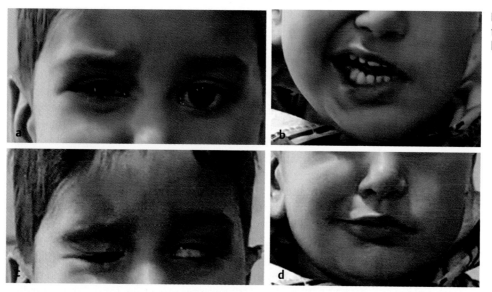

Fig. 16.34 (a–d) Iatrogenic facial palsy of grade VI on the left side.

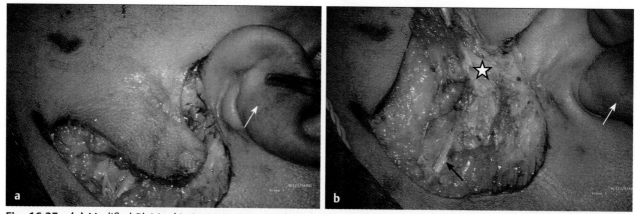

Fig. 16.35 (a) Modified Blair's skin incision given on the left side and cervical subplatysmal flap lifted. **(b)** A lot of fibrosis encountered at the previously operated surgical site (*white asterisk*). Great auricular nerve exposed in neck (*black arrow*). Lobule is shown with *white arrow*.

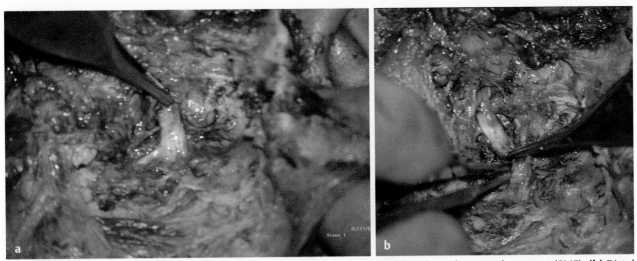

Fig. 16.36 **(a)** Proximal stump of the facial nerve identified just after its exit from the stylomastoid segment (SMF). **(b)** Distal stump of the facial nerve identified just before its bifurcation in parotid.

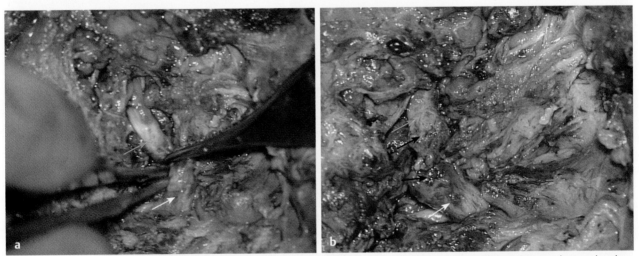

Fig. 16.37 **(a)** Both the proximal (*white arrow*) and distal (*blue arrow*) stumps brought close and approximated to each other. **(b)** Fibrosis and collagenization around the cut ends of the facial nerve are noted (*black arrows*). Proximal stump (*white arrow*) and distal stump (*blue arrow*) can be visualized.

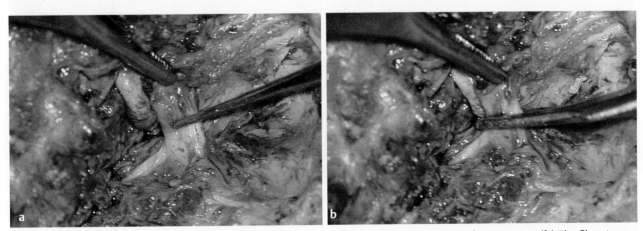

Fig. 16.38 **(a)** The level marked few millimeters beyond the fibrotic end of proximal stump for trimming. **(b)** The fibrotic part being excised with a sharp scissors. *(Continued)*

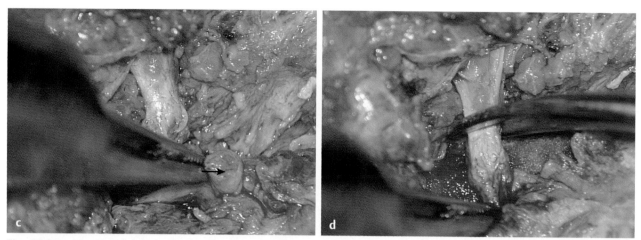

Fig. 16.38 *(Continued)* **(c)** The healthy facial nerve fibers visible through the cut end of the proximal stump (*black arrow*). **(d)** The unhealthy part of the distal stump also trimmed.

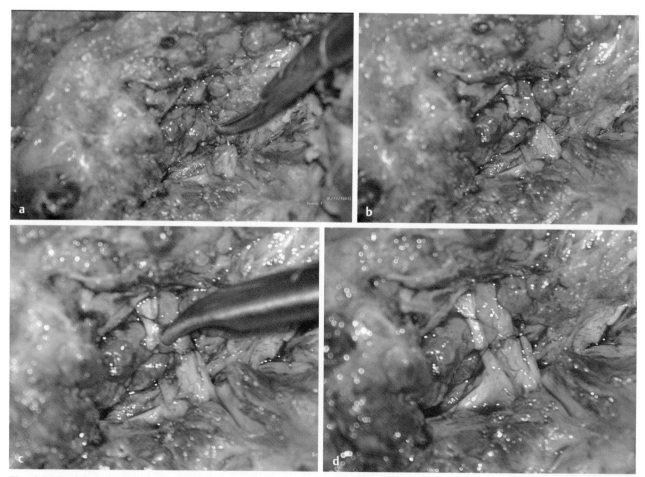

Fig. 16.39 **(a)** End-to-end anastomosis between two cut ends is performed after trimming by applying sutures with 8-0 monofilament (perineurium to perineurium). **(b)** The first suture applied. **(c, d)** The second suture being applied. *(Continued)*

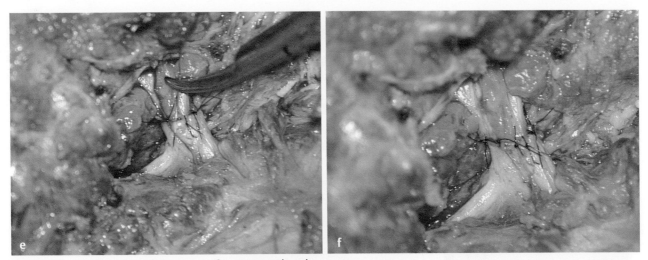

Fig. 16.39   *(Continued)* **(e, f)** Maximum five sutures placed.

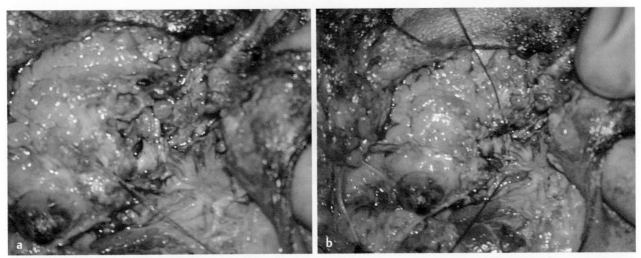

Fig. 16.40   **(a, b)** Parotid tissue being sutured back to sternocleidomastoid muscle in the neck. It is providing protection as well as vascularity to the anastomotic site.

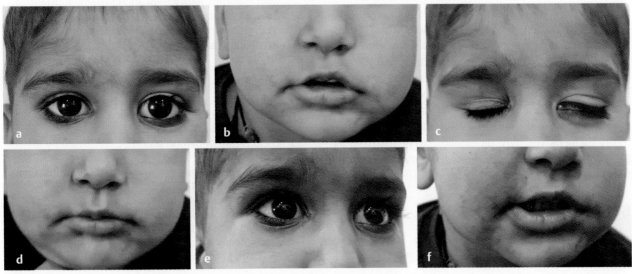

Fig. 16.41   **(a–f)** After 6 months of surgery facial nerve recovery is up to grade III.

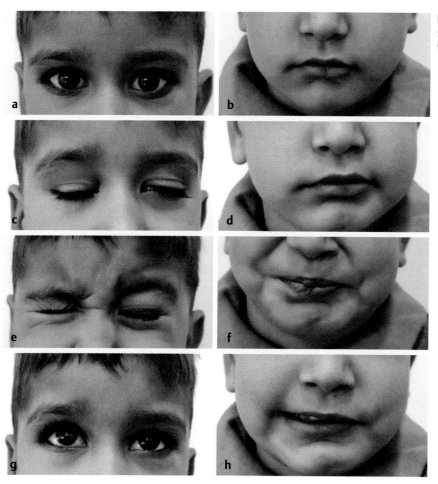

Fig. 16.42 **(a–h)** After 9 months of surgery the facial nerve recovery is up to grade II.

Conclusion

A number of situations are there where extratemporal segment of the facial nerve is at risk. Trauma in any form like blunt trauma, penetrating injury, crush injury, or iatrogenic injury can easily involve this segment of the facial nerve causing grave consequences. These cases should be taken up immediately to avoid complications in the long term. Tumors of parotid gland and tumors of facial nerve itself can involve the facial nerve in its extratemporal segment. By choosing the right approach carefully and following certain practical guidelines, the injury to the facial nerve can be avoided. In case the injury happens, the right technique is to be followed as early as possible to restore the facial nerve function to normal or at least minimize the resulting deformity.

Bibliography

1. Lim CY, Chang HS, Nam KH, Chung WY, Park CS. Preoperative prediction of the location of parotid gland tumors using anatomical landmarks. World J Surg 2008;32(10):2200–2203

2. Imaizumi A, Kuribayashi A, Okochi K, et al. Differentiation between superficial and deep lobe parotid tumors by magnetic resonance imaging: usefulness of the parotid duct criterion. Acta Radiol 2009;50(7):806–811

3. Shawn T. Joseph, Shetty Sharankumar, C.J. Sandya, Vidhyadharan Sivakumar, Peter Sherry, Thankappan Krishnakumar, Iyer Subramania. Eur Arch Otorhinolaryngol DOI 10.1007/s00405-016-3916-6 HEAD AND NECK

4. Quer M, Guntinas-Lichius O, Marchal F, et al. Classification of parotidectomies: a proposal of the European Salivary Gland Society. Eur Arch Otorhinolaryngol 2016;273(10):3307–3312

5. Localization of parotid lesions. Last revised by Andrew Murphy on July 21, 2017

6. Thoeny HC. Imaging of salivary gland tumours. Cancer Imaging 2007;7(1):52–62

7. Fujii H, Fujita A, Kanazawa H, Sung E, Sakai O, Sugimoto H. Localization of Parotid Gland Tumors in Relation to the Intraparotid Facial Nerve on 3D Double-Echo Steady-State with Water Excitation Sequence. AJNR Am J Neuroradiol 2019;40(6):1037–1042

17 Management of Facial Nerve in Lateral Skull Base Surgery

Vestibular Schwannoma—Enlarged Translabyrinthine Approach

Following a cortical mastoidectomy, the mastoidal segment of the facial nerve is identified in the fallopian canal without exposing the nerve. A large size burr with liberal irrigation is used to exenterate all the cells over the mastoidal segment of the fallopian canal (**Fig. 17.1a**).

As labyrinthectomy is performed, the bone of the lateral semicircular canal is drilled as close as possible to the second genu of the facial nerve. This helps in good visualization of the vestibule medial to it (**Fig. 17.1b**). The vestibule represents the lateral end of internal auditory meatus (IAM).

Translabyrinthine approach gives the benefit of early identification of the facial nerve at the lateral-most end of IAM. For this, the superior ampullary nerve is to be identified and preserved as it innervates the ampullary ends of lateral and superior semicircular canal. The superior ampullary nerve is hooked and dissected medially as it continues to the superior vestibular nerve. At the lateral-most end of IAM, the facial nerve is protected by the vertical crest also called as Bill's bar (**Fig. 17.1c**). Hence, by starting the dissection far laterally, the chances of injury to the facial nerve is avoided and the facial nerve is identified conclusively and early. Dissection of tumor from the facial nerve is done gently without traction on the nerve. Care is taken to avoid suction directly over the nerve. To achieve this, Brackmann suction cannulas with side holes are used, and suctioning is performed away from the facial nerve. Bipolar cautery is avoided in the close vicinity of the facial nerve. Preservation of the arachnoid layer helps to preserve vascularity of the facial nerve. Tumor is debulked and the capsule is dissected away from the facial nerve. If, however, the capsule is closely adherent to the facial nerve, it is left in place to preserve facial function. In larger tumors, the facial nerve could be splayed on the anterior surface of the tumor. Facial nerve monitoring is routinely used by the author and is specifically useful in these cases to avoid injury to the splayed facial nerve fibers. At the conclusion of tumor removal, the facial nerve close to its origin at the brainstem (**Fig. 17.1d**) is stimulated with a 0.05 mV current. A robust response observed on

neuromonitoring is an encouraging event and prognosticates a normal postoperative facial function.

In case of interruption of the facial nerve, every attempt should be made to repair the nerve during the primary surgery itself. If two ends of the interrupted facial nerve can be approximated, fibrin glue is used to hold the anastomosis. However, if there is loss of segment of the facial nerve, a sural nerve graft is harvested and used as an interposition graft between the transected ends of the facial nerve. The proximal site of anastomosis in the cerebellopontine angle is held in place with fibrin glue since it is not feasible to suture this part of the nerve due to absence of epineurium. The distal site of anastomosis can be approximated with monofilament sutures or with fibrin glue.

If the proximal facial nerve at brainstem is not available for anastomosing an interrupted nerve, then an early facio-hypoglossal anastomosis or a facio-masseteric anastomosis is planned. These procedures have been described in detail in Chapter 8 titled "Short Duration Flaccid Facial Palsy with Proximal Stump Unavailable."

Vestibular Schwannoma—Middle Cranial Fossa Approach

The middle cranial fossa approach is used for vestibular schwannomas that are primarily intracanalicular or not extending more than 0.5 cm into the cerebellopontine angle with serviceable hearing.

The facial nerve lies in the anterosuperior compartment of the IAM. On incising the dura of the IAM, the facial nerve is immediately seen anteriorly while the superior vestibular nerve is seen posteriorly (**Fig. 17.2a**). Facial nerve monitoring is used to additionally confirm the position of the facial nerve. Since majority of the vestibular schwannomas arise from the inferior vestibular nerve, the superior vestibular nerve is hooked out to visualize the schwannoma (**Fig. 17.2b**). Care is taken not to cause any undue stretch of the facial nerve during excision of the schwannoma. Also, there should be no direct suctioning over the nerve. At the end of schwannoma excision, the facial nerve is once again stimulated with 0.05 mV current. A good robust response suggests normal facial function postoperatively.

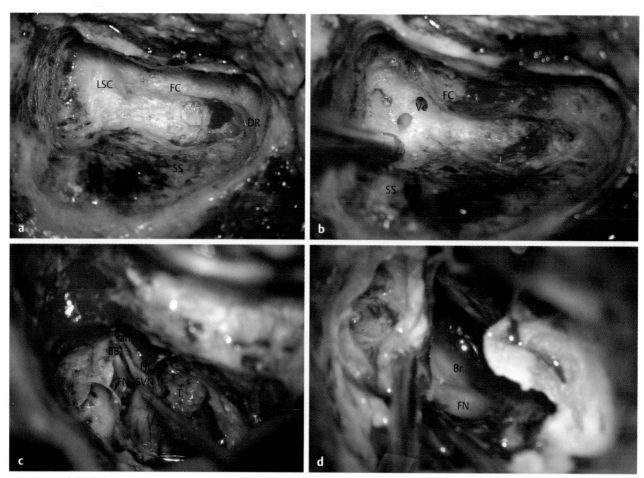

Fig. 17.1 **(a)** All the cells over the mastoidal segment of the fallopian canal exenterated. **(b)** Labyrinthectomy performed (Ve is opened vestibule; FC is fallopian canal of mastoid segment). **(c)** The superior ampullary nerve (san) is hooked and dissected medially as it continues to the superior vestibular nerve (SVN). The facial nerve (FN) at the fundus of internal auditory meatus (IAM) is protected by the Bill's bar. **(d)** After complete tumor removal, the facial nerve (FN) close to its origin at the brainstem (Br) can be visualized. BB, Bill's barDR, digastric ridge; FC, fallopian canal; HC, Horizontal crest; LSC, lateral semicircular canal; SS, sigmoid sinus; T, Tumor.

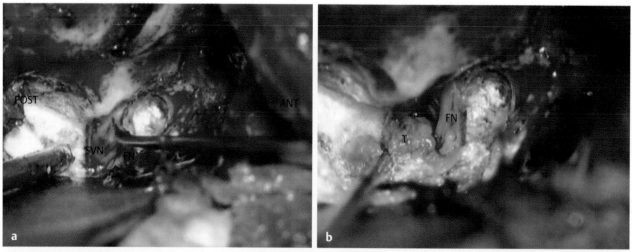

Fig. 17.2 **(a)** Middle cranial fossa approach on the left side. The facial nerve (FN) can be visualized in the anterosuperior compartment while the superior vestibular nerve is seen posteriorly. POST, Posterior; ANT, Anterior. **(b)** The superior vestibular nerve (SVN) has been hooked out to visualize the tumor (T) of the internal auditory meatus (IAM).

Glomus Jugulare Surgery—Infratemporal Fossa Approaches

Anterior transposition of the facial nerve is very important to gain unrestricted access to the jugular foramen. For this, the facial nerve is identified at its exit from the stylomastoid foramen and traced beyond the bifurcation into upper and lower divisions. The facial nerve in its intratemporal course is skeletonized from the geniculate ganglion up to the stylomastoid foramen. The nerve is decompressed in 180 degrees without any damage to the myelin sheath of the nerve. The nerve is then lifted off the fallopian canal. Adhesions to the bed of the fallopian canal are cut sharply to release the nerve from its bed. Periosteum is left around the nerve at the stylomastoid foramen, and the nerve is mobilized from distal to its bifurcation into upper and lower divisions up to geniculate ganglion (**Fig. 17.3a, b**). Failure to mobilize the nerve distally in the parotid as described causes a stretch and stress on the nerve in the anterior transposition position. A tunnel is created in the anterior epitympanic bone to place the anteriorly transposed nerve which is held in place with fibrin glue (**Fig. 17.3c**). The periosteum sleeve around the nerve at stylomastoid foramen is sutured to parotid tissue to hold the nerve in an anteriorly transposed position.

Glomus jugulare tumors are often seen on the medial surface of the mastoidal segment of facial nerve. It is very important to study the high-resolution computed tomography (CT) scans to assess the bony fallopian canal erosion as a preoperative clinical facial nerve paresis could signify facial nerve involvement with the tumor. Every attempt is made to identify the normal facial nerve on either side of the suspected area of involvement and thereafter continue to take the tumor off the nerve. The tumor is dissected off the myelin sheath of the facial nerve. In case of involvement of the perineurium, a decision to resect the involved segment of the nerve is taken.

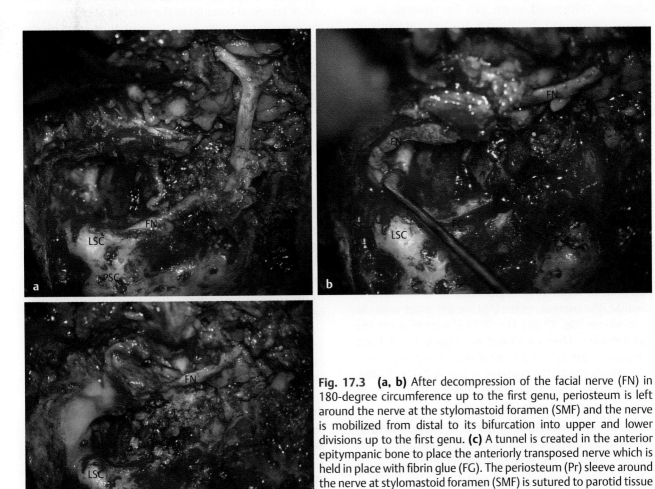

Fig. 17.3 **(a, b)** After decompression of the facial nerve (FN) in 180-degree circumference up to the first genu, periosteum is left around the nerve at the stylomastoid foramen (SMF) and the nerve is mobilized from distal to its bifurcation into upper and lower divisions up to the first genu. **(c)** A tunnel is created in the anterior epitympanic bone to place the anteriorly transposed nerve which is held in place with fibrin glue (FG). The periosteum (Pr) sleeve around the nerve at stylomastoid foramen (SMF) is sutured to parotid tissue to hold the nerve in an anteriorly transposed position. FC, Fallopian canal; LSC, lateral semicircular canal; PSC, posterior semicircular canal; T, tumor.

Although partial transposition of the nerve has been described for C1 and C2 lesions, my early experience made me realize that, although feasible, the facial nerve remains at great risk of iatrogenic injury during the procedure. Hence, I personally do not prefer limited mobilization but perform a full anterior transposition for even C1 and C2 lesions. I have had majority of the cases returning to Grade 2 facial function (House-Brackmann grading system) in 6 to 9 months following surgery with others having Grade 3 facial function, provided that the integrity of the facial nerve has been maintained.

In case the nerve is involved with the tumor, the involved segment is transected. A greater auricular or sural nerve graft is harvested and placed between the proximal and distal uninvolved segments of the facial nerve. Two or three 8-0 monofilament sutures are placed on each approximated end to ensure perfect approximation.

In infratemporal fossa B and C approaches, the anteriorly transposed nerve can be replaced in its normal course and drilling can proceed anteriorly at the root of the zygoma toward the nasopharynx or the sphenoid sinus.

Petroclival Lesions—Transcochlear Approach

Petroclival lesions mandate a transcochlear approach with posterior transposition of the facial nerve.

The facial nerve is skeletonized and exposed in it mastoidal and tympanic segments up to the geniculate ganglion (**Fig. 17.4a**). The greater superficial petrosal nerve (GSPN) is identified from the geniculate ganglion going anteriorly along the base of the temporal lobe. A labyrinthectomy is performed and the facial nerve identified from its labyrinthine segment all along its course in the IAM. The contents of the IAM are left intact with the dural sleeve (**Fig. 17.4b**). The GSPN is sectioned and the facial nerve is lifted off its bed from the mastoidal and tympanic segments. The nerve is then rerouted posteriorly together with the contents of the IAM (**Fig. 17.4b**). The cochlea is then drilled (**Fig. 17.4c**) as also the bone toward the petrous apex (**Fig. 17.4d**).

Posterior transposition of the facial nerve results in an eventual Grade 4 or Grade 3 facial function 6 to 9 months after the procedure. Facial nerve grafting gives a postoperative Grade 3 function in most cases. Hence, if the facial nerve is involved with tumor, the involved segment is transected, and a facial nerve grafting is performed without much hesitation.

Petrous Cholesteatomas—Transotic Approach

In extensive congenital temporal bone cholesteatomas, depending upon the location of the lesion, a transotic approach is often indicated. In this the facial nerve is kept intact in the fallopian canal with a sleeve of bone around it while the labyrinth and cochlea are drilled out (**Fig. 17.5**). Similarly, the contents of the IAM are preserved with a thin shell of bone around it except when cholesteatoma itself has destroyed the bone. Drilling is performed in the infrafacial area, that is, the area medial to the mastoidal segment of the facial nerve.

The transotic approach gives a wide access to the entire temporal bone up to the petrous apex. However, the only disadvantage is the "partial blind area" on the anterior face of the IAM. It is very important not to leave behind some epithelium in this area which could potentially lead to recidivism of the cholesteatoma. However, given this limitation of the approach, it still is an approach which preserves normal facial function which is very vital given the younger age group of these subjects.

The preoperative grading of the facial function with duration of weakness and radiological involvement of the facial nerve is used to counsel the subject about possible scenarios. In case of normal facial function, with the cholesteatoma just adjacent to the nerve without involving it, it can be dissected off the nerve keeping the myelin sheath of the nerve intact. However, if the subject has a facial paresis, it could be due to toxins released by the cholesteatoma or the matrix itself giving pressure on the nerve. In these cases, again, it is often not difficult to find a plane between the cholesteatoma matrix and the facial nerve and peel the matrix off the nerve. In case the subject has longstanding facial palsy where the nerve is fibrosed or atrophic, the nerve is resected, and an interposition graft used between two normal ends of the nerve. However, in case of duration of preoperative facial palsy beyond 2 years, even grafting would probably not give the desired result. In these cases, a facio-hypoglossal or facio-masseteric anastomosis is planned accordingly.

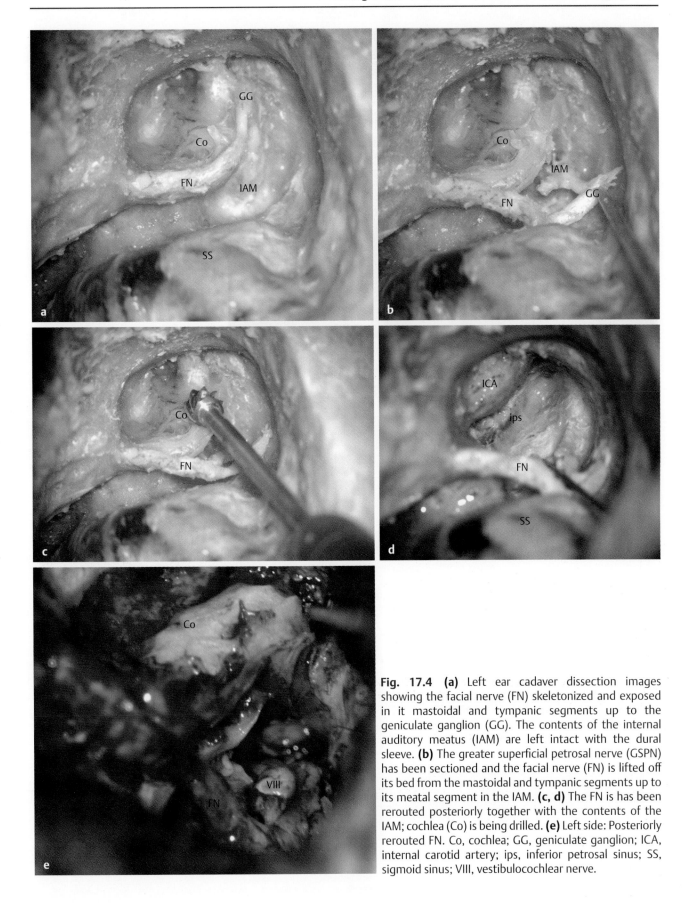

Fig. 17.4 **(a)** Left ear cadaver dissection images showing the facial nerve (FN) skeletonized and exposed in it mastoidal and tympanic segments up to the geniculate ganglion (GG). The contents of the internal auditory meatus (IAM) are left intact with the dural sleeve. **(b)** The greater superficial petrosal nerve (GSPN) has been sectioned and the facial nerve (FN) is lifted off its bed from the mastoidal and tympanic segments up to its meatal segment in the IAM. **(c, d)** The FN is has been rerouted posteriorly together with the contents of the IAM; cochlea (Co) is being drilled. **(e)** Left side: Posteriorly rerouted FN. Co, cochlea; GG, geniculate ganglion; ICA, internal carotid artery; ips, inferior petrosal sinus; SS, sigmoid sinus; VIII, vestibulocochlear nerve.

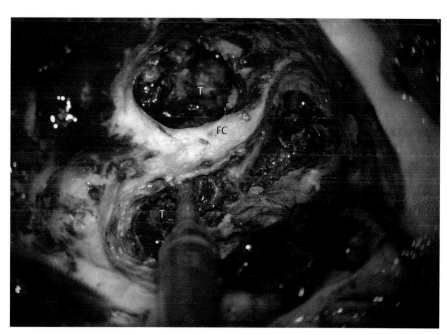

Fig. 17.5 Transotic approach on the left side. FC, Fallopian canal; T, Tumor.

18 Facial Nerve in Cochlear Implantation

Introduction

Cochlear implant surgery is currently an accepted treatment for bilateral severe to profound hearing loss. As in any other otologic surgery, there is a potential risk of damage to the facial nerve. About 20% of pediatric patients with congenital hearing loss, undergoing cochlear implants, have been reported to have inner ear malformation. The possibility of aberrant facial nerve course is higher in such cases, leading to the likelihood of facial nerve injury. It is, therefore, important for the surgeon to be aware of the normal variation of the facial nerve and facial nerve abnormalities usually associated with inner ear malformation.

The most widely performed approach in cochlear implant surgery is the transmastoidectomy posterior tympanotomy approach which entails drilling near the facial nerve. The facial nerve, therefore, is a crucial landmark in performing posterior tympanotomy and accessing the round window niche. Despite the potential of facial nerve injury, cochlear implantation can be performed safely by following standard surgical steps and protocols. Careful evaluation of preoperative imaging studies can alert the surgeon about the abnormal course of the facial nerve and prevent accidental damage to the nerve.

Facial Nerve Anomalies

Aberrant facial nerve can be defined as a variation in shape or course of the facial nerve in the temporal bone with respect to specific anatomic landmarks (i.e., round window, oval window, and lateral semicircular canal) on high-resolution computed tomography (HRCT) and during surgery. Some of the common variations are shown in **Fig. 18.1**.

Normal development of the inner ear structures, the cochlea, and the vestibular labyrinth to a great extent determines the position and course of the facial nerve. If there is a malformation or absence of these structures, then the chances of abnormal course of the facial nerve are quite high. Some malformations in the course of the facial nerve are displacement of:

- The labyrinthine portion more anteromedially
- The tympanic segment anteriorly and medially, hence descending lower in the middle ear
- The second genu to a lower position
- The vertical canal of the facial nerve more anteromedially, sometimes running over the promontory, or at times even across the round window (**Fig. 18.1**). The topic has been described in details in Chapter 1 titled 'Embryology of Facial nerve'.

A proper study of the HRCT of the temporal bone before the surgery will demonstrate these malformations, and adequate precautions can be taken to ensure that the nerve is not damaged. Facial nerve monitoring is recommended in cochlear implant surgery, even more so in cases with inner ear malformations. While using facial nerve monitoring, the anesthetist is informed not to use a long-acting paralyzing agent for the patient.

Facial Nerve Injury in Cochlear Implant Surgery

The facial nerve has an intricate course in the temporal bone. The facial canal may display congenital bony dehiscence and it may show variations and anomalies from its usual course as described above.

The facial recess approach was described by House (1994) and is the standard approach in cochlear implant surgery. The preferred incision is postauricular, a few millimeters behind the postaural groove. In children below 1 year of age, the mastoid process tip is rudimentary or absent and the facial nerve is very superficial. Hence, the facial nerve can be damaged even while taking a postaural skin incision. Therefore, the incision should be moved a little posteriorly as it approaches the tip area, and the incision should not extend beyond the mastoid tip.

Posterior tympanotomy is a triangle-shaped opening bounded superiorly by fossa incudis, medially and posteriorly by the facial nerve, and anteriorly and laterally by the chorda tympani nerve. To get good access to the posterior tympanotomy area, an adequate cortical mastoidectomy should be performed and the posterior canal wall should be carefully thinned out (**Fig. 18.2**).

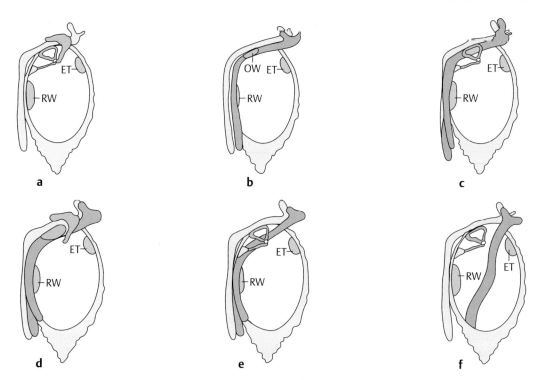

Fig. 18.1 Schematic representation of facial nerve anomalies (clockwise from top left): **(a)** Normal facial nerve, **(b, c)** anteriorly placed nerve, **(d)** bifurcation of the vertical portion of the facial nerve, **(e)** antero-medial displacement of the tympanic segment of the facial nerve, and **(f)** facial nerve running over promontory. ET, Eustachian tube; OW, oval window; RW, round window. Normal facial nerve is yellow coloured and abnormal facial nerve is orange coloured.

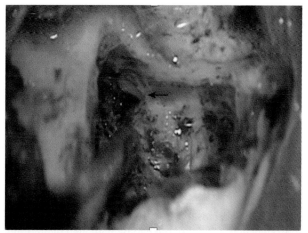

Fig. 18.2 Cortical mastoidectomy showing short process of incus (*black arrow*).

A narrow surgical field and anatomical variation in the facial nerve can increase the risk of nerve injury. Before proceeding for posterior tympanotomy, following landmarks are identified:

- Adequate exposure of fossa incudis and visualization of the short process of the incus should be achieved. The incus guides the surgeon to estimate the position of the facial nerve. An imaginary line drawn through the body of incus extending downwards along the posterior canal wall usually corresponds to the location of the facial nerve.

- The lateral semicircular canal is a good landmark for the facial nerve. The second genu of the facial nerve is medial and inferior to the lateral semicircular canal.

- *Identification of facial nerve*: The drilling in the posterior tympanotomy area is done initially with a cutting burr but subsequently a diamond burr is used closer to the facial nerve. In trying to define the facial nerve, direction of drilling is parallel to the facial nerve and perifacial and retrofacial cells are slowly exenterated till the pink hue of the facial nerve bony canal is seen. It is common to encounter blood vessels just superficial to the bony canal of the facial nerve and it is an important pointer in the correct location of the facial nerve. Use of a diamond burr and copious irrigation is advocated to minimize bleeding and improve visualization. While drilling, it is advisable to stay lateral to the incus and lateral semicircular canal to prevent injury to the facial nerve. Once the facial nerve bony canal is identified and delineated, chances of damage to the nerve are minimized. A diamond burr is used to gradually widen the posterior tympanotomy by drilling parallel to the facial nerve. Sometimes, while delineating the vertical facial bony canal, the nerve sheath may get exposed. The facial nerve function is unlikely to be affected as long as the sheath is intact.

- The fourth landmark is the identification of chorda tympani. The posterior canal wall is further thinned inferiorly until chorda tympani is identified. Once the facial nerve and chorda tympani are identified, widening of the posterior tympanotomy is done without fear of injuring the nerves.

The posterior tympanotomy is widened in both directions, that is, chorda tympani to the facial nerve and from the fossa incudis to the chorda–facial angle. The triangle of the posterior tympanostomy has its base toward the fossa incudis. It is a good practice to design this base in such a way that half of it is in front of the short process of the incus and half of it behind. This will prevent the surgeon from accidentally damaging the annulus anteriorly and facial nerve posteriorly. The external auditory canal is filled with betadine solution while preparing the ear of the patient. This will help in the timely identification of the breach in the external auditory canal while thinning the posterior canal wall by the leaking betadine solution.

After performing the posterior tympanotomy in full dimensions, the structures that can be identified are the incudostapedial joint, the stapedius tendon, the promontory, the round window niche, and the hypotympanic cells. Occasionally, hypotympanic cells may be mistaken for round window by a novice surgeon. Therefore, it is advisable to drill away the bony overhang superior to the round window (operculum) to expose and identify the round window membrane (**Figs. 18.3** and **18.4**). While drilling the round window niche, care should be taken to avoid the shaft of the burr touching the bony canal of the facial nerve as this may result in facial paresis/palsy due to heat injury. Therefore, adequate irrigation and drilling in short bursts are advisable to prevent facial nerve damage.

At times, even after delineating the facial nerve it might be difficult to visualize the round window niche due to unfavorable orientation or angulation of the cochlea. The surgeon can resort to some of the steps mentioned below.

Instillation of normal saline into the middle ear may help visualize the round window niche due to refraction of light and help determine the site for cochleostomy.

Widening of the posterior tympanotomy (extended posterior tympanotomy) by decompressing or even sacrificing the chorda tympani nerve and/or removing the incus buttress may help visualize the round window niche.

Using a 2.7-mm, 30-degree endoscope through the posterior tympanotomy may also help.

Anterior advancement of the posterior wall of the bony external auditory canal to get a wider exposure of the middle ear can be achieved by two osteotomies in the thinned-out canal wall. After completing the cochlear implant insertion, this bony canal wall with the attached external canal skin is reposited in its normal anatomic position and supported by a pack in the external auditory meatus.

A subtotal petrosectomy approach with fat obliteration of the cavity and blind sac closure (cul de sac closure) can be done for better visualization of the round window niche.

A retrofacial approach can be achieved by drilling between the vertical segment of the facial nerve and the posterior semicircular canal to access the round window.

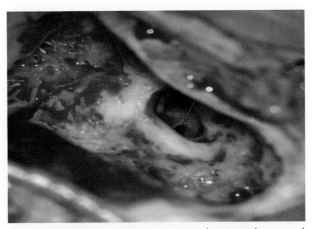

Fig. 18.3 Posterior tympanotomy showing the round window niche (*red arrow*).

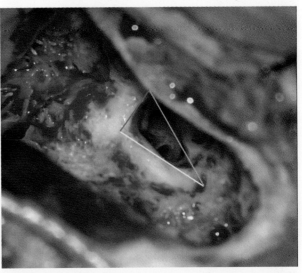

Fig. 18.4 Facial recess or posterior tympanotomy triangle is shown. The trianglular area is limited anterolaterally by the chorda tympani (*green line*) posteromedially by facial nerve (*yellow line*) and superiorly at its base is fossa incudis or incus bridge (*blue line*).

Management of Facial Nerve Injury

The incidence of facial paralysis in cochlear implant surgery with the posterior tympanotomy approach is quite low. Facial paresis/palsy could be immediate or of delayed onset. Immediate-onset paralysis is usually seen in the operating theater after extubation. Delayed onset can be seen a few hours to days after the surgery.

Immediate facial palsy is usually due to direct surgical trauma to the nerve. If during surgery the facial nerve sheath is damaged resulting in bulging of the facial nerve, adequate decompression of the nerve should be done before placing the implant.

The second possibility of injury to the facial nerve is thermal damage by the shaft of the burr while drilling the posterior tympanotomy or defining the round widow to create a cochleostomy (**Fig. 18.5**).

Third, there is a possible mechanism of vasospasm causing ischemia of the nerve. However, in rare instances, there is delayed presentation of facial palsy over a few days to a few weeks. The probable hypothesis is the reactivation of the herpes virus which may have existed in the temporal bone. The transection of the chorda tympani nerve during posterior tympanotomy may lead to reactivation of the herpes virus and can probably explain the cause of delayed facial palsy.

This is a hypothesis that is difficult to prove since most delayed palsies are treated conservatively and almost all of them recover.

If there is immediate facial palsy seen on extubation, the surgeon should go through the steps of surgery or through the video recording of the surgery to identify any injury to the facial nerve.

If the surgeon finds the facial nerve sheath opened and the nerve bulging intraoperatively, a re-exploration and decompression of the facial nerve should be done. Care should be taken to place the electrode array in such a way that it does not come in contact with the exposed area of the facial nerve.

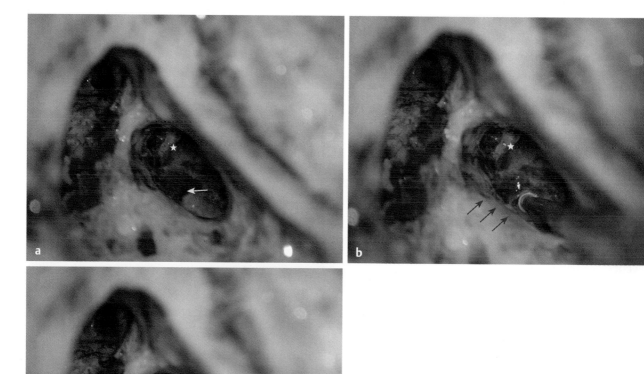

Fig. 18.5 (a) Right ear, cortical mastoidectomy with posterior tympanotomy performed. Round window niche (*yellow arrow*) to be drilled. (b) avoid touching the shaft of moving burr to the exposed fallopian canal (*red arrows*). (c) round window niche drilled and round window membrane exposed (*black arrow*). Incudostapedial joint (*yellow asterisk*).

In various studies, the incidence of facial palsy has been reported to be 0.3 to 3%. Preoperative imaging for assessment of the course of the facial nerve and its variations cannot be overemphasized. Meticulous adherence to the standardized steps of surgery mentioned above especially the identification of the facial and chorda tympani nerves before proceeding with posterior tympanotomy will minimize the risk of facial nerve injury. Any damage to the facial nerve noticed during surgery should be adequately addressed before placing the implant.

Bibliography

1. Jackler RK, Luxford WM, House WF. Congenital malformations of the inner ear: a classification based on embryogenesis. Laryngoscope 1987;97(3 Pt 2, Suppl 40):2–14

2. Alzhrani F, Lenarz T, Teschner M. Facial palsy following cochlear implantation. Eur Arch Otorhinolaryngol 2016;273(12):4199–4207

3. Fayad JN, Wanna GB, Micheletto JN, Parisier SC. Facial nerve paralysis following cochlear implant surgery. Laryngoscope 2003;113(8):1344–1346

4. Mandour MF, Khalifa MA, Khalifa HMA, Amer MAR. Iatrogenic facial nerve exposure in cochlear implant surgery: incidence and clinical significance in the absence of intra-operative nerve monitoring. Cochlear Implants Int 2019;20(5):250–254

5. Thom JJ, Carlson ML, Olson MD, et al. The prevalence and clinical course of facial nerve paresis following cochlear implant surgery. Laryngoscope 2013;123(4):1000–1004

6. Hsieh HS, Wu CM, Zhuo MY, Yang CH, Hwang CF. Intraoperative facial nerve monitoring during cochlear implant surgery: an observational study. Medicine (Baltimore) 2015;94(4):e456

Index